Cutting-edge Vitreoretinal Surgery

Astha Jain • S. Natarajan
Sandeep Saxena
Editors

Cutting-edge Vitreoretinal Surgery

Springer

Editors
Astha Jain
Aditya Jyot Foundation for Twinkling
Little Eyes
Aditya Jyot Eye Hospital
Mumbai
India

S. Natarajan
Aditya Jyot Foundation for Twinkling
Little Eyes
Aditya Jyot Eye Hospital
Mumbai
India

Sandeep Saxena
Department of Ophthalmology
King George's Medical University
Lucknow
Uttar Pradesh
India

ISBN 978-981-33-4167-8 ISBN 978-981-33-4168-5 (eBook)
https://doi.org/10.1007/978-981-33-4168-5

This Springer imprint is published by the registered company Springer Nature Singapore Pte Ltd.
The registered company address is: 152 Beach Road, #21-01/04 Gateway East, Singapore 189721, Singapore

This book is dedicated to our families with thanks for their constant support and motivation.

Foreword

Three internationally renowned experts present in this book, in 11 parts and 43 chapters, a comprehensive overview of the current knowledge in vitreoretinal surgery. The book reflects the authors' lifelong experience and dedication to the technique, skill, and development of modern retinal surgery. I feel the author's commitment and attention to the details necessary for this surgical text. The chapters have been contributed by experts in their respective fields from across the world. Their book gives both, general principles and specific technical details for the retinal surgeon. Thus this book is a treasure grove by the clinical relevance of its selected content, the experience and the scholarship of the authors.

Since 1970, Robert Machemer and others have created a new surgical field with their pioneering work. The principles, techniques, and instruments of retinal surgery are competently presented in this volume. A part describes the latest techniques of visualization and robotic surgery. Several chapters have been devoted to special disease entities such as vascular and proliferative diseases, foveal diseases, trauma and endophthalmitis, ROP and uveitis, each of which requires special methods and knowledge.

The book covers the full spectrum of vitreoretinal diseases and makes the current knowledge about the pathogenesis and management of retinal diseases accessible. The tables and photographs complement the text and give a quick overview. Finally, the book emphasizes and clarifies the critical decision points in surgery. Sometimes there are several methods leading to success, which differ in safety, patient acceptance, and effectiveness. The surgeon selects the method with which he has the greatest success; therefore, this overview of the multiple techniques is important. To choose the most appropriate and least invasive form of several techniques is what I call minimal maximal surgery. The authors try to highlight these possibilities and controversies and the underlying evidence and point out where further research is needed.

Thus this book is useful for every retinal surgeon and ophthalmologist, both as an instructor of residents and fellows and as an independent learner. The learning surgeon will be able to treat vitreoretinal diseases, including traumatology, safely through the precise description of clinically proven techniques. However, every year new methods appear and traditional techniques change. We all learn throughout our lives. That is why I find the chapter, "Self-education in Vitreoretinal Surgery," extremely important. Good surgery is based on the cumulative knowledge of our predecessors and own experience, but this alone is no longer enough. Because progress is so fast today, even such a comprehensive book can only provide the basis for continuous self-learning. Some prefer to look at videos to learn surgery. The argumentative strength and well-organized information of a well-edited book lead to more clarity and a better-integrated view and understanding and will remain a comprehensive authoritative resource.

Retinal specialists, medical or surgical, share a common fascination for the retina, a unique and wonderful tissue that is essential for vision. I am grateful to the authors for sharing their enthusiasm and knowledge. It will benefit surgeons and their patients and hopefully will enable a new generation of surgeons and ophthalmologists to better understand and treat surgical retinal diseases.

Peter Wiedmann
University Eye Hospital Leipzig
Leipzig, Germany

Preface

Vitreoretinal surgery is a highly advanced and specialized field of ocular surgery which is ever-evolving. Since the introduction of vitreoretinal surgery by Machemer, several advances have been made in surgical techniques and instrumentation. This book tries to provide insight into the current concepts of the latest technologies in vitreoretinal surgery. The book is authored by 108 authors of international repute from across the globe.

The book covers the management of all common and uncommon vitreoretinal surgical procedures. There are 11 parts focusing on imaging, instrumentation, techniques of retinal detachment surgery, management of retinal vascular disorder, macular surgery, ocular trauma, endophthalmitis, uveitis, and other retinal disorders. There is a separate part on gene therapy and its surgical technique for inherited retinal disorders. Recent advances such as 3D vitrectomy and robotic surgery have been covered extensively.

The book is written in a lucid manner for a better understanding of the surgical technique and is supported by more than 200 colored figures. Videos of some aspects of the surgery have also been added.

The target audience of the book are the resident and fellows under training as well as practicing vitreoretinal surgeons so that they can be abreast with the newer techniques.

Mumbai, India — Astha Jain
Mumbai, India — S. Natarajan
Lucknow, India — Sandeep Saxena

Contents

Part IV Retinal Detachment: Surgical Techniques

Part V Retinal Vascular Disorders

Part VI Macular Surgery

About the Editors

Astha Jain is a vitreoretinal surgeon. She completed her MD in ophthalmology from King George's Medical University, Lucknow, followed by a fellowship in vitreoretinal surgery from H V Desai Eye Hospital, Pune. She worked as a vitreoretinal surgeon at Narayana Nethralaya, Bangalore before joining Aditya Jyot Foundation. She has several international publications to her credit and is a reviewer for several journals. She is the recipient of Prof. Yasuo Tano Travel Grant for APAO 2013 and also a recipient of Sir Ratan Tata and Sir JRD Tata scholarships for excelling in academics. She is actively involved in the training of vitreoretinal fellows at her center. Her areas of interest include diabetic retinopathy, retinal detachment, retinopathy of prematurity, posterior uveitis, and diagnostics in retinal disorders.

S. Natarajan is a vitreoretinal surgeon and is the chairman and managing director of Aditya Jyot Eye Hospital, Mumbai. He is a Charter Inductee in the Retina Hall of Fame. He is the president of Organized Medicine Academic Guild (OMAG) and Asia Pacific Ophthalmic Trauma Society (APOTS) and past president of All India Ophthalmological Society (AIOS) and Ocular Trauma Society of India (OTSI). He is also the secretary general of Global Eye Genetics Consortium (GEGC) and Board Member of Retina World Congress (RWC) and International Society of Ocular Trauma (ISOT).

The Prestigious International Council of Ophthalmology (ICO) has appointed him as ICO Board of Trustees for 2018–2020. He was conferred with the prestigious Padma Shree award in the year 2013, and he was the first Indian to receive the Gusi Peace Prize. He was also awarded the Asia Pacific Academy of Ophthalmology Achievement Award by APAO. He has more than 100 publications and has edited two books. His areas of interest are ocular trauma, retinal detachment, age-related macular degeneration, inherited retinal disorders, and diabetic retinopathy.

Sandeep Saxena is professor and chief of retina service, Department of Ophthalmology, King George's Medical University, Lucknow, India. After his postgraduation from King George's Medical University, Lucknow, he completed two vitreoretinal postdoctoral fellowships at Barnes Retina Institute and Anheuser Busch Eye Institute, St. Louis, USA and NewYork-Presbyterian Hospital, New York, USA. He has been a DAAD fellow, Bonn,

Germany and a visiting fellow at Oxford University, UK and Harvard Medical School, USA. He is on the editorial board of several journals and has 23 books, 40 book chapters, and over 150 publications to his credit. He also designed "Saxena Retinal Grid 428 and 520" (Ocular Instruments, USA) for measuring retinal lesions.

Part I

Introduction to Vitreoretinal Surgery

1 History of Vitreoretinal Surgery

S. Natarajan, Sonali Verma, and Astha Jain

1.1 Introduction

Jules Gonin, in 1920, was the first to recognise that retinal breaks are responsible for retinal detachment. It is due to this that the history of retinal surgery is mainly divided into pre-Gonin (before 1920) and post-Gonin era.

1.1.1 Pre-Gonin Era

In the pre-Gonin era, management of retinal detachment was attempted using a lot of theories and methods, but the prognosis of a patient with retinal detachment remained poor. James Ware, in 1805, attempted the first surgery for retinal detachment by draining the subretinal fluid through puncturing the sclera with a knife [1].

In 1851, a German physiologist, Herman von Helmholtz, invented direct ophthalmoscope [2]. Coccius in 1853 and von Graefe in 1854 portrayed the course of retinal detachment and observed the first retinal tear [3, 4]. Von Graefe modified the method attempted by Ware by creating a second hole in retina to drain the subretinal fluid in the vitreous cavity in 1863. Martin advised the use of thermocautery in 1881 and de Wecker in 1882 [5, 6]. De Wecker also advocated the use of trephination for permanent drainage of subretinal fluid. Gronholm advocated sclerotomy in 1921 [7].

Grossman, in 1883, suggested the injection of hypertonic saline in subconjunctival space for absorption of subretinal fluid by osmotic action [8, 9].

One of the theories was abnormal leakage of the choroid leading to subretinal fluid for which various procedures such as subretinal fluid drainage and retinopexy were suggested. Another theory that was postulated was to increase the intraocular pressure to settle the retina. Carbone suggested the injection of gelatin in the anterior chamber in 1925 [10]. The other method suggested was to inject material in the vitreous cavity to push the retina back. Leber and Nordenson put forward another vital theory about the role of vitreous traction forces in the pathogenesis of retinal detachment [11].

Stellwag and Donders advised the usage of certain non-surgical measures such as bed rest and immobility of eye [12, 13]. Samelsohn, in 1875 [14], further modified the measures advised by Stellwag and Donders, to bandaging of eye to exert pressure on the eye. A low salt diet was also advised to promote absorption of subretinal fluid.

The rate of success of retinal detachment repair was very low till 1912, approximately 1 in 100,0 [15].

S. Natarajan (✉) · S. Verma
Aditya Jyot Eye Hospital, Mumbai, India

A. Jain
Aditya Jyot Eye Hospital, Mumbai, India

Aditya Jyot Foundation for Twinkling Little Eyes, Mumbai, India

A. Jain et al. (eds.), *Cutting-edge Vitreoretinal Surgery*,
https://doi.org/10.1007/978-981-33-4168-5_1

1.1.2 Post-Gonin Era

In the 1920s, a Swiss ophthalmologist, Jules Gonin recognised the role of retinal breaks in retinal detachment and proposed the sealing of retinal breaks that could help settle the retinal detachment. Gonin proposed 'ignipuncture', where accurate localisation of the break and drainage of subretinal fluid via thermocautery around the tear through sclera was done [16–18]. Amsler and Dubois devised the fundus chart in 1928, which is used till date, in modified form for mapping the extent of retinal detachment, breaks and other lesions in the retina. Many procedures following Gonin's procedure were a modification of it. Methods for cauterisation were either thermal or chemical. Diathermy was either surface, penetrating and partial penetrating or surface diathermy with penetrating application. The use of intraocular air and experimentation with scleral resection provided the base for scleral buckling [19]. In Gonin's era, the success rate of surgery for retinal detachment exceeded 50%.

A year later, after the development of a direct ophthalmoscope, Christian Ruete modified the design and introduced indirect ophthalmoscopy. In 1946, Charles Schepens modified this design and introduced head-mounted binocular indirect ophthalmoscopy as what we know today, which brought about a significant contribution in recognition of breaks in the retina.

1.2 Scleral Buckling

In 1951, Charles Schepens, 'Father of Modern Retinal Surgery', introduced encircling scleral buckling procedure for the management of retinal detachment. The procedure included lamellar scleral placement of the buckle made of polyethylene tube, along with subretinal fluid drainage and thermocautery.

In 1958, Harvey Lincoff travelled to Dusseldorf, Germany, where he observed the use of polyviol explant over the break with a single mattress suture and non-drainage technique of scleral buckling being performed by Ernst Custodis (though he had devised the technique in 1949). He brought back the technique to New York, USA. He observed that the rate of infection with this explant was high, so in consultation with Dow Corning, he developed a soft silicone sponge to buckle retinal tears. It was also observed by him, that the scleral necrosis was more due to the use of diathermy. He noted the use of carbon dioxide pencil to indolent skin lesion at a dermatologist clinic. He then pioneered the use of cryopexy transclerally for sealing breaks in retinal detachment with the help of probe developed by John Mclean. It was also later noted by him that cryopexy could be used for destroying cells in retinoblastoma. Besides this, he also designed spatula-shaped needles to sew the sponge to the wall of the eye, which help reduce the incidence of accidental perforation. Harvey Lincoff learnt that placement of buckle episclerally had far less incidence of inflammation and infection. He adopted this technique and found the same results.

In 1971, through the publication, 'Finding the Retinal Hole', Harvey Lincoff shared the information with the world about finding the position of a primary break in a rhegmatogenous retinal detachment. Today, this set of rules, known as 'Lincoffs rule' are taught to ophthalmologists under training all over the world [20].

1.3 Vitreoretinal Surgery

Robert Machemer, better known as the 'Father of Modern Vitreoretinal surgery', was inspired by a colleague's, David Kashner's first open sky vitrectomy in 1961. He devised VISC (vitrectomy, infusion, suction, cutter) with Jean Marie Parel. After experimenting and succeeding in removing the egg albumin through the motorised instrument via 17 gauge ports, in order to improve the visibility, he later added fibre optic light pipe for endoillumination. In 1970, he obtained good results in cases of vitreous haemorrhage and poor results in case of proliferative vitreoretinopathy [21]. Machemer realised that the best area to approach vitreous was pars plana, as here RPE and ciliary epithelium were so firmly adherent that an opening could be made here without causing retinal detachment.

In 1974, Connor O Malley and Ralph Heinz introduced 20 gauge, three-port pars plana vitrectomy [22]. Gholam Peyman introduced Guillotone vitrectomy cutter. In 1976, Steve Charles introduced linear and delta suction controlled system where suction pressure could be set from 0 to 400 mm Hg. This advancement permitted surgeons to work very close to the retina without the fear of causing iatrogenic retinal tear. Steve Charles also introduced fluid air exchange, flute needle, internal drainage of SRF and endophotocoagulation techniques. He was instrumental in the development of proportional or linear mode in vitrectomy, which is the basis of the machines available today [22]. Though it was Ohm who advised the use of intravitreal gas for pneumoretinopexy, in 1911, Edward W.D. Norton devised the use of sulphur hexafluoride (SF6) as a tamponade agent [19, 23]. Lincoff and Vyagantas pioneered the use of the straight-chain perfluorocarbon gases for the management of complicated detachments. Subsequently, they demonstrated that intraocular gas was not entirely benign and could be the precursor of pre-retinal proliferation [24]. Silicone oil was introduced by Cibis et al. Zivojnovic pioneered the use of silicon oil to treat proliferative vitreoretinopathy and as a tamponade [25].

Modern vitreoretinal surgery has refined over the years. One of the significant advances in retinal surgery was the development of smaller vitrectomy probes, which allowed the transition to the microincision vitrectomy system (MIVS), introduced in 2002 by Fujii et al. using 25-gauge instruments [26], followed by Eckardt in 2005 [27], with 23-gauge cutters and 27 gauge system by Oshima in 2010 [28].

Another significant advancement has happened in the viewing system. Conventional viewing systems included lens such as the Goldman lens, Landers lens, Peymans lens, which were placed on the cornea, provided a limited field of view, and required suturing to be held in position during surgery. Development of wide-angle viewing systems led to an increase in the field of view, but the view was inverted. Stereoscopic diagonal inverter (SDI) developed by Spitnaz and Riever was used to reinvert the image for the surgery. Non-contact wide-field viewing systems such as BIOM (Binocular indirect Ophthalmomicroscope) with SDI, EIBOSS (Erect indirect binocular indirect ophthalmomicroscope system), were developed which have controls for fine focusing integrated into the foot pedal. Chandelier assisted viewing system allows bimanual surgery in complicated retinal detachments and trauma cases.

1.4 Learnings from the Past

History repeats itself and here are some examples of the same. Macular buckling first described in 1957 by Charles Schepens [29] is again in use for appropriate cases of macular hole, macular detachment or foveoschisis associated with posterior staphyloma in pathological myopia.

Poole and Sudarsky introduced the concept of suprachoroidal buckling in 1986 as suprachoroidal implantation for treatment of peripheral retinal breaks in retinal detachment. In 2013, Oshima, Rayes et al. designed a catheter to inject and place long-lasting hyaluronic acid in the suprachoroidal space, indenting the choroid alone to close the retinal tear through the suprachoroidal space. The mechanism is to indent the choroid and create a suprachoroidal buckling effect to close tears or support the retina and can be used instead of suturing a scleral buckle. This method was also suggested for the management of myopic macular traction [30].

Autologous retinal pigment epithelium and choroid transplantation for the treatment of exudative and atrophic maculopathies has been suggested by Parolini et al. in 2019 [31]. Mark Humayun co-invented the Argus series retina implants, also known as the bionic eye, which is a visual prosthesis to improve vision in patients with severe retinitis pigmentosa. He is one of the investigators working on research for replacement of retinal pigment epithelial cells with stem cells for the management of age-related macular degeneration [32].

1.5 Conclusion

Vitreoretinal surgery has been undergoing a lot of refinement and history not only provides us with the knowledge of the past theories and procedures and evolution of a new technique or a machine but also helps us learn from others' experiences. It helps us to have information to form a base, a foundation to build upon and maybe provide an opportunity to work on an idea, to modify or to invent procedures that might be useful in improvement of conditions that we still do not have answers to.

References

1. Ware J. Chirurgical observations related to the eye. London: J Mawman 1805; 2 (2): 238.
2. von Helmholtz HLF. Beschreibung eines Augen-Spiegels. Berlin: A Förstner' sche Verlagsbuchhandlung; 1851.
3. Coccius A. Über die Anwendung des Augen-Spiegels nebst Angabe eines neuen Instruments. Leipzig: Immanuel Muller; 1853. p. 130–1.
4. von Graefe A. Notiz ueber die im Glaskoerper vorkommenden Opacitaeten. Arch f Ophthalmol. 1854;1:351.
5. Martin G. VII Int Cong Med. 1881;3:110.
6. de Wecker M. Ann Oculist Paris. 1882;87:39.
7. Groenholm. Von Graefes Arch Ophthalmol. 1921;105:899.
8. Grossman K. On the mechanical treatment of detached retina. Ophthalmic Rev. 1883;2:289.
9. Mellinger JB. Augenheilanstalt in Basel. 1893;32:79.
10. Carbone. Atti Cong Soc Oftal Ital. 1925:301.
11. Gloor BP, Marmor MF. Controversy over the etiology and therapy of retinal detachment: the struggles of Jules Gonin. Surv Ophthalmol. 2013;58(2):184–95.
12. Stellwag C. Lehrbuch der praktischen Augenheilkunde. Vienna: Wilhelm Braumueller; 1861.
13. Donders. Die Anomalien der Refraction und Accomodation des Auges. Wie; 1866.
14. Samelsohn J. Ueber mechanische Behandlung der Netzhaut-abloesung. Zentrablatt fuer die Medizinischen Wissenschaften. 1875;49:833.
15. Vail DT. An inquiry into results of the established treatment of detachment of the retina and a new theory. Trans Am Acad Ophthalmol Otolaryngol. 1912;17:29.
16. Gonin J. Ann Oculist Paris. 1919;156:281.
17. Gonin J. Pathogenie et anatomie pathologique des decollements retiniens. Bull Soc Franc Ophtal. 1920;33:1.
18. Gonin J. The treatment of detached retina by sealing the retinal tears. Arch Ophthalmol. 1930;4:621.
19. Wilkinson CP, Rice TA. Michels retinal detachment, vol. 2. St Louis: Mosby; 1997. p. 241–333.
20. Lincoff H. The evolution of retinal surgery: a personal story. Arch Ophthalmol. 2009;127(7):923–8. https://doi.org/10.1001/archophthalmol.2009.164.
21. Blodi CF, David Kasner MD. The road to pars Plana vitrectomy. Ophthalmol Eye Dis. 2016;8(1):1–4. https://doi.org/10.4137/OED.S40424.
22. Charles S. The history of vitrectomy: innovation and evolution. Retina Today. 2008:27–9.
23. Rezaei KA, Abrams GW. The history of retinal detachment surgery: primary retinal detachment: options for repair, vol. 1. Berlin: Springer; 2005. p. 1–25.
24. Lincoff H, Gieser R. Finding the retinal hole. Arch Ophthalmol. 1971;85(5):565.
25. Zivojnovic R. Silicone oil in vitreoretinal surgery (Martinus Nijhoff/Dr W junk). Dordrecht: Springer; 1987. p. 25–8.
26. Fujii GY, De Juan E Jr, Humayun MS, Pieramici DJ, Chang TS, Awh C, et al. A new 25-gauge instrument system for transconjunctival sutureless vitrectomy surgery. Ophthalmology. 2002;109:1807–12.
27. Eckardt C. Transconjunctival sutureless 23-gauge vitrectomy. Retina. 2005;25:208–11.
28. Oshima Y, Wakabayashi T, Sato T, et al. A 27-gauge instrument system for transconjunctival sutureless microincision vitrectomy surgery. Ophthalmology. 2010;117:93–102.
29. Schepens CL, Okamura ID, Brockhurst RJ. The scleral buckling procedure. I. Surgical technique and management. AMA Arch Ophthalmol. 1957;58(6):797–811.
30. El Rayes EN. Suprachoroidal catheter for suprachoroidal buckling with and without vitrectomy to treat uncomplicated rhegmatogenous retinal detachment. Retina Today. 2013:71–6.
31. Parolini B, Grewal SD, Mahmoud TH. Combined autologous transplantation of neurosensory retina, retinal pigment epithelium and choroid free grafts. Retina. 2018;38(1):S12–22. https://doi.org/10.1097/IAE.0000000000001914.
32. Michael Jumper J. FDA approves world's first artificial retina—Retina Times talks with Argus® Ii developer, Mark Humayun. ASRS. Retina Times; 2013. https://www.asrs.org/publications/retina-times/details/131/fda-approves-world-first-artificial-retina.

Part II

Surgical Anatomy, Imaging and Anaesthesia in Vitreoretinal Surgery

2 Surgical Anatomy of Vitreous

J. Ben Margines, John Nesemann, and J. Sebag

2.1 Introduction

Vitreous is an enigmatic tissue which is important in many ophthalmic conditions treated with posterior segment surgery. Fascinating scientists for centuries and causing controversy regarding its structure, vitreous poses a unique dilemma regarding the study of its structure, for how is one to study a tissue which has been pressured by evolution to remain invisible? (Fig. 2.1) [1, 2]. Published research has consistently shown its relevance to the development of many common retinal pathologies including Proliferative Diabetic Retinopathy (PDR), exudative age-related macular degeneration (AMD), and via Anomalous Posterior Vitreous Detachment (APVD) retinal detachment (RD), macular holes, and macular pucker. As such, an understanding of vitreous anatomy is crucial to improving surgical approaches and techniques to optimize patient outcomes.

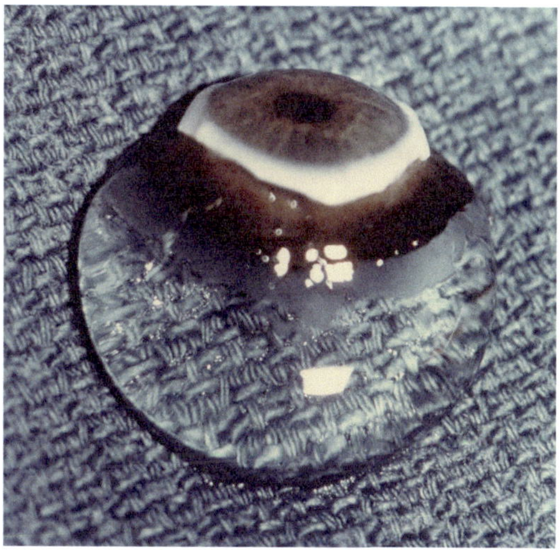

Fig. 2.1 Human vitreous with sclera choroid and retina peeled off. The specimen is situated on a surgical towel in room air, yet maintains its shape due to the firmly gelatinous consistency of the vitreous body in this 9-month-old child. (Cover Photo—Sebag J: The Vitreous – Structure, Function, and Pathobiology, Springer-Verlag, New York, 1989)

2.2 Embryology

Development of the eye starts around day 22 of gestation when the forebrain evaginates to become optic peduncles. They proliferate laterally until day 27 when they become large, single layer vesi-

J. B. Margines · J. Nesemann
David Geffen School of Medicine at UCLA, Los Angeles, CA, USA
e-mail: BMargines@mednet.ucla.edu; JNesemann@mednet.ucla.edu

J. Sebag (✉)
David Geffen School of Medicine at UCLA, Los Angeles, CA, USA

Doheny Eye Institute at UCLA, Los Angeles, CA, USA

VMR Institute for Vitreous Macula Retina, Huntington Beach, CA, USA
e-mail: jsebag@VMRinstitute.com

A. Jain et al. (eds.), *Cutting-edge Vitreoretinal Surgery*,
https://doi.org/10.1007/978-981-33-4168-5_2

cles called the primary optic vesicles that are connected to the developing brain contiguous with the third ventricle through the optic stalk. The primary optic vesicles expand outwards, and upon contacting the surface ectoderm induce the formation of the lens primordia. On day 29, a groove in the optic stalk appears, called the retinal fissure (also known as the choroid or optic fissure); it incorporates both mesenchymal cells and the hyaloid artery and vein by day 33 which vascularizes the optic stalk and optic vesicle. Invagination and fusion of the optic vesicle results in a double-walled structure called the optic cup or secondary optic vesicle. Development of the secondary optic vesicle and optic stalk continues throughout gestation [3].

The same mesenchyme that infiltrated through the optic fissure begins to form the primary vitreous body which has been described by Balazs as a "cellular, loose connective tissue containing blood vessels" [4]. These vessels are the network of fetal hyaloid vasculature, which originate from the optic nerve head and feed the primary vitreous and lens through its three distinct sections: the vasa hyaloidea propria, the branches in vitreous closest to the retina; the tunica vasculosa lentis, which covers the posterior hemisphere of the lens; and the pupillary membrane, which covers the more anterior part of the lens [5] (Fig. 2.2). The retinal fissure begins to close at 37 days and completely encloses the primary vitreous body at 47 days when the anterior portion of the fissure closes, thus sealing the optic cup. Vitreous plays an important role at this stage by exerting internal swelling pressure, influencing the size of the growing eye. Abnormalities in this process might play a role in the pathogenesis of myopia. The primary vitreous then undergoes conversion to the acellular secondary vitreous via the synthesis of new collagen fibrils [4]. Hyaloid vessels reach maximal development by the ninth week of gestation, and persist until the around 3 months of gestation when the vessels begin to atrophy [6]. After atrophy of the hyaloid artery and the vasa hyaloidea propia, the vitreous body does not undergo further cellular remodeling.

Anomalies in regression of the fetal vasculature play a role in the syndrome of persistent fetal vasculature, which causes 5% of infantile blindness, and probably also plays a role in retinopathy of prematurity [5]. Furthermore, regression of the fetal hyaloid vasculature gives rise to Eisner's tracts which are the same structures as Worst's cisterns, described below. Remnants of the fetal hyaloid vasculature might also be the origin of the "glass noodle" floaters that appear later in life, especially in patients with myopic vitreopathy, at times sufficiently severe to cause *Vision Degrading Myodesopsia* [61].

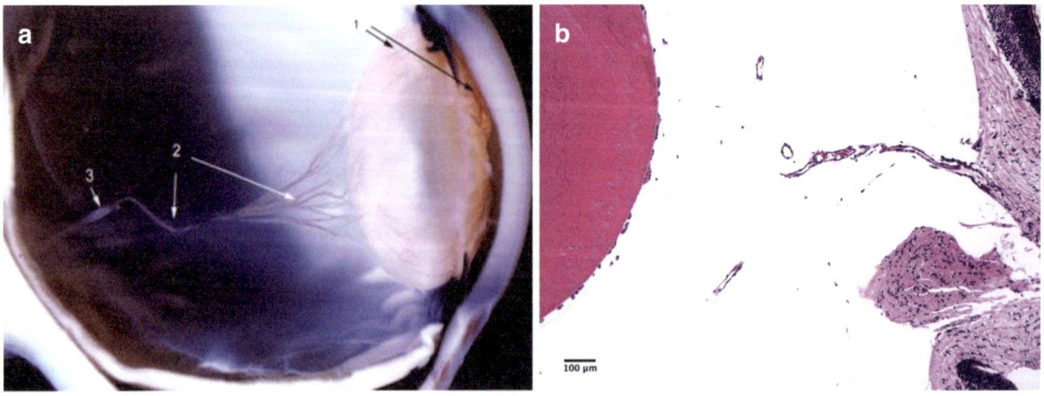

Fig. 2.2 (**a**) Embryologic vasculature of human vitreous during early embryogenesis demonstrates the hyaloid artery arising from the optic disc (left; 3), branching to form the vasa hyaloidea propria in the vitreous body (center; 2), and anastomosing with the tunica vasculosa lentis surrounding the crystalline lens (right; 1). (**b**) Histology of embryonic fetal vitreous vasculature. The crystalline lens is on the left

2.3 Vitreous Anatomy

The vitreous body occupies a spherical space surrounded by the retina, lens, and pars plana of the eye. It can be divided into the central vitreous, basal vitreous, and vitreous cortex. In an emmetropic eye, the vitreous body has an axial length of approximately 16.5 mm with a depression just posterior to the lens named the patellar fossa. Figure 2.3 demonstrates the classic description of significant structures within the vitreous body. The hyaloideocapsular ligament of Weiger is a ring-like attachment of the anterior vitreous body to the lens, measuring 8 mm in diameter and 1 mm in width. "Erggelet's or "Berger's" space is at the center of the hyaloideocapsular ligament. Arising from this space and coursing posteriorly through the central vitreous is the Canal of Cloquet, which is the former site of the hyaloid artery in the primary vitreous. The former lumen of the artery is devoid of vitreous collagen fibrils and is surrounded by fenestrated sheaths that were previously the basal laminae of the hyaloid artery wall. Posteriorly, Cloquet's canal opens into a funnel-shaped region anterior to the optic disc known as the area Martegiani. Jongebloed and Worst described the premacular bursa as an anatomical area of liquid vitreous anterior to the macula (Fig. 2.4) [7].

2.3.1 Vitreous Base and Central Anterior Vitreous

The vitreous base is a 3-dimensional structure in the peripheral anterior vitreous that is shaped like a doughnut or tire straddling the ora serrata, attaching 1–2 mm anterior and 1–2 mm posterior to the ora, as well as extending several mm into the vitreous body. Collagen fibers of the peripheral vitreous project perpendicularly into the ciliary epithelium and peripheral retina, which causes the vitreous base to be the strongest point of vitreo-retinal adhesion [8]. With

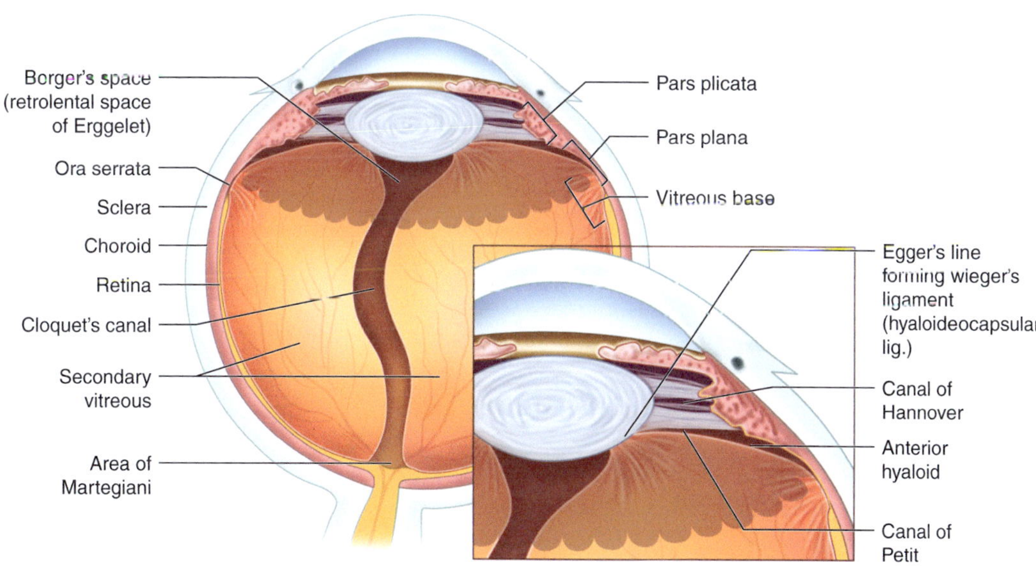

Fig. 2.3 Schematic of classic vitreous anatomy, where structures bear the names of the anatomists (from Sang D: Embryology of the Vitreous. In: The Vitreous and Vitreo-Retinal Interface (Schepens, Neetens, eds). Springer, New York, p 20)

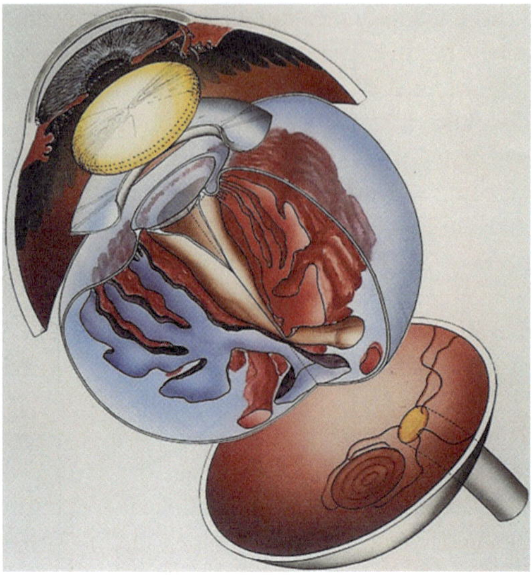

Fig. 2.4 Schematic diagram depicting the cisterns of Worst visualized by injection of India ink. The two structures of import are the Bursa Premacularis (light blue) and Cloquet's Canal (tan-colored). (From Jongbloed WL, Worst JGF: The cisternal system of the vitreous body. Doc Ophthalmol 67:183–96, 1987)

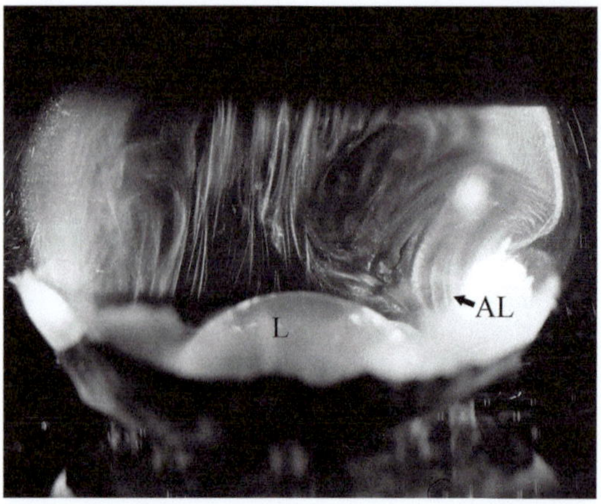

Fig. 2.5 The anterior loop of the human vitreous base ("AL") straddles the ora serrata and is the substrate surface upon which cells migrate and proliferate during anterior proliferative vitreo-retinopathy (PVR). Due to this anatomy, contraction of pathologic PVR membranes causes peripheral retinal detachment as well as ciliary body detachment with hypotony, sometimes also iris retraction

aging, there is a widening of the vitreous base with posterior migration of the posterior border temporally [9]. This unequal migration creates an undulating border that may contribute to the pathogenesis of retinal tears causing peripheral rhegmatogenous retinal detachment, which occur more often temporally [10]. The anterior portion of the vitreous base features the "anterior loop" of vitreous fibrils inserting to the pars plan a ciliaris (Fig. 2.5). This structure is important as it provides the substrate upon which cells migrate and proliferate in the formation of anterior proliferative vitreo-retinopathy (PVR), a major cause of failed retinal detachment surgery.

In anterior PVR, fibronectin and other extracellular matrix components are deposited in the anterior vitreous, allowing for cell migration and proliferation. These cells are myofibroblast-like but can derive from astrocytes and retinal pigment epithelial cells. Normal vitreous inhibits cellular invasion into the vitreous body, thus it is not clear how this is altered to permit cell migration and proliferation in PVR. Contraction is transmitted through the collagen fibers of the anterior loop that straddle the ora serrata to the anterior retina which causes it to "roll" forward. Since the anterior loop also inserts anterior to the ora serrata (Fig. 2.5), severe traction can also pull on the pars plana and detach the ciliary body, causing hypotony. To cure advanced cases, it is often necessary to excise the vitreous base by creating extensive circumferential retinectomies. However, recent studies have shown that treating primary rhegmatogenous retinal detachment by vitrectomy with intraoperative infusion of heparin and 5-FU significantly reduces the incidence of postoperative PVR, which may herald a new era of intraoperative pharmacologic adjuncts to vitreo-retinal surgery [11].

2.3.2 Posterior Vitreous Cortex

The posterior vitreous cortex is a thin, membranous structure continuous from the ora serrata to the posterior pole. Two round holes are present, one in prepapillary region, which is a true hole (see below), and one in the premacular area, which is not a true hole but a dehiscence of the very thin cortex in this region (Fig. 2.6). While the vitreous cortex comprises the entire peripheral shell of the vitreous body, the posterior vitreous cortex

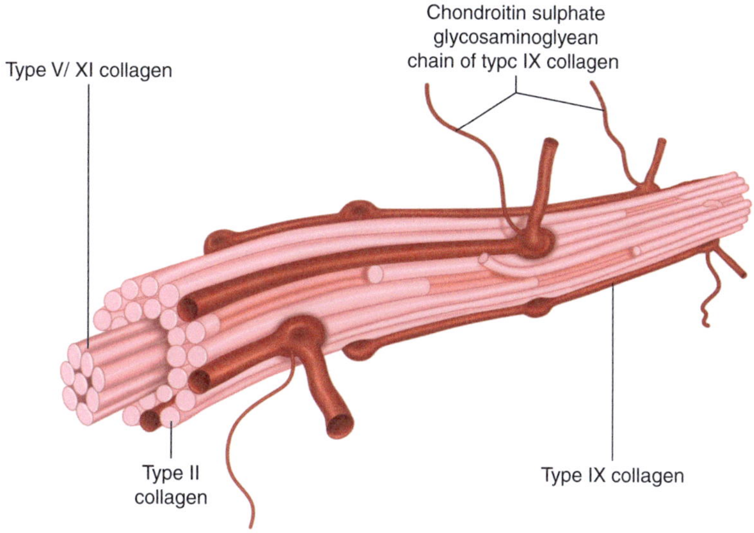

Fig. 2.6 Schematic diagram of vitreous collagen fibril organization, d'apres Bishop. The central core is a hybrid of types V and XI, surrounded by type II collagen (the most prevalent collagen type in human vitreous), with type IX collagen on the surface of the fibril

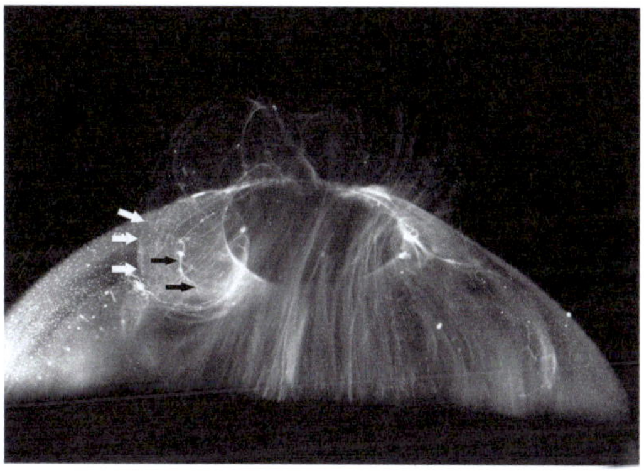

Fig. 2.7 Dark-field slit microscopy of adult human posterior vitreous anatomy after dissection of the sclera, choroid, and retina demonstrates the hole in the prepapillary posterior vitreous cortex (black arrows) with extruding gel vitreous (white arrows). The large circular dehiscence to the right is not a true hole *in situ*, but has the appearance of a "hole" in this dissection due to dehiscence of the very thin premacular posterior vitreous cortex (From Sebag J: The Vitreous – Structure, Function, and Pathobiology. Springer-Verlag, New York, 1989, p 48)

is of great importance to vitreo-retinal surgeons due to its membranous, sheet-like attachment to the retina, focal attachment to the optic disc and fovea, and linear attachments along retinal blood vessels. There is no vitreous cortex directly over the optic disc, and the thinnest area of posterior vitreous cortex is located directly posterior to the premacular bursa of Worst. The posterior vitreous cortex (often incorrectly referred to as the "hyaloid," a term that should be reserved for the embryonic artery of the vitreous body) is 110–110μm thick, and has a lamellar organization of densely packed collagen fibrils composed of various collagen types, primarily type II [12] (Fig. 2.7). The lamellar organization of the posterior vitreous cortex can complicate the induction of PVD during vitreo-retinal surgery, since there can be iatrogenic splitting between the layers of the posterior vitreous cortex, known as *vitreoschisis*, leaving the outermost layer of vitreous attached to the retina [13]. The result could be persistent pathology requiring reoperation [13]. Intraoperative OCT could mitigate against this complication, but simple awareness of the underlying anatomy should alert the surgeon to pay heed.

2.3.2.1 Hyalocytes

Hyalocytes are mononuclear phagocytes that derive from monocyte/macrophage lineage and are distinct from glial cells or retinal pigment epithelium cells, which they can sometimes resemble (Fig. 2.8) [14]. Located in a monolayer 20–50μm anterior to the retina, hyalocytes are postulated to be replaced continuously from bone marrow precursors, but may also undergo mitosis to regenerate. Based on rabbit and bovine studies, hyalocyte density is highest at the vitreous base and the posterior pole, and lowest at the equator [14]. The function of these cells may be to maintain synthesis and metabolism of glycoproteins (including HA), and to promote vitreous clarity by removing fibrin and associated molecules. As members of the reticuloendothelial system found throughout the body (e.g., lung and kidney), hyalocytes act as sentinel cells on the lookout for noxious stimuli, such as trauma, blood, infection and chemical injury. Given their location near the retina, hyalocytes are the first cells to respond to injury or insult in this critical location, and they do so by eliciting an inflammatory/immune response as well as becoming phagocytes for antigen processing and immune mobilization. Hyalocytes have also been shown in bovine models to respond to hypoxia-inducible factor-1 by secreting VEGF [15]. These mechanisms represent typical wound healing which can unfortunately have untoward consequences within the eye, in this case by creating macular pucker, PVR, etc.

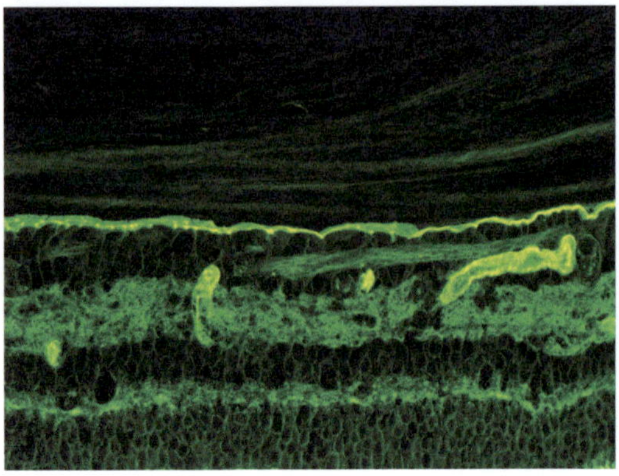

Fig. 2.8 Immunohistochemistry of the surgical anatomy of the posterior vitreous cortex in the monkey demonstrates a lamellar organization of the posterior vitreous above the Inner Limiting Membrane, which is the brightly staining line in the center (Courtesy of Greg Hageman, PhD)

Macular Pucker

If the entire posterior vitreous cortex separates away from the retina, PVD is innocuous. However, in anomalous PVD, there can be splitting between the layers of the posterior vitreous cortex (Fig. 2.9), known as *vitreoschisis* [16]. If

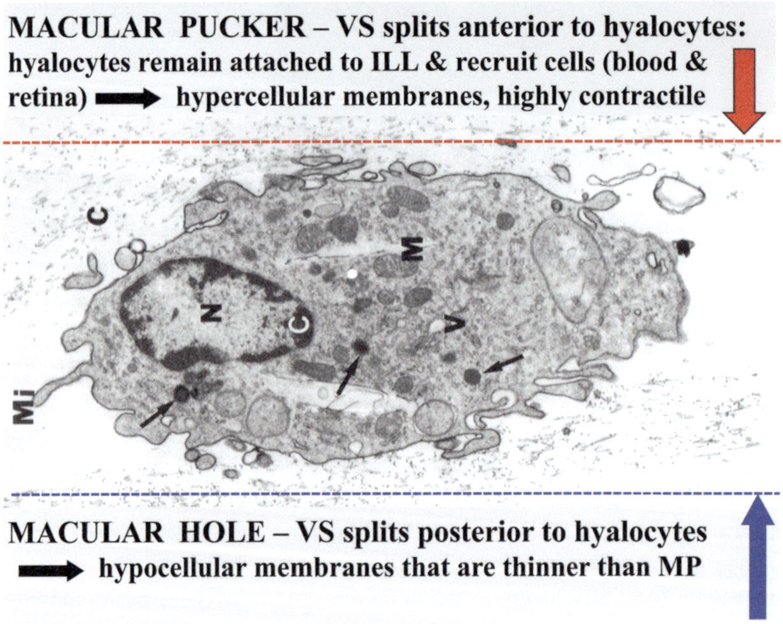

Fig. 2.9 Transmission EM of human hyalocyte embedded in the collagenous posterior vitreous cortex. The anterior segment is above, and the posterior pole is below in this image. During anomalous PVD, vitreoschisis (VS) can split anterior to the level of hyalocytes (red line), leaving them on the retinal surface and promoting contractile membrane formation with macular pucker. VS posterior to the level of hyalocytes leaves a thinner, hypocellular membrane that is commonly found in macular holes. *ILL* internal limiting lamina, *MP* macular pucker

the split occurs anterior to the level of the hyalocyte monolayer, these cells remain attached to the retina and the aforementioned cytokines can lead to cell proliferation forming a hypercellular membrane and membrane contraction, which can cause macular pucker via centripetal (inward toward the fovea) tangential traction. Figure 2.9 demonstrates hyalocytes and their location relative to the level of the split during anomalous PVD with vitreoschisis. It is important that when operating on a patient without PVD, the entire full-thickness of the posterior vitreous cortex is removed, lest the outer layer (with hyalocytes) remains attached to the retina, which would risk the development of postoperative (recurrent) macular pucker.

2.4 Molecular Structure

Vitreous is essentially a bimolecular network primarily consisting of water (98%), and macromolecules (2%), specifically collagen and hyaluronan. In youth, these are homogeneously distributed throughout the vitreous body to form a solid clear gel that is firmly adherent to the retina posteriorly and the lens anteriorly. The interaction of collagen and HA with each other as well as with other extracellular matrix components of the vitreous body is critical to the maintenance of a solid clear gel within the center of the eye, but the exact nature of their association is unknown. Electrostatic interactions between these molecules might play a role, as HA is negatively charged while collagen is positively charged [17]. Whereas it was previously thought that HA and collagen are randomly distributed throughout the vitreous body, it is more likely that there is a highly ordered arrangement to achieve both the gel state (important for shock absorption and physiologic functions described below), and the maintenance of transparency within the vitreous body to allow unhindered photon transmission to the retina.

2.4.1 Collagen

The primary structural macromolecule of vitreous is collagen, of which Type II is the predominant type (75%). Minor forms include types V, IX, and XI, which occur in a molar ratio of 75:15:10, and type XVIII, for which its progenitor (endostatin) is a powerful antiangiogenic molecule, likely important in promoting avascularity and transparency in the center of the eye [18]. These collagen molecules are formed into fibrils containing a central core of hybrid types V/XI, surrounded by type II, with type IX on the surface [19] (Fig. 2.10). Aging and hyperglycemia promote cross-linking of these fibrils with consequent vitreous gel liquefaction and syneresis (collapse) of the vitreous body, which contributes to various vitreo-retinal pathologies [20].

2.4.2 Hyaluronan

Hyaluronan (HA) is a large, negatively charged, non-sulfated glycosaminoglycan, which is produced shortly after birth and throughout life, possibly by hyalocytes [4, 6]. Molecules of HA are intertwined with the collagen matrix providing visco-elastic properties and transparency to the vitreous body [6]. The elasticity of vitreous is responsible for damping the rotational force produced by ocular saccades and head movement.

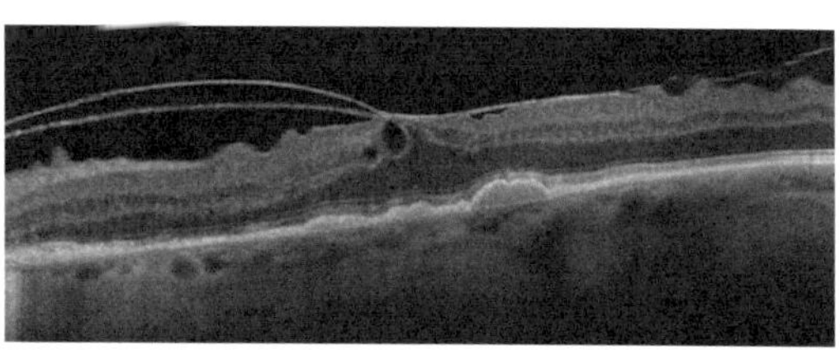

Fig. 2.10 OCT of vitreoschisis in a patient with macular drusen and a macular cyst demonstrates the rejoining of the split posterior vitreous cortex just anterior to the cyst (courtesy of Jay Duker, MD)

As different regions within the vitreous body have differing concentrations of macromolecules, viscoelasticity is heterogenous throughout. A recent study on the rheology of the vitreous gel has hypothesized that the molecular components manifest themselves in the response of the vitreous to shear stress, such that rotational forces are first dampened by the collagen structure, and later by the microfibrils and HA network [21]. The increased distance between the optic disc and the superotemporal retina is speculated to allow for greater strain relief in the inferonasal area and be related to the higher incidence of retinal tears superotemporally, although evidence has not yet shown this. Further, HA within the vitreous body behaves as a polyelectrolyte which is sensitive to ionic changes that alter the compression or extension of the molecule. Thus, changes in ionic milieu in diabetes can cause expansion and compression of the entire vitreous. As new blood vessels grow from the optic disc and retina into the posterior vitreous cortex in proliferative diabetic retinopathy (PDR), the ionic and fluid fluxes will periodically expand and contract the vitreous body, exerting traction anywhere vitreous is attached. In ischemic retinopathies such as PDR, this could stimulate further growth of new blood vessels that are attached to the posterior vitreous cortex and rupture them causing vitreous hemorrhage.

2.4.3 Other Molecular Components

Ascorbate is transported into the vitreous body by a sodium-dependent ascorbate transporter (SLC23A2) such that ascorbate levels are 33–40 times higher in vitreous than blood [22]. As an antioxidant, ascorbate protects the retina, lens, and trabecular meshwork from oxidative stress [22]. Excess oxygen from the highly vascularized retina and choroid is limited from moving anteriorly by the vitreous gel, and it is eliminated in the overlying cortex by the ascorbate. This effect is blunted in liquified vitreous and vitrectomized eyes, such that oxygen diffuses more freely under the influence of head or eye movement, thereby increasing oxidative stress. This is postulated to be a primary reason for the development of nuclear sclerotic cataract (convincingly) [23] and open-angle glaucoma (less certainly) [24] in vitrectomized eyes. Thus, an important consideration when performing vitrectomy is how much vitreous to remove. This depends upon the problem being treated. Vitreo-maculopathies and Vision Degrading Myodesopsia do not need removal of as much vitreous as retinal detachment and diabetic retinopathy. It is therefore worth considering a limited approach in selected cases wherein a surgical PVD is not induced and anterior vitreous cortex is left intact, since studies have shown a lower incidence of cataract surgery following limited vitrectomy [25].

Other molecular components of vitreous (not covered in this chapter) include chondroitin sulfate, fibrillins, and opticin [26, 27]. Other aspects of the role(s) of vitreous in ocular anti-oxidant activities has recently been reveiwed [63].

2.5 Vitreo-Retinal Interface

2.5.1 Inner Limiting Membrane

The Inner Limiting Membrane (ILM), which is the basement membrane of Müller cells, is composed predominantly of type IV collagen, organized in three layers: the lamina rara externa (adjacent to Müller cell footplates, 0.03–0.06μm thick), the lamina densa (thinnest at the fovea, 0.01–0.02μm, and thickest in the posterior pole, 0.5–3.2μm), and the lamina rara interna (a uniform inner layer) [1]. Peeling ILM is often done during vitrectomy surgery for membranous vitreo-maculopathies causing macular holes and macular pucker. Studies suggest that ILM peeling can improve visual outcomes, decrease post-operative cystoid macular edema and lower the rate of secondary premacular membrane development necessitating repeat vitrectomy, thereby providing cost benefit [28–30]. This is because ILM peeling assures the removal of all pathologic vitreous, the true cause of the problem [31]. However, if full-thickness ILM is removed,

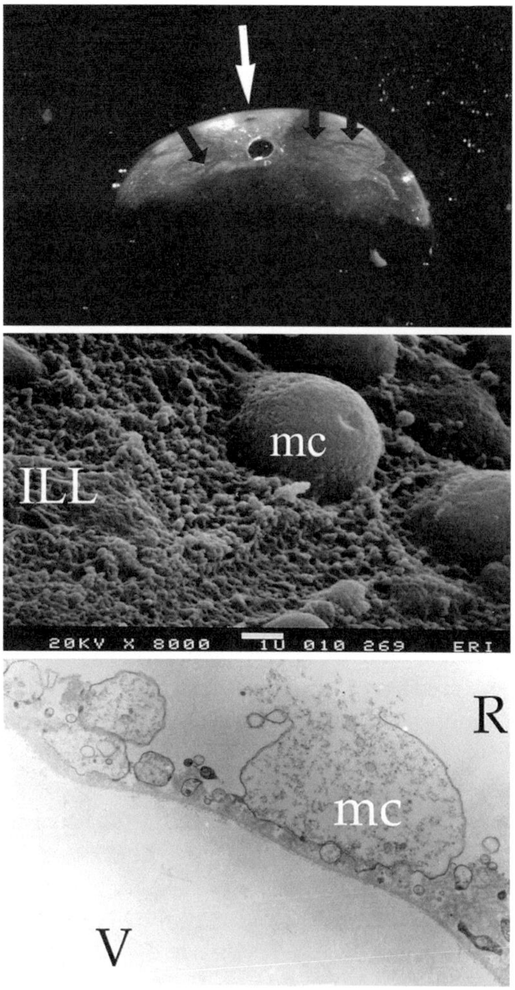

Fig. 2.11 Strong vitreo-retinal adhesion in youth is demonstrated by the persistent adherence of the ILM and footplates of Mueller cells to the posterior vitreous cortex after peeling the retina off the vitreous body. *MC* Mueller cell footplates, *V* vitreous, *R* retina (From Sebag J: Age-related differences in the human vitreo-retinal interface. Arch Ophthalmol 109:966–71, 1991)

there might be damage to the inner retina, specifically Mueller cell footplates (Fig. 2.11). This has indeed been reported but apparently without untoward effects on vision [32]. Other studies, however, found that ILM peeling during reoperations can damage the inner retina and cause secondary optic neuropathy with profound vision loss, a condition termed inner retinal optic neuropathy (IRON) [33]. The recommendation of those studies was to delay reoperation for 6 months, allowing enough time for regeneration of the ILM and safer surgery.

2.5.2 Intervening Extracellular Matrix

Between the posterior vitreous cortex and the ILM of the retina is an Extracellular Matrix (ECM), which is possibly formed by hyalocytes and perhaps Mueller cells as well. This ECM is composed of fibronectin, laminin, and other components including opticin, which is believed to contribute adhesive as well as anti-angiogenic properties [14]. At the sites of strongest vitreo-retinal adhesion, chondroitin sulfate enhances the adhesion, forming the rationale for pharmacologic vitreolysis using avidin–biotin complex chondroitinase [34]. Because of this firm adhesion, caution should be exercised during membrane peel surgery in these locations. In diabetics, the thickening of the vitreo-retinal interface via protein glycosylation, occurring especially in the ECM can contribute to the growth of proliferating new vessels into the posterior vitreous cortex [35], which further increases vitreo-retinal adhesion at these sites, promoting rupture of the new vessels with vitreous hemorrhage, and iatrogenic retinal breaks during surgery. It would be beneficial to target the vitreo-retinal ECM with new pharmacologic vitreolysis agents to assist during surgery, or to be used preventatively to induce PVD prophylactically prior to the onset of advanced disease requiring surgery [36].

2.5.3 Retinal Blood Vessels

The ILM is thinnest over the major retinal blood vessels, featuring pores within the ILM overlying the vessels. Through these pores run strands of vitreous collagen which extend onto and surround the blood vessels. These vitreo-retinovascular bands may explain the adhesion between vitreous and retinal blood vessels, which might contribute to hemorrhagic events when vitreous traction overcomes vessel wall strength [1]. Estimates of the incidence of vitreous hemorrhage during PVD vary from 8% (when considered solely as PVD without retinal tear) to 21–23% (for PVD with retinal tears) [37–39]. Indeed, it is important to consider that non-diabetic patients with acute vitreous hemorrhage that obscures a view of the fundus have a 67% prevalence of retinal tears and a 39% prevalence of retinal detachments [40].

In diabetic patients, the ILM thickens and there are changes to the posterior vitreous cortex that increase vitreo-retinal adhesion. There are also biochemical and structural changes within the vitreous body (see below), that may predispose to anomalous PVD with vitreoschisis, vitreous hemorrhage, and retinal neovascularization [35]. Indeed, diabetic patients with a complete PVD have a lower risk of progressive retinopathy, whereas those with attached and especially partially detached posterior vitreous have the highest risk of progression to more severe forms of diabetic retinopathy [41]. Furthermore, proliferative diabetic retinopathy (PDR) is frequently associated with the development of blood-filled vitreoschisis cavities, both via a tractional event (created by vitreoschisis formation) which ruptures a new blood vessel, or by the blood from a ruptured blood vessel dissecting a plane and creating a schisis cavity. As a consequence, it is important when dissecting fibrovascular vitreoretinal membranes in PDR that both anterior and posterior walls of the vitreoschisis cavity are excised.

2.5.4 Vitreomacular Interface

Macroscopic studies of the vitreo-macular interface identified that the posterior vitreous cortex is thin in a circular area 4–5 mm in diameter, within which the vitreous is attached in an irregular annular zone of 3–4 mm diameter [13]. Ultrastructural studies with scanning electron microscopy of PVDs with vitreous cortical remnants attached to the fovea suggested that there are bands of strong vitreo-retinal attachment at 500μm and 1500μm from the fovea [42]. It is unclear, however, how these areas of thin posterior vitreous cortex and firm vitreo-retinal adhesion relate to the pathogenesis of full-thickness and lamellar macular holes. Indeed, there are various theories regarding the origin of vitreous traction in the pathogenesis of MH formation. One theory claims that during rotation of the eye, dynamic tractional forces are generated by posterior cortical vitreous movement. With OCT imaging, it has been shown that there are greater movement and duplication of the posterior cortical vitreous in patients with advancing stages of MH [43, 44]. This hypothesis seems to be based upon circumstantial evidence and is thus difficult to test experimentally. It is alternatively hypothesized that because of eccentric foci of macula pucker and persistent adhesion to the optic disc, the posterior vitreous cortex exerts centrifugal (outward from the fovea) tangential traction, creating a dehiscence in the central macula [45, 46]. The absence of an animal model with which to test these and other hypotheses makes drawing conclusions difficult. Clinically, however, vitrectomy with chromodissection [47] of the pathologic premacular membrane that is attached to the optic disc is highly effective in curing full-thickness macular holes, while surgery for lamellar macular holes is more effective in tractional than degenerative forms [48].

2.5.5 Vitreopapillary Interface

As the ILM approaches the optic disc, it terminates at the rim, but the basement membrane continues and is known as the inner limiting membrane of Elschnig [13]. This structure is 50 nm thick and thought to be the basal lamina of the astroglia in the optic nerve head. At the central portion of the disc, the membrane thins to 20 nm and follows the irregularities of the underlying cells. Here, it is composed only of glycosaminoglycans and no collagen. This portion is called the central meniscus of Kuhnt. Since the ILM helps prevent the passage of cells into the center of the eye, its absence at the disc as well as the thinness and chemical composition of this central area may account for frequent cell proliferation from or near the optic disc [13].

Vitreo-papillary adhesion (VPA) seems to be important in the pathophysiology of full-thickness macular holes (FTMH) and to a lesser extent lamellar macular holes (LMH), but not at all in macular pucker (MP). Using ultrasound and OCT of the optic disc and macula, Wang et al. found PVD in 92.9% of eyes with MP, 54.5% of eyes with lamellar hole ($P < 0.05$), but only 25% of eyes with macular hole ($P < 0.00001$) [49]. VPA was present in 87.5% of eyes with FTMH, 36.4% of eyes with LMH ($P < 0.05$), and only 17.9% MP eyes ($P < 0.00005$). Intraretinal cysts were present in 4/5 (80%) MP eyes with VPA but only 4.3% of MP eyes without VPA ($P < 0.005$). The investigators concluded that VPA has an important influence over the vector(s) of tangential traction in patients in certain vitreo-maculopathies (FTMH), but not all. Intraretinal cysts in MP are more likely due to traction than exudation (Fig. 2.12).

As described above, the molecular morphology of the vitreous body consists of a meshwork of collagen fibrils and coiled HA molecules interacting with each other and chondroitin sulfate as well as other extracellular matrix molecules. Electrostatic and other interactions between these molecules maintain transparency and the gel state. However, this complex molecular arrangement changes with aging and disease.

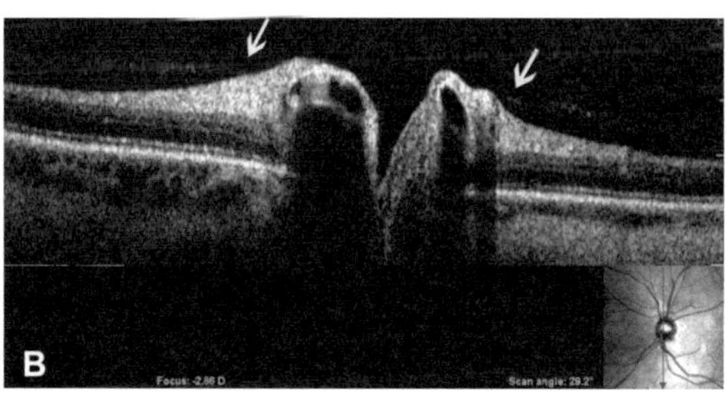

Fig. 2.12 OCT of Vitreo-Papillary Adhesion demonstrates persistent adhesion of the posterior vitreous cortex to the optic disc (arrows) (From Wang MY, Nguyen D, Hindoyan N, Sadun AA, Sebag J: Vitreo-papillary adhesion in macular hole and macular pucker. Retina 29:644–50, 2009)

2.6 Age-Related Changes

In youth, the aforementioned molecular interactions result in central transparency and only the dense collagen matrix in the posterior and peripheral vitreous cortex can be imaged on dark-field slit microscopy. (Fig. 2.13, top). The predominant site of liquefaction is the central vitreous, which has a low density of collagen during youth. Liquid vitreous appears at the early age of 4 years, but the process is accelerated in myopic eyes and with inflammatory conditions, in all cases increasing sharply after 40 years of age [50]. In the adult, there appears to be a reorganization of vitreous macromolecules so that the hydrophilic HA is displaced and forms liquid vitreous (synchysis), ultimately resulting in pockets of liquid vitreous, called lacunae (Fig. 2.13, bottom). The pathogenesis of liquefaction likely involves multiple mechanisms. Theories about this most often involve enzymatic or ROS-mediated destruction of the collagen or degradation and changes in the conformation of collagen and HA leading to cross-linking, aggregation, and displacement of fibrils [8].

During aging, vitreous collagen fibrils cross-link and form visible fibers that course in an anteroposterior direction from the vitreous base anteriorly to the vitreous cortex posteriorly (Fig. 2.13, middle). Anteriorly, these packed fibers branch out anterior and posterior to the ora serrata to form the anterior loop (see above and Fig. 2.5). Posteriorly, they travel circumferentially in the periphery and parallel to Cloquet's canal centrally. They insert into the vitreous cortex at the posterior pole, but do not insert into the Inner Limiting Membrane (ILM). When the spacing between these fibers is disrupted and structures arise in the central vitreous that scatter light and induce myodesopsia, or floaters [51]. In youth, this occurs only in myopic eyes, and patients with type I diabetes, while fibrous degeneration and liquefaction of the vitreous body are commonly found in age-related vitreous degeneration [52].

The transition from a clear gel to fibrous structures in the adult progresses with increased thickening and tortuosity of vitreous fibers in old age

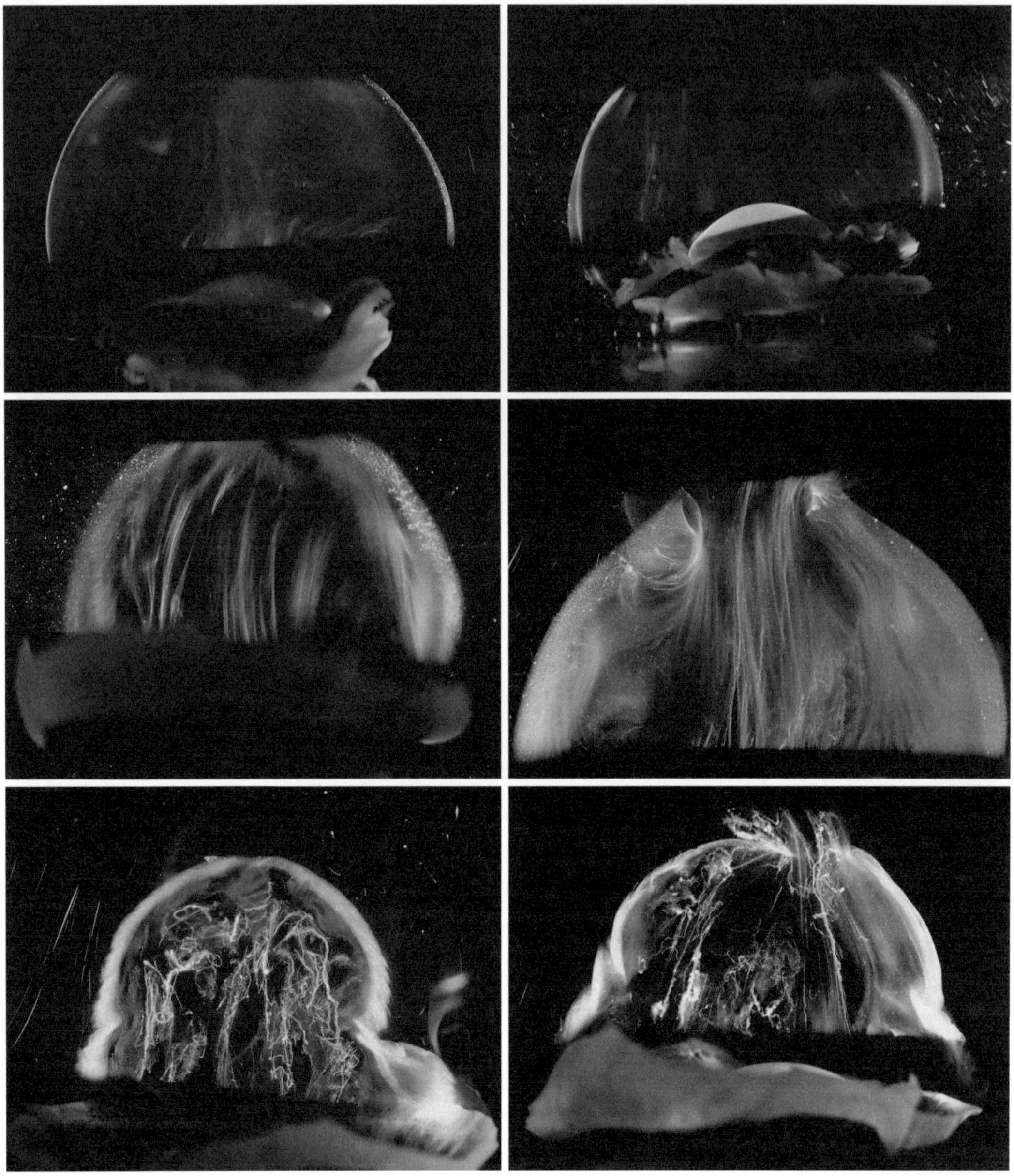

Fig. 2.13 Dark-field slit microscopy of dissected human vitreous demonstrates different morphology at different ages from relatively clear in children (top panel), to a fibrous structure in adults (middle panel), to tortuous aggregates of collagen with adjacent liquefaction in old age (bottom panel)

(Fig. 2.13, bottom). Eventually, destabilization by loss of gel and replacement by liquid vitreous results in collapse of the vitreous body, known as PVD. It is likely that the dissolution of posterior vitreous cortex-ILM adhesion at the posterior pole allows liquid vitreous to enter the retrocortical space. Thereafter, rotational eye movement contributes to the collapse of the vitreous body. Liquefaction is also important for surgical technique: one could mistake entry into a large pocket of liquid vitreous as entry into the retro-cortical space created after PVD. Likewise, surgical entry into a vitreoschisis cavity could be misinterpreted as entry behind the posterior vitreous cortex.

2.7 Vision Degrading Myodesopsia

At the time of PVD, most patients notice the onset of floaters, which are often not bothersome. However, many individuals are significantly bothered by vitreous floaters, due to light scattering by structures with the vitreous body, as well as the dense collagen matrix within the posterior vitreous cortex, as well as folding of this structure. Studies have shown that there can be a significant negative impact on quality-of-life [53, 54]. The reason for this profound dissatisfaction with vision is that vitreous opacification degrades contrast sensitivity function (CSF). Prospective studies found a 54% reduction in CSF following PVD [55]. Subsequent studies discovered that even after PVD there is progressive increase of vitreous density, as measured by quantitative ultrasound [56], and further degradation in CSF with increasing age [57]. These abnormalities can be readily cured with limited vitrectomy [58, 59]. The incidence of cataract surgery following this procedure is 16.9% (mean follow-up = 32 months), which is far superior to that with extensive vitrectomy [20]. Lastly, the treatment of Vision Degrading Myodesopsia with limited vitrectomy is highly cost-effective, more so than cataract surgery [60].

Although YAG lasers have been employed in patients with vitreous floaters, there are no definitive studies showing efficacy [8, 61]. A recent comprehensive review of the subject is in press [62].

References

1. Sebag J. Surgical anatomy of the vitreous and the vitreoretinal interface. In: Tasman W, editor. Duane's clinical ophthalmology. Philadelphia: Lippincott Williams & Wilkins; 1994. p. 1–36.
2. Sebag J, Silverman RH, Coleman DJ. To see the invisible: the quest of imaging vitreous. In: Sebag J, editor. Vitreous: in health and disease. New York: Springer; 2014. p. 193–219.
3. Hoar RM. Embryology of the eye. Environ Health Perspect. 1982;44:31–4.
4. Balazs EA. Fine structure of the developing vitreous. Int Ophthalmol Clin. 1975;15:53–63.
5. Chen C, Xiao H, Ding X. Persistent fetal vasculature. Asia Pac J Ophthalmol (Phila). 2019;8:86–95.
6. Balazs EA, Toth LZ, Ozanics V. Cytological studies on the developing vitreous as related to the hyaloid vessel system. Graefes Arch Clin Exp Ophthalmol. 1980;213:71–85.
7. Jongebloed WL, Worst JF. The cisternal anatomy of the vitreous body. Doc Ophthalmol. 1987;67:183–96.
8. Milston R, Madigan MC, Sebag J. Vitreous floaters: etiology, diagnostics, and management. Surv Ophthalmol. 2016;61:211–27.
9. Wang J, McLeod D, Henson DB, Bishop PN. Age-dependent changes in the basal retinovitreous adhesion. Invest Ophthalmol Vis Sci. 2003;44:1793–800.
10. Wilkinson CP. Prophylaxis and cure of rhegmatogenous retinal detachment. In: Sebag J, editor. Vitreous—in health & disease. New York: Springer; 2014. p. 713–29.
11. Sebag J. Shaken not stirred (guest editorial). Ophthalmology. 2001;108:1177–8.
12. Gal-Or O, Ghadiali Q, Dolz-Marco R, Engelbert M. In vivo imaging of the fibrillar architecture of the posterior vitreous and its relationship to the premacular bursa, Cloquet's canal, prevascular vitreous fissures, and cisterns. Graefes Arch Clin Exp Ophthalmol. 2019;257:709–14.
13. van Overdam K. Vitreoschisis-induced vitreous cortex remnants: missing link in proliferative vitreoretinopathy. Acta Ophthalmol. 2019;98(2):e261–2.
14. Sakamoto T, Ishibashi T. Hyalocytes: essential cells of the vitreous cavity in vitreoretinal pathophysiology? Retina. 2011;31:222–8.
15. Hata Y, Sassa Y, Kita T, Miura M, Kano K, Kawahara S, et al. Vascular endothelial growth factor expression by hyalocytes and its regulation by glucocorticoid. Br J Ophthalmol. 2008;92:1540–4.
16. Sebag J. Vitreoschisis. Graefes Arch Clin Exp Ophthalmol. 2008;246:329–32.
17. Comper WD, Laurent TC. Physiological function of connective tissue polysaccharides. Physiol Rev. 1978;58:255–315.
18. Sebag J. Vitreous and vitreoretinal interface. In: Schachat AP, Wilkinson CP, Hinton DR, Sadda SR, Wiedemann P, editors. Ryan's retina. 6th ed. Edinburgh: Elsevier; 2018. p. 544–81.
19. Bishop PN. Structural macromolecules and supramolecular organisation of the vitreous gel. Prog Retin Eye Res. 2000;19:323–44.
20. Sebag J, Niemeyer M, Koss MJ. Anomalous PVD and vitreoschisis. In: Sebag J, editor. Vitreous—in health & disease. New York: Springer; 2014. p. 265–86.
21. Sharif-Kashani P, Hubschman JP, Sassoon D, Kavehpour HP. Rheology of the vitreous gel: effects of macromolecule organization on the viscoelastic properties. J Biomech. 2011;44:419–23.
22. Holekamp NM. The vitreous gel: more than meets the eye. Am J Ophthalmol. 2010;149:32–6.

23. Holekamp NM, Shui YB, Beebe DC. Vitrectomy surgery increases oxygen exposure to the lens: a possible mechanism for nuclear cataract formation. Am J Ophthalmol. 2005;139:302–10.
24. Siegfried CJ, Shui YB. Intraocular oxygen and antioxidant status: new insights on the effect of vitrectomy and glaucoma pathogenesis. Am J Ophthalmol. 2019;203:12–25.
25. Yee KMP, Tan S, Lesnik Oberstein SY, Filas B, Nguyen JH, Nguyen-Cuu J, et al. Incidence of cataract surgery after vitrectomy for vitreous opacities. Ophthalmol Retina. 2017;1:154–7.
26. Bishop PN. Vitreous proteins. In: Sebag J, editor. Vitreous—in health & disease. New York: Springer; 2014. p. 3–12.
27. Crafoord S, Ghosh F, Sebag J. Vitreous biochemistry and artificial vitreous. In: Sebag J, editor. Vitreous—in health & disease. New York: Springer; 2014. p. 81–94.
28. Guber J, Pereni I, Scholl HPN, Guber I, Haynes RJ. Outcomes after epiretinal membrane surgery with or without internal limiting membrane peeling. Ophthalmol Therapy. 2019;8:297–303.
29. Lois N, Burr J, Norrie J, Vale L, Cook J, McDonald A, et al. Internal limiting membrane peeling versus no peeling for idiopathic full-thickness macular hole: a pragmatic randomized controlled trial. Invest Ophthalmol Vis Sci. 2011;52:1586–92.
30. Yannuzzi NA, Callaway NF, Sridhar J, Smiddy WE. Internal limiting membrane peeling during pars plana vitrectomy for rhegmatogenous retinal detachment: cost analysis, review of the literature, and meta-analysis. Retina. 2018;38:2081–7.
31. Yooh HS, Brooks HL Jr, Capone A Jr, L'Hernault NL, Grossniklaus HE. Ultrastructural features of tissue removed during idiopathic macular hole surgery. Am J Ophthalmol. 1996;122:67–75.
32. Pichi F, Lembo A, Morara M, Veronese C, Alkabes M, Nucci P, et al. Early and late inner retinal changes after inner limiting membrane peeling. Int Ophthalmol. 2014;34:437–46.
33. Pan BX, Yee KM, Ross-Cisneros FN, Sadun AA, Sebag J. Inner retinal optic neuropathy: vitreomacular surgery-associated disruption of the inner retina. Invest Ophthalmol Vis Sci. 2014;55:6756–64.
34. Sebag J. Pharmacologic vitreolysis. In: Sebag J, editor. Vitreous—in health & disease. New York: Springer; 2014. p. 799–816.
35. Nawaz IM, Rezzola S, Cancarini A, Russo A, Costagliola C, Semeraro F, et al. Human vitreous in proliferative diabetic retinopathy: characterization and translational implications. Prog Retin Eye Res. 2019;72:100756.
36. Sebag J. Pharmacologic vitreolysis—premise and promise of the first decade. Retina. 2009;29:871–4.
37. Spraul CW, Lang GE. Vitreous hemorrhage and macular edema with loss of vision. Ophthalmologe. 2005;102:396–8.
38. Coffee RE, Westfall AC, Davis GH, Mieler WF, Holz ER. Symptomatic posterior vitreous detachment and the incidence of delayed retinal breaks: case series and meta-analysis. Am J Ophthalmol. 2007;144:409–13.
39. Bond-Taylor M, Jakobsson G, Zetterberg M. Posterior vitreous detachment—prevalence of and risk factors for retinal tears. Clin Ophthalmol. 2017;11:1689–95.
40. Sarrafizadeh R, Hassan TS, Ruby AJ, Williams GA, Garretson BR, Capone A Jr, et al. Incidence of retinal detachment and visual outcome in eyes presenting with posterior vitreous separation and dense fundus-obscuring vitreous hemorrhage. Ophthalmology. 2001;108:2273–8.
41. Akiba J, Arzabe CW, Trempe CL. Posterior vitreous detachment and neovascularization in diabetic retinopathy. Ophthalmology. 1990;97:889–91.
42. Kishi S. Vitreous anatomy and the vitreomacular correlation. Jpn J Ophthalmol. 2016;60:239–73.
43. Mori K, Gehlbach PL, Kishi S. Posterior vitreous mobility delineated by tracking of optical coherence tomography images in eyes with idiopathic macular holes. Am J Ophthalmol. 2015;159:1132–41.
44. Bikbova G, Oshitari T, Baba T, Yamamoto S, Mori K. Pathogenesis and management of macular hole: review of current advances. J Ophthalmol. 2019;2019:3467381.
45. Sebag J. Anomalous posterior vitreous detachment: a unifying concept in vitreo-retinal disease. Graefes Arch Clin Exp Ophthalmol. 2004;242:690–8.
46. Nguyen JH, Yee KMP, Nguyen-Cuu J, Sebag J. Structural and functional characteristics of lamellar macular holes. Retina. 2018;2(9):881–7.
47. Haritoglou C, Sebag J. Indications and considerations for chromodissection. Retina Phys. 2014;11:34–9.
48. Figueroa MS, Govetto A, Steel DH, Sebag J, Virgili G, Hubschman JP. Pars plana vitrectomy for the treatment of tractional and degenerative lamellar macular holes: functional and anatomical results. Retina. 2018;39(11):2090–8.
49. Wang MY, Nguyen D, Hindoyan N, Sadun AA, Sebag J. Vitreo-papillary adhesion in macular hole and macular pucker. Retina. 2009;29:644–50.
50. Balazs EA, Denlinger JL. The vitreous. In: Davson H, editor. The eye. London: Academic Press; 1984. p. 533–89.
51. Khoshnevis M, Rosen S, Sebag J. Asteroid hyalosis-a comprehensive review. Surv Ophthalmol. 2019;64:452–62.
52. Sebag J. Abnormalities of human vitreous structure in diabetes. Graefes Arch Clin Exp Ophthalmol. 1993;231:257–60.
53. Wagle AM, Lim WY, Yap TP, Neelam K, Au Eong KG. Utility values associated with vitreous floaters. Am J Ophthalmol. 2011;152:60–5.
54. Sebag J. Floaters and the quality of life. Am J Ophthalmol. 2011;152:3–4.
55. Garcia GA, Khoshnevis M, Yee KMP, Nguyen-Cuu J, Nguyen JH, Sebag J. Degradation of contrast sensitiv-

ity function following posterior vitreous detachment. Am J Ophthalmol. 2016;172:7–12.
56. Mamou J, Wa CA, Yee KM, Silverman RH, Ketterling JA, Sadun AA, et al. Ultrasound-based quantification of vitreous floaters correlates with contrast sensitivity and quality of life. Invest Ophthalmol Vis Sci. 2015;56:1611–7.
57. Garcia GA, Khoshnevis M, Yee KMP, Nguyen JH, Nguyen-Cuu J, Sadun AA, et al. The effects of aging vitreous on contrast sensitivity function. Graefes Arch Clin Exp Ophthalmol. 2018;256:919–25.
58. Sebag J, Yee KM, Wa CA, Huang LC, Sadun AA. Vitrectomy for floaters: prospective efficacy analyses and retrospective safety profile. Retina. 2014;34:1062–8.
59. Sebag J, Yee KMP, Nguyen JH, Nguyen-Cuu J. Long-term safety and efficacy of limited vitrectomy for vision degrading vitreopathy resulting from vitreous floaters. Ophthalmol Retina. 2018;2:881–7.
60. Rostami B, Nguyen-Cuu J, Brown G, Brown M, Sadun AA, Sebag J. Cost-effectiveness of limited vitrectomy for vision-degrading Myodesopsia. Am J Ophthalmol. 2019;204:1–6.
61. Nguyen JH, Nguyen-Cuu, Mamou J, Routledge B, Yee KMP, Sebag J: Vitreous structure and visual function in myopic vitreopathy causing Vision Degrading Myodesopsia. Am J Ophthalmol. 2020: S0002-9394(20)30511-0. https://doi.org/10.1016/j.ajo.2020.09.017.
62. Sebag J. Vitreous and vision degrading myodesopsia. Prog Retin Eye Res. 2020;6:100847.
63. Ankamah E, Sebag J, Ng E, Nolan JM. Vitreous antioxidants, degeneration, and vitreo-retinopathy: Exploring the links (review). Antioxidants. 2019;9(1):7. https://doi.org/10.3390/antiox9010007.

Investigations Aiding in Vitreoretinal Surgery

3

Xihui Lin, Christopher Adam, and Asheesh Tewari

3.1 Introduction

Instrumentations in vitreoretinal surgery have evolved significantly over the past 40 years for pars plana vitrectomy. The rotating cutting mechanism of the VISC has been replaced by guillotine cutters capable of cut rates of over 10,000 cuts per minute while instrumentation size has shrunk from 18 gauge to 27 gauge. A variety of other surgical tools such as chandelier lighting, perfluorocarbon liquid, and membrane dyes have allowed the surgeon to tackle complex vitreoretinal situations.

Parallel to the advancement in vitreoretinal instrumentation is the development and improvement of diagnostic modalities. Specifically, two modalities that provide valuable information for the vitreoretinal surgeon are optical coherence tomography (OCT) and ophthalmic ultrasound. We rely on OCT and its intraoperative adaptation for important anatomic information on the vitreomacular interface and macular membranes. Meanwhile, ophthalmic ultrasound gives surgeons gross anatomic clues in situations of poor media view to better plan for surgery. The focus of this chapter is on how these modalities can be applied in specific vitreoretinal surgical situations and its future potential.

X. Lin · C. Adam
Kresge Eye Institute, Detroit, MI, USA

A. Tewari (✉)
Michigan Retina Center, Ann Arbor, MI, USA
e-mail: atewari@michretina.com

3.2 Ophthalmic Ultrasound

The diagnostic application of ultrasound to the field of medicine dates back to 1942 with investigation of the therapeutic properties even earlier. The biologic effects of ultrasound on the eye were first investigated by Zeiss in 1938 [1]. Donn in 1955 attempted to utilize ultrasonic vitreous liquefaction for the treatment of vitreous hemorrhage but the ultrasonic energy required for visualization at the time caused irreversible ocular damage [2]. Purnell and Sokollu in 1964 investigated the chorioretinal effects of focused high-intensity ultrasound and postulated its application for the destruction of intraocular lesions [3, 4]. Mundt et al. in 1956 is credited with publishing the first paper on ophthalmological diagnosis using ultrasound [5]. Shortly thereafter, Oksala and Lehtinen published a series of papers over the next decade providing an extensive review of ophthalmic intraocular pathology and its clinical applications [6]. In the same year, Baum and Greenwood produced some of the earliest high-resolution B-mode images of the eye [7]. Current ophthalmic ultrasound uses probes with frequency up to 12 MHz (compared to 3.5 MHz for

A. Jain et al. (eds.), *Cutting-edge Vitreoretinal Surgery*,
https://doi.org/10.1007/978-981-33-4168-5_3

abdominal ultrasound) for high-resolution views of intraocular structures [8].

Ultrasonic evaluation of ocular structures, specifically the retina, is necessary to perform a complete ophthalmic evaluation when direct visualization is compromised. Although more advanced radiologic imaging modalities such as magnetic resonance imaging and computed tomography can provide gross structural information in an eye where corneal or media opacities prohibit the examination of the posterior segment, ophthalmic ultrasound is still the only practical modality for posterior segment surgical planning. This is due to its higher resolution and ability to observe the dynamic behavior of intraocular structures. The most common situations resulting in decreased visualization in which ultrasound plays a critical role are trauma, advanced corneal or lens opacities, dense vitreous hemorrhage, extensive uveitic inflammation resulting in synechiae, membrane formation, or dense vitreous haze. Furthermore, the evaluation of suspected chorioretinal lesions, posterior foreign bodies, sub-Tenon's space, scleral wall, and deeper retrobulbar pathology are exquisitely imaged with ultrasound. Not all situations of small pupil or media opacity require an ultrasound. Many times a partial assessment can be obtained with the combination of a high diopter slit lamp biomicroscopy lens, optical coherence tomography, and ultrawide field imaging. Specifically ultrawide field imaging technology utilizing confocal scanning lasers can penetrate media opacities well and generate a wide field despite small pupils. If a satisfactory assessment still cannot be obtained with those means, ultrasound can provide vital adjunctive information and can play a key role in the diagnostic workup and therapeutic management of many ophthalmic conditions.

The main purpose of presurgical ultrasound is to give the vitreoretinal surgeons an estimate of the posterior segment pathology to allow for surgical planning. One key question for media opacity cases is the status of the retina. Frequently, ruling out a retinal detachment is relatively straightforward as the retina appears as a high signal hyperechoic membrane-like structure. However, in cases with dense chronic vitreous hemorrhage, the posterior hyaloid face can have a similar appearance to the retina. The two can sometimes be differentiated by observing the membrane movement in dynamic ultrasound and its attachment posteriorly to the optic nerve head. The hyaloid face generally has significant after-movement captured dynamically after a saccadic eye movement whereas detached retina is generally less mobile. If the membrane demonstrates less echogenicity, disappears on lowering of the gain <50 dB, has <100% amplitude of echo, shows significant after movement, has no posterior attachment to the optic nerve head, and is avascular on doppler, a retinal detachment can generally be ruled out. However, attachment of the membrane to the optic nerve does not always signal a retinal detachment as there can be cases of partial posterior vitreous detachment in diabetic retinopathy. In proliferative diabetic retinopathy, a posterior vitreous detachment is less common with dense vitreous hemorrhage and with significant co-existing preretinal membranes. A thickened, blood-stained posterior hyaloid is frequently still attached to the optic nerve due to neovascularization of the disc. Another clue is to look at the distribution of the hemorrhage. Although not always apparent, if there is diffuse hemorrhage of similar consistency anterior and posterior to the membrane, the membrane is likely not retina and represents a vitreous and subhyaloid hemorrhage. In rare occasions, subretinal hemorrhage can occur in diabetic retinopathy but generally, most of the hemorrhage is pre-retinal.

In rhegmatogenous retinal detachment cases, the macula status that predominantly drives surgical timing and decision-making, can usually be quite reliably assessed by the ophthalmic ultrasound by locating the optic nerve shadow and evaluating the retina temporal to it in various axial, longitudinal, and tangential planes. In the hands of an experienced ophthalmic ultrasonographer, the retinal breaks and sites of vitreoretinal traction can also frequently be identified. Although most rhegmatogenous detachments with hemorrhage would be treated with pars plana vitrectomy, the information from the ophthalmic ultrasound can be very useful.

Preoperative imaging can determine safe locations for placement of the trocar-cannula system over attached retina and whether or not an adjunctive scleral buckle should be placed by localizing which quadrant has the greatest pathology and need of support. This decision is surgeon dependent. The authors tend to place a buckle in cases where there is extensive pathology or breaks inferiorly.

The role of the ophthalmic ultrasound in diabetic vitrectomy is multi-faceted. The main goal is to determine the amount and location of the traction obscured by the vitreous hemorrhage. The presence of significant tractional detachment, extent of macular involvement, and a potential rhegmatogenous component are all important (Fig. 3.1). These factors can give the surgeon an estimate of case time, anesthetic options, lens management, instrumentation, and amount of dissection required. It is the preference of the authors to work under general anesthesia for severe cases of diabetic tractional detachment as case time is usually longer and patient agitation can sometimes be an issue. Some surgeons prefer pseudophakia if the patient has a significant cataract with the severe tractional detachment and would recommend a staged cataract surgery prior to vitrectomy. Cataract surgery can be done concurrently with the vitrectomy but in complex and prolonged diabetic cases, postsurgical inflammation can sometimes be severe and cause anterior segment inflammatory complications such as posterior synechiae formation, lens capsular opacification, or in severe cases iris bombe formation. Axial length measurements and meeting desired refractive targets are also more variable in cases of tractional detachment and inappropriate intraocular lens choice can be an issue if the instillation of silicone oil or extensive postoperative inflammation were not anticipated by the surgeon. Therefore, the authors generally prefer separating the cataract and vitrectomy surgery in these cases. Lastly, the location of the tractional detachment and macular status can help planning in terms of safety when administering preoperative intravitreal injections and targeting locations of potential access sites for dissection planes between the epiretinal fibrovascular membranes and retina.

In suspected oncology cases, ultrasound allows evaluation for the presence of a suspected tumor, measurement of the lesion dimensions and depth, internal reflectivity characteristics, and potential biopsy sites. Lastly, ultrasound is very useful in cases of serous or hemorrhagic choroidal detachments (Fig. 3.2). The architecture and shape of the detached tissue, internal reflectivity of fluid, and especially attachment points to the vortex veins and anterior extent to the ciliary body are key diagnostic differences when ruling out a retinal detachment. Ultrasound

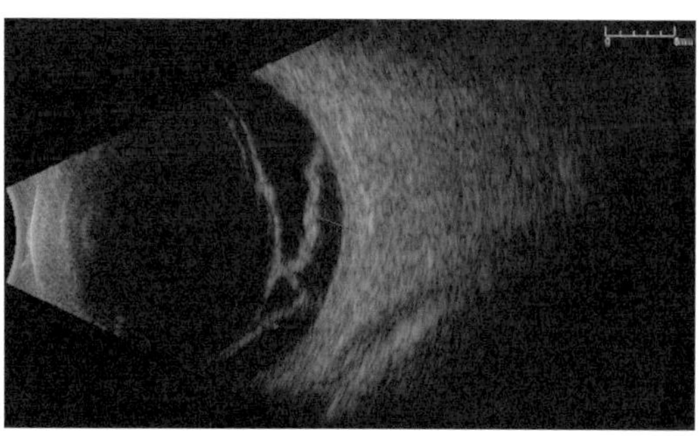

Fig. 3.1 Ophthalmic brightness amplitude scan (B-scan) ultrasound of a combined tractional and rhegmatogenous retinal detachment. B-scan demonstrating a macular involving retinal detachment with rhegmatogenous (arrow) and tractional (arrowhead) components with associated attachment points to the posterior hyaloid face (asterisks) in a patient with proliferative diabetic retinopathy

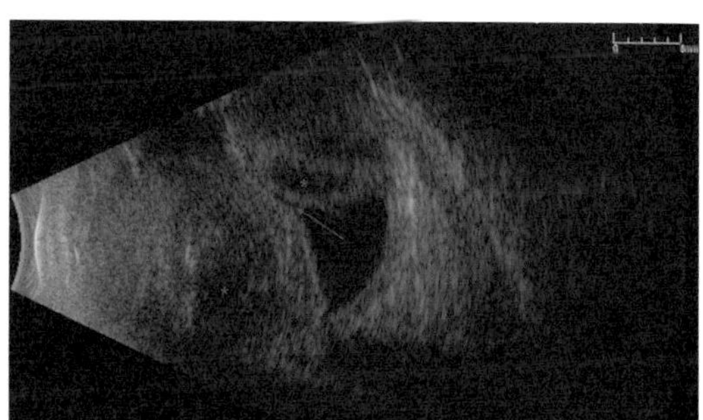

Fig. 3.2 Ophthalmic brightness amplitude scan (B-scan) ultrasound of a hemorrhagic choroidal. B-scan demonstrating kissing (arrow) hemorrhagic choroidals, which occurred during phacoemulsification cataract surgery. At day seven, there is evidence of clot liquefaction (asterisks) which was critical when planning the timing of surgical choroidal drainage

guidance is also critical when planning the timing of surgery based on liquefaction of the clot and which quadrants to safely perform external drainage to avoid iatrogenic and intraoperative complications.

As highlighted above, the importance and utility of ophthalmic ultrasound in providing a qualitative and quantitative assessment for diagnostic and therapeutic management of vitreoretinal disease cannot be overstated. It is the unique ability to image the vitreoretinal tissue dynamically in real time, through media opacities, using nonionizing radiation, and providing multiplanar sections, biometric measurements, evaluation of tissue characteristics, all in a portable bedside manner, that make this modality so attractive and valuable to the field of vitreoretinal surgery.

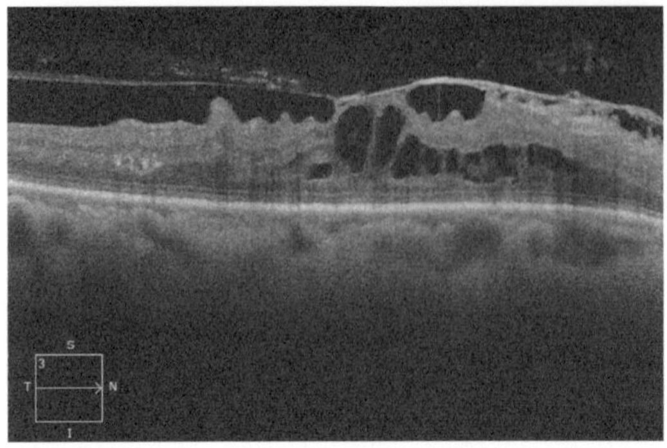

Fig. 3.3 Optical coherence tomography (OCT) of an epiretinal membrane (ERM) causing vitreomacular traction (VMT) and intraretinal cystic changes. Preoperative OCT demonstrating variability in ERM morphology including an area of firm membrane adherence to the retinal surface (arrow), area of membrane elevation with space between the ERM and retina (double arrow), and tractional intraretinal cystic changes (asterisk)

3.3 Optical Coherence Tomography

First invented and utilized for the eye in the early 1990s, modern spectral domain OCT machines have achieved resolutions of as high as 4 um or less while increasing tissue penetration with advancements such as enhanced depth imaging or swept source [9–13]. Although traditionally mostly a tool for evaluating macular pathology, newer wide field OCT technology allows evaluation to the near periphery [14–17]. Most commercially available OCT machines, however, are designed for macular evaluation. Although most presurgical information obtained from the OCT relates to the macula, useful information can be obtained from the OCT for almost all vitreoretinal surgeries.

In macular epiretinal membrane surgeries, the OCT can reliably determine whether a posterior vitreous detachment has occurred. Frequently, the B scan images can delineate interfacial spaces between the epiretinal membrane and the retina (Fig. 3.3). These areas usually are good starting locations for the membrane peel, especially if a sharp instrument will be utilized to initiate the flap. Prognosis can be estimated by observing the status of the external limiting membrane. The integrity of the external limiting membrane and recovery of the external limiting membrane can be an early predictor of visual recovery [18, 19]. Additionally, reduplication of the inner layers underneath an epiretinal membrane is frequently correlated with greater vision improvement after surgery. Post operatively, serial OCT's are useful for monitoring recurrence of epiretinal membrane as well as evaluation of any areas concerning for iatrogenic macular hole formation.

Current staging of macular holes is almost entirely reliant on a macular OCT. Any question about whether a hole is full thickness can be clarified by the macular OCT. The two most important factors to evaluate are the status of the posterior hyaloid and hole size. Part of the staging process of macular holes depends on the degree of posterior vitreous separation. In stage 2 holes, the vitreous attachment on the edge of the hole can be visualized on the B scan OCT whereas the posterior vitreous skirt is usually completely out of the view of the OCT B scan image for stage 4 holes. The inner hole diameter can be directly measured by measuring tools in the OCT analysis software or can be estimated by comparison to the adjacent non-edematous retina, which is around 250 μm. Small holes less than 250 μm have high closure rate with vitrectomy, gas, and no additional procedures. Larger holes frequently require the peeling of internal limiting membrane for closure. Very large holes (>500 μm) on OCT have lower closure rate and frequently require additional techniques such as internal limiting membrane flap, hydrodissection of the macula, or autologous retina transplant. Additional important prognostic factors are the presence of epiretinal membrane and lamellar hole-associated epiretinal proliferation. In these cases, there are significant radial tangential forces maintaining the hole, and hole closure rate is much lower without peeling the membranes.

In rhegmatogenous retinal detachment cases, OCT can be helpful in determining the status of the macula in shallow detachments. Also, OCT can clarify whether a posterior vitreous detachment has occurred in cases where there is no bullous detachment of the macula. It is also the preference of this author to evaluate the posterior hyaloid status of the contralateral eye of giant retinal tear detachments. If a posterior vitreous detachment has not occurred on OCT in these eyes, our practice pattern is to perform prophylactic 360° laser posterior to all areas of white without pressure.

Similar to macular pucker cases, OCT prior to surgeries for diabetic tractional detachment can delineate space between the fibrovascular membrane and the retina to identify potential areas to initiate the dissection. The OCT can also differentiate areas of tractional detachment from tractional schisis or diabetic membrane. In diabetic vitreous hemorrhage cases with documented previous center involving macular edema on OCT, internal limiting membrane peel during the surgery may be helpful.

Although not as frequently performed, subretinal surgery relies on the information provided by the macula OCT (Fig. 3.4). The most common situation relates to acute large sub-macular hemorrhage in the setting of exudative age-related macular degeneration or polypoidal choroidal vasculopathy. The OCT is helpful in identifying the location of the hemorrhage: preretinal, subretinal, or sub-pigment epithelium. The former two are amenable to displacement procedures for the hemorrhage such as intravitreal gas, tissue plasminogen, or surgical displacement of the hemorrhage. The success of displacement procedures is much lower if the hemorrhage is predominantly beneath the pigment epithelium as the blood is trapped in a sponge-like material and cannot be easily evacuated even with submacular surgery.

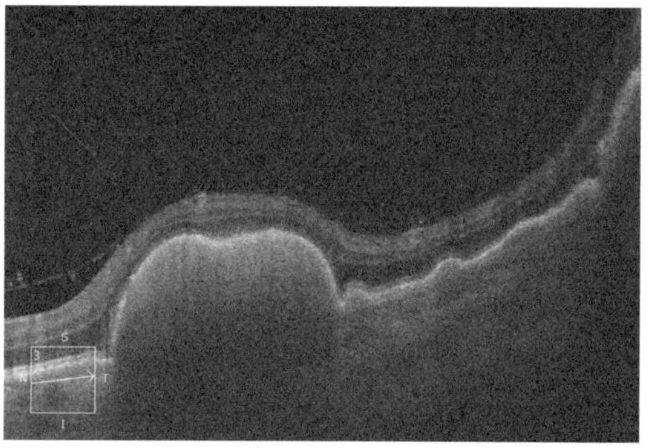

Fig. 3.4 Optical coherence tomography (OCT) of primary vitreoretinal lymphoma (PVRL). OCT demonstrating a large PVRL subretinal lesion (asterisk) causing elevation of the overlying retina and adjacent smaller satellite lesions (arrow heads). There is also evidence of mild vitreous cells (arrow). The OCT was instrumental in preoperative planning of subretinal biopsy sites

3.4 Intraoperative Optical Coherence Tomography

In the last several years, OCT technology has been gradually incorporated into the operating room. The operating room OCT can be in the form of a handheld portable device or an OCT integrated into the operating microscope with the latter having a clear advantage in terms of easier intraoperative utilization (Fig. 3.5). Overall, the intraoperative OCT technology has not been widely adopted due to the additional cost of the machine that could not be fully justified for many nonacademic surgical centers.

The technology is especially useful in vitreomacular traction, epiretinal membrane, macular hole (Fig. 3.6), and diabetic tractional detachment cases [20–23]. In situations with the presence of a thick posterior cortical vitreous still attached to the macula, it sometimes is difficult to confirm if the epiretinal membrane has been peeled. Intraoperative OCT can provide guidance for the surgeon in these cases. Confirmation

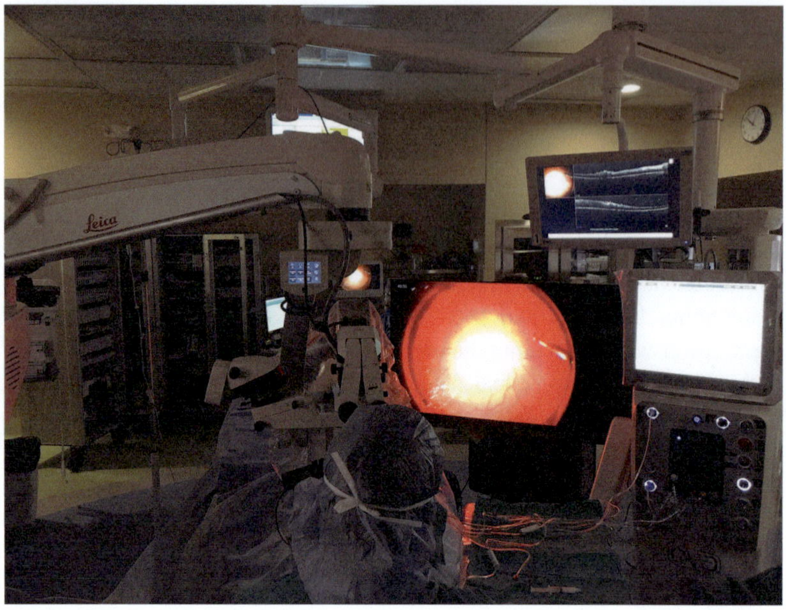

Fig. 3.5 Modern vitreoretinal surgery intraoperative theater. Vitrectomy surgical platform, Heads-up 3D visualization system, Leica Enfocus intraoperative OCT system on Proveo 8 microscope

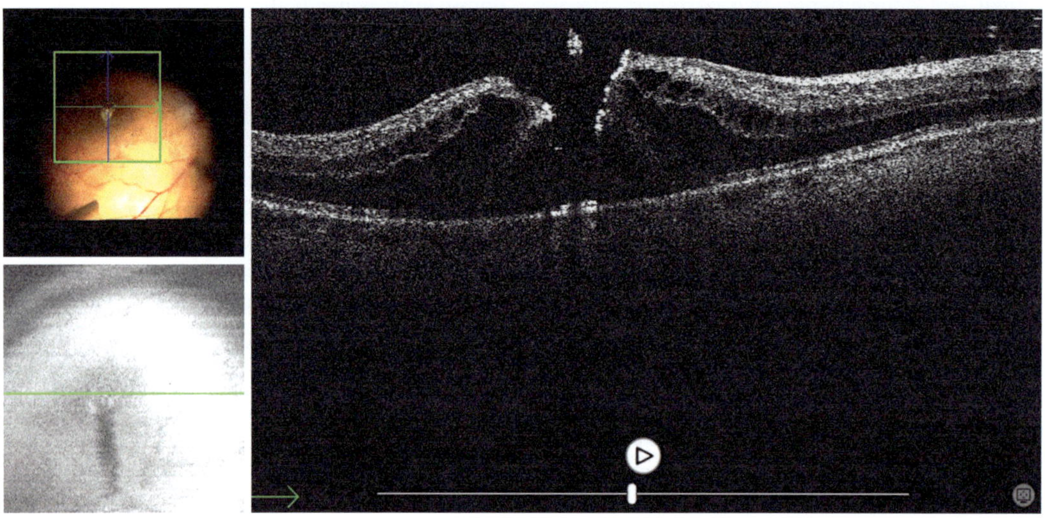

Fig. 3.6 Intraoperative optical coherence tomography of macular hole. Intraoperative color fundus microscopic view with green and blue grid lines indicating the locations of horizontal and vertical OCT B-scans respectively (upper left panel). Horizontal raster line (green line) corresponding to "real time" OCT scan (lower left panel) depicting a full-thickness macular hole moments before performing an OCT-guided internal limiting membrane peel (right panel)

of adequate internal limiting membrane peel in macular hole cases can be done with intraoperative OCT without stainings such as indocyanine green or brilliant blue dye. This is generally suggested by the appearance of dissociated nerve fiber layer seen after internal limiting membrane peel. This is less reliable than assessing the success of epiretinal membrane peel. In tractional diabetic cases, intraoperative OCT can be very helpful in periodically identifying new planes for dissection and distance between the membrane and retina. This can lead to decreased risk of iatrogenic breaks and surgical time.

At this point, real-time OCT-guided surgery is not fully practical as it requires separate controls to move the B scan location and shadowing is a significant problem when the instrument is in view of the B scan. In an electromagnetic wave-based imaging modality such as OCT, the shadowing effect of an instrument will likely always be a problem when the OCT is parfocal with surgeon's view. The biggest problem with such a shadowing effect is the surgeon cannot visualize the actual contact area of the instrument to the retina and must rely on B scans of the adjacent area to gauge instrument location relative to the retina surface. At this time, intraoperative OCT can be used for periodic reassessment of surgical progress rather than for true real-time surgical guidance.

3.5 Conclusion

Perioperative imaging has become an important part of surgical planning for the modern vitreoretinal surgeon. Ophthalmic B scan ultrasound provides gross anatomic information in which media opacity impedes visualization of the posterior segment. This allows the retinal surgeon to estimate surgical complexity. In situations of posterior segment malignancy, important decisions such as the need for enucleation are made based on ultrasound information. Office-based OCT and intraoperative OCT guide surgeons' decisions in macular surgery and detachment surgeries involving the macula. The intraoperative OCT has the potential to give retinal surgeons the ability for intraoperative assessment of surgical progress and differentiate retina from fibrous tissues. Together, these modalities can provide valuable information to increase surgical success rate.

References

1. Zeiss E. Ueber Linsenveraenderungen an heransgenommenen Rindeflinsen durch Ultraschalleinwirkung. v Graefes Arch Ophthalmol. 1938;139:301–22.
2. Donn H. Ultrasonic wave liquefaction of the vitreous humor in living rabbits. AMA Arch Ophthalmol. 1955;53:215–23.
3. Purnell EW, Sokollu A. Production of focal retinitis by ultrasound. Am J Ophthalmol. 1964;58:953–7.
4. Purnell EW, Sokollu A, Torehia R, Tanes N. Focal chorioretinitis produced by ultrasound. Invest Ophthalmol. 1964;3:657–64.
5. Mundt GH, Hughes WF. Ultrasonics in ocular diagnosis. Am J Ophthalmol. 1956;41:488–98.
6. Oksala A. Observations on choroidal detachment by means of ultrasound. Acta Ophthalmol. 1958;36:651–7.
7. Baum G, Greenwood I. The application of ultrasonic locating techniques to ophthalmology. Part II. Ultrasonic slit-lamp in the ultrasonic visualization of soft tissues. AMA Arch Ophthalmol. 1958b;60:263–79.
8. Byrne SF, Green RL. Ultrasound of the eye and orbit. 2nd ed. St. Louis: Mosby; 2002.
9. Huang D, Swanson EA, Lin CP, Schuman JS, Stinson WG, Chang W, Hee MR, Flotte T, Gregory K, Puliafito CA, Fujimoto JG. Optical coherence tomography. Science. 1991;254:1178–81.
10. Fercher AF, Hitzenberger CK, Drexler W, Kamp G, Sattmann H. In vivo optical coherence tomography. Am J Ophthalmol. 1993;116:113–4.
11. Spaide RF, Koizumi H, Pozzoni MC. Enhanced depth imaging spectral-domain optical coherence tomography. Am J Ophthalmol. 2008;146(4):496–500.
12. Yasuno Y, Madjarova VD, Makita S, et al. Three-dimensional and high-speed swept-source optical coherence tomography for in vivo investigation of human anterior eye segments. Opt Express. 2005;13:10652–64.
13. Choma M, Sarunic M, Yang C, Izatt J. Sensitivity advantage of swept source and Fourier domain optical coherence tomography. Opt Express. 2003;11:2183–9.
14. Povazay B, Hermann B, Hofer B, et al. Wide-field optical coherence tomography of the choroid in vivo. Invest Ophthalmol Vis Sci. 2009;50:1856–63.
15. McNabb RP, Grewal DS, Mehta R, Schuman SG, Izatt JA, Mahmoud TH, Jaffe GJ, Mruthyunjaya P, Kuo AN. Wide field of view swept-source optical coherence tomography for peripheral retinal disease. Br J Ophthalmol. 2016;100(10):1377–82.
16. Klein T, Wieser W, Eigenwillig CM, Biedermann BR, Huber R. Megahertz OCT for ultrawide-field retinal imaging with a 1050 nm Fourier domain mode-locked laser. Opt Express. 2011;19(4):3044–62.
17. Kolb JP, Klein T, Kufner CL, Wieser W, Neubauer AS, Huber R. Ultra-widefield retinal MHz-OCT imaging with up to 100 degrees viewing angle. Biomed Opt Express. 2015;6(5):1534–52.
18. Wakabayashi T, Oshima Y, Fujimoto H, Murakami Y, Sakaquchi H, Kusaka S, et al. Foveal microstructure and visual acuity after retinal detachment repair: imaging analysis by Fourier-domain optical coherence tomography. Ophthalmology. 2009;116(3):519–28.
19. Landa G, Gentile RC, Garcia PMT, Muldoon TO, Rosen RB. External limiting membrane and visual outcome in macular hole repair: spectral domain OCT

analysis. Eye (Lond). 2012;26(1):61–9. https://doi.org/10.1038/eye.2011.237.
20. Ehlers JP, Goshe J, Dupps WJ, et al. Determination of feasibility and utility of microscope-integrated optical coherence tomography during ophthalmic surgery: the DISCOVER study RESCAN results. JAMA Ophthalmol. 2015;133:1124–32.
21. Ehlers JP, Khan M, Petkovsek D, et al. Outcomes of intraoperative OCT-assisted epiretinal membrane surgery from the PIONEER study. Ophthalmol Retina. 2018;2:263–7.
22. Bruyère E, Philippakis E, Dupas B, et al. Benefit of intraoperative optical coherence tomography for vitreomacular surgery in highly myopic eyes. Retina. 2017;38:2035–44. https://doi.org/10.1097/IAE.0000000000001827.
23. Ehlers JP, Tao YK, Srivastava SK. The value of intraoperative OCT imaging in vitreoretinal surgery. Curr Opin Ophthalmol. 2014;25(3):221–7. https://doi.org/10.1097/ICU.0000000000000044.

4 Anaesthesia for Vitreoretinal Surgery

Multan M. Sharma
and Jaichandran Venkatakrishnan Vepary

4.1 Introduction

Anaesthesia for vitreoretinal (VR) surgery has gone sea changes in the last three decades. We have moved from 100% general anaesthesia (GA) to almost 80–90% regional anaesthesia and from hospital care to day care. All this has happened due to improved surgical techniques, instrumentation and not the least new anaesthetic drugs and better monitoring.

4.2 Preoperative Evaluation and Preparation

Most VR surgery patients can be treated as day-care patient in the present scenario. Preoperative assessment protocol can be designed according to individual institutions depending on facilities available. Preoperative assessment should be done in a month's period prior to surgery and pre-operative examination should be done by anaesthesiologist on the day of surgery.

4.3 Preoperative Instructions

4.3.1 Instructions Related to Systemic Medications

Instruction should be given very clearly about each medication patient is taking. Patient should take all morning doses of medicines for diseases like thyroid, hypertension, asthma etc. Anti-platelets or anti-coagulants should be stopped and resumed according to cardiologist advice.

4.3.2 Fasting Regimen

Patients are asked to fast 5 h prior to surgery, but clear fluid like water can be taken till 2 h prior to surgery. Diabetics should be taken earliest possible for surgery.

4.4 Regional Anaesthesia

Regional anaesthesia is commonly preferred for VR surgery especially for older and sick patients due to reduced stress response to surgery as well as reduced complications such as postoperative confusion, nausea, vomiting, and urinary retention.

The different techniques of regional anaesthesia are mentioned below.

M. M. Sharma
Aditya Jyot Eye Hospital, Mumbai, India

J. V. Vepary (✉)
Sankara Nethralaya, Chennai, India
e-mail: drvvj@snmail.org

A. Jain et al. (eds.), *Cutting-edge Vitreoretinal Surgery*,
https://doi.org/10.1007/978-981-33-4168-5_4

4.4.1 Intraconal (Retrobulbar) Block

In the modern retrobulbar block, a 23-G, 31-mm long needle is inserted through the skin or conjunctiva in the inferotemporal quadrant as far lateral as possible below the lateral rectus muscle. The initial direction of the needle is tangential to the globe, it then passes below the globe and once it is past the equator, as gauged by the axial length of the globe, it is allowed to go upwards and inwards to enter the central space just behind the globe. The globe is continuously observed during the needle placement. 4–5 mL of local anaesthetic agent is injected slowly. Majority of patients develop good anaesthesia and akinesia but some will require a supplementary injection.

4.4.2 Extraconal (Peribulbar) Block

In the modern peribulbar block, the injection is deliberately made outside the cone. A 23-G, 25-mm long needle is inserted through the conjunctiva as far laterally as possible in the inferotemporal quadrant. Once the needle is under the globe, it is not directed upwards and inwards, but is directed along the orbital floor. 5 mL of local anaesthetic agent is injected slowly. More than 60% of patients require a supplementary injection usually a medial peribulbar block.

4.4.3 Medial Peribulbar Block

The medial peribulbar block is usually performed to supplement the inferotemporal retrobulbar or peribulbar injection, particularly when akinesia is not adequate. A 26-G needle is inserted in the blind pit between the caruncle and the medial canthus to a depth of 15 mm. 3–5 mL of local anaesthetic agent is usually injected slowly.

4.4.4 Sub-Tenon's Block

Sub-Tenon block is performed using a blunt curved cannula. This block can be performed as a primary block technique or as a supplementary block to augment needle block performed as a primary method of anaesthesia. This block is also used to reduce postoperative pain in a patient who had undergone general anaesthesia. Performing a sub-Tenon's block in patients who have undergone previous repeated surgery may not be feasible or sometimes impossible due to scarring and ocular perforation has been reported in a patient with a previous scleral buckle.

4.5 Choice of Local Anaesthetic Agents

The duration of VR surgery is usually longer than routine anterior segment surgeries. Two percent lignocaine hydrochloride has a shorter duration of action. Hence, it is not an ideal choice of a local anaesthetic agent. Anaesthesia can be achieved with 0.5% bupivacaine alone or 0.75% ropivacaine solution.

Local anaesthetic mixture containing equal volume of 2% lignocaine hydrochloride and 0.5% bupivacaine is no more advocated for clinical use. Mixing 2% of these agents in an 1:1 ratio dilutes the anaesthetic mixture to 1% lidocaine and 0.25% bupivacaine resulting in a possible reduction in efficacy of both agents. Since both of them are amide group of local anaesthetic solutions, they compete for the same receptors when used simultaneously so exhibiting shorter duration of action with more rapid onset of action [1].

Recommended dose of 2% lignocaine hydrochloride is 3–5 mg/kg body weight and 0.5% bupivacaine 1–2 mg/kg body weight.

4.5.1 Adjuvants

Hyaluronidase is an enzyme, which reversibly liquefies the interstitial barrier between cells by depolymerization of hyaluronic acid to a tetrasaccharide, thus increases the diffusion of molecules through tissue planes. It is available as a powder and is readily soluble. Hyaluronidase has been shown to improve the efficacy and quality of the needle block. The amount of hyaluronidase used in published studies varies from 5 to150 IU/mL and we recommend 10–15 IU/ml.

4.6 General Anaesthesia

General anaesthesia is usually indicated in paediatric patients, patients with dementia, and high levels of anxiety and in open globe injuries. Local anaesthetic techniques are usually avoided in open globe injuries as it may be associated with an increase in intraocular pressure which can lead to vitreous loss.

4.6.1 Premedication

Premedication is not used routinely for eye surgery but a short-acting benzodiazepine such as temazepam may be given orally to anxious patients [2].

4.6.2 Induction

Propofol is used widely because of its short duration of action, pleasant induction and reduced postoperative nausea. Thiopental is still a satisfactory alternative for induction in both adults and children. Inhalational induction with sevoflurane is another alternative and has largely superseded halothane for gaseous induction in children.

4.6.3 Maintenance of Anaesthesia

Most anaesthesiologists use a gold standard balanced anaesthesia technique (intravenous induction, opioid and a non-depolarizing muscle relaxant), secure the airway with an endotracheal tube and intermittent positive pressure ventilation, for intraocular surgery. Moderate hyperventilation reduces P_aCO_2 and provides excellent operating conditions. Use of lower amount of anaesthetic drugs aids in early recovery from anaesthesia at the end of the surgery. Spontaneous ventilation may need deeper levels of anaesthesia, leading to CO_2 retention and hypotension, which may cause slow recovery.

The laryngeal mask airway is increasingly used for intraocular surgery. Insertion is easier and the problems associated with intubation like postoperative coughing, straining and laryngospasm are virtually eliminated. Care should be taken to maintain sufficiently deep anaesthesia so that the laryngeal mask is not rejected. The laryngeal mask is unsuitable for patients at risk of aspiration. This group includes the morbidly obese, those with gastro-oesophageal reflux and patients with hiatus hernia. In these patients, preoperative administration of an H_2-receptor antagonist and antacid therapy should be considered and a cuffed tracheal tube is recommended to protect the airway. Preoxygenation with the head elevated and cricoid pressure reduces the risk of aspiration. Muscle relaxants are required for intubation and maintenance of anaesthesia.

Before starting the procedure, the surgeon should be encouraged to infiltrate a long-acting local anaesthetic by the sub-Tenon's route. This should successfully eliminate variations in anaesthetic requirements from the surgical stimulus and provide a stable anaesthetic with a reduction in the amounts of general anaesthetic agent required. If topped up towards the end of the procedure, excellent postoperative analgesia can be produced without other analgesic drugs.

4.6.4 Extubation

After extubating endotracheal tube, patient can have straining, bucking or coughing, restlessness and breathe holding [3]. Tracheal extubation thus may cause a marked rise in the IOP and coughing can even increase the IOP up to 50 mmHg [4]. The Valsalva effect produced by coughing can lead to vessel wall rupturing due to a sudden increase in the venous pressure thus resulting in suprachoroidal haemorrhage (SCH). SCH is a serious complication following eye surgery [5]. Cases of delayed non-expulsive type of SCH have been reported after eye surgery following straining at the time of extubation [6].

Intravenous administration of lignocaine or topical spray of lignocaine on vocal cords is used to diminish cough reflex during extubation. Recent studies have shown that smooth emergence from GA could be obtained by filling the ETT cuff with buffered lidocaine [7]. The cough receptors in the tracheal mucosa are blocked by the non-ionized form of the drug which diffuses across the hydrophobic polyvinyl chloride walls of the ETT cuff [8, 9].

4.7 Special Considerations in General Anaesthesia

4.7.1 Intravitreal Gases and Nitrous Oxide

Intravitreal injection of inert gases such as sulphur hexafluoride (SF_6) or perfluoroproprane (C_3F_8) mixed with air is used to tamponade the retina against the choroid. When these gases are injected into the vitreous cavity, soluble N_2O (if used during GA) will diffuse from blood and tissues into vitreous cavity much more rapidly than SF_6 can diffuse out. This increases the volume of the gas bubble causing an increase in IOP. If IOP rises above the perfusion pressure of central retinal artery (around 70 mmHg), then its occlusion may occur leading to permanent blindness. Hence it is advisable to turn off N_2O at least 15 min before the injection of intraocular gases. It is important to provide analgesia with alternative drugs such as fentanyl or by increasing the inspired concentration of the volatile anaesthetic agent.

Intravitreal gases may remain for as long as 3–6 weeks. A risk of re-expansion of intravitreal gases [10] is always there if a second anaesthesia is planned for ophthalmic or non-ophthalmic surgery within that period. If anaesthesia is required, N_2O should be avoided and a regional block should be considered in these patients.

4.7.2 VR Surgery Combined with Penetrating Keratoplasty or "Open Sky Situations"

In cases of combined VR surgery and penetrating keratoplasty, it is very important to prevent any acute rise in the IOP. Any coughing or bucking may lead to expulsion of vitreous or choroidal haemorrhage. IOP is normally controlled by hyperventilation of the lungs. Hypocarbia caused by hyperventilation produces choroidal arterial vasoconstriction with concomitant decrease in the IOP. Proper neuromuscular monitoring is advisable. It is anaesthesiologist's responsibility to ensure that the patient is in deeper plane of anaesthesia at this stage.

4.7.3 VR Surgery Combined with Glaucoma Surgery

VR surgery is occasionally performed with glaucoma surgery (trabeculectomy). Anaesthetic drug such as ketamine increases IOP and should be avoided. Straining/coughing/bucking during intubation and extubation should be avoided.

4.7.4 Combined General Anaesthesia and Regional Anaesthesia for VR Surgery

Orbital block administered during GA may decrease the incidence of oculocardiac reflex, surgical bleeding, postoperative pain and analgesic requirements, and postoperative nausea and vomiting [11, 12].

4.8 Postoperative Care

4.8.1 Pain Relief

Pain following vitrectomy is usually mild or moderate and usually settles with simple analgesics like paracetamol and NSAID. However, cryo-buckle procedure may be associated with moderate to severe pain because of the globe being pulled and traction effect on the extraocular muscles. NSAID as a sole analgesic agent may not be enough and should be supplemented with an opioid (multimodal approach) [13, 14].

Previous study demonstrated a beneficial role of pre-emptive analgesia using regional anaesthetic blocks in VR surgery [15]. It is always a good clinical practice to give a sub-Tenon's injection with local anaesthesia just before closure of the conjunctiva. Pre-emptive analgesia with intravenous ketorolac not only helps in decreasing the pain but also reduces the incidence and severity of postoperative nausea and vomiting [16]. Ketorolac is a potent NSAID (30 mg is equivalent to 10 mg morphine) if given by intramuscular injection. It has a relatively slow onset of action (30 min) but has a long duration of action with a half-life of over 7 h. In children, it can be administered at a dose of 0.5–0.75 mg/kg IV or IM.

4.8.2 Postoperative Nausea and Vomiting

The aetiology of Postoperative Nausea and Vomiting (PONV) is complex and is dependent on patient characteristics, type of surgery, anaesthetic techniques and postoperative course. PONV usually occurs as a result of the manipulation of the extraocular muscles and by alterations in the IOP by volume expansion within the orbit. Patients who undergo either scleral buckling or combined vitrectomy and scleral buckling require extensive manipulation of all the rectus muscles during surgery in contrast to patients who undergone vitrectomy without buckling. Hence the incidence of PONV is quite higher in these patients. PONV may lead to rupture of suture, loss of vitreous, iris prolapse and intraocular haemorrhage. Intravenous ondansetron is found to be effective in preventing PONV if given prior to the reversal of GA at the end of the procedure. Also, PONV can be managed by the use of multimodal anti-emetic approach (ondansetron 0.1–0.15 mg/kg and dexamethasone 200–300 μg/kg) towards the end of surgery [17]. Local infiltration of the surgical site with 0.5% bupivacaine helps decrease PONV as well as provides postoperative analgesia [18]. It is important to note that the surgeon should exclude a rise in the IOP level in patients with persistent vomiting along with severe eye pain and headache.

4.9 Monitored Anaesthesia Care and Conscious Sedation

Monitored Anaesthesia Care (MAC), also known as twilight anaesthesia or conscious sedation is a type of anaesthesia where sedatives are provided to keep the patient calm while allowing the patient to remain awake and responsive. It is used in conjunction with local or regional (peri-bulbar) anaesthesia to keep patients pain free. During MAC continuous monitoring of vitals is mandatory. It is beneficial to use nasal O_2 insufflation. Monitored anaesthesia care is preferred for patients with cardiac disease [19].

References

1. Jaichandran VV, Raman R, Gella L, Sharma T. Local anesthetic agents for vitreoretinal surgery: no advantage to mixing solutions. Ophthalmology. 2015;122(5):1030–3.
2. Aitkenhead AR, Smith G, Rowbotham DJ. Textbook of anaesthesia. Edinburgh: Churchill Livingston; 2007.
3. Huang CJ, Hsu YW, Chen CC, Ko YP, Rau RH, Wu KH, et al. Prevention of coughing induced by endotracheal tube during emergence from general anaesthesia—a comparison between three different regimens of lidocaine filled in the endotracheal tube cuff. Acta Anaesthesiol Sin. 1998;36:81–6.
4. Ersanli D, Meric L, Orga Y, et al. A comparative study of the effects of laryngeal mask vs endotracheal tube on intraocular pressure during general anaesthesia. Med Bull Istanbul. 1998;31:2.
5. Obuchowska I, Mariak Z, Stankiewicz A. Massive suprachoroidal haemorrhage during cataract surgery: case report. KlinOczna. 2002;104(5–6):406–10.
6. Ariano ML, Ball SF. Delayed non-expulsive suprachoroidal haemorrhage after trabeculectomy. Ophthalmic Surg. 1987;18(9):661–6.
7. Jaichandran VV, Bhanulakshmi IM, Jagadeesh V. Intracuff buffered lidocaine versus saline or air—a

comparative study for smooth extubation in patients with hyperactive airways undergoing eye surgery. SAJAA. 2009;15(2):11–4.
8. Camporesi EM, Mortola JP, Sant'Ambrogio F, Sant'Ambrogio G. Topical anesthesia of tracheal receptors. J Appl Physiol. 1979;47:1123–6.
9. Huang CJ, Tsai MC, Chen CT, et al. In vitro diffusion of lidocaine across endotracheal tube cuffs. Can J Anesth. 1999;46:82–6.
10. Lee EJK. Use of nitrous oxide causing severe visual loss 37 days after retinal surgery. Br J Anaesth. 2004;93(3):464–6.
11. Williams N, Strunin A, Heriot W. Pain and vomiting after vitreoretinal surgery: a potential role for local anaesthesia. Anaesth Intensive Care. 1995;23(4):444–8.
12. Ghali AM, El Btarny AM. The effect on outcome of peribulbar anaesthesia in conjunction with general anesthesia for vitreoretinal surgery. Anaesthesia. 2010;65(3):249–53.
13. Kokki H, Purhonen S, Terasvirta M, Ylonen P. Ketoprofen for add-on pain treatment to paracetamol after strabismus surgery in children. Clin Drug Investig. 2004;24:237–4.
14. Jaichandran VV, Bhanulakshmi I, Jagadeesh V, Sujatha R, Kavitha Devi J, Manimaran N. A multimodal approach to post-operative pain relief in children undergoing ambulatory eye surgery. Indian J Anaesth. 2008;52(6):794–9.
15. Morel J, Pascal J, Charier D, De Pasquale V, Gain P, Auboyer C, et al. Preoperative peribulbar block in patients undergoing retinal detachment surgery under general anesthesia: a randomized double-blind study. Anesth Analg. 2006;102(4):1082–7.
16. Vlajkovic G, Sindjelic R, Stefanovic I. Ketorolac as a pre-emptive analgesic in retinal detachment surgery: a prospective, randomized clinical trial. Int J Clin Pharmacol. 2007;45(5):259–63.
17. Lord J. Anaesthesia for eye surgery in paediatrics. Eyes Anaesth Intens Care Med. 2007;8(9):393–6.
18. Shende D, Sadhasivam S, Madan R. Effects of peribulbar bupivacaine as an adjunct to general anaesthesia on peri-operative outcome following retinal detachment surgery. Anaesthesia. 2000;55(10):970–5.
19. Brian Frugoni MD, Annette Mizuguchi K. Essentials of cardiac anesthesia for noncardiac surgery. Amsterdam: Elsevier; 2019.

Part III

Techniques and Instrumentation in Vitreoretinal Surgery

Vitreoretinal Surgery Instruments 5

Diego Ruiz Casas

5.1 Introduction

During the last decade there has been an important evolution in vitreoretinal surgery instruments.

The advent of wide-angle visualization systems allows controlled surgical maneuvers on the whole retinal area, due to a field of view of up to 130°.

Currently, vitrectomy is usually performed with transcleral 23, 25 or 27G valved microcannulas that improve vitrectomy fluidics and intraocular pressure control. The most common surgical platforms: Constellation (Alcon), EVA (DORC) and Stellaris PC/Elite (Bausch and Lomb) permit microincision vitrectomy surgery (MIVS) and phacoemulsification surgery. A 4-port microincisional vitrectomy setting with chandelier light and non-contact wide visualization system is shown in Fig. 5.1.

The new vitreoretinal surgical devices have a better flow control and reduced retinal traction due to new pumps, increased cut per minute rates and reduced size. It is important to understand vitrectomy fluidics to be able to set vitrectomy parameters to perform an efficient and safe vitrectomy.

D. R. Casas (✉)
Retinal Department Hospital Ramón y Cajal, Madrid, Spain

A. Jain et al. (eds.), *Cutting-edge Vitreoretinal Surgery*,
https://doi.org/10.1007/978-981-33-4168-5_5

5.2 Basic Physics to Understand Vitrectomy Fluidics, Pumps and Vitreous Cutters

Pressure is the amount of force applied at the surface of an object per unit area. Pressure is due to the particles inside a container pushing against its walls. Vacuum is negative gauge pressure, a pressure lower than atmospheric pressure. Gradient of pressure is the difference of pressure between two containers. When two recipients are connected at different pressures, particles will move from the most pressurized continent (with more particles) to the less pressurize continent.

Flow is the volume of fluid which passes per unit of time through a pipe. According to Poiseuille's law, flow is directly proportional to the gradient of pressure and inversely proportional to resistance.

Resistance to flow depends on the length of the tubing (the longer, the more resistance), the viscosity of the fluid and, specially, the diameter of the tubing.

The main resistances in a vitrectomy system (bottle of infusion-tubing-microcannula-eye-microcannula-vitrectome shaft-fluid recipient-pump) are the infusion microcannula and the vitrectome shaft because they have the smallest diameters in the system. This is the reason for lower flow rates in small gauge vitrectomy. Low flow rates are helpful when performing vitrectomy on detached retina to reduce vitreoretinal traction,

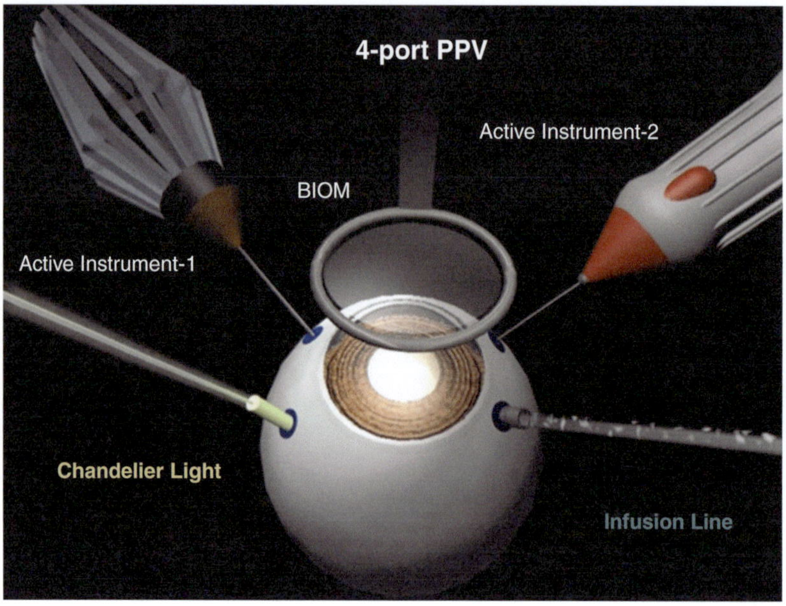

Fig. 5.1 A 4-port microincisional vitrectomy setting with chandelier light and non-contact wide visualization system

but smaller gauges reduce flow and make surgery longer. However, the most important factor in vitrectomy efficiency is surgical technique and not fluidics. Even with 27G vitreous cutter with regular blade and a vitreous flow rate of 1 cc/min, all vitreous could be removed in 4–5 min if the vitreous cutter tip is continuously engaging the vitreous.

If flow is constant in a tubing system, the continuity law says that the fluid speed is faster in narrower sections of the tubing and slower in wider. In narrower sections fluid speed is faster, but pressure is lower according to Bernoulli's equation and this explains the Venturi effect.

Venturi effect is the way venturi pumps generate vacuum, they have a fast fluid flow in a narrow tubing section which is connected to the vitrectomy system and venturi effect generates negative pressure.

5.3 Vitrectomy Pumps

Venturi pumps are the most common pumps in vitreoretinal surgery. They use a venturi system to create vacuum. They control vacuum directly and the outflow will depend on the viscosity of the fluid.

Venturi pumps have a fast response, work well with liquids and gas and can control flow indirectly limiting it through the cutter port.

Peristaltic pumps move fluid inside a tubing compressing the tubing with rollers. The flow is directly controlled by the pump instead of vacuum. Flow control of peristaltic pumps is advantageous because flow will not depend on the viscosity of the fluid (provided the generated vacuum is high enough to generate the set flow), but tubbing compression induces flow pulsations, surge and they have a slower response than venturi pumps, with a rise time to get the preset vacuum. Peristaltic pumps work worse if a mixture of fluid and gas is present inside the tubing.

EVA's vacuflow valve timing intelligence pump is a new pump, which generates negative pressure with tubing expansion by pistons and controls flow with valves. This new system controls vacuum and flow directly with no flow pulsations or surge and allows changing between flow and vacuum control in every step of phacoemulsification or vitrectomy [1].

5.4 Vitrectomy Outflow

Newtonian fluids are substances that deforms continually under an applied shear stress, but vitreous is not a Newtonian fluid. Vitreous is a heterogeneous structure (collagen, hyaluronic acid and water) with viscoelastic properties (it is

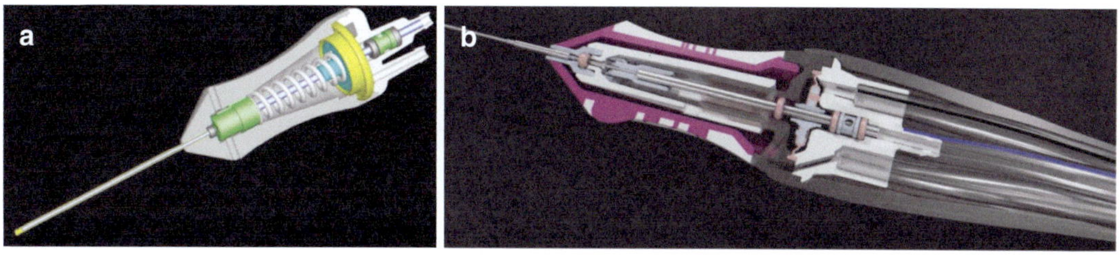

Fig. 5.2 Spring (**a**) vs dual pneumatic (**b**) cutters (Image courtesy of Alcon)

elastic and deformable) and shear thinning (its viscosity decreases under shear strain).

The fluid removed from the vitreous cavity during vitrectomy is a triphasic structure of vitreous, water and air (due to cavitation) and the flow of the mixture is not linear flow, it is turbulent flow, called slug flow.

Slug flow is the kind of flow of a fluid with a suspension of particles. If vitreous particles are large the flow is not laminar but turbulent and the amount of fluid is reduced, however, if vitreous particles are smaller the flow is more linear, and the amount of fluid removed is increased. This is the reason for larger vitreous outflow when using high cut per minute (cpm) settings and the explanation of vitreous shear thinning. However, cut rates over 2000 cpm do not increase flow anymore, probably because the vitreous chunks size is close to collagen molecules size.

Vitreous is a continuous structure connected to vitreous base. During vitrectomy, vitreous is removed trying to reduce retinal traction. Increasing vitrectomy cpm not only increases vitreous flow, but also reduces vitreo–retinal traction. Traction is also reduced with smaller gauges and closed duty cycle that decreases the size of vitreous chunks removed during vitrectomy. Small gauge cutters limit vitreous and aqueous flow due to increased resistance to flow [2–5].

5.5 Vitreous Cutters

The principle of a vitreous cutter is an extrusion line with a blade to segment vitreous and reduce vitreo–retinal traction.

Gauge is the diameter of the vitreous cutter shaft. 23, 25 and 27G cutters are called microincisional vitrectomy (MIVS), compared to 20G cutters, but the main difference is that 20G cutters usually do not have microcannulas. Smaller gauges have lower outflow and are not as stiff as larger G cutters, but they allow the surgeon more delicate maneuvers and can be used as multifunctional instruments.

The size of vitreous cutter port modify outflow, the maximum outflow is obtained when vitreous cutter port is the size of the inner diameter of the vitreous cutter lumen. The smaller the vitreous cutter port the lower is the outflow.

Cuts per minute are the number of cuts generated by the blade in a minute. The higher the cut rate the bigger is the vitreous outflow (shear thinning), the lower is the water outflow (more time closed) and the lower is vitreoretinal traction.

Duty cycle (DC) is the percentage of time the vitreous cutter port is opened in each cut cycle. Spring cutters DC is 50% but it tends to be reduced at high cpm rates. Dual pneumatic cutters (Alcon) can control duty cycle as opened (80%), 50/50 (50%) or closed (20%), however at the highest cpm rates DC tends to be 50% no matter the DC selected (Fig. 5.2). Two-dimensional cutter (TDC, DORC) and Bi-blade (B&L) have a fixed 90–92% DC which is not modified with cpm rate. These cutters have the port opened all the time increasing flow rate; however, they cannot control flow with the port anymore, making flow control needed in larger gauges (smaller gauges have port limiting control due to their size) [2–5].

5.6 Fluid Dynamics

The sphere of influence (SI) is the volume of water around the vitreous cutter port influenced by its fluid dynamics, the distance of tissue attraction around the cutter. SI depends directly on vacuum or flow, but it can be reduced with smaller gauge cutters, reduced vitreous cutter port size, reduced duty cycle and high cpm rates. The surgeon will need smaller SI when performing vitreous shaving in detached retina, and larger SI when trying to aspirate blood, lens fragments or other elements in the attached retina. Vitrectomy cutter gauge is the most important factor to reduce the SI with a fixed vacuum or flow.

The sphere of influence area is a sphere, every tissue around the cutter can be attracted if is close enough to the cutter in water. However, once the vitreous is engaged, it is a continuous structure, and vitreous will be attracted towards the vitreous cutter with a vortex shape, the direction of this vortex depends on the kind of vitreous cutter and cpm. In regular blade cutters at low cpm the vortex shape is perpendicular to the vitreous cutter port, and it forms an acute angle at high cpm. TDC cutters create a vortex shape with an obtuse angle towards the vitreous cutter tip [6–8].

Port flow control is the way vacuum pumps can reduce and control flow indirectly using vitreous cutter tip. Flow will be reduced with a fixed vacuum if the vitreous cutter tip is reduced, the cpm rate increased, the DC reduced, and the gauge is smaller. Vacuum control with port flow control is faster than flow control with peristaltic pumps.

Instant flow is the variation of flow induced by the friction of the blade at the column of fluid. Despite we control average flow with pumps, cpm rate, DC and gauge, flow variation due to instant flow can be 10 times larger than average flow. Instant flow is directly proportional to fluid viscosity, blade speed, inner vitreous cutter surface and the length of the blade excursion and inversely proportional to the inner blade radius, thus instant flow can be reduced with smaller gauge cutters [9].

5.7 Most Common Vitrectomy Systems

5.7.1 Constellation Vision System (Alcon)

Constellation controls IOP directly with flow sensors at the cassette to maintain a set pressure (Fig. 5.3). This IOP control combined with EdgePlus trocars and valved microcannulas makes surgery safer. It uses a venturi pump with vacuum up to 650 mmHg.

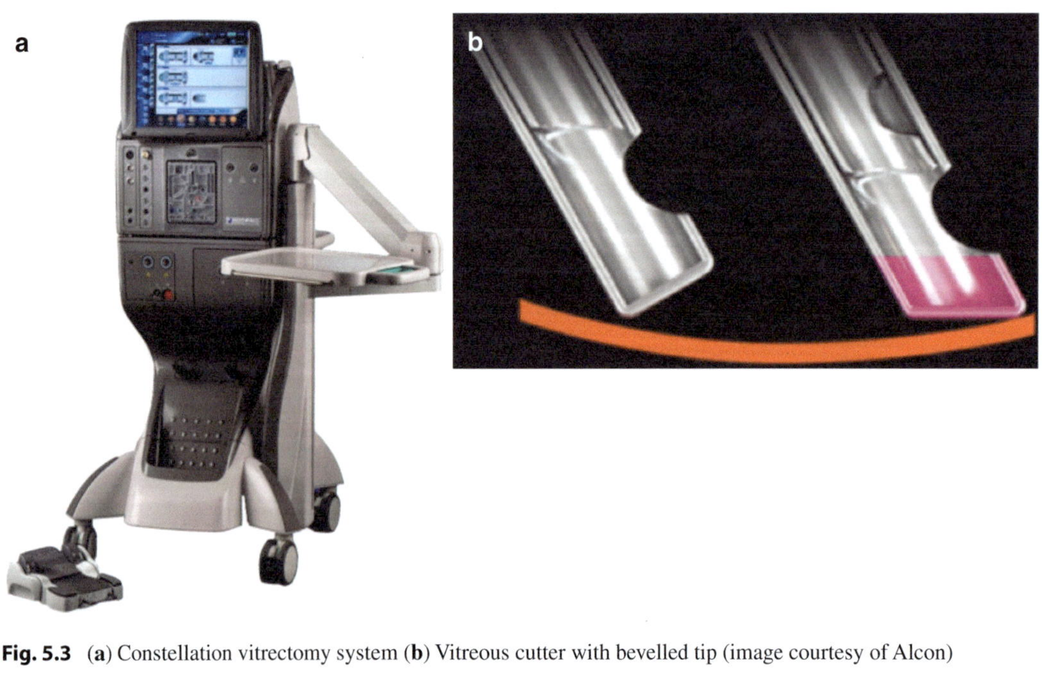

Fig. 5.3 (**a**) Constellation vitrectomy system (**b**) Vitreous cutter with bevelled tip (image courtesy of Alcon)

Vitreous cutters are moved by a dual pneumatic system that allows a cpm rate up to 10,000 cpm with duty cycle control. DC can be set as core (port biased open), 50/50 and shave (port biased closed). Vitreous cutters are optimized with ports close to the end of the tip and beveled to give a closer distance to the tissue and help in dissection maneuvers (Fig. 5.3b).

Constellation uses a Xenon light source which regulates automatically the intensity of light based on gauge size.

Fluid–air exchange can be performed directly in Constellation with the footswitch.

The Constellation Viscous Fluid Injection system can inject and remove 1000 and 5000cs easily with 23 and 25G.

5.7.2 EVA Vitrectomy System (DORC)

EVA's vacuflow VTI pump is the most advanced vitrectomy pump (Fig. 5.4). It provides flow and vacuum control adjustable for each surgical step setting. Flow can be adjusted from 0 to 90 cc/min and vacuum from 0 to 680 mmHg.

Vitreous cutters have twin duty cycle technology (TDC) with another port in the inner shaft leading to double cut rate and a constant duty cycle of 92%. These cutters provide an outflow four times larger than normal cutters in 27G, making surgery faster (Fig. 5.4b, c).

Flow control at 3–4 cc/min with VTI pump makes peripheral vitrectomy on a mobile retina safer.

Laser can be performed with the same footpedal. The footpedal can be activated as dual-linear.

EVA's LED light can be titrated.

5.7.3 Stellaris Elite Vision Enhancement System (B&L)

Stellaris Elite is a venturi pump system. Stellaris Elite has adaptive fluidics that continuously tracks vacuum flow rate to improve anterior chamber stability during phacoemulsification and Attune energy management for phacoemulsification energy (Fig. 5.5).

Stellaris Elite can use single port vitrectomy cutters in 20, 23 and 25G at 7500 cpm and Bi-blade dual port cutters in 25 and 27G at 15000 cpm × 2. The most special feature of the system is the option to use Vitesse hypersonic vitrectomy to liquify the vitreous around the tip with a 100% DC. However, the efficacy and

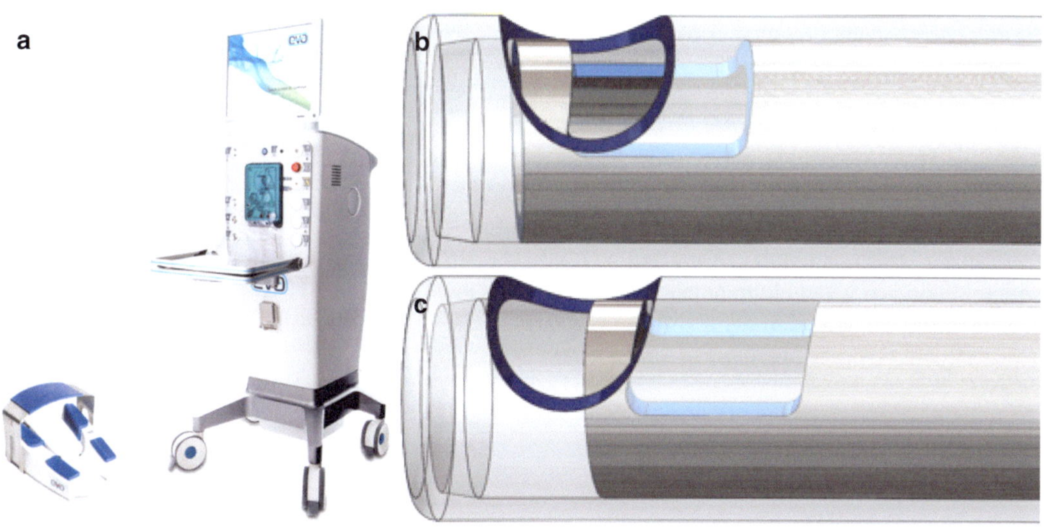

Fig. 5.4 (**a**) EVA vitrectomy system. (**b** and **c**) Vitreous cutter with two dimensional cutting with another port in the inner shaft(Image courtesy of DORC)

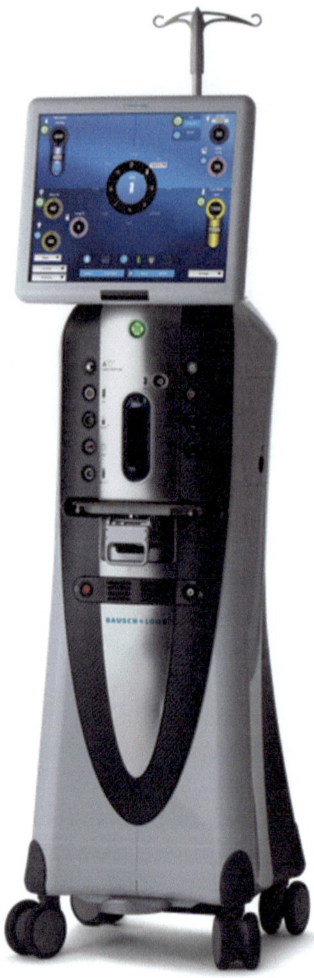

Fig. 5.5 Stellaris Elite vitrectomy system (Image courtesy of Bausch and Lomb)

safety of this hypersonic vitrectomy are not established yet.

Stellaris has a bright xenon light with three filters: yellow, green and amber. They can be used with midfield and widefield light patterns.

Endolaser can be used with the footpedal. This footpedal can also be used in a dual linear way.

5.8 Conclusion

New vitrectomy systems allow vitrectomy with small gauges. Small gauges and new pumps and cutters make vitrectomy safer and more efficient, but it is necessary to understand fluidics to set optimal parameters in each surgical scenario. New cutters with beveled tips make the vitreous cutter a multifunctional tool, TDC cutters enhance outflow and ultrasonic vitrectomy might be a new approach in the future.

References

1. de Oliveira PR, Berger AR, Chow DR. Vitreoretinal instruments: vitrectomy cutters, endoillumination and wide-angle viewing systems. Int J Retina Vitreous. 2016;2:28.
2. Rossi T, Querzoli G, Angelini G, Malvasi C, Rossi A, Morini M, Esposito G, Micera A, di Luca NM, Ripandelli G. Hydraulic resistance of vitreous cutters: the impact of blade design and cut rate. Transl Vis Sci Technol. 2016;5(4):1.
3. Rossi T, Querzoli G, Angelini G, Malvasi C, Iossa M, Placentino L, Ripandelli G. Fluid dynamics of vitrectomy probes. Retina. 2014;34(3):558–67.
4. Charles S. Fluidics and cutter dynamics. Dev Ophthalmol. 2014;54:31–7.
5. Steel DH, Charles S. Vitrectomy fluidics. Ophthalmologica. 2011;226(Suppl 7):27–35.
6. Dugel PU, Abulon DJ, Dimalanta R. Comparison of attraction capabilities associated with high-speed, dual-pneumatic vitrectomy probes. Retina. 2015;35(5):915–20.
7. Dugel PU, Zhou J, Abulon DJ, Buboltz DC. Tissue attraction associated with 20-gauge, 23-gauge, and enhanced 25-gauge dual-pneumatic vitrectomy probes. Retina. 2012;32(9):1761–6.
8. Romano MR, Stocchino A, Ferrara M, Lagazzo A, Repetto R. Fluidics of single and double blade guillotine vitrectomy probes in balanced salt solution and artificial vitreous. Transl Vis Sci Technol. 2018;7(6):19.
9. Rossi T, Querzoli G, Angelini G, Rossi A, Malvasi C, Iossa M, Ripandelli G. Instantaneous flow rate of vitreous cutter probes. Invest Ophthalmol Vis Sci. 2014;55(12):8289–94.

Wide-Angle Viewing System and Endoillumimnation

6

Kazuhito Yoneda and Yusuke Oshima

6.1 Wide-Angle Viewing Systems

For performing MIVS comfortably, wide-angle viewing systems (WAVs) including wide-angle illumination are a useful device for vitreous surgery, which has been continually developed from the late 1980s to the present based on the indirect ophthalmoscopic principle [1–9]. The WAVs not only offer a panoramic view of the surgical fields but also improve the safety and efficiency of the surgical procedures [10, 11]. Surgeons can easily evaluate the fundus status and the location of retinal pathologies through the panoramic view, and engage the peripheral retina without requiring excessive rotation of the eyeball during surgery as was necessary when viewing the fundus through conventional floating prismatic lenses.

In addition, the use of WAVs in conjunction with wide-angle illumination, like a chandelier lighting, allows easier bimanual maneuvers because they can provide a view of all inside the ocular globe without eye rotation, eliminating concerns regarding fragility of small-gauge instruments [12].

These tools play a part in the more widespread use of small-gauge vitrectomy, especially with a 27-g system, for a variety of vitreoretinal pathologies.

At the same time, recently a variety of WAVs has been newly developed or upgraded from the previous version along with the recent widespread use of MIVS.

To obtain a sufficient view of the posterior segment, it is necessary to use a high refractive lens (60D, 90D, and 120D), which is placed in front of the lens of the surgical microscope comparable to indirect ophthalmoscopes. This results in an inverted image. By flicking a reversal system (so-called inverter) into the parallel beam path of the operating microscope, an upright image is created. There are two types of WAVs, contact type and non-contact type.

6.1.1 Contact WAVs

The contact type WAVs includes some kinds of surgical highly refractive lens provided from Volk. Figure 6.1 shows the current commercially available contact wide viewing systems. The angle of view, magnifying power, weight, diameter, and surface reflex are different in each lens. There is a trade-off relation between the width of surgical field and the resolution. The two lenses, Central Retinal Vitrectomy lens (Volk) and Clarivit lens (HOYA) are suitable for macular

K. Yoneda (✉)
Department of Ophthalmology, Subarukai Eye Center, Subarukai Medical Corporation, Higashiohmi-shi, Shiga, Japan
e-mail: kazuyone@koto.kpu-m.ac.jp

Y. Oshima
Vitreoretina and Cataract Surgery Center, Oshima Eye Clinic, Takatsuki, Osaka, Japan

A. Jain et al. (eds.), *Cutting-edge Vitreoretinal Surgery*,
https://doi.org/10.1007/978-981-33-4168-5_6

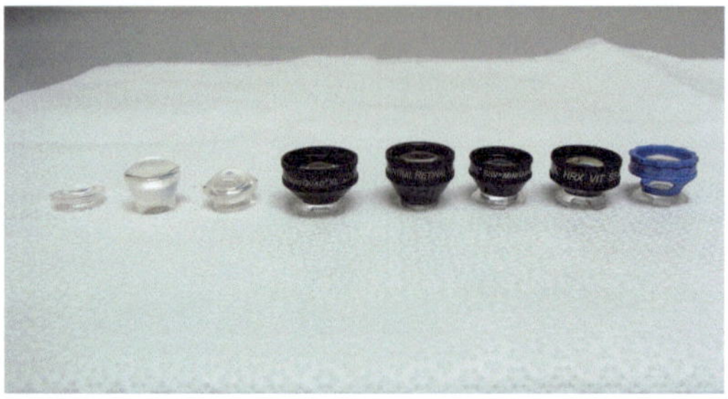

Fig. 6.1 Variety of contact type wide-angle viewing lenses. From left to right, Panoraview (HOYA), central type of ClariVit (Volk), wide type of ClariVit (Volk), MiniQuadXL (Volk), Central Retinal Vitrectomy lens (Volk), MiniQuad (Volk), HRX (Volk), MiniQuad ACS (Volk). Each lens has different features such as the size, shape, weight, and field of view

surgical procedures, such as ILM peeling as they have an excellent resolution but the surgical field of it is narrower than the others. MiniQuad XL has the widest surgical field, but the resolution of it is worse than the other two lenses (Fig. 6.2). The surgeon should choose the type of lens according to the situation. The contact type WAVs are directly attached to the cornea and provide better resolution and stereopsis than the non-contact type as they allow correction of the corneal aberrations. The major drawback is that it requires good assistance. Incomplete attachment of the contact lens during rotation of the eye causes decreased visibility of the fundus.

6.1.2 Non-Contact WAVs

With regard to the non-contact type WAVs, the Oculus BIOM can be used with all microscopes, but the Resight viewing system can only be used with a Zeiss microscope (Fig. 6.3), and the EIBOS viewing system can only be used with a Leica microscope. The other systems available are Merlin, OFFSIS (optic fiber free intravitreal surgery system), and Peyman-Wessels-Landers (PWL) lens. Every system offers excellent optical images with a variety of different magnifications and fields of view ranging from 120 to 130 degrees. By changing the distance between the lens and the cornea, the field of view can be adjusted. Lens condensation can cause inconvenience while using the non-contact type WAVs, which can be overcome by appropriate draping. The corneal surface should be coated with viscoelastic material to prevent corneal dehydration, which can decrease fundus visibility.

6.2 Endoillumination

Various advances have been made in the illumination system to include different types of light sources and use of various filters. To compensate for the insufficient illumination through small-gauge light probes with conventional halogen light bulbs, improved light sources, i.e., xenon and mercury vapor light bulb, were introduced. The increased lumens of xenon light sources are substantial, even with 25-g optic fibers or smaller, and the intraocular illumination is equal to or brighter than the illumination achieved with 20-g probes and conventional halogen or metal halide light bulbs. There are several stand-alone xenon light illuminators that are commercially available, such as Photon (Synergetics Inc.), Accurus High Brightness Il-luminator (AHBI, Alcon Laboratories Inc.), and Bright Star (DORC). In addition, xenon light bulbs are the standard illuminating systems in the next-generation vitrectomy machines, such as the Constellation Vision System (Alcon Laboratories) and the Stellaris PC (Bausch + Lomb), indicating that small-gauge optic fibers with powerful light sources will be the standard for pars plana vitrectomy for the foreseeable future.

On the heels of widespread adoption of WAVs and new light sources during vitrectomy, several new light probes have been developed to achieve wide-angle endoillumination and to minimize wide-angle illumination induced glare [13]. Most of the recently developed light probes offer a more than 100°field of view.

6.2.1 Phototoxicity

Powerful endoillumination has increased the risk of retinal light toxicity. The retinal threshold time is the theoretical time the surgeon can illuminate

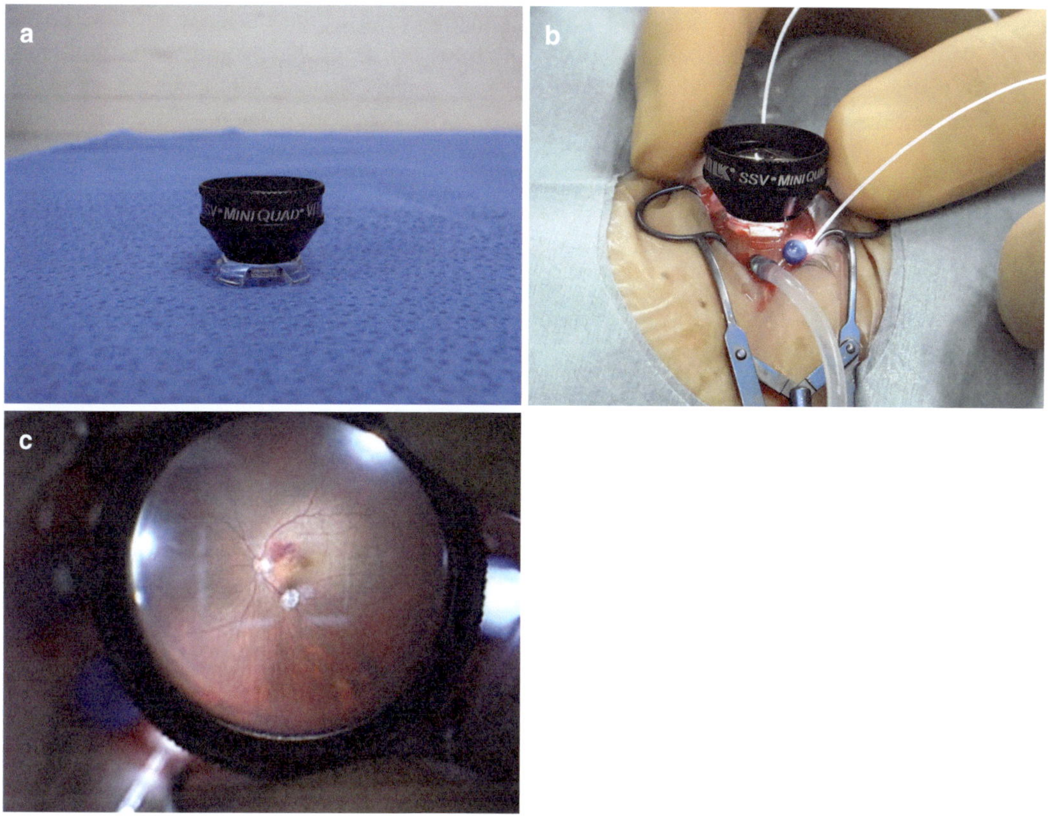

Fig. 6.2 (**a**)–(**c**) MiniQuad XL lens applied on the eye with the surgical field of view. This lens has the widest surgical field, but with low resolution

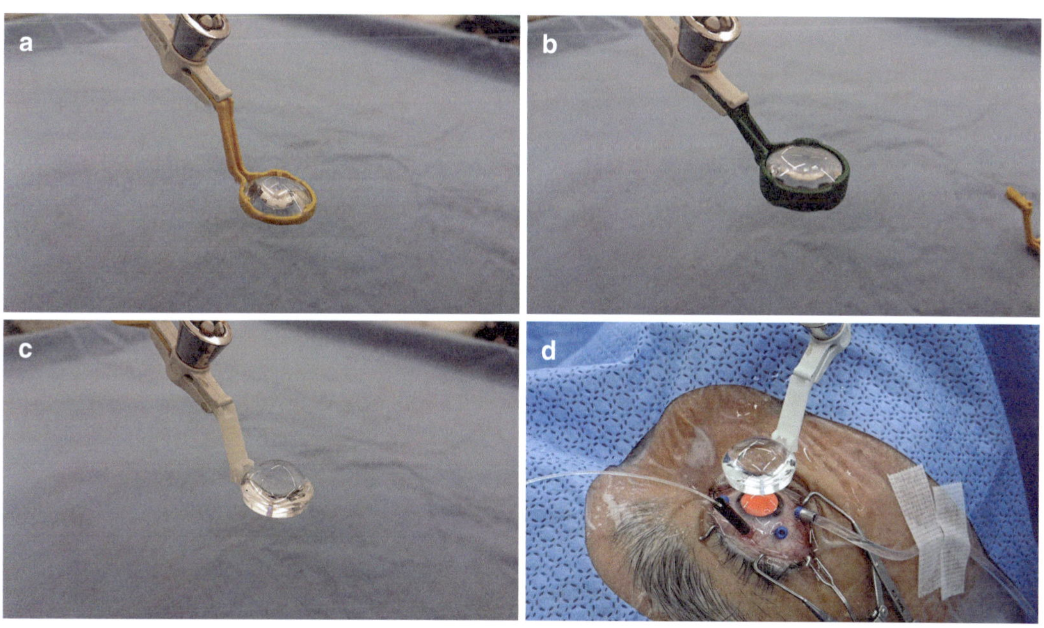

Fig. 6.3 The Resight system comes with different lenses that provide a trade-off relation between the width of the surgical field and the resolution. (**a**) The 128D lens providing a wider surgical field. (**b**) The 60D lens providing high resolution for macular surgeries. (**c**) and (**d**) show the use of disposable lenses

the retina under given settings. The retina threshold time incorporates the aphakic hazard sum, the working distance, brightness, cone of illumination used, and the industry standard for toxicity of 25 J/cm^2. Van den Beisen et al. reported that the permissible exposure time to endoilluminators during vitrectomy can be increased from 1 min to up to 13 min by using an additional 475 nm long pass filter, light levels below 10 mW, and maintaining a distance of at least 10 mm between the light probe and the retina which means that the area illuminated should be larger than the temporal arcades which has a diameter of 10 mm [14]. There has been concern raised over possible retinal phototoxicity with xenon light sources because the spectral distribution of xenon light involves the theoretical phototoxic hazard area in aphakic human eyes. Therefore, current commercially available xenon illuminators feature lower wavelength filters (at least <420 nm), cutting off ultraviolet and blue light to reduce phototoxicity with higher hazard efficiency. Yellow filters have been used to improve tissue safety.

Vital dyes such as idocyanine green, trypan blue, and brilliant blue can interact with the light source and exert further retinal and RPE damage. An overlap between the emission spectrum of the light source and absorption spectrum of the dye can lead to increased release of free radicals causing retinal damage.

6.2.2 Chandelier Endoillumination

Chandelier endoillumination itself is not a new concept. Many surgeons have used the Torpedo Mini Lights chandelier endoilluminator with single optic fiber or multiple optic fibers. However, because of insufficient brightness, either with a conventional halogen or metal halide bulb, this chandelier fiber failed to catch on. In contrast, thanks to the recently developed light sources, the optic fibers for the new chandelier endoilluminators have been developed in a variety of designs and gauges. In addition to the wide field of view, chandelier endoillumination can free up a surgeon's hand from holding a light probe, thus allowing true bimanual manipulation during surgery. In case of retinal detachment, surgeons can perform scleral indentation by themselves to achieve more controlled and smooth peripheral vitreous base shaving, rather than them done by an assistant. For membrane dissections in challenging cases, such as diabetic tractional retinal detachment or proliferative vitreoretinopathy, the freed hand is helpful for holding a forceps to grasp the membranes for separation from the retina or dissection using scissors or a cutter with the other hand.

Currently, the gauge of choice ranges from 25-g to 27-g for single-fiber chandelier and 27-g to 29-g dual-fiber systems [15–19]. All fibers are designed to be self-retaining after transconjunctival insertion, with or without the use of a trocar-cannula system. To obtain sufficient brightness, some surgeons prefer to choose larger-gauge single fibers, i.e., a 25-g fiber rather than a 27-g fiber or smaller. However, unlike the oblique incision technique required to insert the cannulas for vitrectomy, a vertical insertion for the 25-g optic fiber directly through the sclera is required to aim the light appropriately at the posterior pole. In addition, chandelier from a single fiber makes it difficult to cover the whole eye homogenously. Therefore, chandelier illumination with two optic fiber is useful for obtaining homogenous and more widespread illumination, thus eliminating the need to reposition the fiber because of the illumination coming from two different directions [15, 18]. Moreover, adjusting the dual tips is possible for optimizing the illumination angle inside the eye and minimizing any glare from the tips. The direction of illumination can change from the posterior pole to the periphery by changing the curvature of the chandelier fiber outside the eyeball (Fig. 6.4).

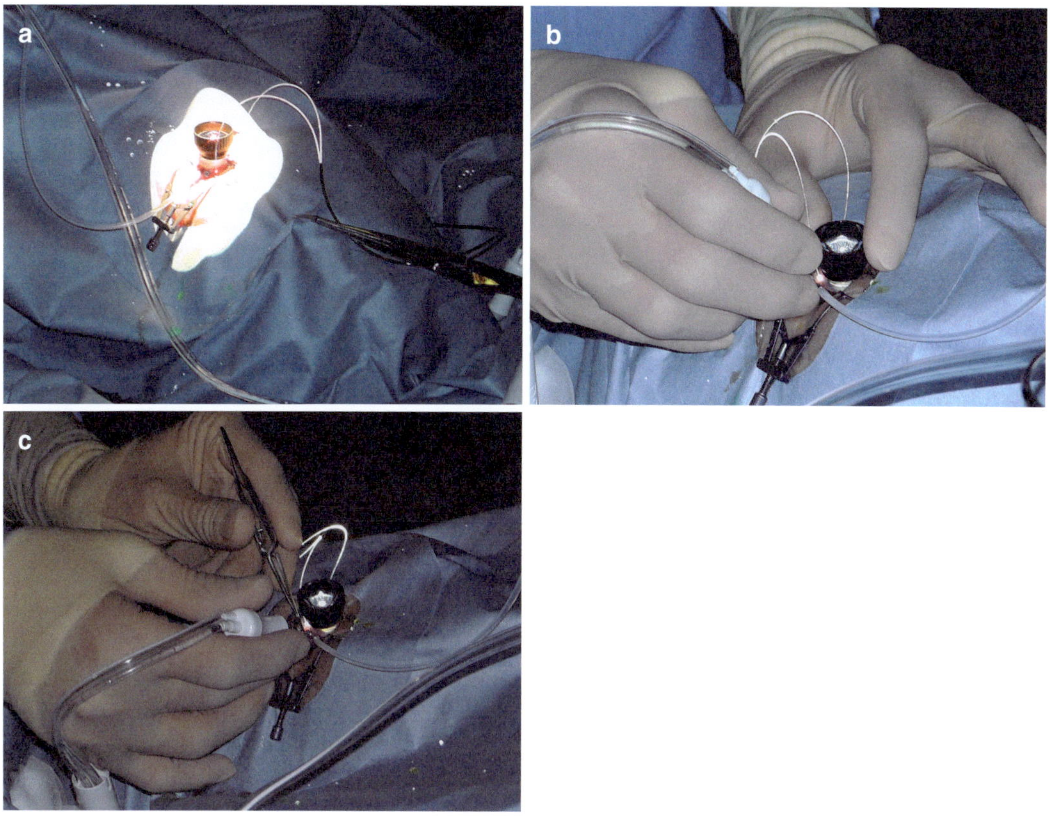

Fig. 6.4 Optimizing and fixing the twin light chandelier direction. (**a**) To control the direction of illumination, it is necessary to use the surgeon's fingers or some device such as a needle holder to fix the chandelier fiber. (**b**) and (**c**) The direction of illumination can change from the posterior pole to the periphery by changing the curvature of the chandelier fiber outside the eyeball

6.3 Conclusion

The use of WAVs and advanced illumination system, provides a better view of the fundus with minimal eye rotation allowing bimanual maneuvers while performing complex vitreoretinal surgeries.

References

1. Spitznas M. A binocular indirect ophthalmomicroscope (BIOM) for non-contact wide-angle vitreous surgery. Graefes Arch Clin Exp Ophthalmol. 1987;225:13–5.
2. Peyman GA. A new wide-angle irrigating contact lens for pars plana vitrectomy. Can J Ophthalmol. 1988;23:150.
3. Bovey EH, Gonvers M. A new device for noncontact wide angle viewing of the fundus during vitrectomy. Arch Ophthalmol. 1995;113:1572–3.
4. Hayashi H, Oshima Y. A wide-field view fundus contact lens for infants. Retina. 1998;18:91–2.
5. Horiguchi M, Kojima Y, Shimada Y. New system for fiberoptic-free bimanual vitreous surgery. Arch Ophthalmol. 2002;120:491–4.
6. Peyman GA, Canakis C, Livir-Rallatos C, Whalen P. Small size pediatric vitrectomy wide-angle contact lens. Am J Ophthalmol. 2003;135:236–7.
7. Landers MB, Peyman GA, Wessels IF, et al. A new, non-contact wide field viewing system for vitreous surgery. Am J Ophthalmol. 2003;136:199–201.
8. Shah VA, Chalam KV. Self-stabilizing wide-angle contact lens for vitreous surgery. Retina. 2003;23:667–9.
9. Nakata K, Ohji M, Ikuno Y, et al. Wide-angle viewing lens for vitrectomy. Am J Ophthalmol. 2004;137:760–2.
10. Kadonosono K. Achieving wide angle view during vitrectomy. Retina Today. 2011;6(1):43–5.

11. Chalam KV, Shah VA. Optics of wide-angle panoramic viewing system-assisted vitreous surgery. Surv Ophthalmol. 2004;49:437–45.
12. Oshima Y, Awh CC, Tano Y. Self-retaining 27-gauge transconjunctival chandelier endoillumination for panoramic viewing during vitreous surgery. Am J Ophthalmol. 2007;143:166–7.
13. Rossi T, Boccassini B, Iossa M, Rossi A, Mutolo A, Tamburrelli C. Wedge-shaped light pipe aperture for pars plana vitrectomy. Retina. 2009;29:1201–6.
14. van den Biesen PR, Berenschot T, Verdaasdonk RM, et al. Endoillumination during vitrectomy and phototoxicity thresholds. Br J Ophthalmol. 2000;84:1372–5.
15. Oshima Y, Chow DR, Awh CC, Sakaguchi H, Tano Y. Novel mercury vapor illuminator combined with a 27/29-gauge chandelier light fiber for vitreous surgery. Retina. 2008;28:171–3.
16. Eckardt C. Twin lights: a new chandelier illumination for bimanual surgery. Retina. 2003;23:893–4.
17. Oshima Y, Awh CC, Tano Y. Self-retaining 27-gauge transconjunctival chandelier endoillumination for panoramic viewing during vitreous surgery. Am J Ophthalmol. 2007;143:166–7.
18. Eckardt C, Eckert T, Eckardt U. 27-gauge Twinlight chandelier illumination system for bimanual transconjunctival vitrectomy. Retina. 2008;28:518–9.
19. Sakaguchi H, Oshima Y, Nishida K, Awh CC. A 29/30-gauge dual-chandelier illumination system for panoramic viewing during microincision vitrectomy surgery. Retina. 2011;31:231–1233.

Sutureless Small-Gauge Vitrectomy

7

Sean Yuan, Vishal S. Parikh, and Gaurav K. Shah

7.1 Introduction

Pars plana vitrectomy (PPV) was first introduced by Robert Machemer in 1972 and has since become the most common procedure for the treatment of posterior segment disease [1]. The original PPV used a single port, 17-gauge vitrectome that Machemer called the vitreous infusion suction vitrectome that required a 2.3-mm scleral incision [1]. In 1974, O'Malley and Heintz introduced a smaller 20-gauge, three-port procedure that became the standard until the early 2000s, when 23-gauge and 25-gauge PPV systems were introduced and widely adopted [2–4]. Most recently, there has been a shift toward smaller gauge vitrectomy with the introduction of the 27-gauge PPV by Oshima et al. in 2010 (Fig. 7.1) [5].

Electronic Supplementary Material The online version of this chapter (https://doi.org/10.1007/978-981-33-4168-5_7) contains supplementary material, which is available to authorized users.

S. Yuan
Washington University School of Medicine, St. Louis, MO, USA
e-mail: sean.yuan@wustl.edu

V. S. Parikh · G. K. Shah (✉)
The Retina Institute, St. Louis, MO, USA
e-mail: mdparikh.vishal@rc-stl.com

A. Jain et al. (eds.), *Cutting-edge Vitreoretinal Surgery*,
https://doi.org/10.1007/978-981-33-4168-5_7

Since its introduction, 27-gauge PPV has become more widespread in clinical practice. The 2017 Preferences and Trends Survey by the American Society of Retina Specialists indicated that 21.9% of vitreoretinal surgeons in the USA had performed 27-gauge PPV in the previous year [6]. As the adoption of small-gauge sutureless PPV becomes more common, it is important to consider its advantages and disadvantages so that each vitreoretinal surgeon can determine its appropriate role in his or her practice. The smaller diameter of the cannulas affects flow rate and cutting efficiency, instrument maneuverability, wound creation, and closure. The implications of these changes will be reviewed in this chapter with a focus on 27-gauge vitrectomy.

7.2 Advantages of Small-Gauge Sutureless Pars Plana Vitrectomy

Vitreoretinal surgeons have pursued small-gauge PPV in the efforts of achieving less traumatic wound construction and closure, less perioperative and postoperative patient discomfort, and comparable risk of endophthalmitis to larger gauges without the need for sutures.

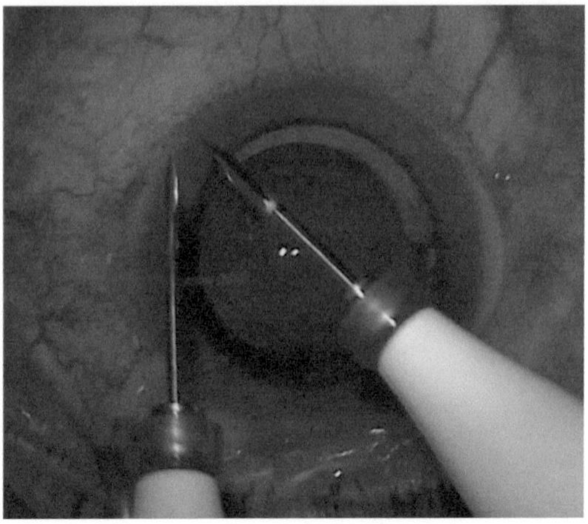

Fig. 7.1 Intraoperative image comparing the smaller 27-gauge trochar and cannula to the larger 23-gauge trochar and cannula

7.2.1 Less Traumatic Wound Construction and Closure

Small-gauge sutureless PPV is advancing toward a reduced need for beveled wound construction and sutures to prevent hypotony, thus resulting in less trauma to the conjunctiva and sclera. Initially, 25G vitrectomy was attempted with straight incisions as better self-sealing was expected with the smaller gauge [7]. However, studies showed better wound closure and reduced hypotony with beveled incisions for 25G [8–10]. With smaller 27-gauge cannulas, the surgeon can perform perpendicular trans-scleral, one-step entry into the vitreous cavity with minimal need for sutures (Fig. 7.2) [11, 12]. As a result, the surgeon may benefit from a reduced technical burden, reduced tissue trauma, and faster start to the procedure (Video 7.1). The smaller sclerotomy diameter and simpler mechanics of instrument passage facilitate postoperative self-sealing and wound-healing due to less wound distortion during surgery (Fig. 7.2) [13].

In addition to more efficient entry, smaller gauge PPV involves less suturing and lower hypotony rates. For 23- and 25-gauge PPV, postoperative hypotony rates have been reported to be 0–10.5% and 0–25.6%, respectively [11, 14]. For 27G PPV, multiple studies have reported minimal to no suturing postoperatively with rates well below 5% of the total sample size [11, 15, 16]. The few cases requiring sutures may have been due to the patient's unique anatomy, such as a taut or thin scleral, or imperfect instrument handling during entry or vitreous removal. Two studies found a 5–6% transient postoperative hypotony rate that may have been due in part to angled incision, which supports the usage of perpendicular incisions [11, 14]. Therefore, it is necessary for the surgeon to remain prepared to suture despite it not being necessary for the majority of small-gauge sutureless PPV.

7.2.2 Less Perioperative and Postoperative Patient Discomfort

With smaller gauge PPV, anesthesia has transitioned from general endotracheal intubation to local retrobulbar or peribulbar anesthesia with or without sedation [11, 12, 14, 15]. However, retrobulbar anesthesia still carries risks including perforation, hematoma, and retrobulbar hemorrhage [17]. With increased use of 27-gauge vitrectomy, surgeons are now performing some cases with topical perioperative anesthesia such as proparacaine or lidocaine jelly with minimal sedation (Video 7.1) [18]. These advances represented a time, cost, and risk improvement over general anesthesia.

Smaller gauge PPV results in minimal postoperative pain management due to less inflammation and faster visual recovery from less traumatic wounds as mentioned previously. Decreased inflammation and pain have been reported comparing 25-gauge systems to 20- and 23-gauge systems [16, 19–21]. Studies comparing 27-gauge PPV to 25-gauge PPV have also showed no instances of significant inflammation postoperatively [16, 22]. More research is necessary to establish if inflammation in 27G is decreased or merely comparable to 25G, but the available data suggests that smaller gauges correlate with decreased inflammation. In addition, absorbable sutures used after larger-gauge procedures rely on inflammation to break down. Small-gauge

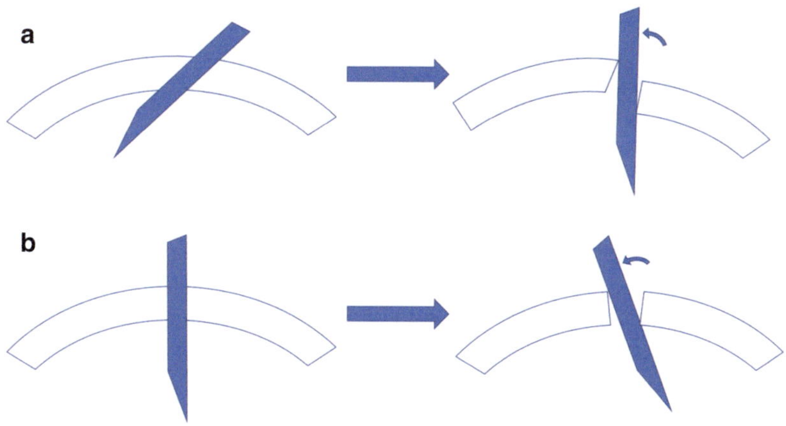

Fig. 7.2 Diagram comparing wound construction techniques. (**a**) Rotating instruments against a beveled cannula wound causes distortion of the sclera, thus making an approximation of the wound edges more irregular during closure. (**b**) With perpendicular cannula wound, the wound edges re-approximate well even with rotation of instruments against the sclera, thus resulting in less suturing with 27-gauge pars plana vitrectomy

sutureless PPV obviates additional inflammation that would be necessary in the healing process.

7.2.3 Comparable Risk of Endophthalmitis to Large-Gauge Vitrectomy

Studies indicate that small-gauge sutureless PPV produces similar postoperative endophthalmitis rates compared to larger gauges that were sutured. The risk of endophthalmitis is directly related to communication between the sterile cavity and the environment. Therefore, there may be a concern that a sutureless wound may increase the risk of endophthalmitis. However, this has not been found to be the case, with several studies showing postoperative endophthalmitis rates of zero and none above 0.3% [14–16].

7.3 Concerns Regarding Small-Gauge Sutureless Vitrectomy

7.3.1 Infusion and Aspiration Flow Rate Limitations on Effective Vitreous Removal

Flow through a vitrectomy probe is affected by aspiration rate, port opening size, cut rate, and the cutter's duty cycle, among other factors [23]. Small-gauge sutureless vitrectomy leads to a decrease in the radius (r) of the lumen of the cannulas, infusion, and vitrectome and thus an increase in resistance (R) in the lumen of the cannulas, infusion, and vitrectome as seen in Eq. (7.1):

$$R = \frac{8\eta L}{\pi r^4} \tag{7.1}$$

where, R = resistance, η = viscosity of fluid, L = length of tube, r = radius of tube.

The fourth-power dependency of radius in this equation means that even a small decrease in radius can produce a large increase in resistance. As resistance increases, flow through the infusion and vitrectome decreases as modeled by Poiseuille's law in Eq. (7.2). To overcome inefficiencies arising from an increase in resistance, vitrectomy platforms and vitrectomes have been improved to increase flow.

$$F = \frac{\Delta P}{R} \tag{7.2}$$

where, F = flow rate, P = pressure (infusion/aspiration), R = resistance.

7.3.1.1 Improved Vitrectome Flow

Flow through the vitrectome is governed by Poiseuille's law. To overcome increased resistance (R), the pressure gradient (ΔP) can be increased in Eq. (7.1) or resistance can be decreased by reducing the viscosity of the vitreous (η) being removed in Eq. (7.2).

The pressure gradient is increased by increasing the aspiration vacuum and the duration over which it works (duty cycle). Small-gauge PPV platforms generally operate at higher aspiration vacuums of 400–650 mmHg to compensate for the smaller vitrectome lumen. Vitrectome design has also been improved to improve the duty cycle to allow for the vitrectomy port to be open longer during the cutting cycle to allow for improved flow. Dual pneumatic drive vitrectomes that actively open the vitrectome have improved duty cycle on traditional guillotine vitrectomes [24]. However, these traditional vitrectomes only cut during the forward motion and blocks aspiration during the backward motion, thus reducing aspiration efficiency. In contrast, the classic vitrectome's inner sleeve is a solid tube. Twin dimensional cutting vitrectomes have improved upon the aforementioned vitrectome with an inner sleeve that contains an additional aperture that allows for cutting during the sleeve's backward motion in addition to forward motion to virtually eliminate a closed port by improving the duty cycle to 92% (Fig. 7.3) [25].

The viscosity of vitreous being removed can be reduced by making the pieces of vitreous being removed smaller. Higher cut rates allow for this to happen. Traditional guillotine vitrectomes are now able to approach 10,000 cuts/min. However, as previously mentioned, the duty cycle can be compromised at high cut rates in traditional vitrectomes. A twin duty cycle vitrectome allows for the effective cut rate to be doubled up to 16,000 cuts/min while still having a 92% duty cycle [26].

7.3.1.2 Improved Infusion Flow

With an increase in aspiration rate due to higher vacuum pressure and an open duty cycle vitrectome, it was necessary to also improve infusion to accommodate high flow to prevent hypotony and globe collapse. Vitrectomy systems now use pressurized infusion systems in contrast to gravity-fed systems to allow for high flow and rapid infusion control [23]. Changes to the infusion tubing itself have also been adapted to allow for increased flow. Instead of a traditional infusion tubing that inserts within the cannula and reduces the lumen of flow to less than the gauge being used, the infusion may be placed in a cap-over fashion so as not to reduce the lumen of the tubing (Fig. 7.4). For example, a traditional 27-gauge infusion may actually have the diameter of a standard 29-gauge tube, whereas the cap-over 27-gauge infusion has no change in diameter (Fig. 7.5).

7.3.1.3 Overall Effect on Operating Time

Taking into account these design changes, average operating times for 27-gauge PPV are similar to or approaching operating times for 23- and

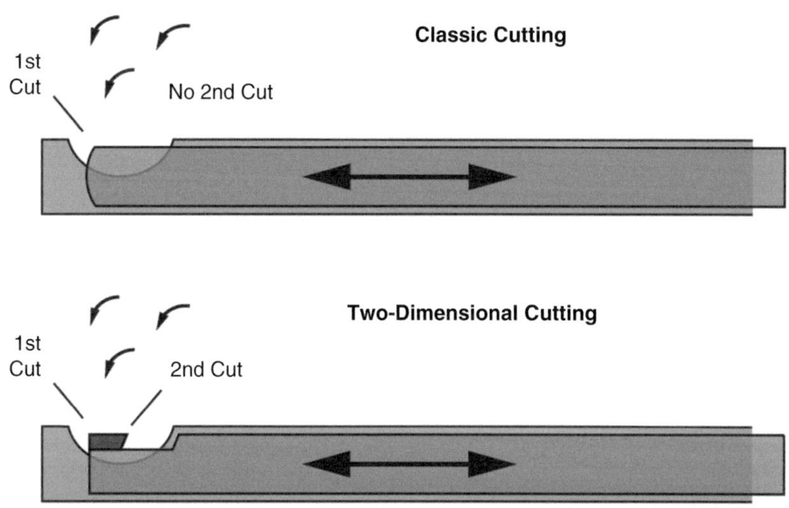

Fig. 7.3 Diagram comparing a classic guillotine vitrectome (**a**) which cuts in a single direction and results in closure of the port when the cutter is down and (**b**) a two-dimensional cutting vitrectome which cuts in both directions and maintains an open port to allow nearly continuous flow of smaller pieces of vitreous

25-gauge. Studies have not shown a consensus but lean slightly toward a longer, but not significant, operating time for 27 gauge [15, 22, 27]. Other studies indicate equivalent operating times [14, 16, 28]. To our knowledge, no studies showed a statistically significant shorter operating time for 27-gauge PPV. However, many studies were pilot studies into 27-gauge vitrectomy and therefore may have been biased by surgeons' learning curves. Longer operating times for 27 gauge, though still a potential concern, do not appear to be significantly different from those of larger gauges and therefore should not dissuade surgeons from considering its adoption.

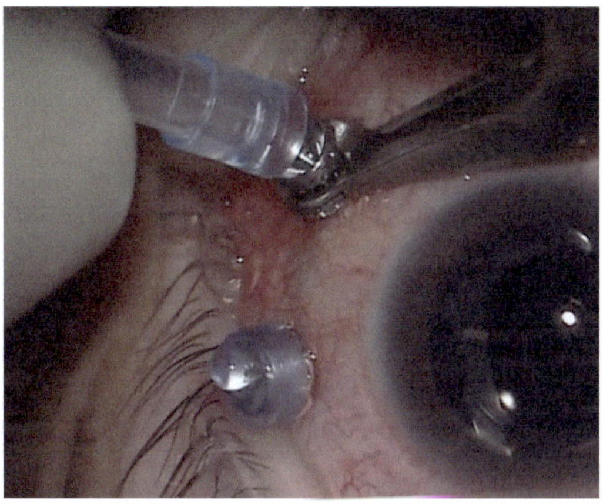

Fig. 7.4 Intraoperative image showing a cap-over infusion line where the valve has been removed from the cannula and the infusion is secured over the cannula to maintain the radius of the cannula lumen

7.3.2 Flexible Instruments Limiting Small-Gauge PPV in Complex Cases

Smaller gauge instruments were and continue to be concerning to some vitreoretinal surgeons due to decreased tensile strength of the shaft, which could lead to damage to the vitrectome, poor tissue handling during membrane dissection, and iatrogenic foreign body introduction. Within the cannula, forceful manipulation of small-gauge instruments can lead to bending and damage to the operating mechanism while performing peripheral vitrectomy. If the shaft of a forceps is bent during operation, then the surgeon may experience decreased control of the forceps while manipulating delicate tissue, such as during a membrane peel.

Changes in instrument design to address flexibility include shortening or supporting the shaft and better alloys for the instruments. Oshima et al. shortened the shaft of their vitrectome from 32 mm to 25 mm to increase shaft stiffness [5]. Rizzo et al. have also reported using a 27-gauge vitrectome with the same length as a 25-gauge one by using a tapered stiffening

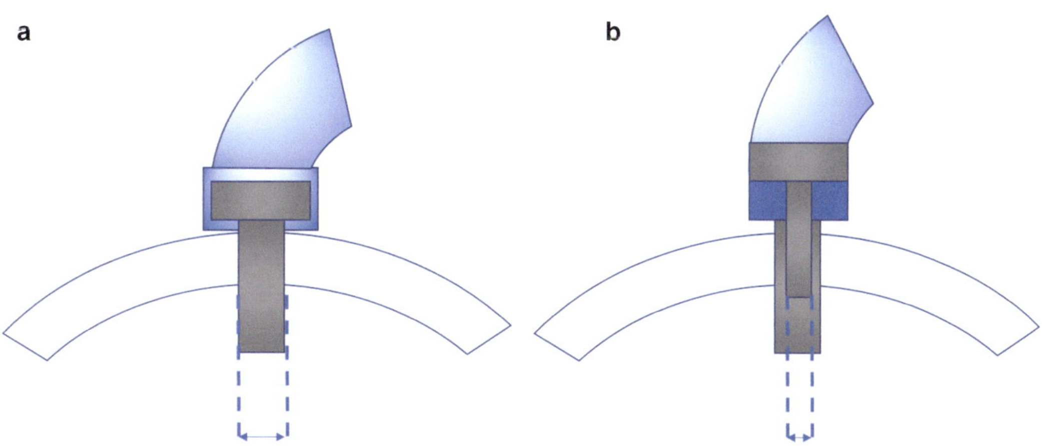

Fig. 7.5 Diagram comparing a cap-over infusion line (**a**) with a traditional infusion line (**b**) where the infusion inserts within the cannula. The traditional infusion may have a smaller diameter (d_2) of a standard 29-gauge tube, whereas the cap-over 27-gauge infusion has no change in diameter (d_1)

sleeve and technique adjustments, namely incising in specific quadrants [12]. The shift to a titanium alloy gives better tensile strength to the shaft. Finally, Khan et al. observed that adverse events related to instrument flexibility may have resulted from the learning curve of adopting a new technique [14]. Increased practice with 27-gauge for particular indications reduces the risk of iatrogenic problems. In short, instrument modifications, reasonable modifications of entry technique, and sufficient practice can alleviate concerns with flexibility.

7.4 Intraoperative Challenges with Small-Gauge Sutureless Vitrectomy and Suggested Technique Modifications

Although vitrectomy platforms and vitrectomes have been adapted for small-gauge sutureless PPV, subtle alterations in technique and approach can help a surgeon overcome challenges related to small-gauge sutureless PPV such as preventing hypotony, inefficient vitreous removal, inducing a posterior vitreous detachment, difficult instrument manipulation, and use of silicone oil.

7.4.1 Preventing Hypotony

With small-gauge sutureless vitrectomy, the eye is sensitive to infusion and aspiration mismatch. The presence of choroidals intraoperatively is an indicator that the eye is not maintaining intraocular pressure well.

In the event that hypotony is an issue during a case, first ensure the infusion cannula is in the vitreous cavity. Next, the integrity of the eye should be ensured by increasing the infusion pressure until the choroidals resolve while still maintaining perfusion of the nerve. Given the sensitive nature of small-gauge PPV, make sure the correct mode is selected for small-gauge PPV on the vitrectomy platform. Next, a systematic evaluation of the infusion line and system should be done: ensure there is an appropriate drip from the infusion bottle, no kinks in the infusion line, and re-confirm that the infusion cannula is in the vitreous cavity. Finally, if the adjustment to infusion and aspiration levels must be made by either increasing the infusion or decreasing the aspiration rate.

Hypotony can be prevented with a thorough evaluation of the infusion line outside the eye prior to operating, confirming placement of the infusion cannula, and the use of a cap-over infusion (Fig. 7.4) to allow for greater infusion flow to compensate for changes in aspiration by the vitrectome.

7.4.2 Inefficient Vitreous Removal

Regardless of improvement in vitrectomy platforms and vitrectome design, a smaller gauge instrument will have a smaller port and adaptations in technique are necessary to improve vitreous removal. Inefficient vitreous removal is identified by the limited movement of the vitreous during core and shave vitrectomy.

With small-gauge PPV, the surgeon needs to be able to readily identify the hyaloid edge and be comfortable with having the vitrectome port face the retina while shaving for efficient vitreous removal. This is unlike 20-gauge and 23-gauge PPV, where holding the vitrectome in place with the port away from the retina will allow for efficient vitreous removal. The use of triamcinolone can aid in finding the vitreous edge and ensuring the vitrectome port is directed at the vitreous, thus leading to more efficient removal.

7.4.3 Inability to Induce Posterior Vitreous Detachment

Traditionally, successful engagement of the hyaloid at the optic nerve leads to optimal posterior vitreous detachment (PVD) by slowly elevating the posterior hyaloid to separate the vitreous from the retina in a centripetal fashion (Fig. 7.6). However, this technique does have its limits in cases with significant vitreoretinal adhesion/traction. When there is difficulty engaging the hyaloid, the initial response is to increase the vacuum. However, this does not always work given the

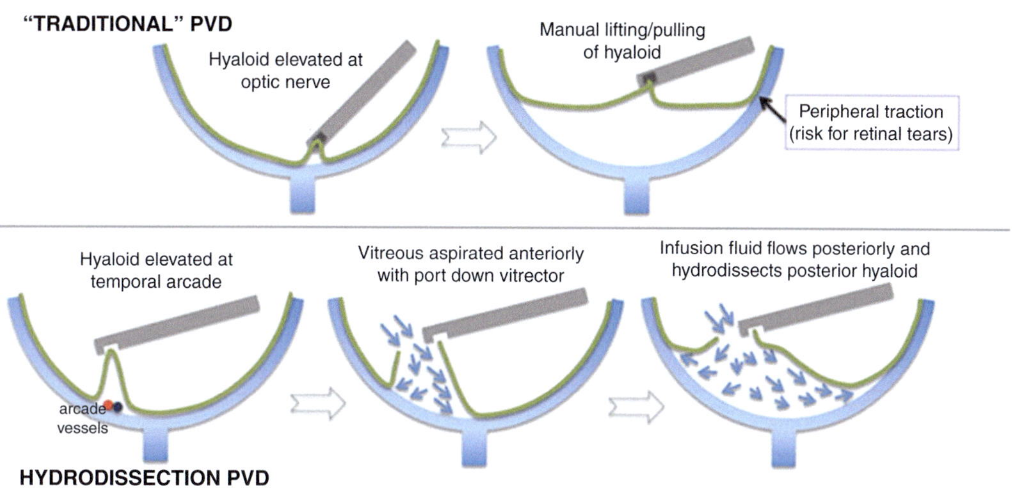

Fig. 7.6 Diagram showing a traditional induction of a surgical posterior vitreous detachment (PVD) (top) and induction of a surgical PVD by hydrodissection (bottom). With a traditional surgical PVD, the hyaloid is pulled off of the retina with traction the vitreoretinal interface. Creating a PVD with hydrodissection involves the infusion fluid flowing into the vitreoretinal interface and push the vitreous off the retina, thereby having no traction on the retina and limiting iatrogenic damage

smaller port opening on the vitrectome and could lead to iatrogenic damage of the retina.

An alternative mechanism by which to surgically induce a PVD without placing traction on the macula and peripheral retina is hydrodissection. This method involves creating an opening in the posterior hyaloid over the superotemporal arcade with the vitrectome port facing down. Using the opening, a 360-degree circumferential vitrectomy at the level of the midperiphery is performed. With the vitreous flowing anteriorly into the vitrectome, the infusion fluid fills the space created posteriorly and hydrodissects the posterior hyaloid face-off of the macula and peripheral retina with minimal to no traction (Fig. 7.6, Video 7.2). Using triamcinolone to identify the posterior hyaloid helps to verify the induction of a PVD.

7.4.4 Inability for Transconjunctival Wound to Close

The primary goal of small-gauge vitrectomy is to have sutureless wounds that improve efficiency and improve patient comfort. The need for sutures in these cases is frustrating.

Cautery can be used to close the overlying conjunctiva and scar the wound closed. Decreasing infusion pressure slightly below the operating level while removing cannulas and then tamponade over the wound can aid in closure. Liquid quick setting sealant is another option.

To prevent a non-sealing wound, straight incisions are suggested to reduce manipulation of the cannula that would damage the surrounding sclera, thus allowing for better wound closure (Fig. 7.2) [11–13].

7.4.5 Difficulty with Instrument Manipulation

Although improvements have been made in the tensile strength of the shaft of small-gauge instruments, adjustments can be made to improve manipulation. Simple techniques involve using a forefinger on the shaft for stability along with oar locking so that the cannula rotates against the sclera instead of the instrument. Adequate vitreous clearance around ports allows for ease of instrument introduction and removal through small cannulas. Finally, for macular work, placing towels on the head and wrist rest to elevate the wrist creates a more downward trajectory toward the macula to limit the bending of the shaft while peeling membranes.

7.4.6 Silicone Oil Insertion or Removal

Silicone oil is used in complex cases when a longer acting tamponade is necessary. Some vitreoretinal surgeons shy away from small-gauge vitrectomy in these complex cases not only because of instrumentation choice but also the time required to insert and remove silicone oil. The use of metal viscous fluid injection tip allows for efficient oil injection at high pressure in around 3 minutes. Oil removal with cap-over high-pressure viscous fluid tubing at high aspiration allows for removal in approximately 5 minutes (Video 7.3). As mentioned previously, improvements in vitrectome design and vitrectomy platform allow for adequate air/fluid exchange to remove residual oil.

7.5 Conclusions

Significant advances have been made with small-gauge sutureless vitrectomy, especially 27-gauge. It possesses numerous benefits that can improve the experience for both surgeon and patient in a variety of cases ranging from vitreous opacities, retinal detachment, and epiretinal membrane to complex detachments with PVR and diabetic tractional retinal detachments. More surgeons are adopting its use every year and trends indicate that it will soon become widely practiced. Each vitreoretinal surgeon should evaluate its role in his or her practice.

References

1. Machemer R, Buettner H, Norton EW, Parel JM. Vitrectomy: a pars plana approach. Trans Am Acad Ophthalmol Otolaryngol. 1971;75:813–20.
2. O'Malley C, Heintz RM Sr. Vitrectomy with an alternative instrument system. Ann Ophthalmol. 1975;7:585–8.
3. Eckardt C. Transconjunctival sutureless 23-gauge vitrectomy. Retina. 2005;25:208–11.
4. Fujii GY, De Juan E Jr, Humayun MS, Chang TS, Pieramici DJ, Barnes A, Kent D. Initial experience using the transconjunctival sutureless vitrectomy system for vitreoretinal surgery. Ophthalmology. 2002;109:1814–20.
5. Oshima Y, Wakabayashi T, Sato T, Ohji M, Tano YA. 27-Gauge instrument system for transconjunctival sutureless microincision vitrectomy surgery. Ophthalmology. 2010;117(1):93.e2–102.e2.
6. American Society of Retinal Specialists. Preferences and trends survey. 2017. www.asrs.org.
7. Fujii GY, de Juan E Jr, Humayun MS, Pieramici DJ, Chang TS, Ng E, Barnes A, Wu SL, Sommerville DN. A new 25-gauge instrument system for transconjunctival sutureless vitrectomy surgery1. Ophthalmology. 2002;109(10):1807–12.
8. Hsu J, Chen E, Gupta O, Fineman MS, Garg SJ, Regillo CD. Hypotony after 25-gauge vitrectomy using oblique versus direct cannula insertions in fluid-filled eyes. Retina. 2008;28(7):937–40.
9. Singh RP, Bando H, Brasil OF, Williams DR, Kaiser PK. Evaluation of wound closure using different incision techniques with 23-gauge and 25-gauge microincision vitrectomy systems. Retina. 2008;28(2):242–8.
10. Taban M, Sharma S, Ventura AA, Kaiser PK. Evaluation of wound closure in oblique 23-gauge sutureless sclerotomies with visante optical coherence tomography. Am J Ophthalmol. 2009;147(1):101–7.
11. Khan MA, Shahlaee A, Toussaint B, Hsu J, Sivalingam A, Dugel PU, Lakhanpal RR, Riemann CD, Berrocal MH, Regillo CD, Ho AC. Outcomes of 27 gauge microincision vitrectomy surgery for posterior segment disease. Am J Ophthalmol. 2016;161:36–43.
12. Rizzo S, Barca F, Caporossi T, Mariotti C. Twenty-seven–gauge vitrectomy for various vitreoretinal diseases. Retina. 2015;35(6):1273–8.
13. Schaal S, Ozkok A, Nesmith B, Eliott D, Scott I. 27-gauge vitrectomy surgery: smaller is better: Retina Today; 2014.
14. Khan MA, Kuley A, Riemann CD, Berrocal MH, Lakhanpal RR, Hsu J, Sivalingam A, Ho AC, Regillo CD. Long-term visual outcomes and safety profile of 27-gauge pars plana vitrectomy for posterior segment disease. Ophthalmology. 2018;125(3):423–31.
15. Rizzo S, Polizzi S, Barca F, Caporossi T, Virgili G. Comparative study of 27-gauge versus 25-gauge vitrectomy for the treatment of primary rhegmatogenous retinal detachment. J Ophthalmol. 2017;2017:6384985.
16. Romano MR, Cennamo G, Ferrara M, Cennamo M, Cennamo G. Twenty-seven-gauge versus 25-gauge vitrectomy for primary rhegmatogenous retinal detachment. Retina. 2017;37(4):637–42.
17. Rubin AP. Complications of local anaesthesia for ophthalmic surgery. Br J Anaesth. 1995;75(1):93–6.
18. Wu RH, Zhang R, Lin Z, Liang QH, Moonasar N. A comparison between topical and retrobulbar anesthesia in 27-gauge vitrectomy for vitreous floaters:

a randomized controlled trial. BMC Ophthalmol. 2018;18(1):164.
19. Thompson JT. Advantages and limitations of small gauge vitrectomy. Surv Ophthalmol. 2011;56(2):162–72.
20. Kellner L, Wimpissinger B, Stolba U, Brannath W, Binder S. 25 gauge versus 20 gauge system for pars plana vitrectomy: a prospective randomized clinical trial. Br J Ophthalmol. 2007;91(7):945–8.
21. Rizzo S, Genovesi-Ebert F, Murri S, Belting C, Vento A, Cresti F, Manca ML. 25-gauge, sutureless vitrectomy and standard 20-gauge pars plana vitrectomy in idiopathic epiretinal membrane surgery: a comparative pilot study. Graefes Arch Clin Exp Ophthalmol. 2006;244(4):472–9.
22. Naruse S, Shimada H, Mori R. 27-gauge and 25-gauge vitrectomy day surgery for idiopathic epiretinal membrane. BMC Ophthalmol. 2017;17(1):188.
23. Steel DH, Charles S. Vitrectomy fluidics. Ophthalmologica. 2011;226(Suppl. 1):27–35.
24. Nagpal M, Paranjpe G, Jain P, Videkar R. Advances in small-gauge vitrectomy. Taiwan J Ophthalmol. 2012;2(1):6–12.
25. Oliveira PR, Berger AR, Chow DR. Vitreoretinal instruments: vitrectomy cutters, endoillumination and wide-angle viewing systems. Int J Retina Vitreous. 2016;2(1):28.
26. Pavlidis M. Two-dimensional cutting (TDC) vitrectome: in vitro flow assessment and prospective clinical study evaluating core vitrectomy efficiency versus standard vitrectome. J Ophthalmol. 2016;2016:3849316.
27. Mitsui K, Kogo J, Takeda H, Shiono A, Sasaki H, Munemasa Y, Kitaoka Y, Takagi H. Comparative study of 27-gauge vs 25-gauge vitrectomy for epiretinal membrane. Eye. 2016;30(4):538.
28. Li J, Zhao B, Liu S, Li F, Dong W, Zhong J. Retrospective comparison of 27-gauge and 25-gauge microincision vitrectomy surgery with silicone oil for the treatment of primary rhegmatogenous retinal detachment. J Ophthalmol. 2018;2018:7535043.

Endoscopic Vitrectomy 8

Rajeev R. Pappuru, Vivek Pravin Dave, and Mudit Tyagi

8.1 Introduction

Retinal surgeons often face clinical situations where there is an operable posterior segment pathology with a compromised anterior segment visualization due to corneal opacities, dense pupillary membranes, thick posterior capsular opacities, or in recent days operated keratoprosthesis. Operating in suboptimal visualization results in incomplete vitreous clearance, missed breaks, incomplete laser, or an incomplete tamponade. The surgical endoscope allows a direct view of posterior segment structures such as the optic disc, the retina, macula, and the blood vessels and helps in overcoming the problems associated with anterior segment opacification and inadequate visualization.

8.2 History

The first ophthalmic application of endoscopy was described in 1934 by Thorpe [1]. He used it for retrieving an intraocular foreign body. Norris et al. in 1978, described a lens and wave-guided viewing system surrounded by a wing of fibers for illumination lodged in a stainless steel sheath of 1.7 mm [2]. This system gave a view of 70° and a magnification of 30×. In 1981, Norris et al. described a series of 18 endoscopic vitrectomy procedures for removing retained foreign bodies and for persistent retinal detachments [3]. They reported a good anatomical outcome with the only complication being a single case of iatrogenic retinal detachment. Volkov et al. in 1990 described the technical characteristics of flexible ophthalmic endoscopes for the first time and described a series of 23 patients operated with endoscopic vitrectomy with good results [4, 5]. Around the same period, Eguchi et al. from Japan described a system of an electronic video endoscope for ophthalmic usage [6]. Uram et al. first described the use of laser ablation via an endoscope in cases of neovascular glaucoma for ciliary process photocoagulation and for retinal photocoagulation during endoscopic vitrectomies [7, 8]. All cases were reported to have good outcomes with no serious adverse effect noted.

8.3 Advantages

The main advantage of the endoscopic vitrectomy technique is that it bypasses media opacities. Hence in conditions of corneal scarring and limited visualization like ocular trauma, endophthalmitis, keratoprosthesis in situ, this technique is invaluable. The flexibility of the endo probe allows visualization of hitherto difficult to visualize areas of the eye such as the ciliary

R. R. Pappuru (✉) · V. P. Dave · M. Tyagi
Kallam Anji Reddy Camous, L V Prasad Eye Institute, Hyderabad, India
e-mail: drmudit@lvpei.org

A. Jain et al. (eds.), *Cutting-edge Vitreoretinal Surgery*,
https://doi.org/10.1007/978-981-33-4168-5_8

sulcus and the ciliary processes [9]. Relatively higher magnification also allows for better identification of small difficult to visualize retinal breaks.

8.4 Instrumentation

An endoscope acts as an optical conduit, capturing light through an objective lens at its distal end and then subsequently transfers the image through an image relay system, that is then viewed on a screen by the operating surgeon.

The authors at this point of time have experience with the E2 and E4 Endoscopy and laser system (EndoOptiks, Inc., Little Silver, Nj, USA). The EndoOptiks E2 Micro Probe™ is the principal component of the entire system. The complete hardware consists of the endo probe console, the foot switch, and the monitor (Fig. 8.1). The camera selection and light intensity are controllable from the front panel while the rear panel has connectors to any video monitor, VCR, or video printer. A 175 Watt xenon light source is used to provide illumination whose intensity can be adjusted from the front panel or the foot switch. Through a 200-μm fiberoptic cable, the treatment laser can generate pulses from 0 to 1200 mW in power and 50 to 2000 ms in width. A charge-coupled device (CCD) camera processes the image procured by the endo probe and displays it on the monitor. The 19.5 gauge endoscope of the E2 system offers 10,000 pixels and a 125° field of view. In 2011, a 23-gauge probe was developed to fit through 23-gauge trocars. This scope delivers 6000 pixels over a 90° field of view and requires the 300 Watt xenon light source for intraocular illumination.

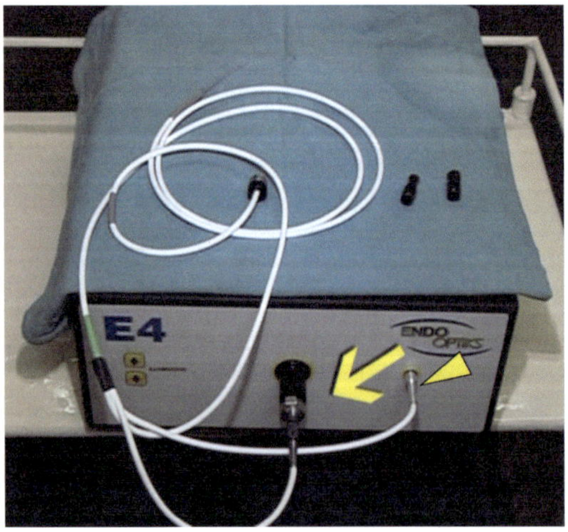

Fig. 8.1 Endoscopic hardware showing the endoscopic probe (yellow arrow) and illumination probe (yellow arrowhead)

8.5 Indications

The commonest indication where endoscopic vitrectomy is used is anterior segment opacities, which interfere with clear visualization of the posterior segment. When faced with posterior segment pathology requiring surgery in presence of gross anterior segment opacities, the conventional practice is to manage the posterior segment pathology conservatively until the anterior segment opacities are treated or they get cleared. The second option possible is to use a temporary keratoprosthesis and operate upon the posterior segment pathology. The disadvantage of waiting till the anterior segment problem is tackled is that often the posterior segment disease is irreversible and time sensitive. Delay can lead to overall reduction of visual potential. The disadvantage of using a temporary keratoprosthesis is the unavoidable requirement of corneal tissue to perform an immediate sequential keratoplasty and can leave the patient with the burden of maintaining a corneal allograft with lifelong immunosuppression. This is especially true for many underdeveloped and developing countries that do not have adequate eye bank facilities [10].

Another emerging application of endoscopic surgery is to diagnose and treat pathology related to the difficult to visualize areas of the eye like the ciliary body, ciliary sulcus, posterior iris epithelium, ora serrata, and the peripheral retina. As against artificially changed relative structural anatomy due to indentation and peripheral optical lens distortions, direct endoscopic visualization allows for understanding the actual in vivo anatomy.

8.6 Clinical Applications

8.6.1 Diagnostic Endoscopy and Prognostication Before Anterior Segment Interventions

In certain clinical situations, the anterior segment opacities that are operable but the surgery is often tedious and can involve multiple interventions, e.g., post-chemical injury limbal stem cell deficit. Penetrating keratoplasty and keratoprosthesis are proven procedures for sight restoration in such cases. These eyes could have other posterior segment disorders and a prior knowledge of these would aid in the proper selection of cases, selection of the surgical procedure, and prognostication of the intervention. In past, direct visualization had not been possible in many eyes with a pre-existing anterior segment opacification. Despite many advances, the B-scan ultrasonography has several limitations of indeterminate readings. The surgical endoscope has allowed a direct view of posterior segment structures such as the optic disc, the retina, macula, and the blood vessels thus proving its superiority over ultrasonography in cases with anterior segment opacifications. These findings have got great clinical and prognostic values.

We had evaluated the role of video-endoscopy in prognosticating the visual outcome in eyes with media opacity obstructing fundus visualization [11]. In our series of 64 eyes, with the help of the stereoscopic picture of the fundus provided by the endoscope, we reported a poor visual prognosis in 17 eyes with retinal detachment and 22 with attached retina. Based on the endoscopic findings 34 of 64 (53%) eyes underwent further complicated procedures. This included 10 (16%) patients with corneal procedure and 24 (37.5%) patients with endoscopic vitreoretinal procedures. In 30 of 64 (46.8%) eyes further complicated procedures could be avoided. Farias and associates had used the endoscope to evaluate the posterior segment and all of the ten patients in their series were considered to be good candidates for KPro surgery based on videoendoscopic examination and subsequently experienced a significant vision improvement after placement of Boston type I KPro [12].

8.6.2 Retinal Reattachment in Hazy Media

Retinal detachments with hazy media and relatively fresh occurrence with minimal proliferative vitreo retinopathy are good candidates for endoscopic vitreous surgery. The high magnification and surface illumination provided by the endoscope is an excellent tool for picking up unseen retinal breaks (Fig. 8.2). Kita et al. in their study showed successful identification of retinal breaks on endoscopy in a series of cases of rhegmatogenous retinal detachment where the preoperative fundus examination failed to pick up retinal breaks [13]. Other studies have reported similar good visual and anatomical outcomes post endoscopic repair [14, 15].

8.6.3 Ocular Trauma

Open globe injuries involving the cornea often have poor visibility once the corneal wound repair heals. These eyes are highly prone to late retinal

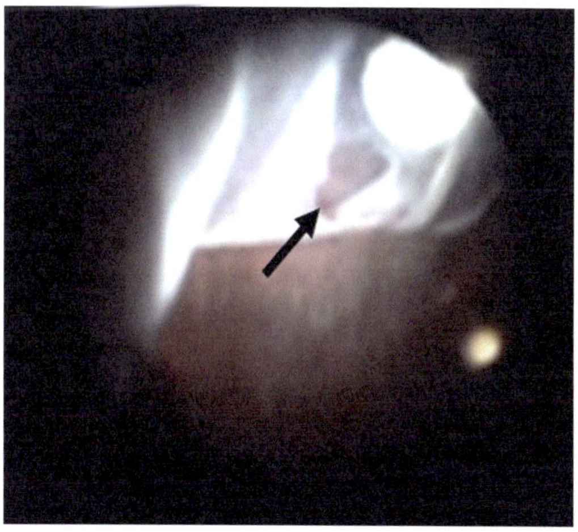

Fig. 8.2 Intraoperative picture depicting the retinal tear (black arrow) with good magnification and illumination in a case of retinal detachment

detachments or traumatic endophthalmitis. Sabti et al. in their case series described 43 eyes that underwent endoscopic vitrectomy for open globe injury-related retinal detachment [16]. They demonstrated a retinal reattachment rate of 91% and improved vision in 81% of cases. Kawashima et al. described a case report of endophthalmitis operated post-globe trauma where intraoperative retrieval of a foreign body was performed, which was not picked up on the preoperative investigations [17].

8.6.4 Retained Intraocular Foreign Bodies

Retrieval of retained intraocular foreign bodies requires adequate visibility to avoid inadvertent iatrogenic retinal tears (Fig. 8.3). Sabti et al. reported a series of cases where endoscopic vitrectomy was used to remove retained foreign bodies [16]. Ten eyes out of the 11 in their series had favorable prognosis.

8.6.5 Endophthalmitis

Endophthalmitis cases usually have poor posterior segment visualization due to corneal edema, corneal tear, or anterior segment inflammatory membrane (Fig. 8.4). Often attempts to peel the membrane to increase visualization can cause iris bleeding and hyphema. Endoscopic visualization in such cases allows for adequate vitrectomy avoiding undue trauma and risk of retinal breaks. Membranes organizing over the ciliary body can also be visualized and if needed, be removed. Favorable anatomical and visual outcomes have been reported by various authors in endoscopic vitrectomy for endophthalmitis [10, 18, 19].

We had described our outcomes of endoscopic vitrectomy in endophthalmitis [20].

In our series of 33 eyes diagnosed as endophthalmitis which were managed with endoscopic vitrectomy. Ten eyes among those with poor visual outcome had a further scope of vision improvement by a future corneal procedure.

8.7 Surgical Nuances

Like any other unconventional surgical methodology, endoscopic vitrectomy has a steep learning curve. Head posture is quite different as compared to what the surgeon is used to usually (Fig. 8.3). Often the head turn is exaggerated depending on the possible location of the camera monitor. Depth perception is nonexistent in endoscopic surgeries because of lack of stereopsis. Unlike a conventional viewing system that offers

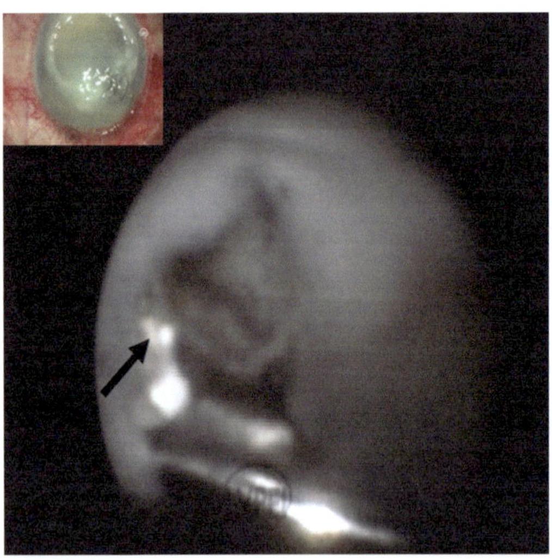

Fig. 8.3 A case of traumatic endopthalmitis (inlet) with retained intraocular foreign body seen (black arrow) in endoscopic view

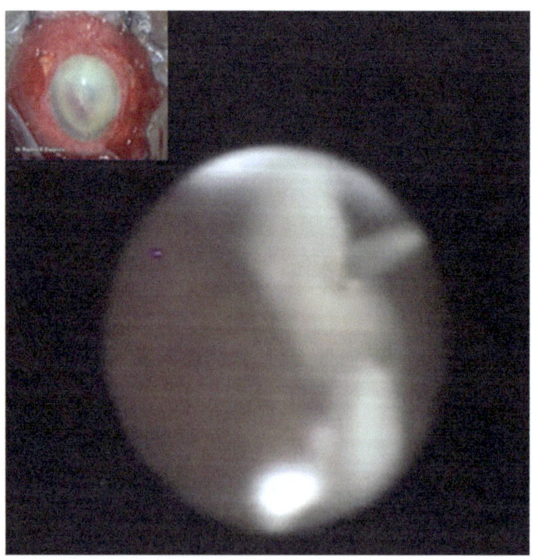

Fig. 8.4 A case of postoperative endopthalmitis (inlet) with dense corneal edema obscuring the posterior segment is visualized well with the help of endoscopy

a bird's eye view of retina, an endoscopy offers a head-on view. As the light source and the camera are in the same axis, there is no shadowing. This eliminates the judgment of the instrument distance from the retina leading to high chances of possible tissue touch and retinal breaks. The overall view is tunnel like, much different from the conventional panoramic view of the retina. Focusing the retina is not controlled on the table but has to be controlled by an assistant on the endoscope machine quite unlike the focusing of a binocular indirect ophthalmic microscope lens. Rotation of the endoscope probe inadvertently causes rotation of the field of view, which can again lead to errors of judgment. Judgmental errors are more common in the peripheral retinal maneuvering because easily identifiable landmarks like the foveal avascular zone and the optic disc are absent in the field of view.

Bimanual surgeries are not possible with an endoscope. Hence advanced diabetic vitrectomies requiring extensive membrane dissection cannot be performed by an endoscope.

Follow-up evaluation remains an unanswered element in very advanced anterior segment opacities.

8.8 Conclusion

Recently, improved vitrectomy instrumentation and cameras provide an exciting background for optimal utilization of endoscopic vitrectomies and now allows the vitreoretinal surgeons to overcome the challenges posed by anterior segment opacities. In spite of the difficulty in mastering the technique, endoscopic vitrectomy is a very fruitful technique to have in a vitreoretinal surgeon's armamentarium.

References

1. Thorpe H. Ocular endoscope: instrument for removal of intravitreous nonmagnetic foreign bodies. Trans Am Acad Ophthalmol Otolaryngol. 1934;39:422–4.
2. Norris JL, Cleasby GW. An endoscope for ophthalmology. Am J Ophthalmol. 1978;85:420–2.
3. Norris JL, Cleasby GW, Nakanishi AS, Martin LJ. Intraocular endoscopic surgery. Am J Ophthalmol. 1981;91:603–6.
4. Volkov VV, Danilov AV, Vassin LN, Frolov YA. Flexible endoscopes. Ophthalmoendoscopic techniques and case reports. Arch Ophthalmol. 1990;108:956–7.
5. Volkov VV, Danilov AV, Vassin LN, Frolov YA. Flexible endoscope for intraocular surgery. Arch Ophthalmol. 1990;108:1037–8.
6. Eguchi S, Araie M. A new ophthalmic electronic videoendoscope system for intraocular surgery. Arch Ophthalmol. 1990;108:1778–81.
7. Uram M. Ophthalmic laser microendoscope ciliary process ablation in the management of neovascular glaucoma. Ophthalmology. 1992;99:1823–8.
8. Uram M. Ophthalmic laser microendoscope endophotocoagulation. Ophthalmology. 1992;99:1829–32.
9. Arroyo J. The role of endoscopy in vitreoretinal surgery today: Retina Today; 2013. p. 54–6.
10. Shen L, Zheng B, Zhao Z, Chen Y. Endoscopic Vitrectomy for severe posttraumatic Endophthamitis with visualization constraints. Ophthalmic Surg Lasers Imaging. 2010;9:1–4.
11. Pappuru RR, Tyagi M, Paulose RM, Dave VP, Das T, Chhablani J, Narayanan R, Saxena RK, Balakrishnan D, Basu S, Sangwan VS. Role of diagnostic endoscopy in posterior segment evaluation for definitive prognostication in eyes with corneal opacification. Am J Ophthalmol. 2017;176:9–14.
12. Farias CC, Ozturk HE, Albini TA, Berrocal AM, et al. Use of intraocular video endoscopic examination in preoperative evaluation of Keratoprosthesis surgery to assess visual potential. Am J Ophthalmol. 2014;158(2):80–6.
13. Kita M, Yoshimura N. Endoscope-assisted vitrectomy in the management of pseudophakic and aphakic retinal detachments with undetected retinal breaks. Retina. 2011;31:1347–51.
14. de Smet MD, Mura M. Minimally invasive surgery endoscopic retinal detachment repair in patients with media opacities. Eye. 2008;22:662–5.
15. Sonoda Y, Yamakiri K, Sonoda S, Uchino E, Doi N, Sakamoto T. Endoscopy-guided subretinal fluid drainage in vitrectomy for retinal detachment. Ophthalmologica. 2006;220:83–6.
16. Sabti KA, Raizada S. Endoscope-assisted pars plana vitrectomy in severe ocular trauma. Br J Ophthalmol. 2012;96:1399–403.
17. Kawashima M, Kawashima S, Dogru M, Inoue M, Shimazaki J. Endoscopy-guided vitreoretinal surgery following penetrating corneal injury: a case report. Clin Ophthalmol. 2010;4:895–8.
18. Comer GM, Stem MS, Saxe SJ. Successful salvage therapy of Fusarium endophthalmitis secondary to keratitis: an interventional case series. Clin Ophthalmol. 2012;6:721–6.
19. De Smet MD, Carlborg EA. Managing severe endophthalmitis with the use of an endoscope. Retina. 2005;25:976–80.
20. Dave VP, Pappuru RR, Tyagi M, Pathengay A, Das T. Endoscopic vitrectomy in endophthalmitis: initial experience of 33 cases at a tertiary eye care center. Clin Ophthalmol. 2019;13:243.

3D Viewing System in Vitreoretinal Surgery

9

Tillmann P. Eckert

9.1 Introduction

For more than 60 years the operating microscope has been an indispensable tool in ophthalmic microsurgery, starting with corneal and cataract surgery in the 1950s and 1960s [1, 2]. In the 1970s, the pioneers of modern vitrectomy had to deal with the limits of the coaxial illumination of the microscopes of that time. With slit lamp illumination and endoillumination probes, they were able to achieve adequate visualization of the delicate intraocular structures [3]. Despite ongoing advances in ophthalmic surgical microscopes, viewing systems, modern light sources, and the development of minimally invasive instrumentation for vitreoretinal surgery nothing fundamental changed in vitreoretinal operating theaters until this decade: The surgeon still looks through the binoculars of the surgical microscope onto the anterior segment and anterior vitreous, or, adding a wide-angle viewing system or a contact lens, into the vitreous cavity.

Electronic Supplementary Material The online version of this chapter (https://doi.org/10.1007/978-981-33-4168-5_9) contains supplementary material, which is available to authorized users.

T. P. Eckert (✉)
Department of Ophthalmology, Klinikum Frankfurt Hoechst, Frankfurt, Germany
e-mail: tillmann.eckert@klinikumfrankfurt.de

A. Jain et al. (eds.), *Cutting-edge Vitreoretinal Surgery*,
https://doi.org/10.1007/978-981-33-4168-5_9

Twenty-five years ago, Japanese groups reported on three-dimensional monitoring systems to perform microsurgery [4, 5]. Attempts to change the conventional microscopic viewing in ophthalmic surgery started 20 years ago. In 1999, Miyake et al. [6] combined a "high-gain avalanche rushing-amorphous photoconductor" (HARP) camera (with a 600 times greater sensitivity than conventional television cameras of that time) and a single camera—3D high-definition television system displaying high-quality 3D images on a stereoscopic display. Observing the display without the need for special glasses they were able to perform cataract surgeries and pars plana vitrectomies in pig cadaver eyes. The illumination intensities could be diminished greatly compared to the intensities required with a conventional microscope. Interestingly, they concluded that such a viewing system does not only reduce the illumination to safer levels regarding possible phototoxic effects on the retina but would also have advantages for the surgical team by delivering identical images to each member. Furthermore, they presumed that this would allow telesurgery and could be effectively used for education [6].

However, the commercially available video technology in the early 2000s was not ready for the development of live 3D digital imaging in vitreoretinal surgery. One typical format available with video cameras attached to surgical microscopes was standard definition (SD) with 720 ×

576 pixels (576i) in PAL. Having operated on an interesting vitreoretinal case and having enjoyed the brilliant resolution of modern microscopes and viewing systems, vitreoretinal surgeons had to face the fact that the quality of the recorded surgical videos did not match with the image quality of the microscopic view. Even after the introduction of high-definition (HD) cameras and HD-ready displays with 1280 × 720 pixels (720p), there was still a significant loss of resolution comparing the surgical view with the recorded videos, let alone the lack of the third dimension. Therefore, the idea to perform intraocular surgery by looking on a three-dimensional TV screen would have seemed unrealistic to most vitreoretinal surgeons. Nevertheless, Bhadri et al. [7] evaluated a stereoscopic camera-based three-dimensional viewing system (Digital Microsurgical Workstation, three-dimensional (3D) Vision Systems, Irvine, USA) for ophthalmic surgery in 2007. The prototype included a stereoscopic camera, a polarized display screen, polarized glasses for the surgeon, and a computer, which captured a three-dimensional real-time video of the surgical field, processed the images, and displayed it on the stereoscopic display screen. Five anterior and five posterior segment surgeons were able to perform standardized microsurgical tasks using the system on porcine eyes. Ergonomics of the system were rated positively. However, the "posterior segment surgeons rated visualization and illumination less favorably, resolution and stereopsis as very limited, and magnification and field of view as equivalent to an operating microscope" [7].

9.2 Heads-Up Surgery with the TrueVision® 3D Viewing System

At that time, TrueVision® 3D Surgical (Santa Barbara, USA) had developed a commercially available platform for 3D imaging with a 3D high dynamic range (HDR) surgical camera. In 2008 the company announced, that "over 2500 ophthalmic, neurological, spine, and otolaryngology (ENT) procedures have been performed using the TrueVision® 3D HD imaging system." The potential of the TrueVision® system for teaching microsurgery was recognized early in otorhinolaryngology [8]. In ophthalmology, cataract surgeons were the first to use the TrueVision® 3D viewing system. The term "heads-up" cataract surgery was introduced [9, 10].

"Heads-up" could be misunderstood. Heads-up displays (HUD) originally developed for military aircraft have become increasingly available not only for pilots but also for modern motorcars. HUD in cars project data such as speed, speed limits, or navigational aids onto the windshield so that the driver can have access to these data while still seeing the traffic in front of him. The term "heads-up" cataract surgery refers to the posture of the surgeon's head while looking on a display in contrast to the conventional "heads-down" posture while looking through the binoculars of a microscope [9, 10].

Arthroscopies in the 1980s were already performed in a "heads-up" manner looking on rather small monitors. In the following years, minimal invasive surgery became popular in many other surgical fields, where endoscopic procedures within body cavities like thorax, abdomen, and pelvis are performed. Since then, surgeons look with their "heads up" on a display to visualize the surgical field and observe and guide their actions. Nowadays, 3D visualization replaces the conventional 2D approach in endoscopic surgery [11, 12]. Microvascular anastomosis can be performed with a 3D system [13–15]. In neurosurgery, where three-dimensional precision is of utmost importance, heads-up surgery with 3D visualization on a large display is possible [16–18]

9.3 Heads-Up Vitreoretinal Surgery

In 2011, Christopher Riemann [19] was the first to report on his experience with the TrueVision® system on a Leica F40 microscope (Leica Microsystems, Heerbrugg, Switzerland) in eight vitrectomies. He used a flat 52-in. LCD panel at a final resolution of 1280 × 972 pixels and found that "visualization was adequate ... but inferior to the microscope oculars" ... and ... "less neck and back strain were noted compared to looking through the microscope oculars in all cases" [19].

As soon as the TrueVision® 3D visualization system became available for Leica ophthalmic microscopes M822 and M844 in the beginning of 2014, Claus Eckardt (Department of Ophthalmology, Klinikum Frankfurt Hoechst, Frankfurt am Main, Germany) started to use the TrueVision® 3D System not only for cataract surgeries but routinely also for vitrectomies. The TrueVision® 3D camera (ICM5) was attached to a Leica M822 microscope via a beam splitter. Thus, the camera received only 50% of the optical beam. This led to a significantly darker image during intravitreal procedures. Therefore, the eyepieces were removed from the microscope and completely replaced by the 3D camera in order to direct 100% of the surgical image to the camera. The increased input of light improved the quality of the 3D digital image significantly [20]. After a short learning period, the 3D visualization system was used for all anterior and posterior segment surgeries. During the live surgery session of the Frankfurt Retina Meeting in March 2014, Eckardt performed a heads-up. This meeting was the starting point for the increasing interest in 3D viewing systems in vitreoretinal surgery.

Eckardt and Paulo [20] evaluated the concept of heads-up vitreoretinal surgery in an experimental and clinical study. Twenty volunteers without experience with surgical microscopy had to perform tasks under the conventional microscope and with the 3D viewing system. The majority preferred the ergonomics of the heads-up display compared to the binoculars.

In the same study, the optical resolution of the microscope was found to be about twice as high than the resolution with the heads-up method. Digital image processing was analyzed. It could be shown that a darker image after reduction of the illumination level could be compensated to a certain amount by increasing the electronic amplification of the signal (increasing the gain) until digital noise became too high. The clinical experience showed that the disadvantage of the lower resolution of the heads-up technique could be offset with a greater magnification. There were no complications that could be related to the heads-up technique. Comparable closure rates after macular hole surgery were obtained with the new technique [20].

In 2016 Alcon (Fort Worth, TX, USA) as a division of Novartis (Basel, Switzerland) launched the NGENUITY® 3D Visualization System in collaboration with TrueVision® 3D Surgical for vitreoretinal surgery and coined the term "Digitally Assisted Vitreoretinal Surgery" (DAVS) [21]. Currently, the NGENUITY® 3D Visualization System is the only commercially available 3D viewing system for vitreoretinal surgery.

Since its introduction in 2014, 3D viewing has become a routine procedure in our hospital. More than 10,000 heads-up cataract surgeries and approximately 5000 heads-up vitrectomies have been performed in Frankfurt since 2014. In addition, other procedures such as glaucoma or corneal surgery are also performed using the 3D system.

In the following parts of this chapter, our approach and the advantages and disadvantages of the current viewing system are discussed before addressing the possible future of 3D viewing in vitreoretinal surgery.

9.4 3D Visualization System Settings in Our Department

The 46-in. high-definition LCD display (JVC GD463D10UQ; JVC; Yokohama, Japan) used in the first months was substituted by a 55-in. ultra-high-definition (UHD or 4K) display (LG 55UB856V; LG; Seoul, South Korea) which improved the resolution. Furthermore, the small but perceptible latency (time lag between surgical action and visualization of this action on the display) seen with the high-definition display decreased and was not disturbing anymore. Since 2015, the author performs all intraocular operations including cataract, glaucoma, corneal and vitreoretinal surgery with a second TrueVision® 3D System. After the acquisition of an

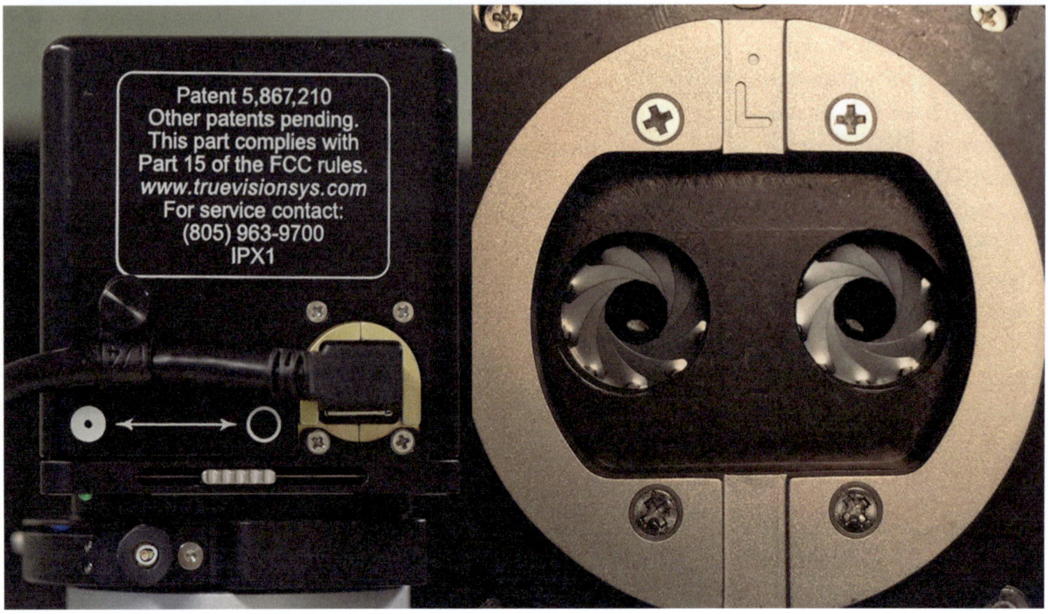

Fig. 9.1 TrueVision® 3D Digital System: mechanically adjustable iris aperture in front of stereoscopic camera ICAM5

NGENUITY® 3D Visualization System at the beginning of 2018, all three surgical theaters in our department are equipped with a digital viewing system.

The main difference between the NGENUITY® 3D Visualization System and its predecessor TrueVision® 3D System is an OLED display (55 in., LG OLED55E6P; LG) and a new software, the 3D camera (TrueVision® ICAM5) is still the same. Both systems can be combined with operating microscopes from Alcon, Zeiss, and Leica.

The ICAM5 has an adjustable iris aperture in front of both objectives which can be altered mechanically (Fig. 9.1). We prefer to open the aperture to about 60%. Working with smaller apertures enhances the depth of field. However, the effect is not pronounced. And the smaller the aperture, the lower is the brightness of the image with a need to increase the illumination level. Additionally, with a small aperture vignetting on the corners of the display can be disturbing, especially in anterior segment surgery.

The 3D camera is attached to the microscope instead of binoculars. Between camera and microscope, a Stereo Diagonal Inverter SDI® 4c (Oculus; Wetzlar, Germany), and a manual safety filter for Leica Microscopes (8005.F2, D.O.R.C.; Zealand, Netherlands) are interposed. An adapter for the Binocular Indirect Ophthalmomicroscope BIOM® 5c (Oculus) is attached underneath the objective of the surgical microscope Leica M822 (Fig. 9.2). We use an objective lens with a working distance of 200 mm. The software of the NGENUITY® 3D Visualization System allows to toggle the orientation of the main view between standard and inverted 180 degrees. Using SDI® 4c this is not necessary. Together with the BIOM® 5c the SDI® 4c allows electronic foot pedal focusing with automatic image inversion.

Macular surgery is always performed with a direct contact lens under high magnification.

The camera is connected via a USB3 cable to the TrueVision® or the NGENUITY® working station with their embedded processing unit (EPU; Fig. 9.3). The working station with the 55-in. 3D display stands on the right side of the operating table approximately 1.5 m from the surgeon and near the inferior half of the operating table. The surgeon, as well as members of the surgical team and observers, wear film-type patterned retarder (FPR) glasses, which are based on circular polarization, and which are also available as clip-ons (Fig. 9.4).

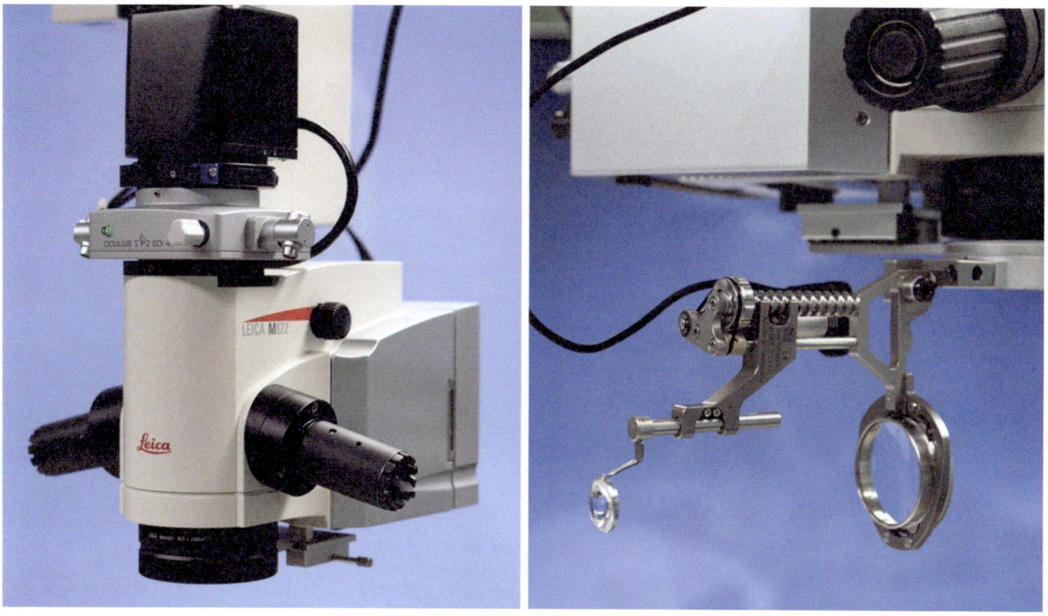

Fig. 9.2 Microscope without oculars (from top to bottom) with ICAM5 (TrueVision), manual safety filter 8005.F2 (D.O.R.C.), Stereo Diagonal Inverter SDI® 4c (Oculus), surgical microscope Leica M822 (left). Adapter and BIOM® 5c (Oculus) under objective (working distance 200 mm) of Leica M822 (right)

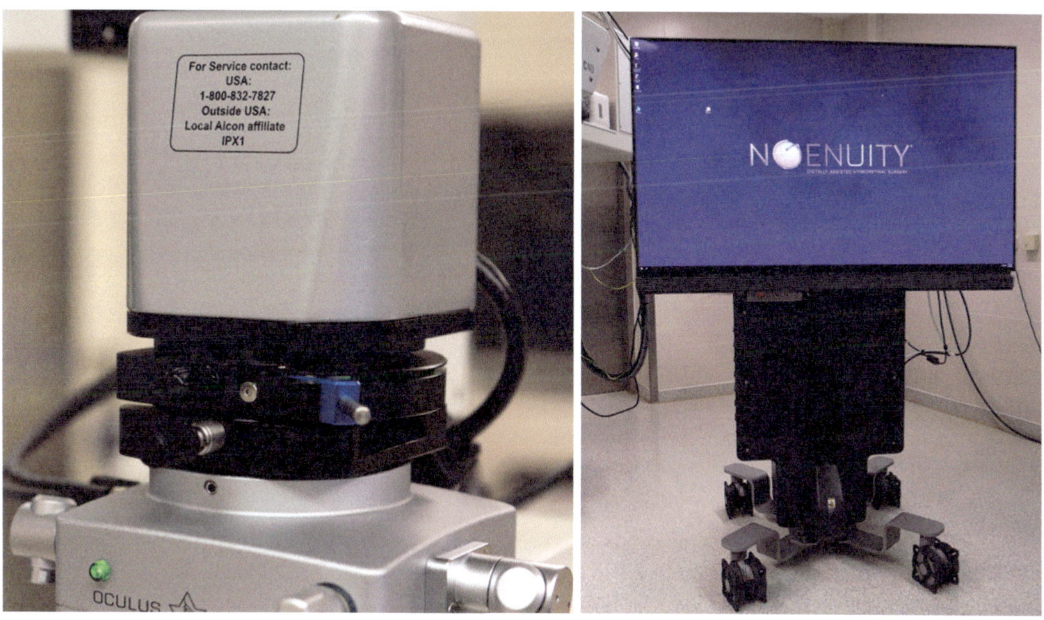

Fig. 9.3 NGENUITY® 3D Visualization System: ICAM5 on Leica M822 (left), OLED 55-inch Panel and working station (right)

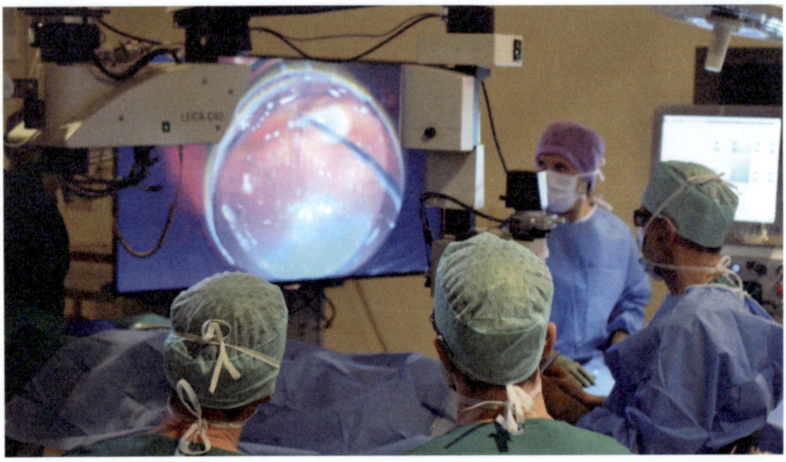

Fig. 9.4 Heads-up surgeon and observers wear film-type patterned retarder (FPR) glasses

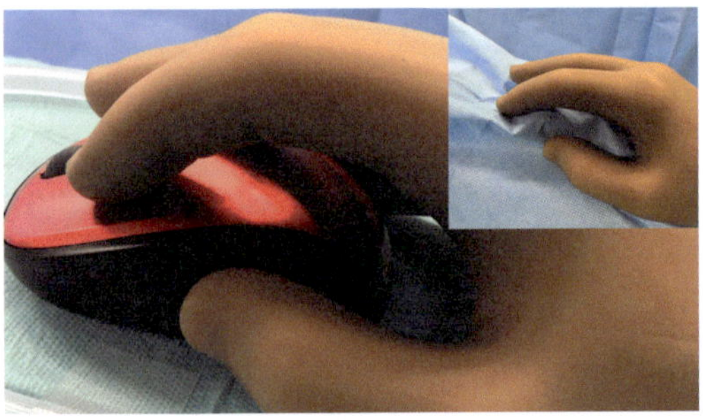

Fig. 9.5 Wireless computer mouse on the armrest of the operating chair used under a sterile surgical draping

Changes in the setting can be made with a wireless keyboard by a nonsterile assistant. The surgeon can use a wireless computer mouse under a sterile surgical draping around the armrest of the operating chair (Fig. 9.5).

Illumination for the anterior segment is provided by the dual illumination system of the Leica M822 combining LED and halogen. The phacovitrectomy system EVA (D.O.R.C.) with its LED Endoillumination Module provides the light for the combined 23-gauge Eckardt Multi-Fiber Endoillumination Probe/Chandelier and the 27-gauge Eckardt TwinLight Chandelier (D.O.R.C.). We routinely perform vitrectomies without the help of an assistant.

9.5 Difference of 3D Viewing with Conventional Analog Microscope Viewing

Starting to perform surgery with a 3D digital viewing system the surgeon will encounter several differences to the conventional analog microscopic viewing:

9.5.1 Surgical Field

Looking through binoculars of an analog microscope, the surgical field is circular. But displays and digital image sensors are rectangular. Therefore, the shape of the surgical field in the anterior segment is also rectangular. In oculoplastic or anterior segment surgery this can be annoying especially while suturing because parts of the suture material, which would be visible through the binoculars, are not visible on the display. This can be compensated by changing the tilting position with the footswitch or by zooming out before grasping the suture and tying a knot.

During vitrectomy, this is not of concern since the circular picture provided by the wide-field viewing system or the contact lens usually fits into the rectangular picture. If the picture is not centered and parts are not displayed on the screen while the eye is tilted to perform procedures in the periphery, the digital picture can be moved partly from the rim toward the center of the display using the computer keyboard.

9.5.2 Colors

In digital photography, a color (white) balance is mandatory to achieve realistic colors. Since the light source of the microscope and the light source of the endoillumination probe and chandelier lights used for vitrectomy have different color temperatures two different settings are required, one for the anterior and one for the posterior segment (Fig. 9.6). The surgeon should adapt his system to the light sources he is using. During surgery, the individual presets for anterior or posterior can be selected using the computer keyboard or a computer mouse. It is advisable to save one's settings on a USB stick in case of an inadvertent reset of the software to standard parameters.

With the OLED display of the NGENUITY® 3D Visualization System colors seem to be more intense compared to the colors on an LED display. The NGENUITY® System offers three different digital "color filters" (blue, red free, yellow). Compared to the standard setting, these adjustments for the color channels may enhance visualization of delicate structures like vitreous and epiretinal membranes. Coppola et al. [22] reported on their initial experience in retinal detachment surgery and stated that digital filters improve the visualization of vitreous remnants. In our experience, the currently available digital filters are not of great benefit (Fig. 9.7).

In the future, colors are likely to be reproduced more natural, especially if the standard red green blue (sRGB) color space will be replaced by the Rec.2020 color space which will require 4K or 8K sensors and displays. If improved color rendering will be of benefit for the surgeon has to be seen.

9.5.3 Resolution

The resolution of the digital image of both TrueVision® 3D System and NGENUITY® 3D Visualization System is still inferior to the resolution of a modern operating microscope with oculars. Eckardt and Paulo [20] (with a Leica 822 and a 46-in. HD LCD display) and Freeman et al.

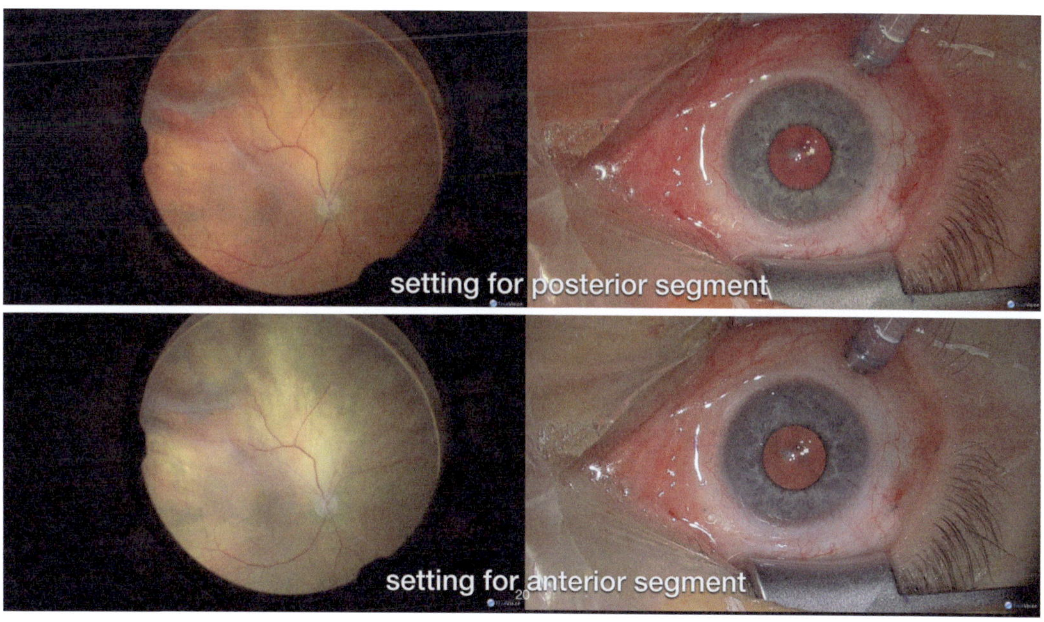

Fig. 9.6 Different color settings for anterior and posterior segment

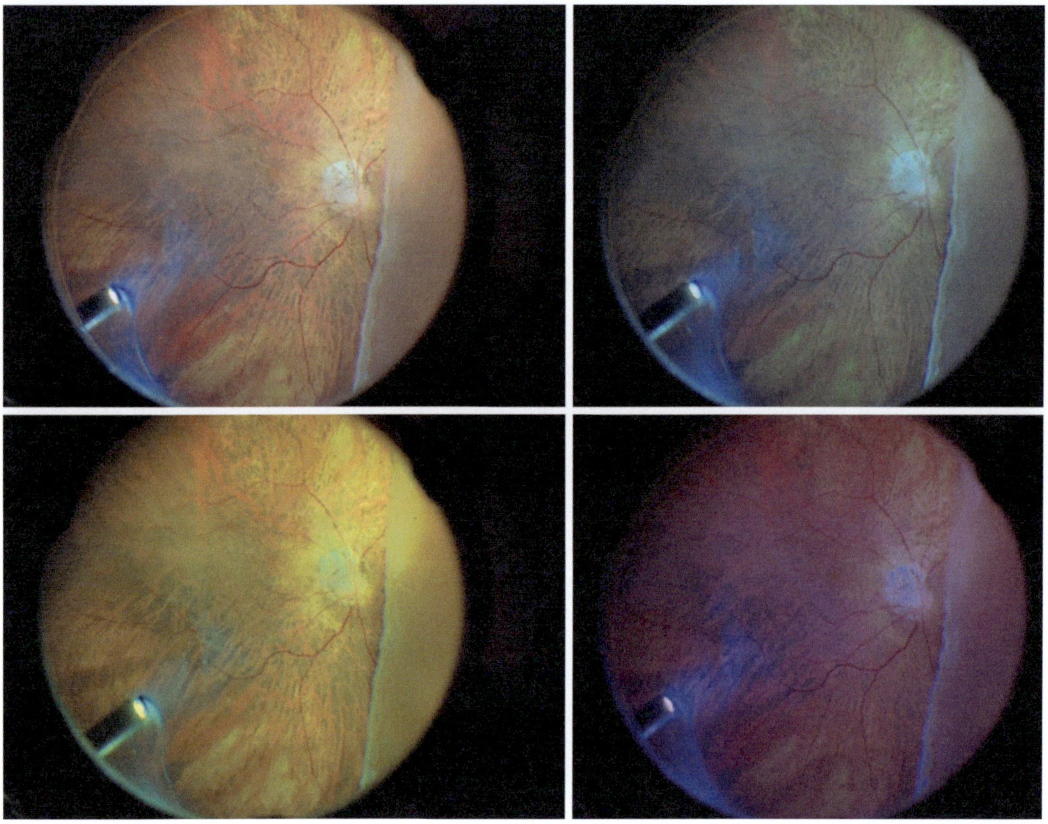

Fig. 9.7 Normal color setting and NGENUITY®'s three digital "color filters" blue, red free, yellow. Visualization of vitreous is not significantly enhanced

[23] (with a Leica 844 and a 50-in. 4K OLED display) used a 1951 Air Force resolution target and found that the resolution of the TrueVision® 3D system was about half of the resolution of the microscope with standard oculars. Since there are no practicable test charts which could be positioned at the level of the retina, a similar comparison of the optical resolution in the posterior segment (combining the optical systems of the microscope, a wide-angle viewing system, or a contact lens and the eye) is not possible, but one can assume that the optical resolution of the digital 3D system is also inferior to the conventional microscope.

However, in clinical practice, the lower resolution of the 3D systems does not play a critical role. In their survey of six retinal surgeons comparing the resolution of the digital 3D system with oculars, Freeman et al. found no significant difference in the surgeons' subjective impressions [23].

The 46-in. high-definition LCD display used in 2014 could only display half of the pixels of the 2K image. With the implementation of a 4K 3D display, which upscales the 2K image obtained by both Full HD sensors of the ICAM5, the difference between analog and digital image has become smaller.

9.5.4 Magnification

When high resolution is needed, the magnification of the microscope should be increased, until the field of interest fills the display completely. The 3D visualization on a large display provides a comfortable view on delicate structures even at high magnifications and facilitates

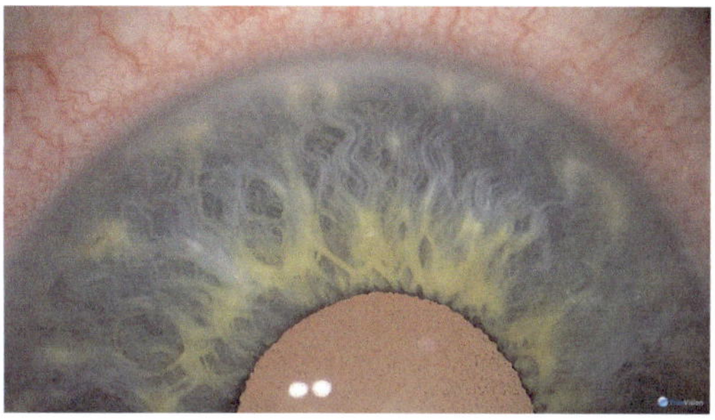

Fig. 9.8 Structure of iris stroma

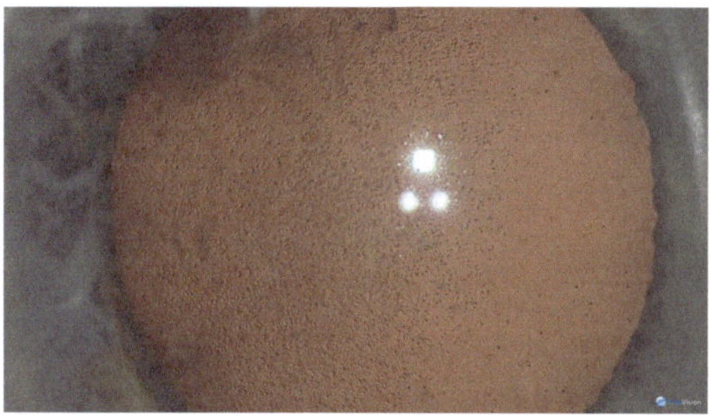

Fig. 9.9 Guttae in Fuchs' endothelial dystrophy

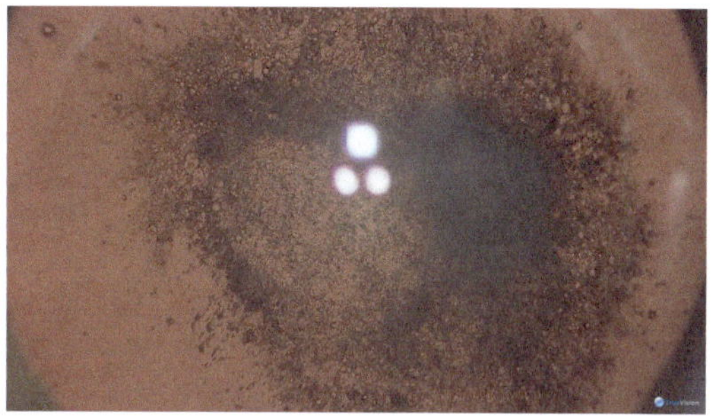

Fig. 9.10 Posterior subcapsular cataract under high magnification

peeling or dissecting membranes and proliferative tissue (Figs. 9.8, 9.9, 9.10, 9.11, 9.12, 9.13, 9.14, and 9.15).

During phacoemulsification under high magnification (routinely sixfold to eightfold), the space within the lens and capsular bag can be visualized truly three-dimensional and has a remarkable depth. During a posterior capsulorhexis (e.g., in combined phacovitrectomy with a bag in the lens-IOL), the author increases the magnification of the microscope to about eightfold until the limbus reaches the horizontal edges of the display. In that way, it is possible to depict the 12-mm diameter of the anterior chamber on the 70-cm high 55-in. 4K display. Each millimeter is displayed on nearly 6 cm of the screen. The large picture enables the surgeon to see small structures in front and behind the posterior capsule.

If the posterior pole between the arcades is shown completely on the 55-in. display while using a macular contact lens like the Lens Macular Window (Advanced Visual Instruments, Inc., New York, NY, USA) with a magnification of the microscope of up to 14-fold, approximately 6 mm of the central posterior pole are depicted on the 70-cm high 55-in. 4K display. Thus, each millimeter of the macula and the perimacular retina is visible on about 11 cm of the screen.

9.5.5 Depth of Field

In our practice, the depth of field during vitrectomy with a wide-angle viewing system like the BIOM® 5 is at least comparable to the analog microscope. We routinely use a reusable 90 D Lens (90°, Oculus) and focus on the central retinal vessels. With both 3D visualization systems, a relatively sharp image can be obtained up to the equator without refocusing. Only if vitreous base shaving or other maneuvers in the periphery are performed, the focus must be changed. This can be done easily with the electronic foot pedal of the BIOM® 5.

In anterior segment surgery, the focus is changed depending on the plane of interest. Freeman et al. [23] measured the depth of field using a millimeter scale mounted on a 45° wedge at low and high magnifications with an aperture of 50%. The depth of field seemed to be higher with the digital 3D system, but this was only significant for the lowest magnification.

Decreasing the aperture increases the depth of field but leads to a darker image. Therefore, we prefer an aperture of about 60%.

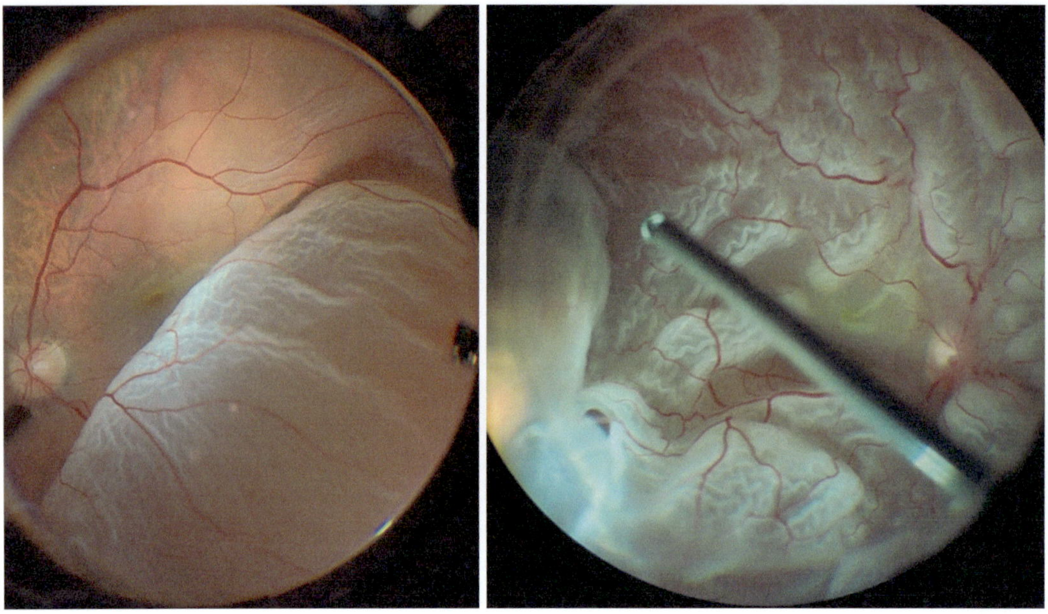

Fig. 9.11 Retinal detachments: wide-angle viewing

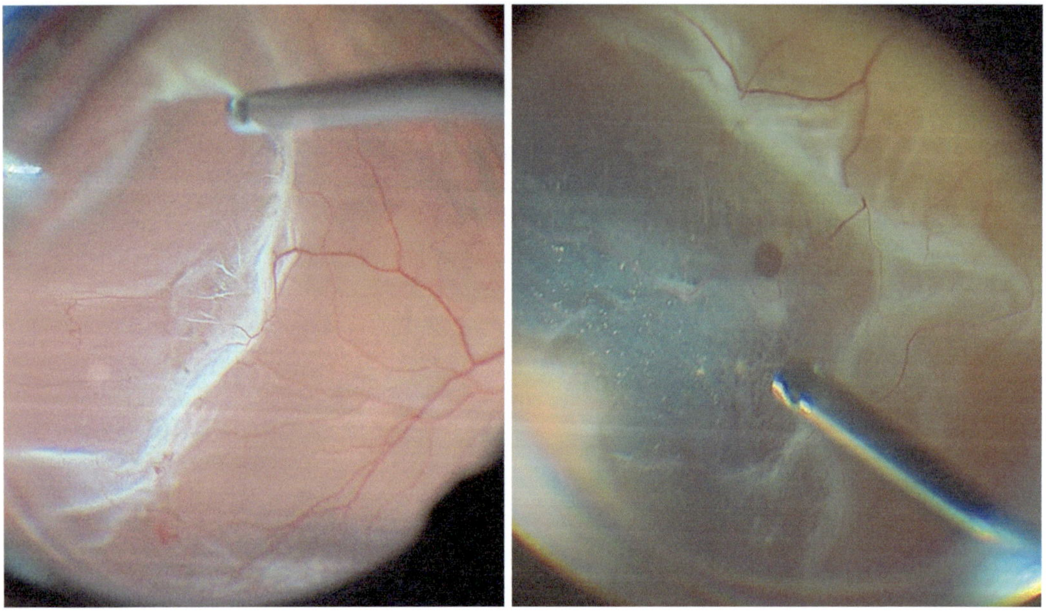

Fig. 9.12 Peripheral retina in retinal detachment: lattice degeneration (left) and round hole within microcystic degeneration (right)

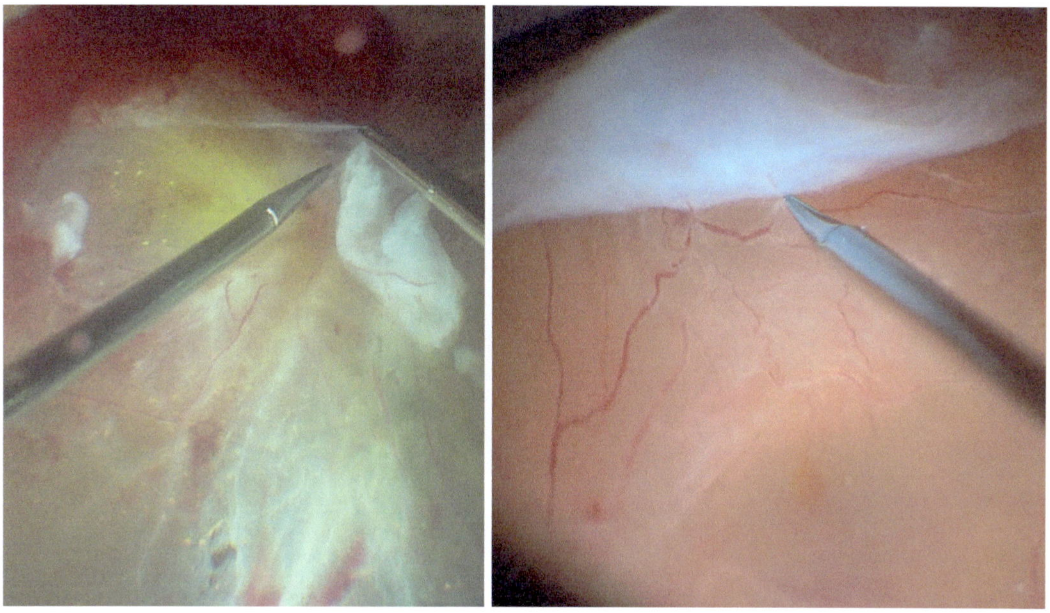

Fig. 9.13 Bimanual dissection of neovascular membranes in PDR

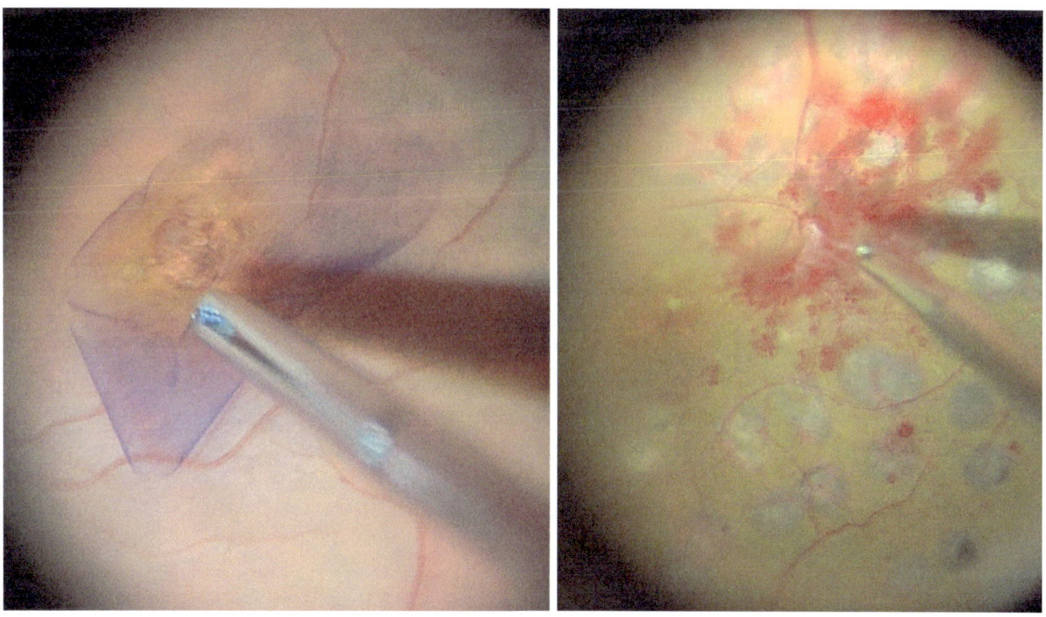

Fig. 9.14 High magnification with lens macular window (advanced visual instruments): preparing a circular ILM flap in a large macular hole (left) and paramacular neovascularization in PDR (right)

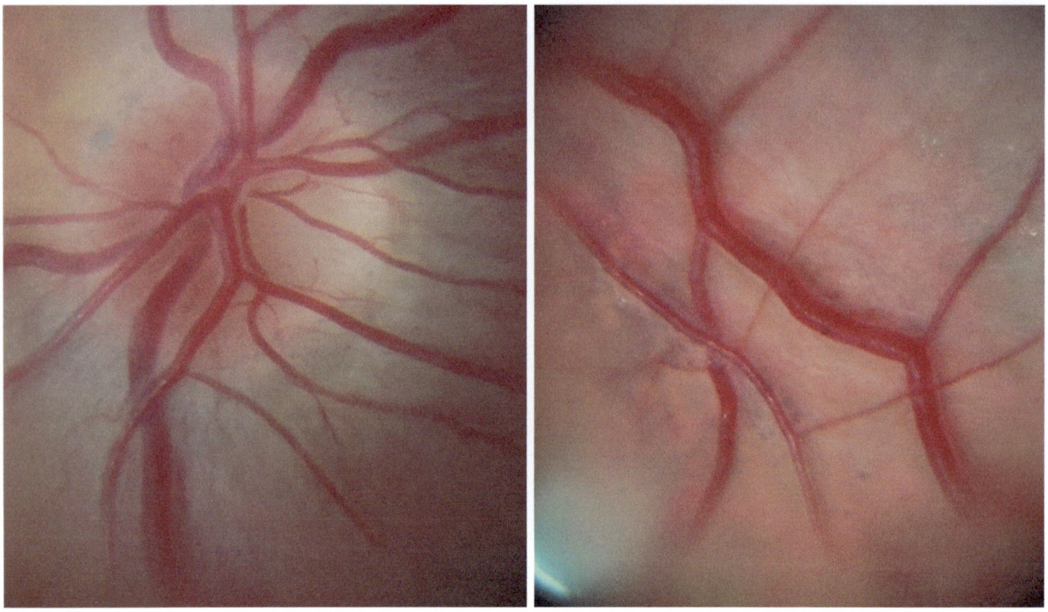

Fig. 9.15 High magnification with lens macular window: optic nerve and central retinal vessels

9.5.6 Illumination

In vitreoretinal surgery, phototoxicity is still an issue [24]. With 3D digital viewing systems (endo)illumination levels can be diminished by increasing the sensitivity (gain) of the image sensors, until picture noise becomes disturbing [20]. The gain can be changed easily within the software of the systems. Illumination level depends also on the iris aperture of the camera. With an aperture of about 60%, the average illumination level of chandelier lights or handheld illumination probes can be set to about 30–50% of the maximum illumination level or less with the EVA (D.O.R.C.) in gain 1 or 2. Increasing the camera gain to 3 or 4, it is possible to reduce the illumination levels to significantly lower levels. This is especially useful in situations with reduced visualization due to dark-pigmented posterior segments, in eyes with dense vitreous hemorrhages, or during 27-gauge vitrectomy.

Todorich et al. [25] described their technique of unassisted vitrectomy and vitreous base shaving using a light pipe for scleral indentation and transillumination. They enhanced the intraocular illumination using the NGENUITY® 3D visualization system with its light amplification settings increased to near-maximal gain.

Adam et al. [26] evaluated the endoillumination levels in ten surgeries using the TrueVision® 3D HUD platform and a Lumera® 700 (Carl Zeiss Meditec AG; Jena, Germany). They found that operations could be performed with only 10% of the maximum output and concluded that this could reduce the risk of retinal phototoxicity during vitreoretinal surgery.

Talcott et al. [27] compared the same 3D HUD surgical platform with the standard operating microscope in a prospective randomized study in 39 patients with macular holes or epiretinal membranes. Minimum endoillumination was significantly lower ($p < 0.001$) with 3D HUD compared with the standard microscope.

Kunikata et al. [28] reported on a heads-up 3D system using the MKC-700HD HD Medical Image and Video Recorder (Ikegami, Tokyo, Japan), a Lumera T (Zeiss) microscope, the Constellation platform, and 27-gauge instrumentation (Alcon). They were able to perform macular surgery in six eyes with the 27-gauge light probe set at only 1% and concluded that phototoxicity for macular retinal cells can be reduced to a minimal degree with excellent intraoperative visualization.

9.6 Learning Curve

Getting comfortable with the current 3D viewing systems usually takes only a few surgeries. Nevertheless, the surgeon must adapt to the different eye–hand coordination with digital systems. Using binoculars, eyes and hands are aimed at one object. In contrast to this nearly "natural" viewing, the head and eyes in 3D digital viewing must be aligned with the display, while the hands are turned in a different direction toward the surgical field. The speed of repetitive surgical actions (e.g., suturing) can be reduced while using a 3D viewing system. However, in vitreoretinal surgery, quick repetitive actions are usually not required, while precise and rather slow actions like vitreous cutting and shaving can be easily performed. Membrane dissection or peeling seems to be easier with the high magnification provided by digital viewing systems.

Romano et al. [29] compared 25 vitrectomies with a three-dimensional heads-up microscope with 25 vitrectomies using a traditional microscope. For the surgeon and observers, the degree of satisfaction was significantly higher with the 3D viewing system.

Interestingly, Talcott et al. [27] found in their prospective randomized study of 39 patients undergoing macular surgery that overall operating time did not differ. Macular peel time was significantly longer (mean about 3 min longer) with the NGENUITY® 3D system compared to a standard operating microscope (Lumera 700 with RESIGHT®, Zeiss), although all three surgeons were experienced with the 3D system. However, they still used a 46-in. HD display instead of a 55-in. 4K display. Despite ILM peeling in all cases, the indirect lens of the RESIGHT® fundus viewing system (Zeiss) was used in about 25% instead of a contact lens.

Babu et al. [30] compared ILM peeling in a prospective randomized trial including 40 patients either operated with an analog operating microscope (Lumera T, Zeiss) using the RESIGHT® 500 (Zeiss) or the NGENUITY® 3D system on the same microscope. They found a small but significant difference in the number of surgical attempts to initiate an ILM flap and a nonsignificant trend to a more difficult ILM peeling under 3D visualization. The slightly increased difficulty to grab a completely attached ILM using the NGENUITY® could be explained by the relatively low magnification used in this study and the lower resolution of the 3D viewing system. It would be interesting to see if the same difference would have been found always using a direct macular contact lens for the ILM peeling.

Kumar et al. [31] performed a prospective randomized single surgeon pilot study comparing the outcomes of 50 patients after vitrectomy with ILM flap technique for full-thickness macular holes. Twenty-five eyes in each group were operated either with a conventional operating microscope (Zeiss) or with the NGENUITY® 3D system. Total surgical time, ILM peel time, and outcomes were similar in both groups.

9.7 Ergonomics

Depending on the focal length of the objective lens, the operating microscope is positioned above the surgical field at a given working distance. The ophthalmic surgeon aligns his hands to the surgical field and looks through the oculars. Often it is necessary to bend the head and neck slightly forward to reach the oculars. In fact, musculoskeletal disorders in ophthalmologists are a known and common problem [32].

Vitrectomies can last for hours, especially in complex surgical situations such as tractional retinal detachments in proliferative vitreoretinopathy (PDR) or proliferative diabetic retinopathy (PVR). During such demanding operations, the surgeon's eyes stick to the eyepieces of the microscope for a long time. This inevitably leads to mechanical stress on the neck and back.

Yu et al. [33] performed a biomechanical analysis and stated that "loads on the neck joint are twice as high in the microscope than the heads-up

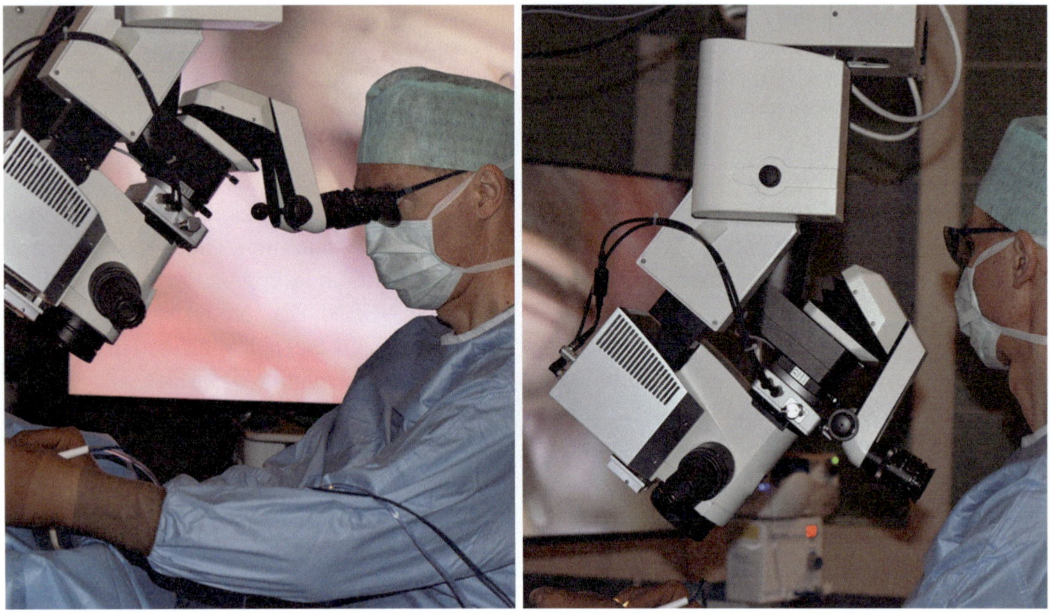

Fig. 9.16 Angle surgery using gonioscope and tilted microscope. Strenuous posture with oculars (left), relaxed position heads-up (right)

displays." Yu et al. [34] compared neck angles and shoulder flexion during microsurgical tasks with microscopes or video displays and concluded that postures improved using video displays.

One main advantage of 3D viewing compared to conventional microscopes is the fact that the surgeon is not forced to bring his upper body into line with the binoculars. Whereas the posture of the ophthalmic surgeon's hands is determined by the position of the eye he is operating on, the posture of the upper body and head are not. The eyes are gazing at the different points of interest on the relatively large display while the upper body and head which are turned to the display can constantly move. It is even possible to lean back on the operating seat. Such dynamic changes are less stressful than the relatively rigid posture looking through oculars of a conventional microscope.

In microinvasive glaucoma angle surgery requiring gonioscopy, it is necessary to tilt the microscope to up to 30 degrees. Using oculars, the posture of the surgeon's neck is quite strenuous. With heads-up surgery, the surgeon can obtain a much more comfortable position (Fig. 9.16).

A kyphosis can cause severe problems for intraocular surgery since the head and eye cannot be postured horizontally. The microscope must be tilted toward the surgeon until the eye can be visualized properly. With a traditional microscope, the surgeon would be forced to lean forward to reach the oculars. 3D Visualization enables the surgeon to remain in a comfortable position [35] (Fig. 9.17).

But there is a drawback of 3D visualization: Whereas the surgeon looks perpendicular to the display, an assistant sitting perpendicular to the surgeon has a different view of the screen. Especially if an assistant sits on the same side as the panel he has to turn his head significantly to the screen and away from the surgical field. Rizzo et al. [36] examined the satisfaction of their surgical team with the 3D viewing system. In fact, they found that the assistant surgeons were somewhat dissatisfied due to their uncomfortable position. A similar observation was made by Zhang et al. [37].

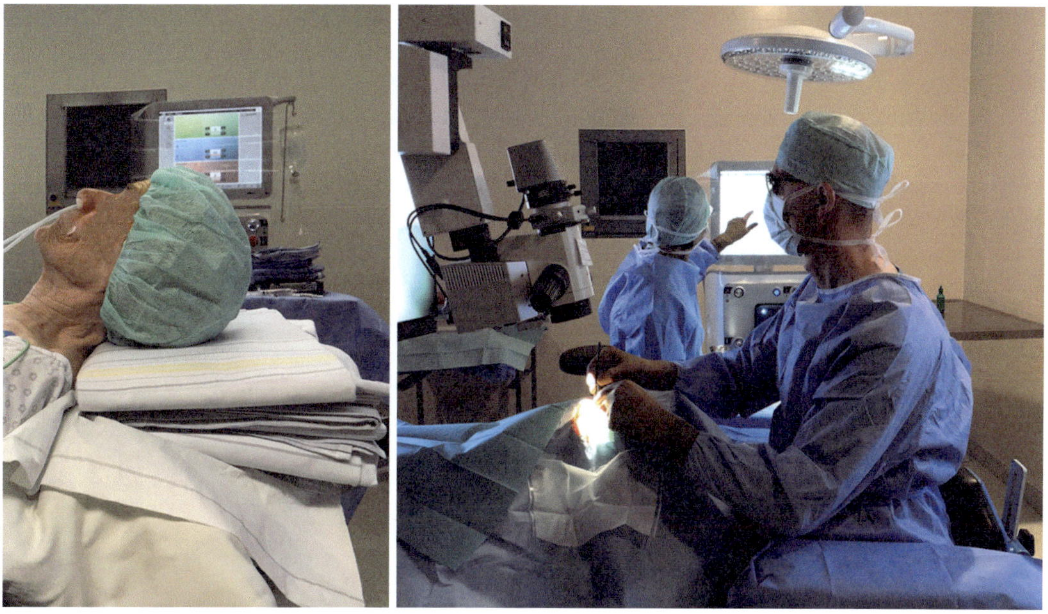

Fig. 9.17 Severe kyphosis preventing a horizontal posture of the patient's head and neck (left) and requiring a significant tilt of the microscope (right). Heads-up surgery enables the surgeon to sit comfortably

9.8 Additional Intraoperative Information

In heads-up surgery, the most relevant information for the surgeon is the microscopic view of the surgical field. For cataract surgeons, tools like "True Guide®" with "incision optimization guidance and IOL alignment templates" already exist [38]. In vitreoretinal surgery, additional data like live intraoperative OCT can be shown simultaneously with the live image on the same display [39].

Alcon has developed the Datafusion™ software [40], which allows the surgeon using the CONSTELLATION® Vision System from Alcon to see the data of the CONSTELLATION® machine on the NGENUITY® 3D Visualization System.

Kita et al. [41] reported on the combination of the NGENUITY® 3D Visualization System with an ocular endoscopic vitrectomy system (FiberTech, Chiba, Japan). The endoscopic view could be simultaneously seen on the 55-in. OLED display.

It seems possible that other simultaneously displayed data will help surgeons to tailor their intraoperative measures (e.g., wide-angle fluorescein angiographies and laser photocoagulation in occlusive retinal vascular diseases like PDR).

9.9 Problems with 3D Displays

In general, looking for hours on a computer display can cause fatigue [42, 43] probably due to a decreased blink rate and amplitude and therefore especially in dry eye syndrome. In addition, viewing three-dimensional displays can lead to conflicts between binocular vergence and accommodation [44, 45], also termed as visual asthenopia [45]. In our experience, conflicts between vergence and accommodation do not seem to be a real issue using modern 3D 4K displays at a distance of at least 1.5 m, regardless of age and presbyopia.

During laser photocoagulation, we use a manual safety laser filter. This avoids the very bright laser flashes seen on the display without a laser filter. Although watching the laser photocoagulation without a filter is harmless for the observing team and the camera, it dazzles the observers. This is especially annoying during panretinal laser photocoagulation. Accordingly, Zhang et al. [37] reported on nausea and dizziness during prolonged laser photocoagulation and wondered if special color filters could soften the disturbing flickering light.

A significant problem is the declining demand for consumer 3D displays. Instead, TV manufacturers are focusing on 2D screens with ultrahigh definition. Therefore, the range of 3D displays available for heads-up surgery is very limited and it is not clear if medical-grade 3D 8K screens will become available.

9.10 Head-Mounted Displays

Head-mounted displays have been already used 20 years ago [46]. A head-mounted display for 3D vitreoretinal surgery seems to be a viable option according to the first experience of two groups [47, 48]. Both groups used the Head-Mounted Display System HMS-3000MT (Sony Corporation, Tokyo, Japan) with two separate OLED displays and a resolution of 1280 × 720 pixels for each display.

The author has no experience with this approach. If such head-mounted monitors (Sony's HMM weighs 480 g) are well tolerated and ergonomic even during long surgeries should be evaluated. In the future, it seems realistic that head-mounted displays with higher resolutions such as 4K for each display will enhance stereoscopic viewing.

9.11 Technical Problems

The more sophisticated a technology is, the more critical is the reliability of the components. In 3D viewing, malfunctioning could occur with the 3D camera, the working station, and the display. In our department, there were only a few technical problems during surgery within 5 years. If there is a problem a reset of the computer should be tried first. However, it is advisable to be able to switch to the oculars if the 3D viewing system fails during an operation.

In future 3D systems, it would be advantageous to improve the surgeon's control of the settings of the viewing system. Nowadays, the surgeon still must ask a nonsterile assistant to change settings within the software, unless an optional footswitch (available for the NGENUITY®) or a wireless computer mouse under a sterile surgical draping is used. A change of the mechanical iris aperture can only be exerted by an assistant but not by the surgeon.

9.12 Teaching

Currently, a conventional analog microscope enables only the surgeon and one assistant to enjoy a three-dimensional image with high resolution. Surgical staff and visitors usually participate while looking at 2D monitors lacking the spatial information of a 3D image. Chhaya et al. [49] examined medical students after viewing 2D and 3D videos of ocular surgeries and found that 3D viewing offered a better understanding of vitreoretinal surgeries. Accordingly, 3D viewing systems provide the same image to the surgeon, surgical staff, and visitors if they look on a 3D monitor with polarizing glasses. In our department, visitors are fascinated by the opportunity to have the same view of the surgical field as the surgeon. Thus, with a 3D viewing system teaching vitreoretinal surgery becomes more effective. A senior surgeon can supervise a novice surgeon sitting or standing a few meters behind the novice while giving him advices. Because senior and novice surgeons have the same 3D image, an intervention during critical steps is possible before complications occur. Without worrying the patient, it is possible for the instructor to communicate with the surgeon discreetly but clearly using a mobile phone and a headset worn by the novice (Fig. 9.18) [50].

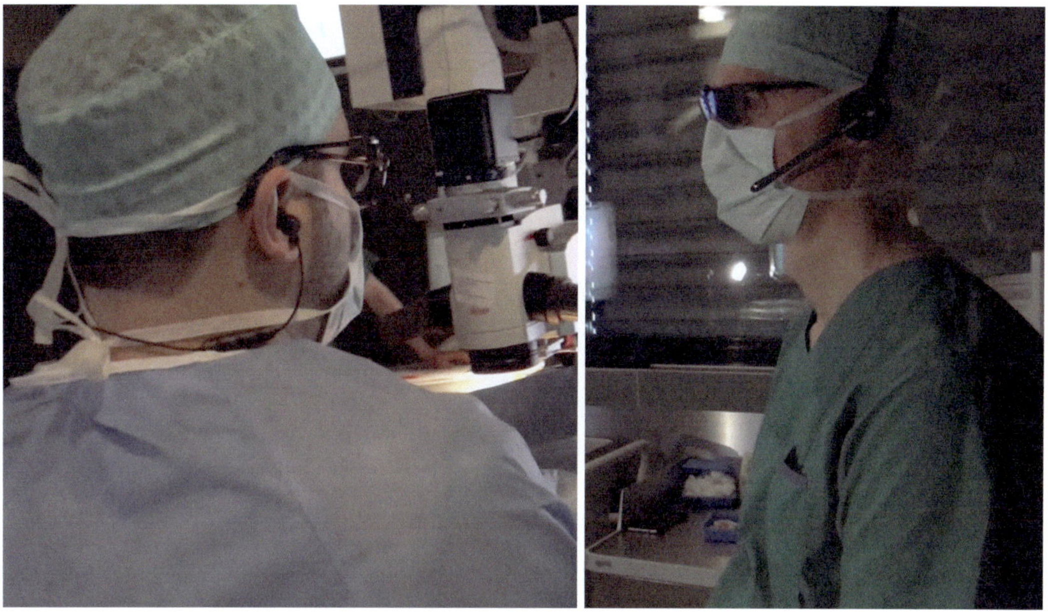

Fig. 9.18 Wireless communication between instructor and surgeon using mobile phones and headsets

9.13 The Future of 3D Viewing Systems

Soon we will see comparable 3D viewing systems for ocular surgery developed by operating microscope companies like Leica and Zeiss. ARRI Medical (Munich, Germany) has already developed a fully digital surgical microscope called ARRISCOPE® [51]. It has no analog optics anymore. TrueVision has announced a rather small "robotic digital surgical microscope" called TrueScope® [52] which will be independent from a conventional operating microscope. The surgeon will be able to look above a robotic arm carrying the 3D camera so that a smaller display could be placed above the patient and nearer to the surgeon.

If autostereoscopic displays [53, 54] will replace the current polarizing 3D displays has to be seen.

As soon as 3D visualization systems with two 4K instead of 2 Full HD image sensors will be available the resolution of digital microscopes will become at least as good or even better than the resolution of analog microscopes. Yamashita et al. [55] already reported on the experimental use of a 2D 8K camera in ophthalmic surgery. It seems possible that even 3D 8K cameras will be available in the next years and that stereoscopic 8K displays will replace the 3D 4K displays currently in use. This would certainly enhance the resolution of the future 3D viewing systems significantly. However, this would require even more powerful EPUs dealing with the immense data sizes, and it remains unclear if such systems would be a valuable improvement for clinical use compared to the present systems. If head-mounted displays will be widely accepted as an alternative visualization method has to be seen [56].

One can assume that 3D digital visualization systems will supersede traditional operating microscopes.

References

1. Barraquer JI. The microscope in ocular surgery. Am J Ophthalmol. 1956;42(6):916–8. https://doi.org/10.1016/0002-9394(56)90666-3.
2. Barraquer JI, Barraquer J, Littman H. A new operating microscope for ocular surgery. Am J Ophthalmol. 1967;63(1):90–7. https://doi.org/10.1016/0002-9394(67)90581-8.

3. Machemer R. Reminiscences after 25 years of pars plana vitrectomy. Am J Ophthalmol. 1995;119(4):505–10. https://doi.org/10.1016/S0002-9394(14)71238-3.
4. Kobayashi H, Hayashi M, Urano H. Three-dimensional videomonitor in microsurgery. Neurochirurgia. 1993;36(4):129–30. https://doi.org/10.1055/s-2008-1053811.
5. Mochizuki R, Kobayashi S. HDTV single camera 3D system and its application in microsurgery. Proc SPIE. 2177:31–4. https://doi.org/10.1117/12.173891.
6. Miyake K, Ocha I, Miyake S, et al. Application of a newly developed, highly sensitive camera and a 3-dimensional high-definition television system in experimental ophthalmic surgeries. Arch Ophthalmol. 1999;117(12):1623. https://doi.org/10.1001/archopht.117.12.1623.
7. Bhadri PR, Rowley AP, Khurana RN, et al. Evaluation of a stereoscopic camera-based three-dimensional viewing workstation for ophthalmic surgery. Am J Ophthalmol. 2007;143(5):891–2. https://doi.org/10.1016/j.ajo.2006.12.032.
8. Ilgner J, Park JJ-H, Labbé D, et al. Using a high-definition stereoscopic video system to teach microscopic surgery. In: Woods AJ, Dodgson NA, Merritt JO, et al., editors. Stereoscopic displays and virtual reality systems XIV. Bellingham, WA: SPIE; 2007. p. 649008.
9. Weinstock RJ, Desai N. Heads up cataract surgery with the TrueVision 3D display system. In: Garg A, Alio JL, editors. Surgical techniques in ophthalmology: cataract surgery. New Delhi: Jaypee Brothers; 2010. p. 124–7.
10. Weinstock RJ, Donnenfeld ED. 3D visualization in ophthalmology: new technology offers a “heads-up” way to perform surgery. Cataract & refractive surgery today. 2008. pp. 62–65. https://crstoday.com/articles/2008-may/crst0508_16-php/?single=true. Accessed 28 Nov 2020.
11. Di Marco AN, Jeyakumar J, Pratt PJ, et al. Evaluating a novel 3D stereoscopic visual display for transanal endoscopic surgery: a randomized controlled crossover study. Ann Surg. 2016;263(1):36–42. https://doi.org/10.1097/SLA.0000000000001261.
12. Smith R, Day A, Rockall T, et al. Advanced stereoscopic projection technology significantly improves novice performance of minimally invasive surgical skills. Surg Endosc. 2012;26(6):1522–7. https://doi.org/10.1007/s00464-011-2080-8.
13. Cheng H-T, Ma H, Tsai C-H, et al. A three-dimensional stereoscopic monitor system in microscopic vascular anastomosis. Microsurgery. 2012;32(7):571–4. https://doi.org/10.1002/micr.22035.
14. Liu J, Chen B, Ni Y, et al. Application of a three-dimensional microsurgical video system for a rat femoral vessel anastomosis. Chin Med J. 2014;127(2):348–52.
15. Mendez BM, Chiodo MV, Vandevender D, et al. Heads-up 3D microscopy: an ergonomic and educational approach to microsurgery. Plast Reconstr Surg Glob Open. 2016;4(5):e717. https://doi.org/10.1097/GOX.0000000000000727.
16. Beez T, Munoz-Bendix C, Beseoglu K, et al. First clinical applications of a high-definition three-dimensional exoscope in pediatric neurosurgery. Cureus. 2018;10(1):e2108. https://doi.org/10.7759/cureus.2108.
17. Belykh E, George L, Zhao X, et al. Microvascular anastomosis under 3D exoscope or endoscope magnification: a proof-of-concept study. Surg Neurol Int. 2018;9:115. https://doi.org/10.4103/sni.sni_36_18.
18. Mascitelli JR, Schlachter L, Chartrain AG, et al. Navigation-linked heads-up display in intracranial surgery: early experience. Oper Neurosurg. 2017;15(2):184–93. https://doi.org/10.1093/ons/opx205.
19. Riemann CD. Machine vision and vitrectomy: three-dimensional high definition (3DHD) video for surgical visualization in vitreoretinal surgery. In: Woods AJ, Holliman NS, Dodgson NA, editors. Stereoscopic displays and applications XXII, vol. 7863. Bellingham, WA: SPIE; 2011. p. 78630K1–8.
20. Eckardt C, Paulo EB. Heads-up surgery for vitreoretinal procedures: an experimental and clinical study. Retina. 2016;36(1):137–47. https://doi.org/10.1097/IAE.0000000000000689.
21. Novartis. Alcon launches the NGENUITY® 3D Visualization System designed to further enhance retinal surgeon experience | Novartis. 2019. https://novartis.gcs-web.com/alcon-launches-the-ngenuity-3d-visualization-system. Accessed 13 Jan 2019.
22. Coppola M, La Spina C, Rabiolo A, et al. Heads-up 3D vision system for retinal detachment surgery. Int J Retina Vitreous. 2017;3:46. https://doi.org/10.1186/s40942-017-0099-2.
23. Freeman WR, Chen KC, Ho J, et al. Resolution, depth of field, and physician satisfaction during digitally assisted vitreoretinal surgery. Retina. 2018;39(9):1768–71. https://doi.org/10.1097/IAE.0000000000002236.
24. Coppola M, Cicinelli MV, Rabiolo A, et al. Importance of light filters in modern vitreoretinal surgery: an update of the literature. Ophthalmic Res. 2017;58(4):189–93. https://doi.org/10.1159/000475760.
25. Todorich B, Stem MS, Hassan TS, et al. Scleral transillumination with digital heads-up display: a novel technique for visualization during vitrectomy surgery. Ophthalmic Surg Lasers Imaging Retina. 2018;49(6):436–9. https://doi.org/10.3928/23258160-20180601-08.
26. Adam MK, Thornton S, Regillo CD, et al. Minimal endoillumination levels and display luminous emittance during three-dimensional heads-up vitreoretinal surgery. Retina. 2017;37(9):1746–9. https://doi.org/10.1097/IAE.0000000000001420.
27. Talcott KE, Adam MK, Sioufi K, et al. Comparison of three-dimensional heads-up display surgical platform to standard operating microscope for macular surgery.

Ophthalmol Retina. 2018;3(3):244–51. https://doi.org/10.1016/j.oret.2018.10.016.
28. Kunikata H, Abe T, Nakazawa T. Heads-up macular surgery with a 27-gauge microincision vitrectomy system and minimal Illumination. Case Rep Ophthalmol. 2016;7(3):265–9. https://doi.org/10.1159/000452993.
29. Romano MR, Cennamo G, Comune C, et al. Evaluation of 3D heads-up vitrectomy: outcomes of psychometric skills testing and surgeon satisfaction. Eye. 2018;32(6):1093–8. https://doi.org/10.1038/s41433-018-0027-1.
30. Babu N, Kohli P, Ramachandran NO, et al. Comparison of surgical performance of internal limiting membrane peeling using a 3-D visualization system with conventional microscope. Ophthalmic Surg Lasers Imaging Retina. 2018;49(12):941–5. https://doi.org/10.3928/23258160-20181203-06.
31. Kumar A, Hasan N, Kakkar P, et al. Comparison of clinical outcomes between "heads-up" 3D viewing system and conventional microscope in macular hole surgeries: A pilot study. Indian J Ophthalmol. 2018;66(12):1816–9. https://doi.org/10.4103/ijo.IJO_59_18.
32. Dhimitri KC, McGwin G, McNeal SF, et al. Symptoms of musculoskeletal disorders in ophthalmologists. Am J Ophthalmol. 2005;139(1):179–81. https://doi.org/10.1016/j.ajo.2004.06.091.
33. Yu D, Sackllah M, Woolley C, et al. Quantitative posture analysis of 2D, 3D, and optical microscope visualization methods for microsurgery tasks. Work. 2012;41(Suppl 1):1944–7. https://doi.org/10.3233/WOR-2012-0412-1944.
34. Yu D, Green C, Kasten SJ, et al. Effect of alternative video displays on postures, perceived effort, and performance during microsurgery skill tasks. Appl Ergon. 2016;53 Pt A:281–9. https://doi.org/10.1016/j.apergo.2015.10.016.
35. Skinner CC, Riemann CD. "Heads up" digitally assisted surgical viewing for retinal detachment repair in a patient with severe kyphosis. Retin Cases Brief Rep. 2018;12(3):257–9. https://doi.org/10.1097/ICB.0000000000000486.
36. Rizzo S, Abbruzzese G, Savastano A, et al. 3D surgical viewing system in ophthalmology: perceptions of the surgical team. Retina. 2018;38(4):857–61. https://doi.org/10.1097/IAE.0000000000002018.
37. Zhang Z, Wang L, Wei Y, et al. The preliminary experiences with three-dimensional heads-up display viewing system for vitreoretinal surgery under various status. Curr Eye Res. 2019;44(1):102–9. https://doi.org/10.1080/02713683.2018.1526305.
38. Truevision. TrueGuide. 2018. http://truevisionsys.com/trueguide.html. Accessed 13 Jan 2019.
39. Ehlers JP, Uchida A, Srivastava SK. The integrative surgical theater: combining intraoperative optical coherence tomography and 3D digital visualization for vitreoretinal surgery in the DISCOVER study. Retina. 2018;38(Suppl 1):S88–96. https://doi.org/10.1097/IAE.0000000000001999.
40. Alcon. Alcon introduces NGENUITY® 3D visualization system with DATAFUSION™ to simplify, customize vitreoretinal surgery | Alcon.com. 2018. https://www.alcon.com/news/media-releases/alcon-introduces-ngenuityr-3d-visualization-system-datafusiontm-simplify.
41. Kita M, Mori Y, Hama S. Hybrid wide-angle viewing-endoscopic vitrectomy using a 3D visualization system. Clin Ophthalmol. 2018;12:313–7. https://doi.org/10.2147/OPTH.S156497.
42. Blehm C, Vishnu S, Khattak A, et al. Computer vision syndrome: a review. Surv Ophthalmol. 2005;50(3):253–62. https://doi.org/10.1016/j.survophthal.2005.02.008.
43. Rosenfield M. Computer vision syndrome: a review of ocular causes and potential treatments. Ophthalmic Physiol Opt. 2011;31(5):502–15. https://doi.org/10.1111/j.1475-1313.2011.00834.x.
44. Hoffman DM, Girshick AR, Akeley K, et al. Vergence-accommodation conflicts hinder visual performance and cause visual fatigue. J Vis. 2008;8(3):33. https://doi.org/10.1167/8.3.33.
45. Wee SW, Moon NJ, Lee WK, et al. Ophthalmological factors influencing visual asthenopia as a result of viewing 3D displays. Br J Ophthalmol. 2012;96(11):1391–4. https://doi.org/10.1136/bjophthalmol-2012-301690.
46. Chen JC, Moffitt K, Levy ML. Head-mounted display system for microneurosurgery. Stereotact Funct Neurosurg. 1997;68(1–4 Pt 1):25–32. https://doi.org/10.1159/000099898.
47. Dutra-Medeiros M, Nascimento J, Henriques J, et al. Three-dimensional head-mounted display system for ophthalmic surgical procedures. Retina. 2017;37(7):1411–4. https://doi.org/10.1097/IAE.0000000000001514.
48. Martínez-Toldos JJ, Fernández-Martínez C, Navarro-Navarro A. Experience using a 3D head-mounted display system in ophthalmic surgery. Retina. 2017,37(7):1419–21. https://doi.org/10.1097/IAE.0000000000001664.
49. Chhaya N, Helmy O, Piri N, et al. Comparison of 2D and 3D video displays for teaching vitreoretinal surgery. Retina. 2018;38(8):1556–61. https://doi.org/10.1097/IAE.0000000000001743.
50. Eckardt C, Ahdab K, Eckert T. Use of mobile phones during heads-up surgery-a new way of teaching cataract and vitreoretinal surgery. Retina. 2019;Suppl 1:S191–3. https://doi.org/10.1097/IAE.0000000000002493.
51. ARRI Medical. Arriscope. 2019. https://www.arri-medical.com/.
52. Truevision. TrueScope digital surgical microscope. 2018. http://truevisionsys.com/truescope.html. Accessed 06 Jan 2019.
53. Christopher LA, William A, Cohen-Gadol AA. Future directions in 3-dimensional imaging and neurosurgery: stereoscopy and autostereoscopy. Neurosurgery.

2013;72(Suppl 1):131–8. https://doi.org/10.1227/NEU.0b013e318270d9c0.
54. Narita Y, Tsukagoshi S, Suzuki M, et al. Usefulness of a glass-free medical three-dimensional autostereoscopic display in neurosurgery. Int J Comput Assist Radiol Surg. 2014;9(5):905–11. https://doi.org/10.1007/s11548-014-0984-1.
55. Yamashita H, Tanioka K, Miyake G, et al. 8K ultra-high-definition microscopic camera for ophthalmic surgery. Clin Ophthalmol. 2018;12:1823–8. https://doi.org/10.2147/OPTH.S171233.
56. Williams GA. Surgical viewing: do you see what I see? Retina. 2017;37(7):1219. https://doi.org/10.1097/IAE.0000000000001721.

10 Robotics in Vitreoretinal Surgeries

Matthew J. Gerber and Jean-Pierre Hubschman

10.1 Introduction

Robotic systems have found widespread use across many surgical applications due to their increased precision, higher maneuverability, and improved visualization over traditional surgical techniques. In 2012, the da Vinci Surgical System (Intuitive Surgical, Inc.) accounted for approximately 450,000 surgical procedures performed including surgeries in the fields of gynecology, urology, and general surgery [1]. However, despite these advances, the adoption of robotic systems to vitreoretinal surgery has lagged behind than in other surgical practices. The delayed adoption can be attributed to the unique advantages of intraocular ophthalmic surgery including the direct three-dimensional and high-magnification view of intraocular structures, the minimally invasive nature of intraocular instrumentation, and the unhindered maneuverability and range of surgical instruments.

The promise of improved safety and efficiency has inspired the development of robotic platforms aimed at performing complete surgeries with incorporated tool exchangers and tightly integrated visualization systems. Visualization modalities such as digital microscopy and optical coherence tomography (OCT) can supersede the current practice of using optical stereo surgical microscopes due to their improved resolution and depth-sensing capabilities. Additional benefits of robotic surgery in ophthalmology include the possibility of more precise surgical manipulations, augmented visual and tactile feedback, full automation, and "teleoperated" surgery.

The purpose of this chapter is to summarize the progress that has been made toward the goal of robotic ocular surgery for clinical patient care. Also discussed are the previous and current intraocular robotic systems and their validation through experimental testing.

10.2 Intraocular Surgical Robotics

In this section, we present a history of robotic systems specifically designed for intraocular surgical procedures.

10.2.1 Early Intraocular Surgical Robotics

One of the first intraocular robotic systems was the "Stereotaxical Micro-telemanipulator" developed in 1989 [2]. This system was composed of a

M. J. Gerber
Department of Mechanical and Aerospace Engineering, University of California, Los Angeles, CA, USA
e-mail: gerber211@ucla.edu

J.-P. Hubschman (✉)
Stein Eye Institute, University of California, Los Angeles, CA, USA
e-mail: hubschman@jsei.ucla.edu

A. Jain et al. (eds.), *Cutting-edge Vitreoretinal Surgery*,
https://doi.org/10.1007/978-981-33-4168-5_10

spherical micromanipulator with three degrees-of-freedom (DOF) mounted on a 3-DOF translational stage. The system successfully performed ocular vitrectomy and radial keratotomy with greater accuracy but slower speed compared to a human surgeon [3]. A similar spherical mechanism was patented in 1998 [4] for intravascular drug delivery, implantation of micro-drainage devices, and the intraretinal manipulation of micro-electrodes. These tasks were successfully executed with minimal tissue damage.

In 1997, through a collaboration between ASA-JPL and MicroDexterity Systems, a teleoperated robotic system "Robot Assisted MicroSurgery" was developed [5]. This system was lightweight, compact, and demonstrated tool-tip positional precision of 10 μm. The control device was integrated with actuators to measure the surgeon's hand motion, but the main limitations were the software complexity and the absence of a mechanically constrained remote center of motion (RCM).

In the same year, a research group from Northwestern University developed a robotic platform to measure the intraluminal of feline retinal vessels (diameters of 20–150 μm) and extract blood samples [6]. The system used a Stewart platform controlled by a handheld trackball and two buttons. The intended direction of tool motion was entered into a computer beforehand. Despite nonintuitive control scheme, the device was successfully used for vein cannulation and acquiring retinal blood samples in anesthetized cats.

With the widespread acceptance of the da Vinci Surgical System in other surgical fields, our team investigated its application to vitreoretinal surgery in 2006 [7]. By attempting to perform pars plana vitrectomy using standard 25-gauge instruments, we demonstrated several deficiencies of the system in posterior segment surgical procedures. A significant shortcoming was that the RCM of the da Vinci Surgical System is preset and located 9 cm away from the corneal incision. Furthermore, the image quality of the endoscope was insufficient and suffered from a limited field of view.

Later, our group sought to modify the da Vinci Surgical System with the addition of a Stewart platform. The combined device was named the Hexapod Surgical System [8]. The main advantage of this system was the ability to place the virtual RCM at the surgical incision using automated software, allowing the system to constantly reposition the RCM as dictated by the surgery. To demonstrate the stability of the RCM, a mounted vitreous cutter was inserted into a postmortem pig eye through a 20-gauge sclerotomy site with minimal observed stress at the site of corneal incision. However, the main limitation was the limited translation and angulation range of motion (an intraocular 30° cone), which were insufficient for general posterior segment intraocular surgery.

In 2009, an early prototype from the University of Tokyo demonstrated initial success with use of a custom micromanipulator prototype [9]. This was a teleoperated robotic system with three-dimensional vision feedback provided to the surgeon, who controlled the robot through a pair of custom joysticks. The mechanical design of the robotic system consisted of a pair of spherical guides to allow for 6 DOF while mechanically constraining the RCM. Ophthalmic surgical instruments were mounted to the robotic system and posterior vitreous detachment, retinal vessel sheathotomy, and retinal vessel micro-cannulation were performed in postmortem pig eyes. Success was reported in all procedures except retinal vein cannulation, which was limited by deficiencies in visualization.

10.2.2 Recent Intraocular Surgical Robotics

10.2.2.1 Johns Hopkins University Steady-Hand Manipulator

The Computational Interaction and Robotics Laboratory at The Johns Hopkins University developed a steady-hand robotic system for microsurgery. This robotic system, described initially in 1999 [10], was developed to extend a human surgeon's ability to perform small-scale intraocular manipulation tasks that required human judgment, sensory integration, and hand–eye coordination. With this system, the surgical instrument was simultaneously held by the surgeon and an actively controlled robot arm. By measuring forces applied on the surgical tool deflections could be corrected and used to provide smooth, tremor-free, precise, and scaled motion of the tool. Initial experiments on chicken egg membranes demonstrated that the system was capable of assisting the surgeon in manipulating tissue within predefined force bounds [11].

In 2012, the same group reported developments of the Steady-Hand Eye Robot for vitreoretinal surgery [12]. By adding a tool holder with a quick-release mechanism and an RCM tilt mechanism, the improved robot was designed to address previous ergonomic and safety limitations. The handheld manipulator enabled bilateral manipulation using a two-robot configuration and could be used by right- or left-handed users. The tool holder enabled fixation of the axial direction while allowing tool rotation about its axis. It was easily attached to the robot arm, facilitating delineation between sterilizable and non-sterilizable parts.

10.2.2.2 University of Utah

In 2016, the Telerobotics Laboratory at the University of Utah developed a compact teleoperated surgical system for retinal surgery that used commercially available instruments [13]. A custom stylus was developed for an intuitive haptic interface to enable ergonomic teleoperation. Tool-tip positional resolution was reported as 0.5 μm and precision as ≤1 μm. Experimental results demonstrated that, using this system, the instrument forces acting on the retina were reduced compared to manually performed surgery.

10.2.2.3 The MICRON

In 2010, with a collaboration between the Robotics Institute at Carnegie Mellon University and Johns Hopkins University, an active handheld micromanipulator was developed [14]. Through image guidance, the device, called the MICRON (Fig. 10.1), reduced hand tremors to

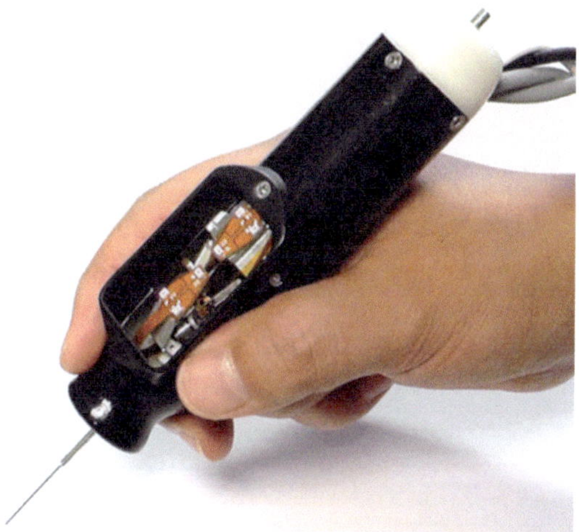

Fig. 10.1 The MICRON from Carnegie Mellon University and Johns Hopkins University; Image source: [15]

provide a smooth, scaled motion during surgical procedures. By tracking the instrument in the microscope view, the MICRON assisted the surgeon during the approach, puncture, and injection stages of retinal vein cannulation. Experiments performed on postmortem pig eyes demonstrated an increase in success rate from 29% to 63% with the use of the MICRON. Handheld testing also demonstrated a maximum reduction in positional error of 52%.

In 2015, the same group further improved the MICRON by increasing its DOF to six [15]. The design incorporated a Gough Stewart platform with a cylindrical workspace and a constrained RCM near the tool tip. The instrument included a custom optical-tracking system used in control feedback. The improved system was evaluated under varying conditions to demonstrate trajectory-following errors of ≤20 μm and a reduction of approximately 90% in hand tremor.

Most recently, in 2017, the same group tested the MICRON using a stretched vinyl membrane [16]. The position of the handle and tool tip were visually tracked at 2 kHz with 4 μm accuracy using active LEDs to provide 6 DOF of the tool-tip orientation and position over a workspace of approximately 1000 × 1000 × 400 μm. By integrating a force-sensing needle into the MICRON, the researchers claimed the system could reliably predict tissue puncture. The group also demonstrated an automated position-holding feature that allowed for switching from tremor-canceling operation mode to full-motion compensation. Thus, the tool tip could be maintained inside an artificial vein for longer periods of time with significantly reduced tool-tip motion after venipuncture. However, these evaluation studies were performed on artificial phantom models and are therefore limited due to the unrealistic nature of the phantoms.

10.2.2.4 Vanderbilt University Intraocular Probe

In 2013, the Advanced Robotics and Mechanism Applications Research Laboratory at Vanderbilt University presented a small (25 gauge) OCT probe for real-time intraoperative ocular imaging [17]. The hand-held probe was complete with an internal scanning system such that it could be held by a surgeon to image target posterior pole and peripheral structures. With a scanning range of 2 mm, an axial resolution of 4–6 μm, and a lateral resolution of 25–35 μm, the probe had sufficient imaging capability to produce clear B-mode images of target intraocular tissues.

Later, the same group developed an 11-DOF robotic platform specifically for retinal microvascular surgery integrated with the B-scan probe [18]. The robot design was based on a 6-DOF Stewart-Gough platform incorporated onto a 2-DOF differential wrist with a 3-DOF actuator. Experimental evaluations of stent deployment and membrane peeling were shown with results verified by OCT imaging. This system was unique in that it allowed for both ocular manipulation and intraocular surgical manipulation. However, the OCT imaging system was never registered to the robot coordinate frame, reducing its usefulness and prohibiting the possibility of automated feedback-based control of the manipulator.

In 2015, the same group incorporated the B-mode OCT probe into custom, handheld micro-forceps to form a unique vitreoretinal surgical system [19]. Developed specifically for epiretinal membrane peeling, the coplanar OCT imaging probe was integrated into the micro-forceps to reduce instrument shadows in the OCT scans (Fig. 10.2). The design also allowed for constant tracking of the membrane surface during peeling operations such that the surface approach (tool-tip to membrane distance) could be known in real time. The team studied the surface approach of a postmortem goat retina with the robotic-controlled forceps. Expectedly, the surgeon's performance was dramatically improved when real-time feedback from the OCT forceps was combined with robot-assisted control of the surgical tool. However, this system was incapable of rotating the tool about its centerline, dramatically reducing its mobility and precluding its use in more realistic surgical manipulations.

Finally, the same team overcame many of the previous deficiencies of their system by devel-

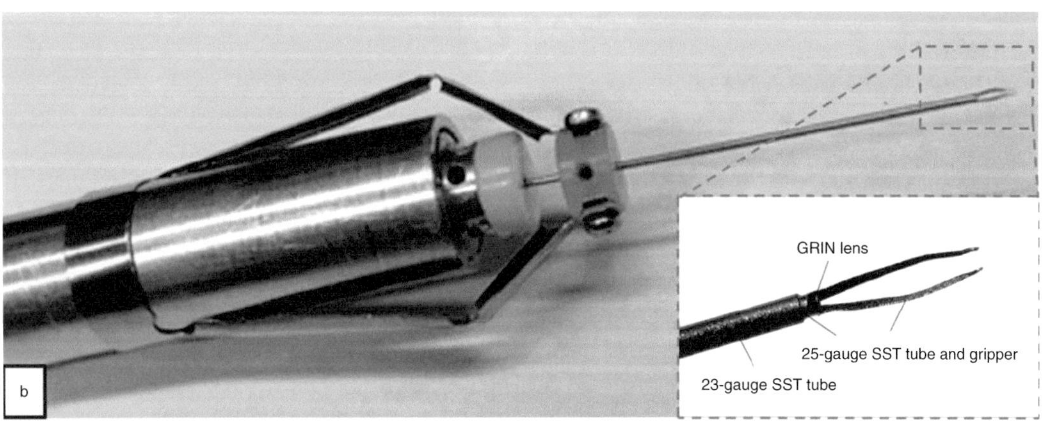

Fig. 10.2 OCT-integrated forceps design; Image source: [19]

oping methods to achieve real-time OCT feedback and assistive robotic control based on B-scan mode OCT imaging [20]. A teleoperated control interface was developed and integrated with the system to allow for intuitive control by the surgeon. The imaging coordinate frame of the OCT probe was registered to the robotic coordinate frame for improved control. A dual-rate control method that used low-frequency OCT feedback combined with high-frequency positional information from encoders was presented and evaluated for accuracy and latency. Three-dimensional assistive virtual fixtures generated from OCT feedback were presented and used to perform subretinal injections into artificial phantom blood vessels. Limitations of the developed system included the slow rate of OCT feedback.

10.2.2.5 University of Leuven, Belgium

In 2014, the Micro- and Precision Engineering Group at the Catholic University of Leuven presented a teleoperated robotic system complete with motion scaling, tremor compensation, and scaled force feedback [21]. This was a co-manipulated robotic system intended to assist a surgeon by offering increased stability and precision during intraocular manipulations by reducing tremor and maintaining a fixed position for prolonged durations. The device was a 4-DOF parallel arm mechanism with a mechanically fixed RCM and controlled via a 4-DOF spherical mechanism (Fig. 10.3).

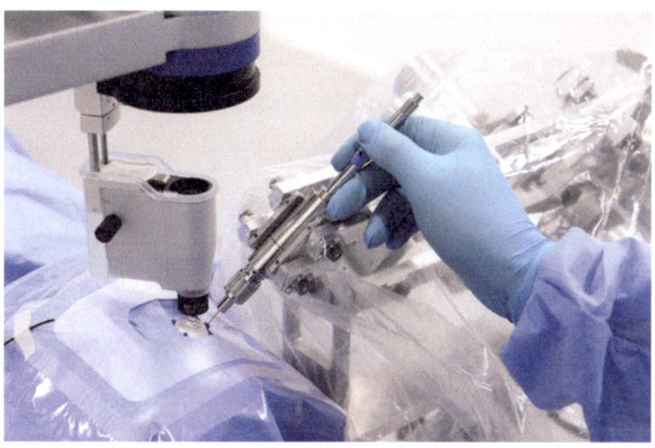

Fig. 10.3 The Belgium group's co-manipulated robotic platform; Image source: [22]

This robot was later used to evaluate the feasibility of robot-assisted retinal vein cannulation for treating retinal vein occlusion [23]. To do so, retinal vein cannulation was performed on in vivo pig eyes using the surgical robot with a mounted microneedle. Complete success was defined as a stable intravenous position of the needle tip for more than 3 min, and was confirmed in 15 out of 18 eyes. No technical failures of the robotic device were reported.

Following this success, the same group reported on the clinical translation of their developed system and the resulting world-first, in-human, robot-assisted retinal vein cannulation [22]. Four patients with retinal vein occlusion were treated at the University Hospital of Leuven in the context of a phase I clinical trial. The trial involved safely injecting an anticoagulant (ocriplasmin) into a targeted 100–150 μm thick retinal vein with injection periods of up to 10 min on human patients. The results demonstrated that it was possible to perform retinal vein cannulation with the aid of robotic technology in a standard operating room environment.

10.2.2.6 Munich

In 2013, the Department of Robotics and Embedded Systems at the Technical University of Munich introduced their arm design of an ophthalmic robotic system [24]. The robot was a unique parallel–serial mechanism composed of prismatic piezoelectric actuators that controlled the movements of four serial segments, two parallel coupled joint elements, and one prismatic joint in the end effector. Compared to other systems, the Munich robot was physically compact (94 ± 28 × 33.5 × 18.5 mm), roughly the size of an average human hand. Furthermore, the system was designed to mount to a patient's head to solve the problem of patient motion by incorporating a goggle-like mounting device integrated with the robotic system. While the intended application was vein cannulation, no clinical evaluation was performed and the system was evaluated only on engineering metrics.

The following year, the same team developed virtual-fixture control methods and experimentally evaluated their results [25]. These virtual fixtures included the virtual constraint of the RCM as well as autonomous RCM adjustment. These additions were evaluated on postmortem pig eyes. The latest work from the Munich group used the same device to develop teleoperated capabilities [26]. Using a controller that featured force feedback, a control scheme for the positional error was implemented. The resulting system allowed the surgeon to perform precise and comfortable micromanipulation.

10.2.2.7 Preceyes Surgical System

The Preceyes Surgical System (Fig. 10.4) is a high-precision device for vitreoretinal surgical procedures. It was developed at the Eindhoven University of Technology in the Netherlands and is currently undergoing clinical evaluation by Preceyes B.V., a spin-off company of the university. The system consists of a joystick-like motion controller used as an input by the surgeon and an instrument manipulator with a mounted surgical instrument that performs the physical operation. The instrument manipulator is rigidly fixed to the operating table by a custom headrest and reproduces the movements of the motion controller. The surgeon monitors and guides the intraocular tool procedure through a standard surgical microscope. The compact design of the instrument manipulator allowed it to unobtrusively fit into the operating room environment.

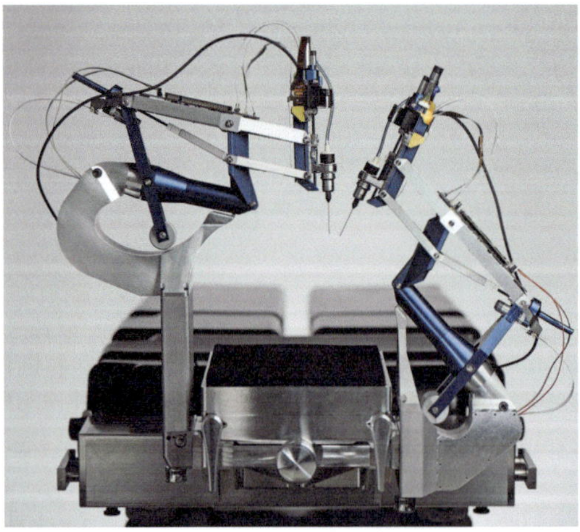

Fig. 10.4 The Preceyes Surgical System; Image source: Preceyes B.V.

The design of the instrument manipulator was based on a parallelogram linkage common to many surgical robots. A counterweight was added to adjust the center of mass, thereby minimizing the required actuator torques and enhancing the system safety (the tool position is fixed even in the event of a power loss). A tool-tip positional resolution of 10 μm was reported. To demonstrate the capabilities of Preceyes, live pigs were anesthetized and venous occlusions created [27].

In 2018, the Preceyes Surgical System was used to perform retinal membrane peeling and subretinal injection in human patients [28]. The objective was to prove the feasibility and safety of using robotic assistance in common retinal procedures. A clinical trial was conducted to compare the robot-assisted surgery to manual surgery in patients requiring the removal of retinal membranes. In the first stage, the robot was used to lift a flap of the retinal membrane from the macula surface using a beveled needle. In the second stage, the robot was used to perform subretinal injection of recombinant tissue plasminogen activator (rtPA) in three patients with central vision loss due to subretinal hemorrhage secondary to age-related macular degeneration.

Twelve patients with macular holes were recruited to perform membrane peeling. The use of the robot was amenable to the standard surgical workflow, with the surgeon and assistant sitting in their usual positions. A high degree of tool-tip positional precision was reported in the direction perpendicular to the retina, which was constrained to small (10 μm) incremental advancements of the tool. Once positioned, a virtual boundary was imposed in the control software to restrict additional depth movement commands and prevent iatrogenic retinal trauma. While the robot-assisted surgical procedures took longer than those manually performed (4 min 55 s compared to 1 min 20 s), the amount of iatrogenic retinal microtrauma during robot-assisted surgeries (defined as retinal touches and microhemorrhages) was decreased.

For the subretinal injection, three patients were placed under local anesthesia. The procedure involved robot-assisted delivery of 0.025–0.10 mL of a rtPA solution under the retina. In one patient, transient intraoperative exacerbation of cataract precluded a clear view of the cannula tip and was manually completed, but the subretinal injections were otherwise successful in all patients.

Despite the robot-assisted surgical procedures being slower than the manually performed ones in all cases, the robot-assisted procedures resulted in fewer inadvertent retinal touches and microhemorrhages, indicative of the robot's safety. Over all procedures, no system malfunctions or technical glitches were encountered and the robotic system was deemed to be unobtrusive within the operating theater. However, the robotic system was equipped with only an emergency retract function to account for unexpected patient head movement. In the interest of safety, precautions were required to minimize this risk: all cases involved the patient's head being taped to the operating table and in the case of membrane peeling, the patients underwent general anesthesia maintained with muscle relaxation and mechanical ventilation to ensure spontaneous respiration was eliminated. Finally, the operation of the system sacrificed speed in favor of surgical safety; i.e., precision was lost with increases in operational speed. In addition, there is an upper limit to the physiological ability of the human surgeon to perceive depth when using the standard surgical microscope.

10.2.2.8 Intraocular Robotic Interventional and Surgical System

With the use of femtosecond laser systems, emerging technological advances have enabled the autonomous completion of specific steps of cataract surgery such as corneal incisions, capsulorhexis, and lens fragmentation. While effective, laser-based technologies are unable to perform physical manipulation of tissue such as the removal of emulsified lens or the insertion of an intraocular lens implant. First presented in 2013, the Intraocular Robotic Interventional and Surgical System (IRISS) was developed through a collaboration between the Stein Eye Institute and the Mechatronics and Controls Laboratory at the University of California, Los Angeles [29].

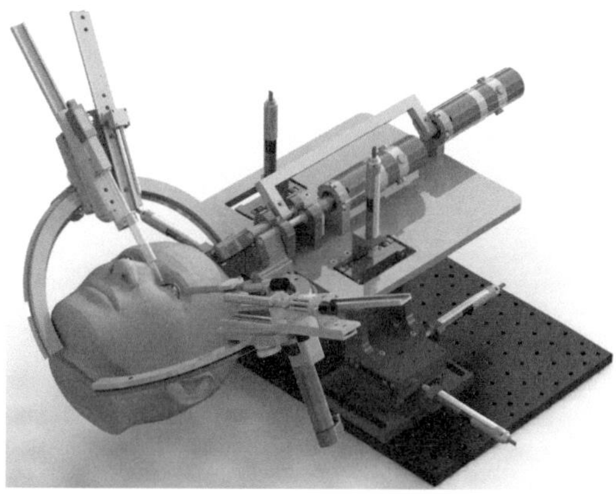

Fig. 10.5 The IRISS system; Image source: [30]

The IRISS (Fig. 10.5) was aimed at remotely operated and fully automated intraocular manipulation and featured a simple tool-change mechanism, a set of low-power lasers for aligning the RCM to the corneal incision, and a range of motion that covered the entire hemisphere and allowed for the simultaneous use of two surgical instruments in close proximity [30].

The clinical requirement of a kinematically constrained RCM formed the basis for the mechanical design of the IRISS. The surgical manipulator included two independently controllable arms, each holding two interchangeable surgical instruments. This configuration allowed for minimal interference with a surgical microscope, allowed the patient's head to be contained within the workspace, and allowed for an intuitive mapping between the control device and the IRISS. A wide array of commercially available microsurgical instruments were adapted for use with the surgical manipulator.

The custom surgical controller was designed as a surgeon-held input device analogous to a standard intraocular surgical instrument. During motion of the surgical controllers, reference commands were generated and modified with an array of motion scaling and tremor reduction to increase the safety and precision of the system. The choice of which surgical instrument to engage as well as the irrigation and aspiration forces for an I/A tool were provided to the system through a graphical user interface and through a foot pedal. The system enabled three-dimensional

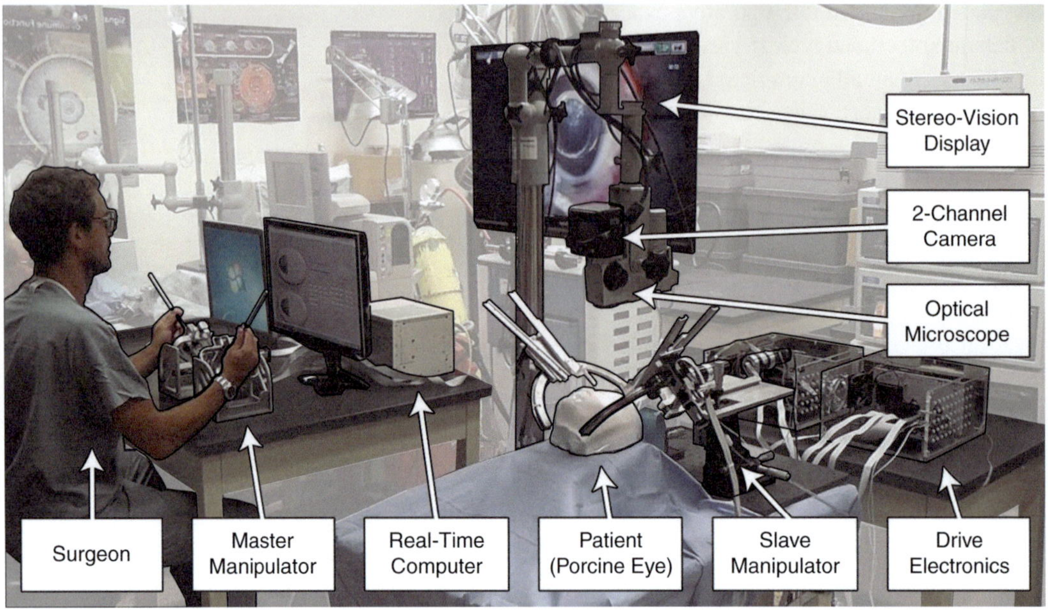

Fig. 10.6 The clinical evaluation of the IRISS system in teleoperation mode; Image source: [30]

visualization through a TrueVision stereo system. Alignment of the mechanical RCM to the corneal incision was accomplished through two low-power lasers mounted onto the tool carriage and aligned through an automated, vision-based method.

The IRISS was used to validate the system on an array of procedures required by cataract surgery and vitreoretinal surgeries (Fig. 10.6). The evaluation was performed on postmortem pig eyes in a standard operating theater with the surgeon seated beside the surgical controllers and the visual displays. The IRISS was able to perform anterior lens capsulorhexis, viscoelastic injection, hydro-dissection, lens aspiration, retinal vein cannulation, and vitrectomy. In particular, retinal vein cannulation was performed to validate the ability of the IRISS to perform precise tasks. Also, in many procedures, the second arm was mounted with an additional tool to demonstrate the unique ability of the IRISS to simultaneously manipulate two surgical instruments inside the eye. Finally, the IRISS was the first robotic system to successfully create a round, curvilinear capsulorhexis and the first to perform an entire cataract surgery from beginning to end.

Following this initial success, our group improved the IRISS for the purpose of performing automated cataract extraction via OCT feedback [31]. Despite cataract surgery being one of the most successful and common intraocular procedures, surgical complications remain due to the physiological limitations of a human surgeon and deficiencies in sensing capabilities. Complications include posterior capsule rupture, incomplete lens removal, and corneal incision leakage. However, cataract extraction remains a manually performed operation despite being the main source of the aforementioned complications.

Automated alignment and tool insertion was achieved through an image-processing algorithm that characterized the corneal incision by location and orientation. Anatomical structures were segmented and modeled through preoperative OCT scans using a custom algorithm that automatically generated a parameterized model. A cataract-extraction trajectory was preoperatively planned by reconstructing the intraocular structures with a trajectory chosen to mobilize lens material and increase surgical efficacy and efficiency. During lens extraction, the predefined trajectory was tracked alongside scheduled aspiration and irrigation forces. To account for the variable surgical environment, intraoperative supervision and manual intervention strategies were provided to the surgeon. Intraoperative OCT scans localized around the tool tip were displayed to the surgeon in real time and allowed for real-time anatomical evaluation. For improved safety, intraoperative diagnostics and intervention methods allowed the surgeon to override or modify the cataract-extraction procedure.

The IRISS was evaluated in a clinical environment using postmortem pig eyes (Fig. 10.7). The objective was to autonomously remove the entire lens without surgical complications. The automated procedure was performed on 30 eyes and preoperative, intraoperative, and postoperative OCT volume scans were acquired for analysis. In addition, microscope-based examination was performed by a trained surgeon to assess the integrity of the tissues and to determine if lens material remained. Results indicated that posterior capsule rupture was avoided in all 30 trials. Complete lens extraction was achieved on 25 of the samples, but in the five remaining cases, minute particles of lens material were discovered after surgery hidden behind the iris where the OCT was unable to image. Therefore, the imperfect success rate was due to limitations of the sensing technology and not to the developed system itself.

10.3 Future of Vitreoretinal Surgical Robotics

In the future, we may see surgical robots with artificial intelligence and the resulting capacity to make surgical decisions without the input of a human surgeon. More likely in coming years, we may see fully automated surgical robots perform a very specific and routine task independently from the surgeon. Such feats will be accomplished with improved feedback from OCT or other image modalities, tightly integrated, and registered into the surgical system. Finally, the possibility of integrating augmented reality displays with the surgical experience is also likely for improved safety and efficacy.

To this end, we are envisioning a surgical system with an augmented-reality cockpit integrated with multisensory feedback to perform complete intraocular procedures. We have recently performed studies in a virtual environment (Fig. 10.8) to establish that haptic feedback improves performance during preretinal membrane peeling procedures. Participants over a range of skillsets were asked to perform virtual preretinal membrane peeling using two modes: (1) haptic and visual feedback enabled and (2) only visual feedback enabled. Results demonstrated a reduction in task-completion

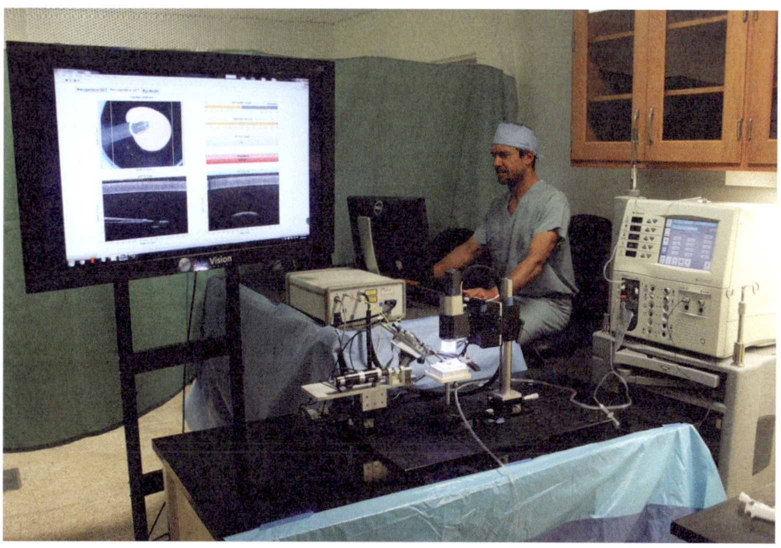

Fig. 10.7 The setup of the IRISS system for automated cataract extraction. The surgeon supervises the extraction and offers guidance; Image Source: [31]

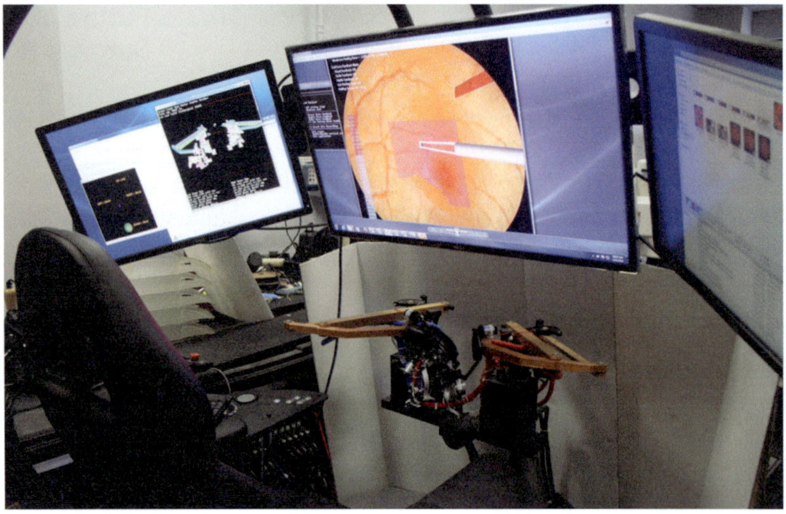

Fig. 10.8 Augmented reality-enabled surgical cockpit for robot-assisted, vitreoretinal surgery located in the Bionics Lab of UCLA; Used with permission from the Bionics Lab at UCLA

time, retinal damage, and other metrics with the full complement of feedback enabled. It is likely that additional systems similar to this one will appear in upcoming years.

10.4 Conclusion

In conclusion, the full potential of surgical robotics in vitreoretinal surgical applications lies in developing sight-saving or sight-improving procedures that are currently impossible using current manual instrument control and sensing. Examples include prolonged cannulation of retinal veins or accurate delivery of stem cells or gene therapy drugs into the subretinal spaces. More broadly, improved tool precision can reduce anatomical damage, improve surgical outcomes, and enable new surgical techniques which are uncommon in current practice. Despite these possibilities, improved optimization of existing systems and their acceptance into general practice are required before vitreoretinal surgical robotic systems can be fully deployed into operating rooms.

References

1. Annual Report 2017. Intuitive Surgical, Inc.
2. Guerrouad A, Jolly D. Automatic analysis of weariness during a micromanipulation task by SMOS. IEEE Conf Proc. 1989;3:906–7.
3. Guerrouad A, Vidal P. SMOS: Stereotaxical microtelemanipulator for ocular surgery. IEEE Conf Proc. 1989;3:879–80.
4. Yu D, Cringle SJ, et al. Robotic ocular ultramicrosurgery. Aust N Z J Ophthalmol. 1998;26:S6–8.
5. Charles S, Das H, Ohm T, et al. Dexterity-enhanced telerobotic microsurgery. In: Proc IEEE Int Conf Adv Robot. 1997; July 5–10.
6. Jensen PS, Grace KW, et al. Toward robot-assisted vascular microsurgery in the retina. Graefes Arch Clin Exp Ophthalmol. 1997;235(11):696–701.
7. Bourla DH, Hubschman JP, et al. Feasibility study of intraocular robotic surgery with the da Vinci surgical system. Retina. 2008;28(1):154–8.
8. Mulgaonkar AP, Hubschman JP, et al. A prototype surgical manipulator for robotic intraocular micro surgery. Stud Health Technol Inform. 2009;142:215–7.
9. Nakano T, Naohiko S, Takashi U, Yasuhiro T, Mamoru M. A parallel robot to assist vitreoretinal surgery. Int J Comput Assist Radiol Surg. 2009;4(6):517.
10. Russell T, et al. A steady-hand robotic system for microsurgical augmentation. Int J Robot Res. 1999;18(12):1201–10.
11. Üneri A, Marcin AB, Handa J, Gehlbach P, Taylor RH, Iordachita I. New steady-hand eye robot with micro-force sensing for vitreoretinal surgery. In: Biomedical robotics and biomechatronics (BioRob), 2010 3rd IEEE RAS and EMBS international conference on; 2010. p. 814–9.
12. He X, Roppenecker D, Gierlach D, Balicki M, Olds K, Gehlbach P, Handa J, Taylor R, Iordachita I. Toward clinically applicable steady-hand eye robot for vitreoretinal surgery. In: ASME 2012 international mechanical engineering congress and exposition. New York: American Society of Mechanical Engineers; 2012. p. 145–53.
13. Manikantan N, Bernstein PS, Abbott JJ. A compact telemanipulated retinal-surgery system that uses commercially available instruments with a quick-change adapter. J Med Robot Res. 2016;1(02):1630001.

14. MacLachlan RA, Becker BC, Tabarés JC, Podnar GW, Lobes LA Jr, Riviere CN. Micron: an actively stabilized handheld tool for microsurgery. IEEE Trans Robot. 2012;28(1):195.
15. Yang S, MacLachlan RA, Riviere CN. Manipulator design and operation of a six-degree-of-freedom handheld tremor-canceling microsurgical instrument. IEEE/ASME Trans Mechatron. 2015;20(2):761–72.
16. Gonenc B, Chae J, Gehlbach P, Taylor RH, Iordachita I. Towards robot-assisted retinal vein cannulation: a motorized force-sensing microneedle integrated with a handheld micromanipulator. Sensors. 2017;17(10):2195.
17. Joos KM, Shen J-H. Miniature real-time intraoperative forward-imaging optical coherence tomography probe. Biomed Opt Express. 2013;4(8):1342–50.
18. Yu H, et al. Design, calibration and preliminary testing of a robotic telemanipulator for OCT guided retinal surgery. In: Robotics and automation (ICRA), 2013 IEEE international conference on. IEEE; 2013.
19. Yu H, et al. Evaluation of microsurgical tasks with OCT-guided and/or robot-assisted ophthalmic forceps. Biomed Opt Express. 2015;6(2):457–72.
20. Yu H, et al. Calibration and integration of b-mode optical coherence tomography for assistive control in robotic microsurgery. Trans Mechatron. 2016;21(6):2613–23.
21. Gijbels A, Vander Poorten EB, Stalmans P, Van Brussel H, Reynaerts D. Design of a teleoperated robotic system for retinal surgery. In: Robotics and automation (ICRA), 2014 IEEE international conference on. IEEE; 2014. p. 2357–63.
22. Gijbels A, Smits J, Schoevaerdts L, Willekens K, Vander Poorten EB, Stalmans P, Reynaerts D. In-human robot-assisted retinal vein cannulation, a world first. Ann Biomed Eng. 2018;46(10):1676–85.
23. Willekens K, Gijbels A, Schoevaerdts L, Esteveny L, Janssens T, Jonckx B, Feyen JHM, et al. Robot-assisted retinal vein cannulation in an in vivo porcine retinal vein occlusion model. Acta Ophthalmol. 2017;95(3):270–5.
24. Nasseri MA, et al. The introduction of a new robot for assistance in ophthalmic surgery. In: 2013 35th annual international conference of the IEEE engineering in medicine and biology society (EMBC). IEEE; 2013.
25. Nasseri MA, et al. Virtual fixture control of a hybrid parallel-serial robot for assisting ophthalmic surgery: an experimental study. In: 5th IEEE RAS/EMBS international conference on biomedical robotics and biomechatronics. IEEE; 2014.
26. Barthel A, et al. Haptic interface for robot-assisted ophthalmic surgery. In: Engineering in medicine and biology society (EMBC), 2015 37th annual international conference of the IEEE. IEEE; 2015.
27. de Smet MD, et al. Release of experimental retinal vein occlusions by direct intraluminal injection of ocriplasmin. Br J Ophthalmol. 2016;100(12):1742–6.
28. Edwards TL, et al. First-in-human study of the safety and viability of intraocular robotic surgery. Nat Biomed Eng. 2018;2(9):649–56.
29. Rahimy E, Wilson J, Tsao TC, Schwartz S, Hubschman JP. Robot-assisted intraocular surgery: development of the IRISS and feasibility studies in an animal model. Eye. 2013;27(8):972–8. https://doi.org/10.1038/eye.2013.105.
30. Wilson JT, et al. Intraocular robotic interventional surgical system (IRISS): mechanical design, evaluation, and master–slave manipulation. Int J Med Robot Comput Assist Surg. 2018;14(1):e1842. https://doi.org/10.1002/rcs.1842.
31. Chen C-W, et al. Intraocular robotic interventional surgical system (IRISS): semi-automated OCT-guided cataract removal. Int J Med Robot Comput Assist Surg. 2018;14(6):e1949. https://doi.org/10.1002/rcs.1949.

Tamponading Agents in Vitreoretinal Surgery

11

Astha Jain, Thirumalesh MB, and Jivitesh Singh

11.1 Introduction

Tamponading agents close the retinal break and keep the neurosensory retina opposed to the RPE whilst retinopexy heals. The surface tension of the tamponading agents helps to seal the retinal break and prevents fluid from moving into the sub-retinal space till the retinopexy forms a permanent barrier. Ohm was the first to introduce air into the vitreous cavity although he did not use the word "tamponade" [1]. Rosengren was the first to use the word "tamponade" and reported successful treatment of retinal detachment with air. Tamponading agents can be divided into liquids and gases [2].

11.2 Physical Properties of Tamponading Agents

The tamponade effect of the vitreous substitutes depends on the arc of contact between the agent and the inner retinal surface, which mainly depends on four physical parameters, namely, specific gravity, buoyancy, interfacial tension, and viscosity [3].

A. Jain (✉)
Aditya Jyot Foundation for Twinkling Little Eyes, Mumbai, India

Aditya Jyot Eye Hospital, Mumbai, India

T. MP · J. Singh
Narayana Nethralaya, Bengaluru, India

A. Jain et al. (eds.), *Cutting-edge Vitreoretinal Surgery*,
https://doi.org/10.1007/978-981-33-4168-5_11

Specific Gravity The specific gravity of the aqueous and vitreous humour is slightly more than water. The specific gravity for any tamponading agent should be less than water to allow it to float in the vitreous cavity.

Buoyancy Buoyancy is the force that keeps any object afloat. Archimedes principle states that any object, wholly or partially immersed in a fluid, is pushed up by a force that is equal to the weight of the fluid displaced by the object. The buoyancy of intraocular gas is more than that of silicone oil as its specific gravity is much less than water. The buoyancy is maximum at the apex of the bubble.

Interfacial Tension When two immiscible agents are used, the interaction that occurs at the surface of the substance is called interfacial tension. A substance with higher interfacial tension tends to remain as a single large bubble with minimal dispersion. Gases have higher interfacial tension compared to liquids such as PFCL and silicone oil.

Viscosity Viscosity of a fluid is defined as resistance to deformation. The lesser the viscosity, the lower is the energy required to deform a large bubble into small droplets. Silicone oil has high viscosity ranging from 1000Ccs to 5000cs preventing its dispersion into small bubbles.

11.3 Types of Tamponading Agents

Tamponading agents can be gaseous or liquid. Commonly used gaseous agents include air, sulphur hexafluoride, and perfluoropropane. Liquid agents include silicone oil which is lighter than water. Perfluorocarbon liquids and heavy silicone oil are liquid tamponading agents which are heavier than water. The gas/water interface surface tension is the greatest and therefore is the most effective in closing retinal breaks (70 erg/cm^2). This is followed by silicone oil/water interface surface tension (50 erg/cm^2) [4].

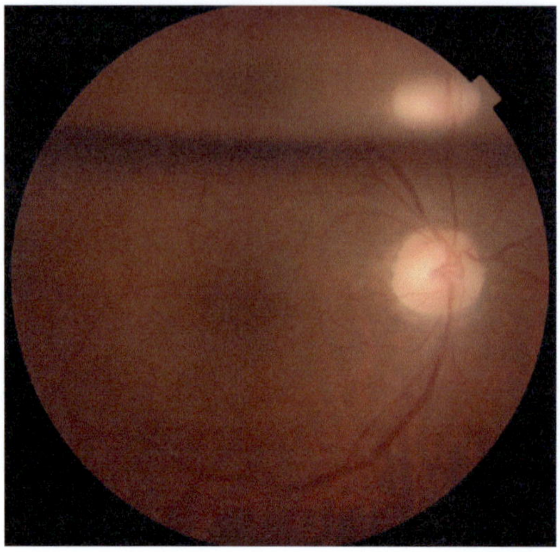

Fig. 11.1 Fundus image of the right eye showing partial gas fill following pars plana vitrectomy

11.4 Gaseous Tamponading Agents

11.4.1 Kinetics of Intraocular Gases

Air Air is colourless, inert, non-expansile, and short-acting gas. It remains in the eyes for a few days and is then replaced by aqueous humour. Air has been successfully used as a tamponading agent in the repair of primary retinal detachment with superior breaks [3]. Superior breaks are isolated from SRF due to gravity and hence retina RPE adhesions form early. Therefore, short-acting tamponade such as air is useful as it leads to early visual recovery. Inferior breaks have also been treated with air if SRF is drained completely [4].

Other Gases Sulphur hexafluoride (SF6) and perfluoropropane (C3F8) are the commonly used gases. C2F6 is also used less commonly. These gases are heavier than air. One hundred percent SF6 doubles in volume in 2 days and is completely absorbed in 10–14 days. Hundred percent C3F8 quadruples in volume in 3 days and lasts for 30–45 days. The gas bubble goes through the phases of expansion, equilibrium, and dissolution. The expansion is due to absorption of nitrogen, oxygen, and carbon dioxide from the surrounding fluid into the bubble. In the equilibrium phase, the diffusion of nitrogen into the bubble is balanced by diffusion of gas into the surrounding fluid. During the dissolution state, gas is ultimately absorbed in the bloodstream [5]. A small volume of pure gas is used in pneumatic retinopexy. Non-expansile air gas mixtures are used as tamponade after vitrectomy. Twenty percent SF6, 14% C3F8, and 16% C2F6 are commonly used to fill the vitreous cavity after vitrectomy (Fig. 11.1).

11.4.2 Preparation of Gas for Injection

A millipore filter is used to maintain the sterility of the gas. A 50-mL syringe is usually used to withdraw gas from the cylinder. The gas is diluted with air to achieve the appropriate concentration of the gas. In cases of pneumatic retinopexy where pure expansile gas is required, a pressure reducing system can be attached to the gas cylinder to withdraw the gas. The gas should not be left in the syringe for long periods as the gas concentration may get altered due to diffusion of gases. For injecting gas after vitrectomy, fluid–air exchange is first performed. Air is then replaced by the desired gas. Infusion is stopped by applying a clamp to the infusion cannula. Gas syringe is then connected to the infusion line, the clamp removed and around 40 mL of gas is slowly injected to replace air.

11.4.3 Contraindication

Air Travel Reduced atmospheric pressure during air travel can lead to expansion of intraocular gas bubble and increase in intraocular pressure. This can lead to pain, decreased vision, vascular occlusion, and in extreme cases wound dehiscence and globe rupture. It is therefore advisable to avoid air travel if there is any intravitreal gas bubble.

Diving During diving, the hyperbaric pressure causes the intraocular gas bubble to decrease in size according to Boyle's law. During the ascent back to the water surface, atmospheric pressure decreases causing expansion of the gas bubble, which can result in vitreous, retinal, or choroidal haemorrhage [6].

Nitrous Oxide Anaesthesia Nitrous oxide in the blood is highly water soluble. It can enter the intraocular gas bubble and lead to increased intraocular pressure. Later when the nitrous oxide returns to the bloodstream, the eye becomes hypotonous. Therefore, nitrous oxide should be discontinued at least 30 min before the injection of intraocular gas to allow its clearance from the bloodstream. Also, the use of nitrous oxide anaesthesia in gas-filled eyes must be avoided.

11.4.4 Complications

Increase in Intraocular Pressure It is one of the most common complications of intraocular gas. It is usually transient due to gas expansion and can be managed by topical and systemic medications. Elevated IOP is more dangerous in eyes with pre-existing optic nerve damage. The gas bubble may expand to push the lens iris diaphragm forward which can lead to angle-closure glaucoma. Gas aspiration from the vitreous cavity may be indicated in such cases. Aphakic eyes are more prone to this complication as the iris can easily move forward.

Cataract Oxidative stress following vitrectomy can lead to cataract. Prolonged contact of intraocular gas with the posterior surface of the lens leads to posterior subcapsular cataract. Poor compliance with post-operative positioning can lead to early development of cataracts.

Gas Migration Gas can migrate into the subconjunctival space, anterior chamber, or sub-retinal space. Subconjunctival migration can occur due to inadequate sclerotomy closure. In most cases no treatment is required. Anterior chamber gas migration can occur even in phakic eyes without any zonular weakness. Intraoperative migration of gas in AC can lead to poor visualization of the posterior segment. Ophthalmic viscoelastic substances can be inserted into AC to remove gas. Long-term presence of gas in AC can lead to corneal decompensation. This is due to decreased endothelial nutrition due to direct contact between the gas and the endothelium. Gas is not directly endotheliotoxic [7]. Sub-retinal migration of gas can occur during fluid–air exchange if the traction on the retina is not adequately relieved. During pneumatic retinopexy, subretinal gas migration can occur if there is fish egging of the gas bubble.

11.5 Silicone Oil

Silicone oil was introduced by Cibis for use as intraocular tamponade [8]. They are particularly useful in cases that require a longer duration of tamponade.

11.5.1 Chemical Property

Silicone oils are hydrophobic polymers of silicone–oxygen bonds called organosiloxane with a variety of side chains. The chemical and physical properties of the silicone oil depend upon the molecular weight, the length of the linear chain, and the chemical structure of the side group. Viscosity of the silicone oil is expressed in centistokes. Increase in the polymer chain length increases the molecular weight of the oil thus increasing its viscosity. Silicone oil that is currently in use has viscosity ranging from 1000cs to 5000cs. Increase in the viscosity of silicone oil lessens the emulsification [9]. The radical side groups determine whether the silicone oil is heavier or lighter than water. The most commonly used silicone oil is polydimethylsiloxane which is lighter than water.

11.5.2 Physical Property

Silicone oil has a buoyant force as the specific gravity of silicone oil (around 0.97) is less than the aqueous and the vitreous humour. This upward force helps in maintaining the reattachment of the superior retina if the traction is adequately relieved. The presence of silicone oil close to the retina can also cause redirection of radial forces to tangential forces, which in turn are less effective. As the posterior retinal surface is covered by only a thin layer of aqueous, the intraocular fluid currents are inadequate to cause retinal redetachment unless the traction is significant [10]. There is always an inferior space filled with vitreous fluid as silicone oil cannot completely fill the eye. This inferior fluid with restricted movement can gradually accumulate proteins and lead to perisilicone proliferation.

The surface tension is responsible to maintain the shape of the bubble, prevent its migration through the retinal hole, and prevent any emulsification. Presence of surgical debris such as blood, viscoelastic solution, lipid, proteins etc. tend to decrease the surface tension and lead to early emulsification. Silicone oil emulsification increases the risk of PVR, retinal redetachment, keratopathy, and secondary glaucoma. Increasing the viscosity decreases the rate of emulsification. However, it has been shown that there is no difference in emulsification between 1000cs and 5000cs oil [11]. This is because apart from viscosity, other factors affect the rate of emulsification, which are content of impurities or low molecular weight siloxane, and absorption of various biological fluids such as blood, protein, lipids etc. Emulsification of silicone oil is also time dependent and most cases emulsify within 1 year [12]. Movement of silicone oil can lead to shear forces which can cause early emulsification. A more complete fill of silicone oil decreases the rate of emulsification.

11.5.3 Indications for Using Silicone Oil

Retinal Detachment Silicone oil is the tamponading agent of choice in cases of RD with PVR, viral retinitis, giant retinal tear, and choroidal coloboma and in chronic uveitis with hypotony [13].

RD with PVR The silicone study group was a randomized multicentre trial to compare silicone oil with long-acting gas (SF6 or C3F8) as the tamponading agent for the management of RD with PVR [14–18]. It was found that silicone oil performed better than SF6 with visual acuity better than 5/200 and attached macula. However, C3F8 had similar results as that of silicone oil. Even in eyes needing relaxing retinotomy, silicone oil was found to be as effective as C3F8. Complications related to IOP and corneal abnormalities were found to be similar to oil and C3F8. Silicone oil is the tamponade of choice in cases of severe anterior PVR, difficulty in postoperative positioning, cases of redetachment, hypotony, and in one-eyed patients for early visual recovery.

Proliferative Diabetic Retinopathy Use of silicone oil in PDR can cause regression of pre-existing iris neovascularisation and prevent post-operative rubeosis by compartmentalizing the eye and preventing the migration of the angiogenic factors anteriorly [19, 20]. Silicone oil can act as a diffusion barrier to oxygen and prevents the decrease in anterior chamber oxygen tension, hence decreases the stimulus for neovascularization [21]. Haemorrhage can lead to reproliferation behind silicone oil, which can be prevented by sealing all the bleeding points. In cases with attached retina with recurrent haemorrhage because of rubeosis iridis, silicone oil injection can lead to useful ambulatory vision. Sophisticated surgical technique combined with silicone oil has shown some success in eyes with very poor prognosis such as those with failed vitrectomy for PDR with advanced PVR [22].

Trauma Retinal detachment following trauma can be associated with severe PVR, retinal incarceration, choroidal detachment, vitreous haemorrhage, unstable scleral wound, and hypotony due to ciliary body detachment. In such situations, silicone oil is useful for long-term tamponade.

11.5.4 Complications with Silicone Oil

Keratopathy Corneal decompensation with bullous or band keratopathy can occur when silicone oil stays in contact with corneal endothelium for a long duration. This usually occurs when emulsified silicone oil migrates into the anterior chamber (Fig. 11.2). Even after oil removal, small oil droplets can migrate into anterior chamber and damage corneal endothelium. The Silicone Study report 7 disclosed an incidence of keratopathy of 27% at 2 years, equal to that of C_3F_8 [23].

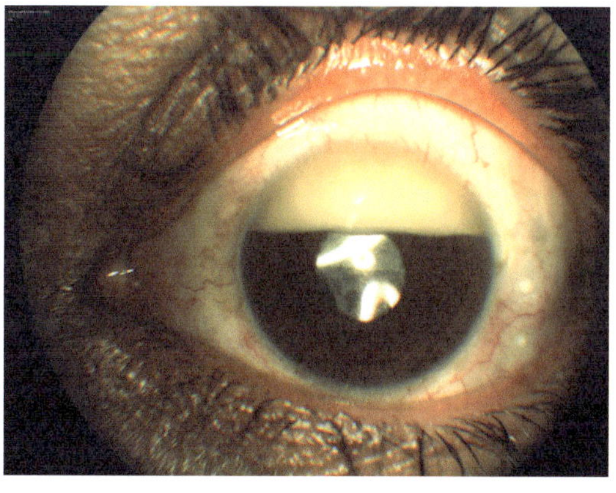

Fig. 11.2 Anterior segment image showing inverse hypopyon due to emulsified silicone oil in anterior chamber

Glaucoma The incidence of silicone oil-induced secondary glaucoma ranges from 11 to 56% [24–26]. In the early postoperative period, the rise in IOP could be due to silicone oil overfill or pupillary block glaucoma. Pupillary block glaucoma is more common in aphakic eyes and is relieved by performing an inferior iridotomy. Chronic elevation of IOP occurs when emulsified oil directly blocks the aqueous outflow through the trabecular meshwork or causes inflammatory cells to impede the outflow. The treatment consists of antiglaucoma medications, topical or periocular steroids, and removal of silicone oil with the removal of oil droplets from the anterior chamber. IOP elevation may persist even after removal of oil as remaining small oil droplets or persistent inflammation may continue to obstruct the trabecular outflow or damage to the trabecular meshwork may be permanent. Glaucoma drainage devices may be used to treat such refractory glaucoma.

Silicone Oil Infiltration of Retina and Optic Nerve Intraretinal oil droplets have been identified using OCT after macular hole surgery with internal limiting membrane (ILM) peel and silicone oil tamponade. The proposed mechanism is an iatrogenic defects in the ILM that may increase the ability of emulsified oil to penetrate retinal tissue [27]. Silicone oil infiltration of the optic nerve has been reported in another study using swept-source OCT, which showed multiple hyper-reflective spaces within the prelaminar optic nerve head and has been confirmed by adaptive optics [28]. Histopathological evidence of silicone oil invasion of the optic nerve has been shown in a patient who underwent RD repair after trauma.

Silicone Oil Adherence to Intraocular Lens (IOL) Silicone oil most significantly adheres to silicone IOL. Small droplets may adhere to the IOL even after removal of silicone oil. This may result in visual disturbances. Simple irrigation of IOL may be partially affective in removing these droplets. Silicone oil may interact with the silicone IOL causing a permanent alteration on its surface.

11.5.5 Silicone Oil Removal

The optimal timing of silicone oil removal is controversial. Removal has been recommended as early as 2 months [29]. Anatomically successfully treated eyes have a likelihood of improved visual acuity after silicone oil removal [30]. The main complication associated with silicone oil removal is retinal redetachment and hypotony. The rate of retinal redetachment varies from 0 to 32% [25]. The duration of silicone oil tamponade does not affect the rate of redetachment [30]. Prophylactic 360-degree laser retinopexy and encircling reduces the incidence of redetachment after oil removal.

11.6 Heavy Silicone Oil

Densiron® 68 and Oxane HD are the available heavy silicone oils. Densiron® 68 (Fluoron Co, Neu-Ulm, Germany) is a solution of perfluorohexyloctane (F6H8) and 5000 cSt silicone oil, characterized by an increased viscosity of F6H8 (from 2.5 to 1387 mPa) and a resulting reduction of the tendency to disperse [31]. Oxane HD is a mixture of 5700-centistoke silicone oil and RMN-3 (a partially fluorinated olefin) with a viscosity of 3300-3500 mPa [32]. The buoyancy pressure in the upper retina with conventional silicone oil was calculated at only 0.05 mmHg. In an eye filled with Densiron, the added pressure (calculation with a specific gravity of 1.06 g/cm^3) is approximately 0.1 mmHg [33].

In severe PVR, especially in cases with previous multiple vitreous surgeries and tenacious RD of the inferior quadrants, there is a high chance of redetachment. Owing to the lighter-than-water density of silicone oil, an accumulation of proliferative cells and mediators, uncovered retinal breaks, and areas of unsupported retina may exist inferiorly in eyes in a slight under-filled situation, which might cause recurrent or persistent retinal detachment. Heavy silicone oil can be a therapeutic option in patients with complex inferior retinal redetachment with PVR. As the density is more than water, it is effective in tamponading the inferior retina.

11.6.1 Complications and Adverse Reactions

Moderate inflammatory reaction with fibrin accumulation (30–40%), epiretinal membrane formation with suspected intraretinal gliosis (30%), persistent elevated IOP, and pseudo-hypopyon due to emulsification of silicone oil are the most common adverse effects seen in one of the studies where Densiron was used. The early emulsification and pseudo hypopyon formation can be explained by the lesser viscosity of Densiron compared to the higher viscosity of the commonly used silicone oil [34]. Redetachments within the posterior staphyloma in highly myopic patients are common during Densiron endotamponade [35].

11.7 Perfluorocarbon Liquids

Perfluorocarbon were developed as a blood substitute for their biologically inert nature and their property of transporting oxygen. The biologic compatibility led to their use as retinal tamponade. Chang et al. were first to study the use of Perfluorocarbon Liquids (PFCLs) in humans [36]. The use of PFCL in retinal surgeries became an important landmark to handle cases that were previously deemed inoperable.

11.7.1 Chemical and Physical Properties

Perfluorocarbon liquids are fully fluorinated synthetic analogues of hydrocarbons containing carbon–fluorine bonds. The straight-chain compounds C_5 to C_9 are liquids, as are most of the cyclic compounds ranging from C_5 to C_{17}. PFCLs are colourless and odourless and possess high density (1.6–2.1 specific gravity) and low viscosity (2–3 centistokes at 25 °C). PFCLs are biologically inert and stable at temperatures up to 400 °C.

PFCLs are optically clear compounds with variable refractive indices different from saline or water. This allows for easy visibility of PFCL in saline intraoperatively. The greater the difference between refractive index, more is the visibility at the interface. Perfluoro-n-octane has a more visible surface interface (refractive index 1.27 vs. 1.33 of water).

The high specific gravity as compared to water is helpful in settling detached retinas by pushing the sub-retinal fluid anteriorly and simultaneously flattening the retina. The tamponade force is higher as compared to silicon oil.

PFCLs have low surface tension and high interfacial tension. This property decreases the likelihood of sub-retinal migration of PFCL. Due to cohesive forces amongst PFCL molecules, it tends to remain in one single bubble. Also, the low viscosity of PFCL (0.8–8.03 centistokes at 25 °C) allows for easy injection and aspiration of fluid. The boiling point of PFCL is greater than water (400–500 °C).

11.7.2 Indications for Use of PFCL

Retinal Detachment with Proliferative Vitreo-Retinopathy The high specific gravity of PFCL allows anterior displacement of sub-retinal fluid and avoids the need to create a posterior drainage retinotomy. This reduces iatrogenic retinal damage. The tamponade force of PFCL stabilizes the retina during membrane peeling. PFCLs are optically clear and do not absorb radiation at wavelengths used for laser. Photocoagulation can therefore be performed in the PFCL-flattened retina.

Giant Retinal Tear PFCL has revolutionized the way giant retinal tears with retinal detachment are treated now. Before the introduction of PFCL, patients had to be kept in a prone position and intra-ocular gas was injected to unfold the giant retinal tear. With the use of PFCL, reattachment rates are up to 90%. PFCL has advantage of gentle manipulation of the retina to unfold the tear.

Dislocated Lens and IOLs PFCL is an ideal tool to remove a spontaneous or traumatic dislocated nucleus, a posteriorly dislocated nucleus fragment or an intraocular lens after cataract extraction. A pars plana vitrectomy is performed, where all vitreous adhesions are freed from the lens or the intraocular lens. PFCL is injected beneath the lens, lens fragment, or IOL. This helps two purposes, first is to keep the lens afloat and second to prevent any damage to the retina by dropping or sudden posterior dislocation.

Ocular Trauma PFCL is helpful in managing cases of traumatic retinal detachments which are complicated by vitreous hemorrhage, traumatic cataract and choroidal hemorrhage. During vitrectomy in cases of ocular trauma, there are high chances of iatrogenic tears due to poor visibility, especially if it is complicated with vitreous haemorrhage. PFCL is injected once the cortical vitreous is cleared. PFCL flattens the posterior retina, dissects through the posterior hyaloid and clears the vitreous haemorrhage from the posterior pole.

Intraocular foreign body may be associated with ocular trauma. Management of foreign bodies becomes easier with the use of PFCL. Foreign bodies with specific gravity less than PFCL such as wooden or plastic foreign bodies can be floated anteriorly and removed.

Sub-macular Haemorrhage For removal of sub-retinal blood, one retinotomy is made near the edge of the bleed, which is away from fovea. PFCL is then injected on the posterior pole in one single bubble. PFCL gradually displaces the liquefied blood away from fovea, which is finally removed from the retinotomy site. A soft-tipped cannula can hasten this process.

PFCL as Tamponading Agent Several studies have used PFCL as a short-, medium-, and long-term tamponade. The physical features of PFCLs make them excellent vitreous substitutes for dealing with inferior retinal pathology, where common tamponades with a density lower than water, like silicone oils or gases, are not so effective.

Use of PFCL as a tamponading agent for a short duration of 6–7 days does not appear to cause any toxic effects. The reattachment rate with PFCL is reported to be high, averaging between 76% and 82% with visual acuity improvement in 50–86% of cases [37–40]. The primary reattachment rates ranged between 86% and 92% with visual acuity improvement in 69% cases when PFCLs were used as a medium-term postoperative tamponade [41–46]. A typical granulomatous inflammatory reaction with precipitates was observed on the posterior lens capsule, retina, optic nerve head, or retinal blood vessels in 28% of patients. The inflammation started between 7 and 10 days after surgery and may impair posterior segment visualization. The inflammatory reaction did not correlate with final visual acuity, retinal attachment, PVR development, or persistently high intraocular pressure.

Few studies have described the use of PFCL for long-term tamponade [47, 48]. An inflammatory reaction develops as early as the third postoperative week in all cases. A white flocculent, flake-like material on various intraocular structures is found on various intraocular structures, such as the posterior lens capsule, the pars plana, the vitreous base, the optic nerve head, and the posterior retina. PFCL also disperses and migrates into the anterior chamber causing corneal endothelial damage.

Heavy silicone oil is an approved and safe tool for treating inferior pathology. Retinal toxicity of PFCL in humans has not been ruled by means of ERG or histological examination. Therefore, PFCL as a tamponading agent should be used with caution and must be removed completely as soon as possible once the retinopexy is complete. PFCL should not be used together with silicone oil as mixing can generate a new fluid known as sticky silicone oil [49].

11.7.3 Complications

Sub-retinal PFCL Small bubbles of PFCL can easily migrate into the sub-retinal space through retinal breaks. To prevent the formation of small bubbles, one must inject PFCL slowly and submerge the tip of the cannula in the formed PFCL bubble to make one large bubble. If one injects PFCL rapidly without submerging the tip of the cannula in the formed PFCL bubble, numerous PFCL bubbles with a fish-egg appearance are easily formed. These bubbles should be removed before the surface of the PFCL reaches the height of the retinal tears. A large retinal break or large peripheral retinotomies are a risk factor for sub-retinal PFCL [50].

PFCL in the Anterior Chamber Residual PFCL in the vitreous cavity may migrate into the anterior chamber post-operatively and cause visual disturbance, corneal endothelial loss, or elevation of intraocular pressure (Fig. 11.3). The effects of PFCL in the anterior chamber depends on the amount of PFCL. High volume of PFCL can cause endothelial damage by blocking its nutrition. Corneal decompensation with the replacement of endothelium with fibrotic tissue can occur 2 weeks after anterior chamber injection [51]. PFCL less than 0.25 mL appears to induce no damage to corneal endothelium but may cause changes in the trabecular meshwork [52].

Thus, if PFCL is found in the anterior chamber, it should be removed using a small-gauge needle at the slit lamp Also, surgeons should take care to remove PFCL completely from the vitreous cavity during vitrectomy.

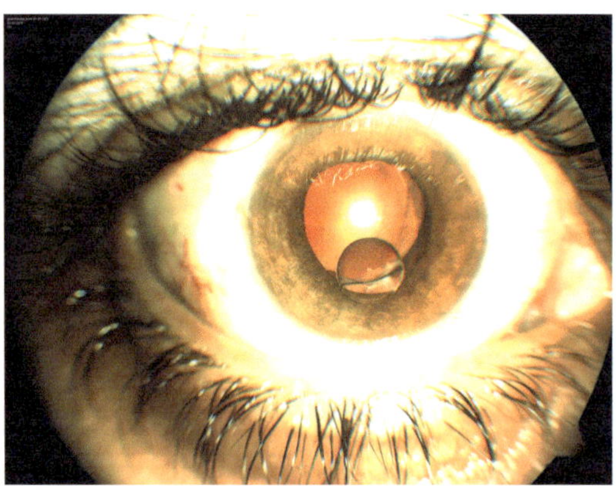

Fig. 11.3 PFCL bubble seen in the anterior chamber in a pseudophakic eye

Ocular Toxicity PFCL cannot be left in vitreous cavity for extended period because of ocular toxicity. Extended use of PFCL as tamponade can cause both chemical and mechanical toxicity. It has been observed in animal models that high specific gravity of PFCL leads to mechanical toxicity due to compression of retina underlying it. PFCL can infiltrate the internal limiting membrane and penetrate deeper through the retinal layers involving the photoreceptor nuclear layer and the outer segment layer producing morphological changes. Atrophy and loss of outer plexiform layer and atrophy of retinal pigment epithelium have been reported. PFCL was not found beyond the Bruch's membrane [53].

Chemical toxicity of PFCL is due to its polar impurities. These impurities cause adsorption of lipoproteins and proteins, causing fibroblastic reaction and formation of pre-retinal membranes. Some PFCLs like perfluorotributylamine have a higher tendency to give this reaction due to its amine group. Toxicity with Perfluoro-n-octane, a straight chain PFCL is the least as studied in rabbit models.

Effectiveness of Various Tamponading Agents The silicone study was a randomized clinical trial comparing 1000 cSt silicone oil to 20% SF6 or 14% C3F8 in cases of RD with PVR. Better anatomic and visual outcomes were reported with silicone oil vs SF_6 at 1 year. No significant differences in anatomic or visual outcomes were found between silicone oil and C_3F_8 [12, 13].

In a retrospective study comparing silicone oil vs C_3F_8 gas in the treatment of RD amongst highly myopic eyes with posterior staphyloma, C_3F_8 was associated with significantly better initial success rates and significantly better visual outcomes [54]. In another retrospective series of 56 eyes with recurrent RD associated with PVR and treated with PPV and retinectomy, silicone oil tamponade yielded significantly higher success rates than gas [55].

No significant differences in anatomical and visual success were noted between 1000 cSt and 5000 cSt silicone oil in a retrospective series of 325 eyes with complex RD [56]. Another retrospective series of 82 eyes with complex RDs reported that the use of 5000-cSt silicone oil was associated with a significantly higher rate of recurrent RD following silicone oil removal [57].

The HSO Study is an RCT comparing Densiron 68 with conventional silicone oil (either 1000 or 5000 cSt per surgeon preference) amongst patients with inferior RD associated with PVR. Forty-six patients treated with HSO were compared to 47 patients treated with standard silicone oil. The interim analysis of this study reported that, at 12 months, there were no significant differences in the anatomic success rates or visual outcomes between HSO tamponade and conventional silicone oil tamponade [58]. Neither non-inferiority nor superiority was shown with regard to final acuity.

In a case series of 12 patients, Densiron 68 was used as a primary endotamponade in patients with complex inferior retinal detachment, where standard procedures would have been unlikely to succeed. Only 4 of 12 patients (30%) showed a stable retinal re-attachment [35]. It seems that even a heavier-than-water tamponade cannot completely displace the PVR stimulating environment from the base of posterior staphyloma resulting in re-proliferation and renewing of tractional membranes.

In another case series, 49 patients affected by complex retinal re-detachment complicated with PVR were recruited. The mean follow-up was 7.6 months. The mean best-corrected visual acuity after Densiron 68 removal was 0.95 logMAR, standard error (SE: 0.068). Retinal reattachment rate was 61.2% after first surgery and 81.6% after second surgery. Nineteen cases (38.8%) had recurrences when intraocular heavy silicon oil was in situ [59].

11.8 Conclusion

Use of gas or silicone oil tamponade has led to favourable outcomes in patients with RD. PFCL is a good intraoperative tool for managing complicated scenarios effectively. Long-term use is restricted owing to its chemical and mechanical toxicity to the retina. HSO is best used in complex RD with PVR changes, especially inferior RD, which uses the physical property of high specific gravity of HSO.

References

1. Ohm J. Über die Behandlung der Netzhautablösung durch operative Entleerung der subretinalen Flüssigkeit und Einspritzung von Luft in den Glaskörper [On the treatment of retinal detachment by surgical evacuation of subretinal fluid and injection of air into the vitreous]. Albrecht Von Graefes Arch Für Ophthalmol. 1911;79(3):442–450 (in German).
2. Rosengren B. Results of treatment of detachment of the retina with diathermy and injection of air into the vitreous. Acta Ophthalmol. 1938;16(4):573–9.
3. Tan HS, Oberstein SYL, Mura M, Bijl HM. Air versus gas tamponade in retinal detachment surgery. Br J Ophthalmol. 2013;97:80–2.
4. Martínez-Castillo V, Verdugo A, Boixadera A, García-Arumí J, Corcóstegui B. Management of inferior breaks in pseudophakic rhegmatogenous retinal detachment with pars plana vitrectomy and air. Arch Ophthalmol. 2005;123:1078–81.
5. Mohamed S, Lai TY. Intraocular gas in vitreoretinal surgery. HK. J Ophthalmol. 2010;14(1):8–13.
6. Butler FK Jr. Diving and hyperbaric ophthalmology. Surv Ophthalmol. 1995;39:347–66.
7. Kanclerz P, Grzybowski A. Complications associated with the use of expandable gases in vitrectomy. J Ophthalmol. 2018;2018:8606494. https://doi.org/10.1155/2018/8606494.
8. Cibis PA, Becker B, Okun E, Canaan S. The use of liquid silicone in retinal detachment surgery. Arch Ophthalmol. 1962;68:590–9.
9. Crisp A, dejuan E Jr, Tiedeman J. Effect of silicone oil viscosity on emulsification. Arch Ophthalmol. 1987;105:546.
10. Saxena S, Gopal L. Fluid vitreous substitutes in vitreo retinal surgery. Curr Ophthalmol. 1996;44:191–206.
11. Scott IU, Flynn HW Jr, Murray TG, Smiddy WE, Davis JL, Feuer WJ. Outcomes of complex retinal detachment repair using 1000- versus 5000-centistoke silicone oil. Arch Ophthalmol. 2005;123(4):473–8.
12. Toklu Y, Cakmak HB, Ergun SB, Yorgun MA, Simsek S. Time course of silicone oil emulsification. Retina. 2012;32(10):2039–44.
13. Azen SP, Scott IU, Flynn HW Jr, et al. Silicone oil in the repair of complex retinal detachments: a prospective observational multicenter study. Ophthalmology. 1998;105(9):1587–97.
14. The Silicone Study Group. Vitrectomy with silicone oil or sulphur hexafluoride gas in eyes with severe proliferative vitreoretinopathy: results of a randomized clinical trial. Silicone study report 1. Arch Ophthalmol. 1992;110:770.
15. The Silicone Study Group. Vitrectomy with silicone oil or perfluoropropane gas in eyes with severe proliferative vitreoretinopathy: results of a randomized clinical trial. Silicone study report 2. Arch Ophthalmol. 1992;110:781.
16. The Silicone Study Group. Postoperative intraocular pressure abnormalities in the silicone study. Silicone study report 4. Ophthalmology. 1993;100:1629.
17. The Silicone Study Group. Relaxing retinotomy with silicone oil or long-acting gas in eyes with severe proliferative vitreoretinopathy. Silicone oil report 5. Am J Ophthalmol. 1993;116:557.
18. The Silicone Study Group. The incidence of corneal abnormalities in the silicone study. Arch Ophthalmol. 1995;113:764.
19. Brourman ND, Blumenkranz MS, Cox MS, et al. Silicone oil for treatment of severe proliferative diabetic retinopathy. Ophthalmology. 1989;96:759.
20. McCuen BW II, Rincoff JS. Silicone oil for progressive anterior ocular neovascularization after failed diabetic vitrectomy. Arch Ophthalmol. 1989;107:677.
21. De Juan E, Hardy M, Hatchell DL, et al. The effect of intraocular silicone oil on anterior chamber oxygen pressure in cats. Arch Ophthalmol. 1986;104:1063.
22. Rinkoff JS, de Juan E, McCuen BW II. Silicone oil for retinal detachment with advanced proliferative vitreoretinopathy following failed vitrectomy for proliferative diabetic retinopathy. Am J Ophthalmol. 1986;101:181.
23. Abrams GW, Azen SP, Barr CC, et al. The incidence of corneal abnormalities in the silicone study. Silicone study report 7. Arch Ophthalmol. 1995;113(6):764–9.
24. Al-Jazzaf AM, Netland PA, Charles S. Incidence and management of elevated intraocular pressure after silicone oil injection. J Glaucoma. 2005;14(1):40–6.
25. De Corral LR, Cohen SB, Peyman GA. Effect of intravitreal silicone oil on intraocular pressure. Ophthalmic Surg. 1987;18(6):446–9.
26. Honavar SG, Goyal M, Majji AB, et al. Glaucoma after pars plana vitrectomy and silicone oil injection for complicated retinal detachments. Ophthalmology. 1999;106(1):169–176, discussion 177.
27. Chung J, Spaide R. Intraretinal silicone oil vacuoles after macular hole surgery with internal limiting membrane peeling. Am J Ophthalmol. 2003;136(4):766–7.
28. Mrejen S, Sato T, Fisher Y, Spaide RF. Intraretinal and intra-optic nerve head silicone oil vacuoles using adaptive optics. Ophthalmic Surg Lasers Imaging Retina. 2014;45(1):71–3.
29. Jiang Y, Li X. The best timing of silicone oil removal. Zhonghua Yan Ke Za Zhi. 1997;33(1):39–41.
30. The Silicone Study Group. The effect of silicone oil removal. Silicone study report 6. Arch Ophthalmol. 1994;112:778.
31. Kim YK, Gunther B, Meinert H. A new, heavier-than-water silicone oil: a solution of perfluorohexyloctane in polydimethylsiloxane. Eur J Ophthalmol. 2019;15(5):627–37.
32. Prazeres J, Magalhães O Jr, Lucatto LF, Navarro RM, Moraes NS, Farah ME, Maia A, Maia M. Heavy

silicone oil as a long-term endotamponade agent for complicated retinal detachments. Biomed Res Int. 2014;2014:136031.
33. Wong D, Williams R, Stappler T, Groenewald C. What pressure is exerted on the retina by heavy tamponade agents? Graefes Arch Clin Exp Ophthalmol. 2005;243(5):474–7.
34. Sandner D, Engelmann K. First experiences with high-density silicone oil (Densiron) as an intraocular tamponade in complex retinal detachment. Graefes Arch Clin Exp Ophthalmol. 2006;244(5):609–19.
35. Sandner D, Herbrig E, Engelmann K. High-density silicone oil (Densiron) as a primary intraocular tamponade: 12-month follow up. Graefes Arch Clin Exp Ophthalmol. 2007;245(8):1097–105.
36. Chang S, Ozmert E, Zimmerman NJ. Intraoperative perfluorocarbon liquids in the management of proliferative vitreoretinopathy. Am J Ophthalmol. 1988;106(6):668–74.
37. Drury B, Bourke RD. Short-term intraocular tamponade with perfluorocarbon heavy liquid. Br J Ophthalmol. 2011;95(5):694–8.
38. Suk KK, Flynn HW Jr. Management options for submacular perfluorocarbon liquid. Ophthalmic Surg Lasers Imaging. 2011;42(4):284–91.
39. Velikay M, Stolba U, Wedrich A, Li Y, Datlinger P, Binder S. The effect of chemical stability and purification of perfluorocarbon liquids in experimental extended-term vitreous substitution. Graefes Arch Clin Exp Ophthalmol. 1995;233(1):26–30.
40. Sirimaharaj M, Balachandran C, Chan WC, et al. Vitrectomy with short term postoperative tamponade using perfluorocarbon liquid for giant retinal tears. Br J Ophthalmol. 2005;89(9):1176–9.
41. Sigler EJ, Randolph JC, Calzada JI, Charles S. 25-gauge pars plana vitrectomy with medium-term postoperative perfluorotamponade for inferior retinal detachment. Ophthalmic Surg Lasers Imaging Retina. 2013;44:34–40.
42. Sigler EJ, Randolph JC, Calzada JI, Charles S. Pars plana vitrectomy with medium-term postoperative perfluoro-n-octane for recurrent inferior retinal detachment complicated with advanced proliferative vitreoretinopathy. Retina. 2013;33:791–7.
43. Sigler EJ, Randolph JC, Charles S. Foreign body response within postoperative perfluoro-n-octane for retinal detachment repair. Retina. 2014;34(2):237–46.
44. Rofail M, Lee LR. Perfluoro-n-octane as a postoperative vitreoretinal tamponade in the management of giant retinal tears. Retina. 2005;25(7):897–901.
45. Rush R, Sheth S, Surka S, Ho I, Gregory-Roberts J. Postoperative perfluoro-n-octane tamponade for primary retinal detachment repair. Retina. 2012;32:1114–20.
46. Singh J, Ramaesh K, Wharton SB, Cormack G, Chawla HB. Perfluorodecalin-induced intravitreal inflammation. Retina. 2001;21(3):247–51.
47. Kirchhof B, Wong D, van Meurs J, et al. Use of perfluorohexyloctane as a long-term internal tamponade agent in complicated retinal detachment surgery. Am J Ophthalmol. 2002;133(1):95–101.
48. Kertes PJ, Wafapoor H, Peyman GA, Calixto N Jr, Thompson H. The management of giant retinal tears using perfluoroperhydrophenanthrene. A multicenter case series. Vitreon collaborative study group. Ophthalmology. 1997;104(7):1159–65.
49. Romano MR, Vallejo-Garcia JL, Parmeggiani F, Vito R, Vinciguerra P. Interaction between perfluorcarbon liquid and heavy silicone oil: risk factor for "sticky oil" formation. Curr Eye Res. 2014;32(2):212.
50. Garcia-Valenzuela E, Ito Y, Abrams GW. Risk factors for retention of subretinal perfluorocarbon liquid in vitreoretinal surgery. Retina. 2004;24(5):746–52.
51. Stolba U, Krepler K, Velikay M, Binder S. Anterior segment changes in rabbits after experimental aqueous replacement with various amounts of different perfluorocarbon liquids. Graefes Arch Clin Exp Ophthalmol. 1999;237(6):501–7.
52. Moreira H, de Queiroz JM Jr, Liggett PE, McDonnell PJ. Corneal toxicity study of two perfluorocarbon liquids in rabbit eyes. Cornea. 1992;11(5):376–9.
53. Figueroa MS, Casas DR. Inflammation induced by perfluorocarbon liquid: intra- and postoperative use. Biomed Res Int. 2014;2014:907816. https://doi.org/10.1155/2014/907816.
54. Mancino R, Ciuffoletti E, Martucci A, et al. Anatomical and functional results of macular hole retinal detachment surgery in patients with high myopia and posterior staphyloma treated with perfluoropropane gas or silicone oil. Retina. 2013;33:586–92.
55. Quiram PA, Gonzales CR, Hu W, et al. Outcomes of vitrectomy with inferior retinectomy in patients with recurrent rhegmatogenous retinal detachments and proliferative vitreoretinopathy. Ophthalmology. 2006;113:2041–7.
56. Scott IU, Flynn HW Jr, Murray TG, Smiddy WE, Davis JL, Feuer WJ. Outcomes of complex retinal detachment repair using 1000- vs 5000-centistoke silicone oil. Arch Ophthalmol. 2005;123:473–8.
57. Soheilian M, Mazareei M, Mohammadpour M, Rahmani B. Comparison of silicon oil removal with various viscosities after complex retinal detachment surgery. BMC Ophthalmol. 2006;6:21.
58. Joussen AM, Rizzo S, Kirchhof B, Schrage N, Li X, Lente C, et al. Heavy silicone oil versus standard silicone oil in as vitreous tamponade in inferior PVR (HSO Study): interim analysis. Acta Ophthalmol. 2011;89(6):e483–9.
59. Caporossi T, Franco F, Finocchio L, Barca F, Giansanti F, Tartaro R, et al. Densiron 68 heavy silicone oil in the management of inferior retinal detachment recurrence: analysis on functional and anatomical outcomes and complications. Int J Ophthalmol. 2019;12(4):615–20.

Part IV

Retinal Detachment: Surgical Techniques

Scleral Buckling and Management of Retinal Dialysis

12

Kim Ramasamy, K. Naresh Babu, Piyush Kohli, and B. Dhipak Arthur

12.1 Introduction

Rhegmatogenous retinal detachment (RRD) is characterized by separation of neurosensory retina (NSR) from the underlying retinal pigment epithelium (RPE) and is caused by a full-thickness retinal break. The two most common surgical approaches for the treatment of RRD are scleral buckling (SB) and pars plana vitrectomy (PPV). Due to its better ergonomic, vitrectomy is gaining popularity worldwide [1–6]. Over the last decade, the number of retina training programs teaching SB has declined considerably [7]. If this dangerous trend is continued, retina specialists will forget the technique of performing buckling and it will become a lost art [1–10].

The anatomical and visual outcomes of SB surgery for the management of primary RRD are comparable to vitrectomy [1–6]. SB continues to have its own place in the armamentarium of RRD surgery. This chapter will highlight the principles, relevant surgical anatomy, nuances of the surgical technique, and intra- and postoperative complications of SB.

K. Ramasamy (✉) · K. Naresh Babu · P. Kohli
B. Dhipak Arthur
Department of Vitreoretina Services, Aravind Eye Hospital and Post Graduate Institute,
Madurai, Tamil Nadu, India
e-mail: kim@aravind.org

A. Jain et al. (eds.), *Cutting-edge Vitreoretinal Surgery*,
https://doi.org/10.1007/978-981-33-4168-5_12

12.2 History

Till the start of the twentieth century, RRD was considered an untreatable disease. In early 1900s, *Jules Gonin* single-handedly changed the landscape of RD surgery forever. He proved that retinal break(s) are the cause, and not the consequence, of RRD. Gonin then laid down the principles of RD surgery and developed the first successful surgery, "*Ignipuncture*" (Table 12.1) [7–9].

The first SB surgery was done by *Ernst Custodis* in 1949, with the help of polyviol exoplant. Later, *Lincoff* (1965) made a number of modifications to the Custodis procedure to make it similar to what is practised today [11]. These modifications included:

1. Replacing polyviol exoplant with silicon sponge
2. Developing spatula needle for safe scleral suturing
3. Replacing diathermy with cryotherapy for creating chorioretional adhesions

12.3 Preoperative Localization of Break

The success of SB surgery depends on the accurate localization of all the breaks. The more time one spends preoperatively localizing all the

Table 12.1 Principles of RD surgery and "Ignipuncture" surgery as given by Gonin

Principles of Gonin	
1	Identification and accurate localization of all retinal breaks
2	Creation of chorioretinal adhesions
3	Creation of appositional closure of retinal breaks by indentation of RPE
Ignipuncture	
1	Accurate pre- and intraoperative localization of retinal breaks
2	2–3 mm long incision in sclera beneath the retinal break (drainage sclerostomy)
3	Drainage of subretinal fluid beneath the retinal break through the drainage sclerostomy
4	Direct thermocautery of the break through the drainage sclerostomy

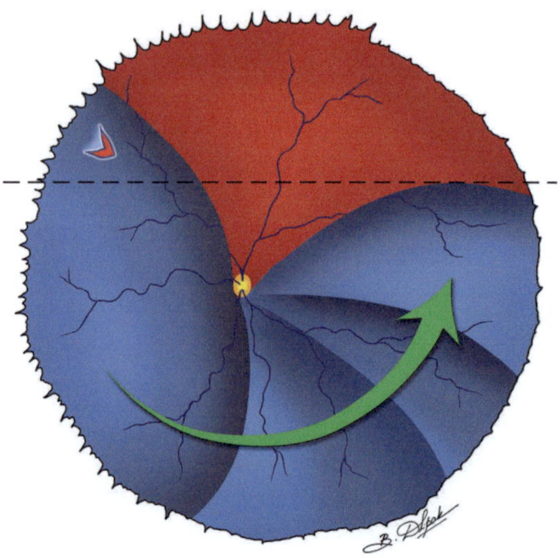

Fig. 12.1 Subretinal fluid spreads inferiorly due to gravity

breaks, lesser one struggles during the surgery. As more than 50% of the detachments have more than one break, a thorough attempt should be made to search all the breaks [12]. Any untreated break(s) can lead to failure of the surgery.

As the spread of subretinal fluid (SRF) is governed by a limited number of anatomical factors and gravity, the location of the primary break can be discerned from the topography of the detachment (Fig. 12.1). Lincoff gave a set of rules for identification of the primary break on the basis of the shape of the detachment (Fig. 12.2) [13, 14].

12.4 Relevant Surgical Anatomy

The following points must be kept in mind during the surgery:

- Ora serrata corresponds to the spiral of Tillaux (Fig. 12.3).
- Superior oblique (SO) muscle travels temporally under the superior rectus (SR) muscle and gets inserted 12–14 mm posterior to limbus. Care must be taken to prevent engaging (and damaging) SO tendon, while hooking the SR muscle (Fig. 12.4).

Fig. 12.2 Location of the primary break can be discerned from the topography of retinal detachment. Figure shows pictorial presentation of the Lincoff rules. (**a**) In case of a total bullous retinal detachment (RD), break will be from 11 to 1'o clock; (**b–d**) in case of a superior RD with detachment going beyond the horizontal meridian on one side, break will be within 1.5 clock hours from 12'o clock on that side; (**e**) in case of temporal RD, break will be within 1.5 clock hours from the highest point of RD; (**f**) in case of a superior RD with another one bullous component, the break will be at the edge of the bullous part; (**g**) in case of a shallow inferior symmetrical RD, break will be at 6'o clock; (**h**) in case of a shallow inferior RD with SRF slightly higher on one side, the break will be located inferiorly on that same side; (**i**) in case of an asymmetric inferior RD crossing the horizontal, the break will be 1.5 clock hours form the highest point of the RD; (**j**) inferior breaks can never cause a bullous RD. In case of a bullous inferior RD, the break has to be superior with fluid tracking down from the break in the periphery. If this track is not visible, the patient can be asked to lie down with head hyperextended; and (**k**) in case of high myopia with posterior staphyloma and RD localized to the posterior pole, the causative break is possibly a macular hole

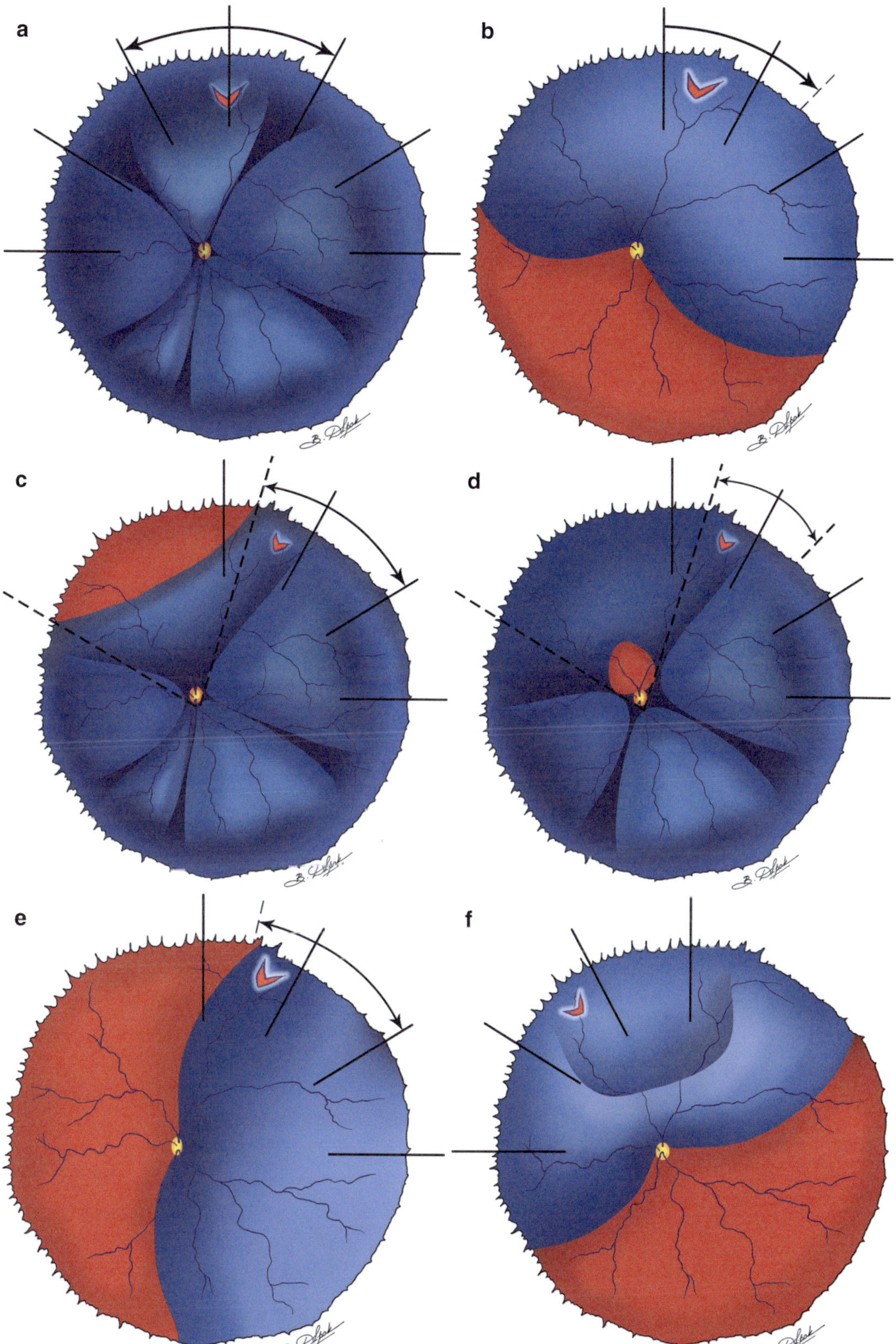

(continued)

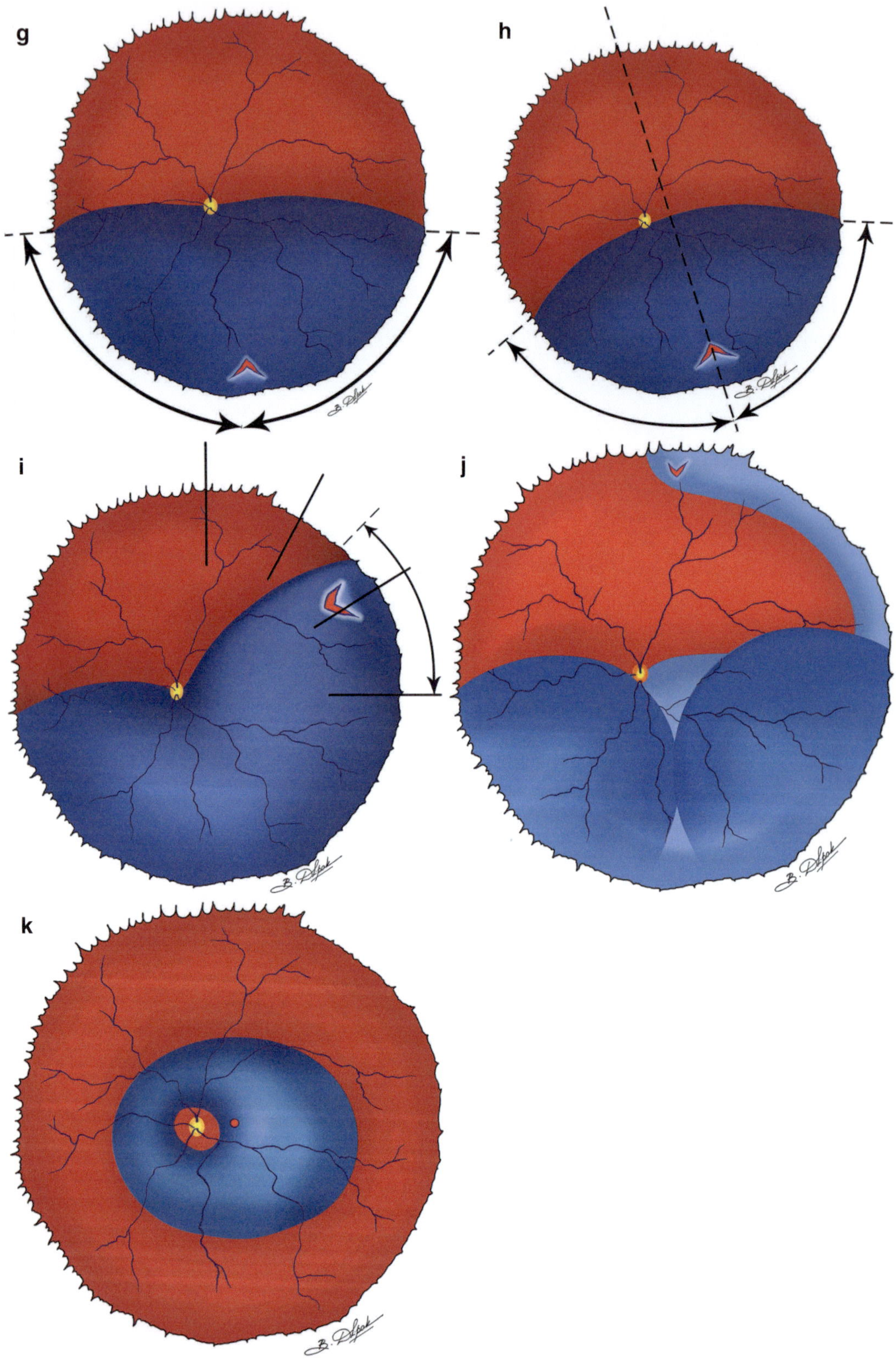

Fig. 12.2 (continued)

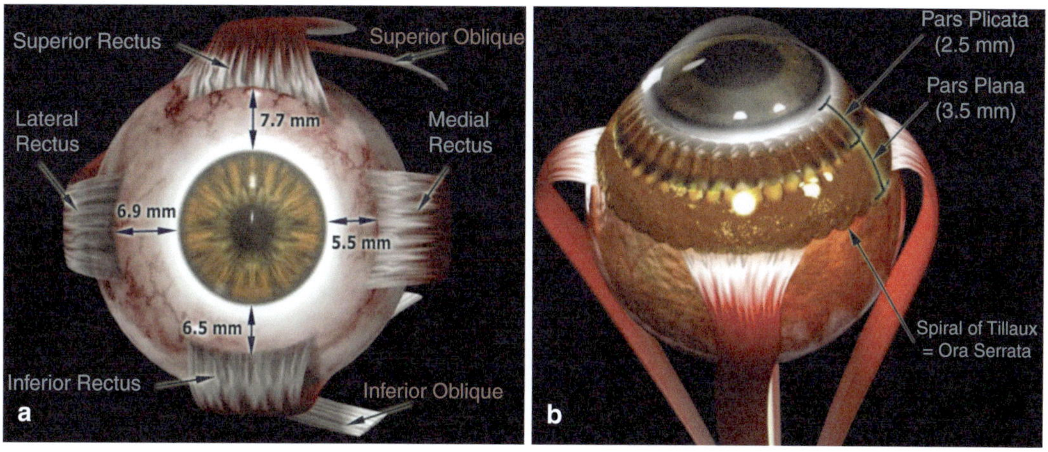

Fig. 12.3 Ora serrata corresponds to the spiral of tillaux (**a**) front view and (**b**) superior view

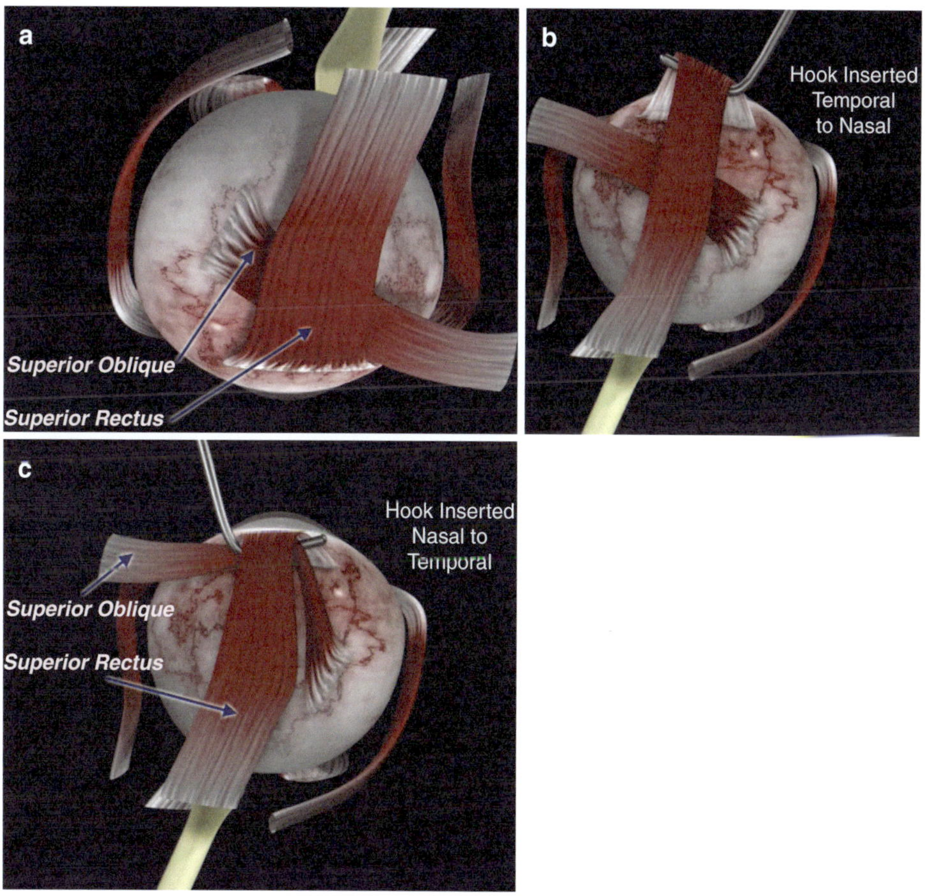

Fig. 12.4 (**a**) Superior oblique (SO) muscle gets inserted under the superior rectus (SR) muscle, (**b**) SR muscle should be hooked from temporal to nasal to avoid damaging SO muscle, and (**c**) In case SR muscle is hooked from nasal to temporal, SO muscle may also be accidentally hooked

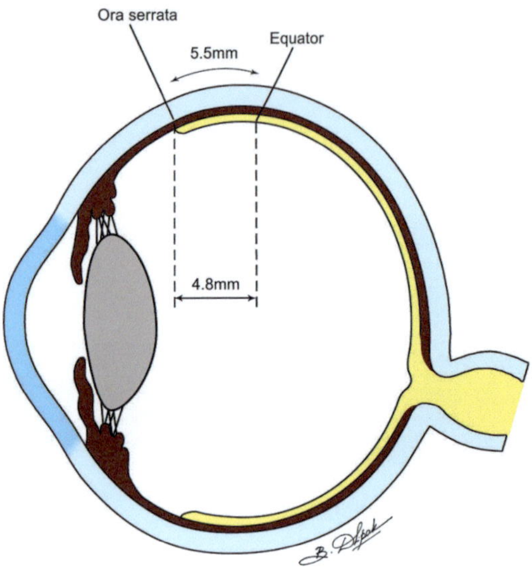

Fig. 12.5 Equator lies 5.5 mm chord length posterior to ora serrata

- Vortex veins are prone to damage while passing buckling material, suturing the explants, and during SRF drainage. There are seven vortex veins with at least one in each quadrant. Four of them exit on either side of the vertical recti at 1, 5, 7, and 11 clock hours, with the supero-temporal quadrant one (beneath the SO tendon) being the most consistent. The veins pass within sclera for 2–4 mm in posterior direction and exit 14–18 mm posterior to limbus. Great care must be taken to hook the muscles pre-equatorially, drain SRF near the horizontal recti and avoid damage to the vein's intrascleral portion during suturing.
- Vitreous base lies 2–3 mm chord length posterior to ora serrata.
- Equator lies 5.5 mm chord length posterior to ora serrata (Fig. 12.5).

12.5 Instrumentation

One needs to know about the cryotherapy machine, the various silicon buckles, and suture material.

12.5.1 Cryotherapy

Chorioretinal adhesions, for the treatment of retinal breaks, can be achieved with either diathermy, cryotherapy, or laser photocoagulation. Diathermy is produced by delivering a high-frequency (*13.56 MHz*) current through the sclera, which generates heat inside it. However, it cannot be used on intact sclera as it causes shrinkage and necrosis of sclera. It was earlier used along with implants, after scleral dissection, and is rarely used now. Laser photocoagulation requires close contact of NSR and RPE to produce adhesions and is the preferred technique for treating retinal breaks in the attached retina.

The best modality for treating retinal breaks during SB surgery is cryotherapy. It is based on Joule-Thompson principle, i.e., if gas is allowed to expand through a narrow aperture, a sudden drop in temperature is noted. This cooling effect is used to produce chorioretinal adhesions by dissolution of cellular membranes. During freezing, intracellular crystals are formed, causing mechanical injury. During thawing, water and electrolytes separate, causing a change in pH with rupture of cell membranes. Nitrous oxide is the most commonly used gas for cryotherapy. It produces a temperature of *−89 °C* when used at a pressure of *600 psi*.

The cryotherapy machine consists of a nitrous oxide cylinder (blue color), a cryoprobe, a pedal to activate the cryoprobe, and a panel for attaching the cryoprobe tubings and a gauge displaying the pressure (Fig. 12.6). Before starting the surgery, the surgeon should always ensure that adequate pressure is being built.

12.5.2 Silicon Buckles

The buckles can be used as either explants or implants. The latter can be placed inside a partial-thickness scleral tunnel made after partially dissecting the overlying sclera. As they are not used now, only exoplants will be described in this chapter.

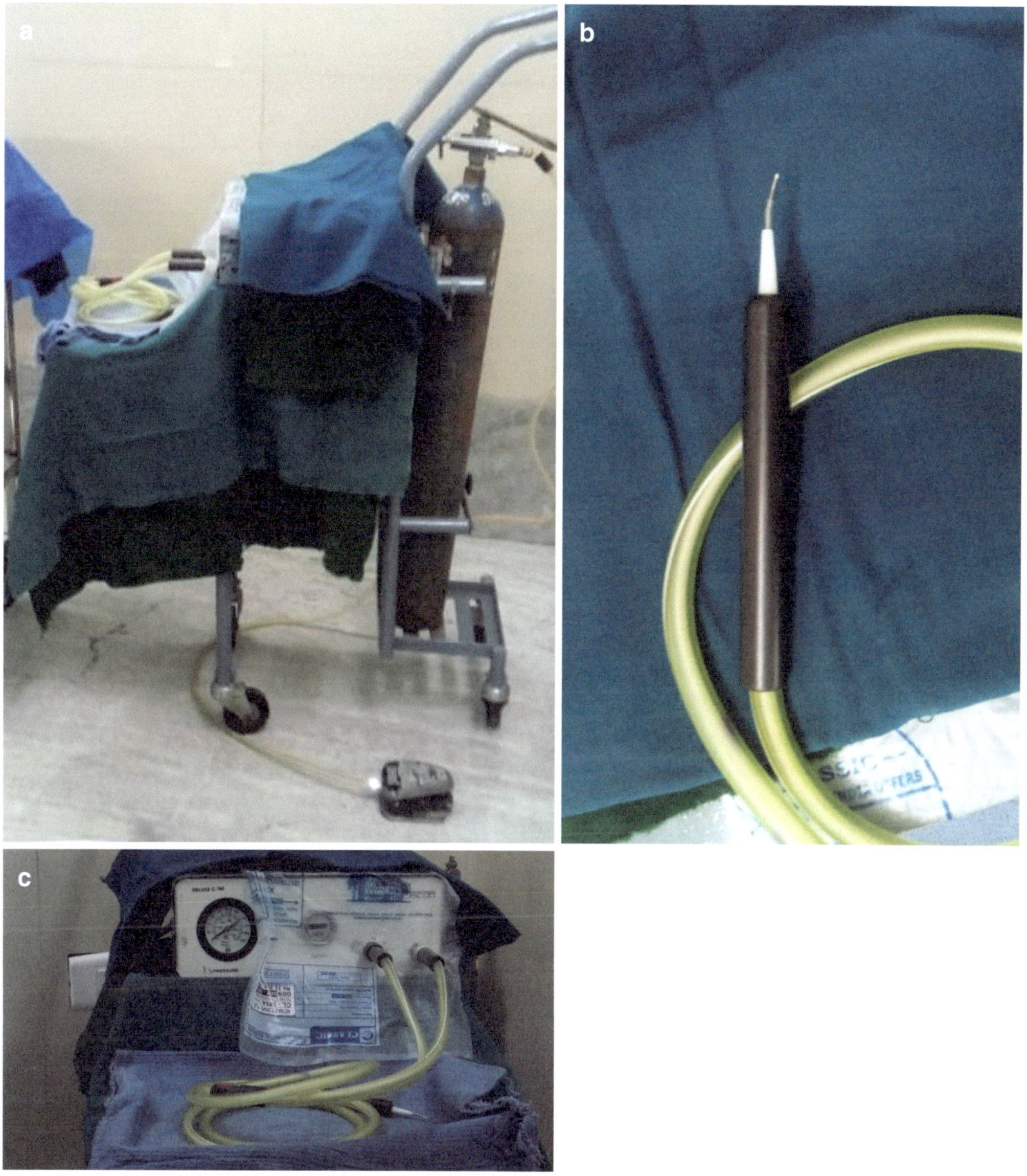

Fig. 12.6 (**a**) The cryotherapy machine consists of a nitrous oxide cylinder (blue color); (**b**) a cryoprobe (note the sleeve on the cryoprobe), a pedal to activate the cryoprobe; and (**c**) a panel for attaching the cryoprobe tubings and a gauge displaying the pressure

The exoplants currently used are made up of modified, cross-linked polydimethyl-silioxane. The advantages of this material include water insolubility, low toxicity, high elasticity, and biological inactivity, i.e., it neither supports bacterial growth nor is carcinogenic. The explants can be either solid or sponge, with the latter containing closed air cells. Although the air cells do not interconnect with each other, they are exposed to the surface in case the sponges are cut open. These open or connected pores may absorb fluid and harbor bacteria, causing infection.

Table 12.2 Type of exoplants

Type	Number	Use
Bands and strips	Sub 100s except 219, 220, 225, and *240*	Encirclage to support vitreous base
Implants and wedges	100s	Rarely used now
Tires	200s	Circumferential segmental buckle to support breaks
Sponges	500s	Mainly radial buckle to support breaks

The exoplants can be classified into four types (Table 12.2). The band and strips are used for 360-degree encirclage, mainly to support the vitreous base. Most commonly used bands are 240 band (2.5 mm width, 0.6 mm height) and 42 band (4.0 mm width, 1.25 mm height). The 240 band is flat on both sides and can be used either way. However, 42 band has one side flat (shiny looking) and other side convex (dull looking) and is sutured with flat side toward the sclera.

The tires have radii of curvature similar to that of the globe and are used to support the break(s). Their one side is grooved while the other side can be either concave or convex. The groove has a width of 2.5 mm, enabling 240 band to fit in. The convex ones (286 is most commonly used) are used for retinal dialysis as the convex curvature supports the vitreous base. The concave ones can either be symmetrical (groove passed through center of the tire) or asymmetrical (groove does not pass through center of the tire). Asymmetrical tires are placed such that the long, slender side goes under the muscle (anterior) so as to decrease the chances of anterior segment ischemia; and the short, hefty side supports the break (posterior) so as to give a higher buckle indent. While symmetrical ones are used to support lattices and atrophic holes, asymmetrical ones are used for supporting horse-shoe tears (HST). The most commonly used symmetrical and asymmetrical tires are 277 (7 mm) and 276 (7 mm), respectively [15, 16].

The sponges are mainly used as radial explants, however, they can also be used as circumferential buckles. The cylindrical sponges are cut lengthwise to half-thickness and the convex side is sutured toward the globe so as to provide a higher indentation.

12.5.3 Sutures

5.0 polybutylate-coated braided polyester needle with a spatulated needle is used. The flat top and flat bottom of the needle ensures that it separates the scleral layers while passing. 3/8 circle needle is most commonly used. However, in case the assess is difficult, like in the case of posterior sutures, 1/2 circle needle can also be used.

12.6 Principle of Buckling

SB helps reattach the retina by counteracting the forces that initially caused it to detach. Normally, the vector forces caused by localized vitreous traction on retina at the edge of posterior vitreous detachment (PVD) are counterbalanced by retinal adherence to the eye wall. However, in case the vitreous traction exceeds the counteracting forces, a retinal tear. The eye wall indentation produced by the buckle (more in case of radial buckles) decreases this vitreous traction by decreasing its magnitude and changing its direction, thus re-establishing the equilibrium. In addition, the circumferential buckles help to decrease the traction by decreasing the diameter and circumference of the vitreous base. This effect can be understood with the help of Hook's law, which states that the force of stretch is directly proportional to the distance the spring is stretched. Circumferential buckle reduces the diameter of the vitreous cavity as well as the vitreous base, thus decreasing the transvitreal traction.

12.7 Indications

SB is best indicated in young patients with anterior breaks, absence of PVR changes, phakic eyes, high myopes, and eyes with no posterior vitreous detachment [17]. SB works the best in case of an RD caused by retinal dialysis [18–21].

Retinal dialysis is defined as a break at the junction of the retina and the pars plana, typically along the course of the ora serrata. It should be carefully distinguished from giant retinal tear (GRT) as the latter is best treated by vitrectomy. However, this topic will be dealt elsewhere.

12.8 Surgical Steps Along with Intraoperative Complication

SB needs proper preoperative planning and careful execution of all the steps. Any step gone wrong can cause the surgery to fail.

12.8.1 Anesthesia

SB can be performed under either local or general anesthesia (GA). In case of children, GA is preferred.

12.8.2 Conjunctival Peritomy

A pair of non-toothed conjunctival forceps and blunt-tipped Wescott scissor is used to perform a 360-degree peritomy. Limited peritomy can be done in case of segmental buckling. The peritomy can be done either at the limbus or 2–3 mm away from it. In case of limbal incision, two radial incisions at 3 and 9'o clock can be given to enlarge the circumference of the conjunctival opening. This will prevent its tearing during retraction while exposing the sclera. In case of the posterior incision, radial incisions are not usually necessary. Blunt-tipped Steven's tenotomy scissors are inserted in the sub-tenon's space between all the two recti in all four quadrants and spread to achieve adequate scleral exposure.

12.8.3 Muscle Bridling

All the four recti are bridled with traction sutures, in order to stabilize and move the eyeball during surgery. Muscle hook is placed on the sclera posterior to the muscle insertion, passed under the muscle in a circumferential direction, and brought anteriorly to engage the muscle. If the hook is completely under the muscle throughout its width, no resistance is felt during this maneuver. However, if resistance is being felt, it means that the hook is not in the correct plane. Applying unnecessary force will lead to splitting of the muscle. In such a case, the hook should be removed and reinserted. Great care must be taken to include full muscle (width and thickness) in the traction suture. In case only a part of the muscle is included in the traction sutures, it can rupture while pulling the sutures.

All the tenon's capsule attachment to the muscles and sclera are then stripped off completely. While bridling, medial rectus (MR) is bridled first followed by inferior rectus (IR), lateral rectus (LR), and then superior rectus (SR). In order to expose the SR tendon, the assistant has to pull both the horizontal recti downward. Care must be taken to prevent scleral perforation with the needle of suture while bridling the muscles. An *inverse suture* can be used in a tangential manner, instead of radial, to prevent muscle injury and scleral perforation. The suture is then thrown into two knots, one close to the muscle and the other away from it. The latter knot is meant for the assistant to hold and pull the muscle, while the former one provides adequate traction to the muscle during the pull. A general rule is that the horizontal muscles are pulled vertically, while the vertical muscles are pulled horizontally.

During muscle manipulations (hooking or pulling), the heart rate should constantly be monitored to look for bradycardia, due to oculocardiac reflex. In case of bradycardia, the muscles should be released instantly. If the bradycardia persists, intravenous atropine may be needed [22].

12.8.4 Inspection

After bridling all the muscles, the surgeon should always *inspect* for any scleral thinning and anomalous vortex veins. In case of extreme scleral thinning, the surgery may be converted to vitrectomy.

12.8.5 Localizing the Breaks

The success of SB surgery depends on the accurate localization and treatment of all the retinal breaks. All the retinal breaks are located and marked on the sclera with the help of gentle diathermy, heated needle head, marker pen, cryoprobe, and specially designed localizers (Gass, O'connor) (Table 12.3). In case of a bullous RD, precise anteroposterior location of the break can be difficult due to parallax effect. Hence, the scleral indentation should be started from the ora in the meridian of the break and then taken posteriorly toward the posterior margin of the break. Another technique is to drain the subretinal fluid (SRF) first, inject intravitreal air to form the globe, and then treat the retinal break. This technique was initially described by *Peyman* and is now called as D-ACE sequence (Drainage-Air, Cryo, Encirclage) [23].

12.8.6 Treating the Retinal Breaks

The cryoprobe can be either straight or curved. The *tip* of the cryoprobe should be used to treat the break. Improper technique can lead to inadvertent posterior freeze. This can be avoided by ensuring that the indentation is caused by the tip and not by the shaft. The shaft of the probe can be covered with a sleeve to prevent inadvertent cryotreatment to the adjacent areas.

Contiguous cryo-spots are given to completely surround each retinal break. Repeat freezing of the same area is avoided. Two rules of thumb for cryotherapy are:

- Treat the breaks in attached retina first
- Treat the anterior margin of break first

On applying cryotherapy, an immediate tissue reaction is seen in form of an ice ball progressively expanding outwards in every direction from the tip of the probe. Cryotherapy is continued for 2–3 seconds after a distinct whitening of the neurosensory retina is observed (Fig. 12.7). In cases of shallow RD, the cryoprobe approximates RPE to retina and both freeze simultaneously. However, in case of a bullous RD, cryo-treatment does not always reach the neurosensory retina. In such cases, an orangish hue within the indented choroid should be taken as the end point. Suspicious lesions should always be treated. In fact, a suspicious retinal break is sometimes identified after cryo-treatment. A retinal break becomes more prominent after cryo-treatment due to the resultant stark color difference, break being red and surrounding retina being white.

The tip of the cryoprobe is allowed to completely thaw before attempting withdrawal. Any attempt to remove the probe while it is still frozen can lead to choroidal hemorrhage and scleral avulsion. While moving the probe from one point to another, care must be taken not to damage the vortex veins. Cryotherapy leads to dispersion of RPE pigments, resulting in ERM formation and proliferative vitreoretinopathy (PVR) [24, 25].

Table 12.3 Technique to mark the retinal break on sclera

Type of break	Technique
Small break	Single spot in the center
Large horse-shoe tear	Three spots—One at the posterior margin and one at each of the two horn
Dialysis	Two ends and the posterior extent of the mid-point

12.8.7 Placing the Exoplants

Buckle indentation is needed to offset the traction in the areas of elevated retinal breaks only. The breaks in attached retina can be treated with cryopexy alone (Table 12.4).

Note: Options for treating RD with extensive lattices and a retinal tear

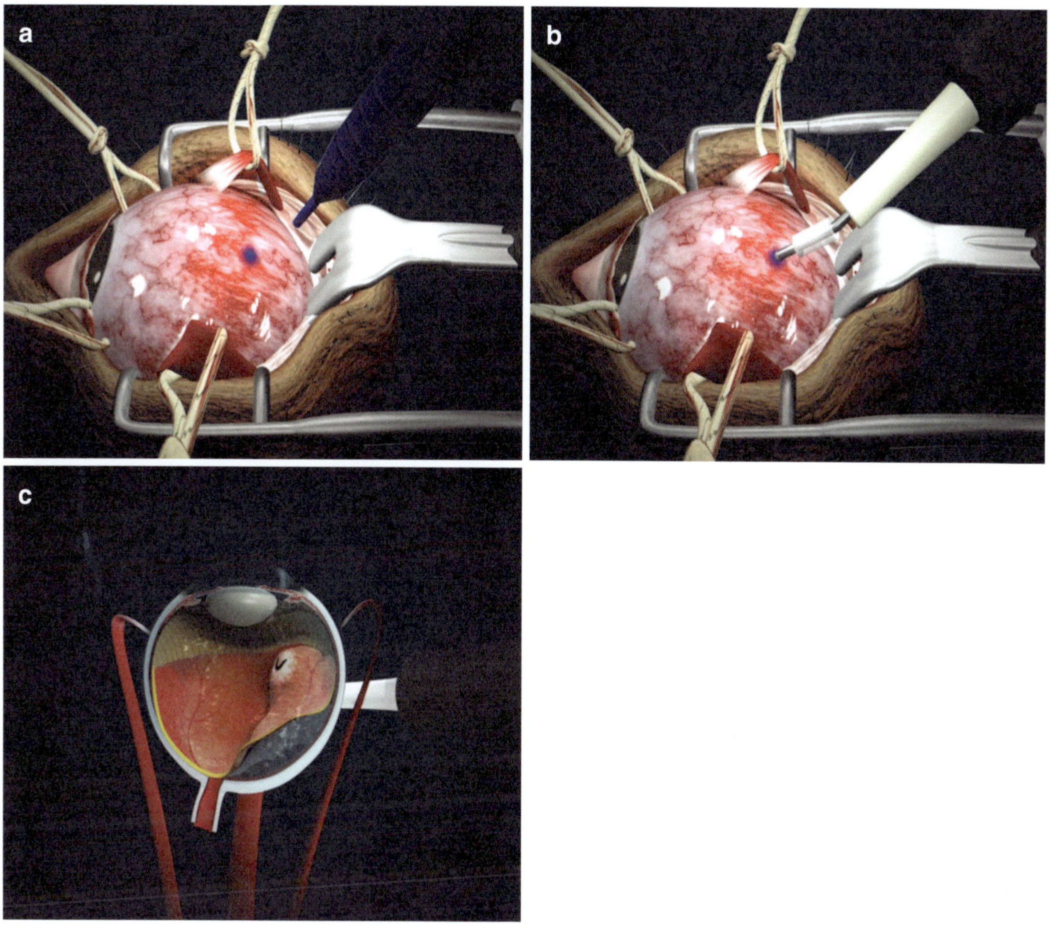

Fig. 12.7 (**a**) The break is localized and marked on the sclera, (**b**) cryotherapy is used to treat the break (note the sleeve on the cryoprobe), and (**c**) tissue reaction due to cryotherapy in form of an *ice ball progressively expanding outwards in every direction* from tip of the probe

Table 12.4 General rules for placing a buckle

Extent	Rule
Lateral	Extend explant for 30° or 1 clock hour on either side of the tear
Antero-posterior	Posterior edge of break is placed on center or anterior crest of buckle
	Extend explant 1–2 mm beyond posterior margin of break

1. Broader band (42 band) to support lattices along with a sponge to support the tear.
2. In case a tire is planned to support the break, the 2.5 mm groove on the explant can be extended with the help of a crescent knife. Extending the groove by half the width of the crescent knife on either side can widen it to the necessary width to accommodate a 4-mm band [26].

12.8.8 Suture Placement

Adequate exposure of sclera is crucial for proper suturing. The assistant has to pull the traction sutures at a widely divergent (obtuse) angle as well as retract the conjunctiva to expose posterior sclera enough to allow suturing of explants at the required place. In order to expose the supero-temporal quadrant, the SR needs to be pulled nasally and LR inferiorly. Similarly, to expose infero-nasal quadrant IR needs to be pulled temporally and MR superiorly. Any laxity on the part of the assistant can lead to scleral perforation while suturing.

Mattress sutures with an intrascleral length of 4–5 mm are placed parallel to the long axis of the explant at half the depth of sclera. The thumb rule for correct depth estimation is that the suture should be visible throughout its course in the sclera. In case there is a vortex vein in the path of the suture, the suture should be straddled into two halves to avoid injury to the vein. In case vortex vein is cut or torn, it is immediately cauterized to avoid prolonged bleeding. Such straddled sutures are useful in case of a scleral thinning and hypotonus globe also.

The technique of suturing is very important. Initially, the tip of needle is placed on sclera such that the tangent of tip is parallel (not banking) to the scleral surface. Gentle downward pressure is applied to create a small indent in sclera. The needle is then advanced keeping tangent of its tip parallel to scleral surface, till the desired depth is achieved. Once the desired depth is reached, no more downward pressure is applied. The needle is then advanced forward till adequate length is achieved. At this point, upward pressure is applied to take the suture out. However, care must be taken not to apply too much pressure posteriorly, which can cause scleral perforation with the heel of the needle (Fig. 12.8). It is better to grasp the needle at its tip and remove the needle along its curve. Once the tip is out of sclera, focus should be shifted from the tip to the heel. The entrance and exit wound should not be too shallow, else they can partially tear out under tension.

While suturing a radial explant, first bite is taken in anteroposterior direction and then in posteroanterior direction. While suturing a circumferential explant, the posterior bite is taken first followed by anterior bite. The surgeon should always work over the cornea to make adequate space for both the assistant and the surgeon. While placing inferior sutures, the posterior bite is taken in the forward direction and anterior bite in a reverse manner. While placing inferior sutures, the surgeon has to fold his/her arm such that hand faces up toward the surgeon, while the elbow faces down toward patient's feet. Then, both the bites are taken in reverse direction. The sutures can either be placed before or after passing the explants. The suture should lie never lie in between the explant and sclera as it increases the chances of scleral erosions.

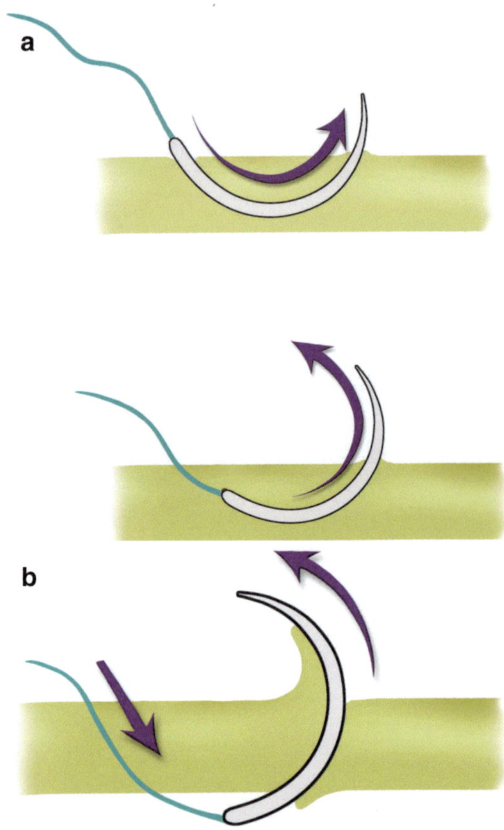

Fig. 12.8 (**a**) While taking out the needle, care must be taken not to apply too much pressure posteriorly, which can cause scleral perforation with the heel of the needle. The needle should be grasped at its tip and removed along its curve. Once the tip is out of the sclera, focus should be shifted from the tip to the heel. (**b**) In case care is not taken, the heel of the needle may cause scleral perforation

The height of buckle can be increased by:

1. Increasing the separation between the sutures: In case of a radial explant (buckle/sponge), the width of the sutures should at least 1.5 times that of the explant. For example, for a break measuring 2DD, a 5-mm sponge is used and the sutures are placed 8 mm apart. While suturing a sponge, assistant has to pull both its ends and hold tightly. Two sutures are placed on either side of the encirclage band. The posterior-most suture should be at least 3mm posterior to posterior margin of break. In case, the suture has to be placed in the far posterior sclera and it is impossible to safely pass the needle in posteroanterior direction, a

double-armed suture can be used so that both the bites can be taken in anteroposterior direction.

While placing a circumferential buckle, the anterior bite is placed at least 1-mm posterior to the muscle insertion to prevent anterior segment ischemia. For a low buckle height, the sutures are placed 2 mm wider than the buckle width, i.e., 1 mm on either side. In order to get a high buckle height, the sutures are placed 3–4 mm wider than the buckle width, i.e., 1.5–2 mm on either side. Hence, to get a high buckle height for a 276/277 circumferential tire:

- Anterior bite is placed 1 mm from muscle insertion
- Buckle is placed 1.5 mm from anterior bite (1 + 1.5 = 2.5 mm from muscle insertion)
- Posterior bite 1.5 mm from posterior margin of buckle (1 + 1.5 + 7 + 1.5 = 11 mm from muscle insertion)

  As suturing a tire alone can provide height to the buckle, segmental buckles (without encirclage) can be used for localized RD, with shallow SRF and without PVR caused by either one break or retinal dialysis or breaks limited to 1–2 clock hours [27].

2. Shortening of encirclage band: Achieving the desired height from shortening of encirclage band alone is targeted in case of a band buckle with vitrectomy. The general rule is:

- *8–10 mm* shortening for *low* buckle height
- *10–20 mm* shortening for *moderate* buckle height
- *>20 mm* shortening for *high* buckle height

One of the major complications during suture placement is scleral perforation. It should be suspected in case SRF, blood or pigments suddenly appear while suturing. In case of such an event, it is very important that the surgeon should not panic. The following protocol should be followed.

- Remove the suture.
- If SRF is being drained, do not allow the eyeball become soft, reform it by injecting saline in vitreous cavity.
- Examine the retina.
- In case of an iatrogenic break, perform cryotherapy around the break and support it by extending the buckle posteriorly.
- In case of bleeding, apply immediate pressure by pulling the traction sutures to tamponade the bleed. Position the eye so as to prevent subfoveal migration of blood.
- After managing the complication, continue suturing with extra care.
- The encirclage band is sutured ends-to-end either with the help of a Watkze sleeve or clove hitch knot (CHK). CHK can be tied and untied easily.

12.8.9 SRF Drainage

Removal of SRF brings the retinal break close to RPE and provides volume for the buckling element. The indication of SRF drainage include:

1. Bullous RD
2. Chronic RD
3. Inferior retinal breaks
4. Old patient (poor RPE function)
5. PVR changes
6. Break(s) not localized
7. High myopes and aphakic
8. Intolerance to high IOP (glaucoma)

The site selection of SRF drainage (SRFD) is very important and the following things should be kept in mind:

1. Sufficient SRF should be present.
2. Should be just above or below the horizontal meridian. Vertical muscles should be avoided to prevent injury to vortex veins.
3. Should be at or slightly anterior to equator as choroid is less vascular.
4. Nasal quadrant is preferred because in case of a subretinal bleed, it is less likely to track under macula.
5. Should be made under the explant, so that any inadvertent retinal break is automatically supported.

6. Areas treated with cryotherapy should be avoided as it causes choroidal congestion and SRFD can cause choroidal hemorrhage.
7. Areas with large break should be avoided to prevent any vitreous drainage through the drainage site.

There are two major *techniques* for SRFD.

1. Traditional "cut down technique": The proposed site of scleral cut down is treated with moderate cautery. A 3-mm scleral incision is made, keeping the blade perpendicular to sclera, till a small knuckle of black colored choroid becomes increasingly visible and finally bulges into the incision (Fig. 12.9). Diathermy is applied to coagulate the choroidal vessels. All pressure on globe is relieved before the choroid is penetrated with a needle. The needle is advanced slowly for about 2 mm till SRF starts draining.
2. Trans-scleral needle drainage: A 26G needle can be used to perforate the sclera to drain the SRF without any cut down [28]. In contrast to the traditional technique, traction sutures are pulled during this technique to increase the globe pressure. The needle is slowly advanced roughly till the hub of the 26G needle, when the resistance suddenly gives away and SRF starts draining. Otherwise, a 26G needle is bent like cystitome of capsulorhexis. Thus, the tip will be perpendicular to sclera and used for perforation, while the shaft will be tangential and act like a guard by preventing the tip to enter beyond 2 mm [29].

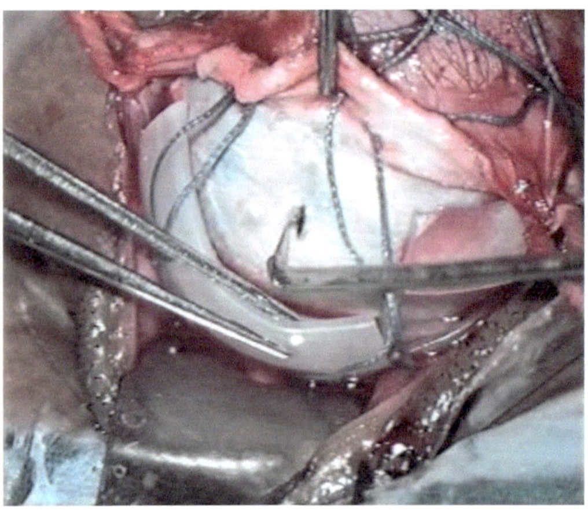

Fig. 12.9 Clinical image showing scleral incision for subretinal fluid drainage in "traditional" cut down technique

As SRF continues to drain, press the sclera anterior to drainage site. Appearance of pigment particles indicates that the drainage is nearing completion. If SRFD does not start or stops prematurely, the drainage site is inspected to exclude:

1. Retinal incarceration, which appears as star-shaped folds radiating from drain site. DO NOT try to reposition the incarcerated retina as this can cause greater damage.
2. Reassess depth of SRF at drain site: If deep SRF is present near the drainage site, globe is gently massaged to distract the sclerostomy edges. If this does not help, a fresh choroidotomy is made.

It is very important that the assistant continuously pulls the traction sutures in order to maintain the ocular pressure. Any laxity of traction sutures, can lead to hypotony, suprachoroidal effusions or hemorrhages, hyphaema, and pupil constriction. Appearance of blood from the drainage site indicates choroidal hemorrhage (needle injury to its vessels). In such a case, the traction sutures are pulled to increase the intraocular pressure till the bleeding stops.

12.8.10 Adjusting the Height of Scleral Buckle

After SRF is completely drained, tighten the loose scleral sutures to achieve an adequate buckle height. In case the eye is excessively soft, it is reformed by injecting saline before tightening the sutures. The sutures may need revision, in case the break(s) are not supported or adequate buckle height is not achieved. The assistant should not leave the traction sutures until the sutures are tightened and globe reformed. After tightening the sutures, the knots are rotated pos-

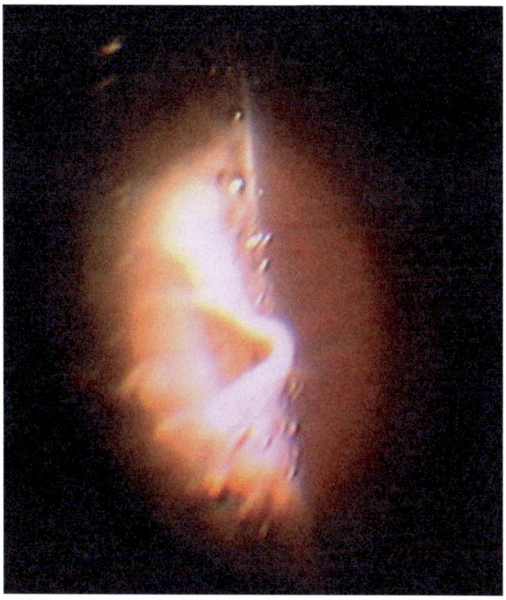

Fig. 12.10 Clinical image showing fish mouthing, due to excessive folds

teriorly to prevent conjunctival erosions. Excessive tightening of the encirclage band is avoided as this can lead to retinal folds and "fish-mouthing" (Fig. 12.10). In case of excessive folds, the encircling band is loosened.

12.8.11 Final Examination

After tightening the suture, retina is examined again to be check:

1. Optic disc perfusion: In case of pale disc or artery pulsations, poor perfusion should be suspected and paracentesis should be performed, especially in case of a non-drainage surgery.
2. The breaks should be well supported by buckle without any fish mouthing.
3. Drainage site must be examined.

12.8.12 Tenon and Conjunctiva Closure

Tenon's capsule and conjunctiva are irrigated with balanced salt solution and broad-spectrum antibiotics (*gentamycin, 40 mg/mL*). Tenon and conjunctiva are sutured in two different layers. An appropriate closure prevents buckle migration, buckle exposure, and subsequent buckle infection.

12.8.13 Documentation

All details regarding the site of breaks and SRFD, type of explant, and position of the sutures and whatzke's sleeve/CHK are correctly documented.

12.8.14 Overview of Surgical Steps

Table 12.5 gives an overview of all the surgical steps.

12.9 Important Postoperative Complications

Table 12.6 describes all the intra- and postoperative complications.

1. *Angle-closure glaucoma*: This occurs due to ciliary body detachment. It is treated with hourly topical steroids and cycloplegics. In case anterior chamber does not form within 7 days, choroidal drainage with anterior chamber may be needed.
2. *Anterior segment ischemia*: This is associated with high buckle height. The patient may present with pain, decreased vision, epithelial and stromal corneal edema, corneal endothelium precipitates, marked uveitis, shallow anterior chamber cataract, lens opacification, excessive buckle height (in extreme cases dumb-bell shaped vitreous cavity). Mild cases respond to topical steroids and cycloplegics, however, severe cases require release of encirclage element.
3. *Persistent SRF*: Sometimes SRF may persist for up to 3 months. In case all the breaks are closed, it can be safely observed. However, SRF with open breaks may need intervention in form of gas injection, laser, or even buckle revision.

Table 12.5 Overview of surgical steps

Give adequate anesthesia
Perform a 360-degree conjunctival peritomy (encirclage planned) or localized peritomy (segmental buckling)
Bride all four recti
Strip off all the tenon's capsule attachment to the muscle insertion and sclera
Inspect the sclera for thinning and the location of vortex veins
Localize and mark all retinal break(s) with the help of indirect ophthalmoscope (IDO)
Perform cryotherapy for all known and suspected breaks
Place the explant under the recti
Place loose temporary sutures around the explants
Drain the subretinal fluid under IDO guidance
Inject saline into the vitreous cavity to form the eyeball
Tighten the temporary sutures
Inspect for adequate buckle height and optic disc for pulsations
Make the suture knots permanent. Rotate the knot so that it is posterior to the buckle
End-to-end tighten the encirclage with Watzke sleeve/ clove hitch knot
Examine the optic disc. Perform paracentesis, if required
Remove the traction sutures
Wash with balanced salt solution and broad-spectrum antibiotics (gentamycin, *40 mg/mL*)
Suture tenon's capsule and conjunctiva in two different layers
Document all important findings

4. *Buckle extrusion and infection*: This is due to inadequate closure of conjunctiva and tenon's capsule. The buckle has to be explanted in these cases.

Table 12.6 Intra- and postoperative complications of scleral buckling

Intraoperative complications	
Step	*Complications*
Anesthesia	Globe perforation, retrobulbar hemorrhage, and central retinal artery occlusion
Muscle bridling	Ocular cardiac reflex, muscle rupture, lost muscle, damage to vortex vein, scleral perforation
Break localization	Damage to vortex vein, scleral perforation
Scleral suturing	Scleral perforation, iatrogenic retinal breaks
Subretinal fluid drainage	Damage to vortex vein, choroidal hemorrhage, retinal incarceration, retinal perforation, vitreous gel incarceration, vitreous hemorrhage, choroidal detachment (serous and hemorrhagic) due to hypotony
Early postoperative complications	
Lid edema	
Periocular infection	
Conjunctival chemosis	
Corneal edema/corneal defect	
Impaired rectus muscle function	
Anterior segment ischemia	
Angle-closure glaucoma	
Open breaks	
Serous choroidal detachment	
Hemorrhagic choroidal detachment	
Persistent SRF	
Late postoperative complications	
Diplopia	
Refractive errors due to axial length changes	
Buckle or suture extrusion and infection	
Trans scleral erosion (intrusion) of sutures or buckling material	
Macular pucker	
Proliferative vitreoretinopathy	
Recurrent retinal detachment	

12.10 Newer Development: Chandelier-Assisted Scleral Buckling

The surgery is very physically demanding as it needs repeated alternate placement of microscope and indirect ophthalmoscope. The latest development of chandelier endoillumination allows the surgeon to perform SB just like vitrectomy. *A noncontact wide*-angle viewing apparatus allows easy identification and treatment of retinal breaks.

Trans-scleral fiber optic-assisted scleral buckling was *first described in 2012 by Aras* et al. [30] They used a *torpedo*-style chandelier light source through an un-cannulated sclerotomy. This technique was later modified by Kita et al. *in 2013* [31]. They used a *25G fiber*-optic chandelier light source through a standard trans-scleral cannula.

This system has multiple advantages. Firstly, it improves the ergonomics of the surgery. Secondly, it improves the visualization of peripheral retinal breaks, decreasing the chances of missing them. Thirdly, it is a good teaching tool as the surgery can be screened live just like a vitrectomy. Fourthly, it improves communication among team members as all of them simultaneously view all aspects of the surgery. As a result, the duration of surgery decreases, while the chances of success increases [32–36].

12.11 Conclusion

SB is an elegant extraocular surgery that enables a surgeon to reattach the retina without disturbing the vitreous. It is significantly less expensive compared to vitrectomy, especially in phakic eyes [37]. Although vitrectomy is a better option for advanced PVR changes, SB gives excellent results in uncomplicated primary RRD. The young retina surgeons should try and acquire the surgical skill, lest the technique will be lost.

References

1. Schwartz SG, Flynn HW. Primary retinal detachment: scleral buckle or pars plana vitrectomy? Curr Opin Ophthalmol. 2006;17:245–50.
2. Heimann H, Bartz-Schmidt KU, Bornfeld N, Weiss C, Hilgers RD, Foerster MH. Scleral buckling versus primary vitrectomy in rhegmatogenous retinal detachment study group. Scleral buckling versus primary vitrectomy in rhegmatogenous retinal detachment: a prospective randomized multicenter clinical study. Ophthalmology. 2007;114:2142–54.
3. Heimann H, Hellmich M, Bornfeld N, Bartz-Schmidt KU, Hilgers RD, Foerster MH. Scleral buckling versus primary vitrectomy in rhegmatogenous retinal detachment (SPR study): design issues and implications. SPR study report no. 1. Graefes Arch Clin Exp Ophthalmol. 2001;239:567–74.
4. Saw SM, Gazzard G, Wagle AM, Lim J, Au Eong KG. An evidence-based analysis of surgical interventions for uncomplicated rhegmatogenous retinal detachment. Acta Ophthalmol Scand. 2006;84:606–12.
5. Park SW, Kwon HJ, Kim HY, Byon IS, Lee JE, Oum BS. Comparison of scleral buckling and vitrectomy using wide angle viewing system for rhegmatogenous retinal detachment in patients older than 35 years. BMC Ophthalmol. 2015;15:121.
6. Sodhi A, Leung LS, Do DV, Gower EW, Schein OD, Handa JT. Recent trends in the management of rhegmatogenous retinal detachment. Surv Ophthalmol. 2008;53:50–67.
7. Seider MI, Nomides RE, Hahn P, Mruthyunjaya P, Mahmoud TH. Scleral buckling with chandelier illumination. J Ophthalmic Vis Res. 2016;11:304–9.
8. Wolfensberger TJ. Jules Gonin. Pioneer of retinal detachment surgery. Indian J Ophthalmol. 2003;51:303–8.
9. Albert DM, Gloor BP, McPherson AR. Why Jules Gonin achieved his "audacious goal initiative" - and why he is a model for the present day. Ophthalmology. 2015;122:1955–7.
10. Schwartz SG, Garoon R, Smiddy WE, Flynn HW Jr. The legacy of Jules Gonin: one hundred years of identifying and treating retinal breaks. Graefes Arch Clin Exp Ophthalmol. 2018;256:1051–2.
11. Lincoff HA, Baras I, McLean J. Modifications to the Custodis procedure for retinal detachment. Arch Ophthalmol. 1965;73:160.
12. Saxena S, Lincoff H. Finding the retinal break in rhegmatogenous retinal detachment. Indian J Ophthalmol. 2001;49:199–202.
13. Lincoff H, Gieser R. Finding the hole. Arch Ophthalmol. 1971;85:565–9.
14. Lincoff H, Kriessig I. Finding the retinal hole in the pseudophakic eye with detachment. Am J Ophthalmol. 1993;117:442–6.
15. DORC products. https://www.dorc.eu/product/scleral-buckling-products-style-240-25mm-circling-band
16. FCI products. https://fci-ophthalmics.com/products/fci-silicone-bands
17. Park SW, Lee JJ, Lee JE. Scleral buckling in the management of rhegmatogenous retinal detachment: patient selection and perspectives. Clin Ophthalmol. 2018;12:1605–15.
18. James M, O'Doherty M, Beatty S. Buckle-related complications following surgical repair of retinal dialysis. Eye (Lond). 2008;22:485–90.
19. Chang JS, Marra K, Flynn HW Jr, Berrocal AM, Arroyo JG. Scleral buckling in the treatment of retinal detachment due to retinal dialysis. Ophthalmic Surg Lasers Imaging Retina. 2016;1(47):336–40.
20. Jan S, Hussain Z, Khan U, Khan MT, Karim S. Retinal detachment due to retinal dialysis: surgical outcome after scleral buckling. Asia Pac J Ophthalmol (Phila). 2015;4:259–62.
21. Stoffelns BM, Richard G. Is buckle surgery still the state of the art for retinal detachments due to retinal dialysis? J Pediatr Ophthalmol Strabismus. 2010;47:281–7.
22. Bosomworth PP, Ziegler CH, Jacoby J. The oculocardiac reflex in eye muscle surgery. Anesthesiology. 1958;19:7–10.
23. Gilbert C, McLeod D. D-ACE surgical sequence for selected bullous retinal detachments. Br J Ophthalmol. 1985;69:733–6.

24. Jaccoma EH, Conway BP, Campochiaro PA. Cryotherapy causes extensive breakdown of the blood-retinal barrier. A comparison with argon laser photocoagulation. Arch Ophthalmol. 1985;103:1728–30.
25. Bonnet M, Fleury J, Guenoun S, Yaniali A, Dumas C, Hajjar C. Cryopexy in primary rhegmatogenous retinal detachment: a risk factor for postoperative proliferative vitreoretinopathy? Graefes Arch Clin Exp Ophthalmol. 1996;234:739–43.
26. Shanmugam PM, Ramanjulu R, Mishra KCD, Sagar P. Novel techniques in scleral buckling. Indian J Ophthalmol. 2018;66(7):909–15.
27. Kreissig I. View 1: minimal segmental buckling without drainage. Br J Ophthalmol. 2003;87:782–4.
28. Azad R, Kumar A, Sharma YR, Rajpal. Modified needle drainage. A safe and efficient technique of subretinal fluid drainage in scleral buckling procedure. Indian J Ophthalmol. 2004;52:211–4.
29. Agarwal MK. Modified needle drainage. A safe and efficient technique of subretinal fluid drainage in scleral buckling procedure. Indian J Ophthalmol. 2004;52:342–3; author reply 343.
30. Aras C, Ucar D, Koytak A, Yetik H. Scleral buckling with a non-contact wide-angle viewing system. Ophthalmologica. 2012;227:107–10.
31. Kita M, Fujii Y, Kawagoe N, Hama S. Scleral buckling with a noncontact wide-angle viewing system in the management of retinal detachment with undetected retinal break: a case report. Clin Ophthalmol. 2013;7:587–9.
32. Cohen E, Rosenblatt A, Bornstein S, Loewenstein A, Barak A, Schwartz S. Wide-angled endoillumination vs traditional scleral buckling surgery for retinal detachment - a comparative study. Clin Ophthalmol. 2019;13:287–93.
33. Assi A, Abdelmassih Y, El-Khoury S. Endoillumination-assisted modified scleral buckling. Retina. 2018;38:320–4.
34. Hu Y, Si S, Xu K, Chen H, Han L, Wang X, Ma Z. Outcomes of scleral buckling using chandelier endoillumination. Acta Ophthalmol. 2017;95:591–4.
35. Narayanan R, Tyagi M, Hussein A, Chhablani J, Apte RS. Scleral buckling with wide-angled endoillumination as a surgical educational tool. Retina. 2016;36:830–3.
36. Jeon GS, Han JR. Effectiveness of scleral buckling with a wide-field surgical microscope and chandelier illumination in retinal detachment repair. Ophthalmologica. 2019;242:31–7.
37. Seider MI, Naseri A, Stewart JM. Cost comparison of scleral buckle versus vitrectomy for rhegmatogenous retinal detachment repair. Am J Ophthalmol. 2013;156:661–6.

Pneumatic Retinopexy

13

Astha Jain, S. Natarajan, Thirumalesh MB,
and Priyanka Singh

13.1 Introduction

The term "Pneumatic retinopexy" was coined by Hilton and Grizzard who were the first to perform the procedure [1]. Pneumatic retinopexy (PR) is a minimally invasive procedure of retinal detachment repair. It consists of injecting an expandable gas bubble in the vitreous cavity followed by appropriate patient positioning and sealing the retinal break using laser photocoagulation or cryotherapy. Advancement in small gauge sutureless vitrectomy with success rate >90% with a single procedure has made it the procedure of choice for many surgeons. A study by Mc Laughlin et al. analysed the vitreoretinal procedure trend from 2000 to 2014 using data from US medicare and found that the preference for retinal detachment repair shifted towards vitrectomy with a distribution of 83% vitrectomy, 5% scleral buckling and 12% pneumatic retinopexy in 2014 [2]. However, PR is still a procedure of choice in selected cases as it is a simple, cost effective and less time-consuming process with a success rate of up to 97% with proper case selection [3].

13.2 Patient Selection

An ideal case to be treated by pneumatic retinopexy is rhegmatogenous retinal detachment without PVR with single break or a group of breaks within 1 clock hour located in the superior 8 clock hours of the fundus. PR may be the procedure of choice in certain cases:

1. Where scleral buckle is not preferable such as those with very thin sclera
2. Single break under the superior rectus where buckle may induce a vertical diplopia
3. Re-detachment following scleral buckling where subretinal fluid accumulates due to an open superior break
4. Patients with a pre-existing filtering bleb or those who may require it in the future
5. Scarred conjunctiva

Phakic patients have shown to do better than aphakic or pseudophakic patients [4, 5]. This may be because aphakic or pseudophakic eyes are more prone to develop tiny breaks in far periphery and in multiple quadrants. Posterior capsular opacification can also limit the view of the peripheral retina. If peripheral retina can be

A. Jain (✉) · S. Natarajan
Aditya Jyot Foundation for Twinkling Little Eyes, Mumbai, India

Aditya Jyot Eye Hospital, Mumbai, India

T. MB
Narayana Nethralaya, Bengaluru, India

P. Singh
Rukmini child and eye care centre, Kanpur, India

A. Jain et al. (eds.), *Cutting-edge Vitreoretinal Surgery*,
https://doi.org/10.1007/978-981-33-4168-5_13

adequately examined, aphakia or pseudophakia is not a contraindication for PR [6].

Patients unsuitable for PR are the following:

1. Proliferative vitreoretinopathy: As PR does not relieve traction, it is unsuitable for treating detachment with PVR graded C or D. However, mild PVR away from the retinal break is not a contraindication for PR.
2. Advanced glaucoma: Patients with severe glaucoma may suffer noticeable damage even with brief fluctuations in IOP which may occur during gas injection.
3. Cloudy media: Identification and treatment of all the retinal breaks is the key to success of PR procedure. Cloudy media may prevent adequate evaluation of retina and hence the risk of missed retinal break making it a contraindication to PR procedure.
4. Inability to maintain posture: Post-procedure positioning is essential to provide adequate tamponade to the retinal breaks. Patients with physical or mental comorbidities who are unable to maintain posture are unsuitable candidates for PR.
5. Inferior breaks: Cases with breaks in the inferior 4 clock hours are difficult to treat with PR as it is difficult to maintain head tilt below horizontal.
6. Extensive lattice degeneration: Extensive lattice degeneration poses a high risk for developing new retinal breaks and hence PR is better avoided. Lattice degeneration extending 3 clock hours or less does not affect the success rate [3].

Pneumatic retinopexy has been considered in certain special cases as mentioned below. However, it is not the procedure of choice in these cases:

1. Break extending more than 1 clock hour: Multiple breaks in multiple quadrants, although difficult to repair by PR, can be done by alternate head positioning [6]. Breaks spanning 3 clock hours pose no particular problem [7].
2. Giant retinal tear and retinal dialysis: Fresh giant tears extending <180° and with mobile flaps have been treated with Pneumatic retinopexy by Irvine and Lahey [8]. Superior retinal dialysis extending at least 3 clock hours have been treated by Melgen et al. in a small case series of four patients [9]. However, these are small case series and PR is not the procedure of choice in these cases.
3. Retinal detachment associated with macular hole: Pneumatic retinopexy has been used to successfully treat retinal detachment associated with macular hole [10, 11]. PR can be the procedure of choice in cases of retinoschisis with very posterior outer layer breaks and RD [7].
4. Retinal detachment associated with choroidal detachment and hypotony: PR can be used as an adjunct in these cases. PR would facilitate an early definitive surgery by restoring IOP and decreasing the extent of detachment [12].

13.3 Technique

A careful preoperative evaluation is essential in planning the surgery. Features that are unfavourable for the procedure such as PVR, media opacity, lattice degeneration etc. should be carefully noted. The procedure consists of retinopexy, gas tamponade and posturing.

13.3.1 Anaesthesia

The procedure can be done under topical, subconjunctival, subtenon or peribulbar anaesthesia. The procedure is performed using aseptic precautions in the operating room or the outpatient department.

13.3.2 Retinopexy

Retinal break is visualised using an indirect ophthalmoscope and transconjunctival cryopexy is applied before the injection of gas. Laser can be used instead of cryo for retinopexy as a two-part procedure. Gas bubble is first injected into the vitreous cavity followed by positioning for 1 or 2 days. Once the break is reattached, laser photocoagulation is applied using an indirect ophthalmoscope after positioning the patient's head to move the gas bubble away from the break. Laser photocoagulation can also be applied through the gas bubble if the bubble is large. However, one must be careful not to overtreat as gas has an insulating effect, conducting heat away from the laser spot at a slower rate, which may lead to retinal necrosis and hole formation [7]. Cryopexy is more convenient as it can be done as a single procedure and it is easier to find the break when they are open.

13.3.3 Paracentesis

A 27-gauge needle is used to withdraw around 0.2 mL of aqueous through the limbus to reduce the intraocular volume to make space for the gas bubble.

13.3.4 Injection of Gas

The selected gas is withdrawn in a 2-mL syringe through a millipore filter in a sterile fashion. The gas should be withdrawn just a few minutes prior to injection because of high risk of gas leakage [13]. The needle is inserted at the pars plana 4 mm posterior to the limbus in phakics and 3.5 mm posterior to limbus in case of pseudophakic eye. The injection site should be away from the site of the break and highly detached retina. Head of the patient should be turned to one side to make the injection site uppermost. The needle is passed into the eye perpendicular to the sclera into the mid vitreous cavity. The needle is then withdrawn to leave around 3 mm in the globe. The tip of the needle should be pointed away from bullous detachment. The entire volume of the gas is injected briskly to prevent multiple small bubbles known as "fish-eggs". One should hold the plunger down until the needle is withdrawn to prevent the escape of gas back into the syringe. A cotton-tipped applicator is used to occlude the perforation site to prevent any gas escape.

13.3.5 Indirect Ophthalmoscopy

Immediately following gas injection, optic nerve head is visualised to assess the perfusion of the central retinal artery. If perfusion appears to be compromised, a second paracentesis is done to bring down the IOP and perfusion reassessed. It is also important to note that a single gas bubble is formed in the vitreous cavity and there are no "fish eggs".

13.3.6 Postop Positioning

The patient is instructed to begin positioning immediately. Head posture is advised in a way such that the meridian with the retinal break lies superior. Steam-roller manoeuvre can be used to prevent tracking of subretinal fluid inferiorly into the macula in cases of macula on RD [14]. In this technique, the patient is first positioned head down and gradually the head is rotated in a way such that the gas bubble rolls over the large elevated break.

13.3.7 Choice of Intraocular Gas

Sulphur hexafluoride (SF6) and perfluoropropane (C3F8) are the most commonly used gases. Filtered air, a non-expansile gas, has also been used with a single operation success rate of 80.5% [15]. Being non-expansile, filtered air causes minimal vitreous disturbance and hence a lower incidence of PVR [16]. Air gets absorbed within a few days. SF6 doubles in volume in reaching maximum size in 36 hours and lasts for around 10–14 days. C3F8 quadruples in volume in 3 days and lasts for around 30–45 days. Air is non-expansile and lasts for 3–5 days [17]. The size of the gas bubble should be such that all retinal breaks are covered for at least 4–5 days. A 0.3-mL gas bubble covers approximately 60° arc of retina and 1.2 mL covers 80–90° [7]. 0.5–0.6 mL of SF6 and 0.3 mL of C3F8 is usually injected. Due to its greater expansion, a smaller amount of C3F8 is required. However, its longevity can cause undue vitreous traction during head movement which may lead to retinal break formation.

13.4 Complications

- *Entrapment of gas in prehyaloid space*: Injection of gas anterior to the anterior hyaloid space into the space of petit may give the appearance of "sausage sign", an oval loculated bubble that usually does not move with the change in head position. As the gas bubble expands, it breaks through the anterior hyaloid face and enters the vitreous cavity without creating new break. If necessary, a large trapped bubble can be removed by passing a 27G needle mounted on a syringe with small amount of saline and plunger removed. The needle is passed into the gas bubble so that it escapes through the needle and bubbles out in the saline [7].
- *Subretinal Gas*: It usually occurs when there is a formation of "fish-egg" at the time of gas injection. The "fish-egg" gas bubble may pass through the existing retinal break giving the retina a pearly dome-shaped refractile sheen [18]. Attempt can be made to remove the bubble by massaging the bubble back into the vitreous cavity using scleral depression and positioning the patient's head. Smaller sub-retinal bubble can be ignored and additional large bubble injected into the vitreous cavity. Large subretinal bubble may require prompt intervention for its removal. This complication can be prevented by posturing the patient so that small bubbles do not come in contact with a large break till the bubbles coalesce. Flicking the globe intraoperatively by a cotton-tipped applicator may also cause the small bubbles to coalesce and form a large bubble thus preventing their subretinal migration.
- *New Retinal Break*: It is one of the most common causes of failure of PR [19]. New retinal break may occur as the expanding gas bubble may cause additional vitreoretinal traction. They are usually located in the superior retina with the majority within 3 clock hours of the original break [20]. They are seen most commonly in the first month following the procedure [21]. Prophylactic 360 peripheral laser retinopexy has been advocated by Tornabe to reduce the risk of new break formation [4]. Giant retinal tear has also been rarely reported [22].
- *Re-opening of the original break*: There is no relief of the vitreoretinal traction with PR. Therefore, the break must be treated adequately with laser or cryopexy to develop strong chorioretinal adhesion to prevent reopening of the break.
- *Proliferative Vitreoretinopathy*: Risk of PVR after PR is found to range between 3 and 13% [20]. Vitreous membranes can form around the gas bubble, which can precipitate PVR [23]. Management involves pars plana vitrectomy.
- *Macular Hole*: The rate of macular hole development is similar to that after PPV ranging from 0 to 3% and can be managed by vitrectomy [20].
- *Cystoid macular edema*: It has been reported in 11% of cases and the risk is more in cases with macular detachment [24].
- *Migration of gas in anterior chamber*: This can occur even in phakic eyes and can cause elevated IOP. Gas from anterior chamber can be evacuated by paracentesis [25].
- *Suprachoroidal gas*: This complication can be prevented by ensuring that the needle tip is well within the vitreous cavity.
- *Cataract progression*: The incidence of cataract formation following pneumatic retinopexy is also very less compared to pars plana vitrectomy· Lenticular changes after pneumatic retinopexy were found in 38% of eyes in a study of 193 eyes [26]. Another study on 33 patients reported no lenticular changes up to 2 years after the procedure [27].

13.5 Outcome

Chan et al. did a comprehensive study of 4138 eyes undergoing PR over a period of 21 years. They reported the average single operation success rate as 74.4% and final operation success rate as 96.1% [28]. Tornambe et al. reviewed 302 consecutive cases of PR with a follow-up of 6 months to 10 years [3]. The single operation success rate was 68% for all 302 cases and 7% for a subgroup of cases. This subgroup had the following criteria: phakic eyes; only one quadrant of retinal detachment; only one retinal break located in the upper two-thirds of the fundus; postoperatively prophylactic 360° PR. The risk of retinal redetachment after PR is highest in the first 3–6 months [29]. Tornambe et al. demonstrated the rate of redetachment beyond 6 months postoperatively to be only 1% [3]. Success with PR depends upon proper case selection and surgical technique. Even with reoperations, PR is a very cost-effectcive method of retinal detachment repair [30].

13.6 Conclusion

Pneumatic retinopexy is a simple, cost effective and less time-consuming procedure associated with good visual recovery and less morbidity. Proper case selection and surgical technique can increase the success rate to 97%. All these make PR the procedure of choice in selected cases.

References

1. Hilton GF, Grizzard WS. Pneumatic retinopexy: a twostep outpatient operation without conjunctival incision. Ophthalmology. 1986;93:626–40.
2. McLaughlin MD, Hwang JC. Trends in vitreoretinal procedures for medicare beneficiaries, 2000 to 2014. Ophthalmology. 2017;124:667–73.
3. Tornambe PE. Pneumatic retinopexy: the evolution of case selection and surgical technique: a twelve year study of 302 eyes. Trans Am Ophthalmol Soc. 1997;95:551–78.
4. Algvere P, Hallnäs K, Palmqvist BM. Success and complications of pneumatic retinopexy. Am J Ophthalmol. 1988;106(4):400–4.
5. Abecia E, Pinilla I, Olivan JM, Larrosa JM, Polo V, Honrubia FM. Anatomic results and complications in a long-term follow-up of pneumatic retinopexy cases. Retina. 2000;20(2):156–61.
6. Tornambe PE, Hilton GF, Kelly NF, Salzano TC, Wells JW, Wendel RT. Expanded indications for pneumatic retinopexy. Ophthalmology. 1988;95(5):597–600.
7. Hilton GF, Das T, Majji AB, Jalali S. Pneumatic retinopexy: principles and practice. Indian J Ophthalmol. 1996;44:131–43.
8. Irvine AR, Lahey JM. Pneumatic retinopexy for giant retinal tears. Ophthalmology. 1994;101(3):524–8.
9. Melgen SE, Michels M. Pneumatic retinopexy for the treatment of giant retinal dialyses. Am J Ophthalmol. 1994;118(6):762–5.
10. Menchini U, Scialdone A, Visconti C, Brancato R. Pneumoretinopexy in the treatment of retinal detachment with macular hole. Int Ophthalmol. 1988;12(4):213–5.
11. Rashed O, Sheta S. Evaluation of the functional results after different techniques for treatment of retinal detachment due to macular holes. Graefes Arch Clin Exp Ophthalmol. 1989;227(6):508–12.
12. Yeung L, Kokame GT, Brod RD, Lightman DA, Lai JC. Pneumatic retinopexy for retinal detachment associated with severe choroidal detachment. Retina. 2011;31(1):87–92.
13. Humayun MS, Yeo JH, Koski WS, Michels RG. The rate of sulfur hexafluoride escape from a plastic syringe. Arch Ophthalmol. 1989;107:853–4.
14. Tornambe PE. Pneumatic retinopexy. Surv Ophthalmol. 1988;32(4):270–81.
15. Yee KMP, Sebag J. Long-term results of office-based pneumatic retinopexy using pure air. Br J Ophthalmol. 2011;95(12):1728–30.
16. Sebag J, Tang M. Pneumatic retinopexy using only air. Retina. 1993;13:8–12.
17. Lincoff H, Mardirossian J, Lincoff A, et al. Intravitreal longevity of three perfluorocarbon gases. Arch Ophthalmol. 1980;98:1610–1.
18. McDonald HR, Abrams GW, Irvine AR, et al. The management of subretinal gas following attempted pneumatic retinal reattachment. Ophthalmology. 1987;94(4):319–26.
19. Gorovoy IR, Eller AW, Friberg TR, Coe R. Characterization of pneumatic retinopexy failures and the pneumatic pump: a new complication of pneumatic retinopexy. Retina. 2014;34(4):700–4.
20. Holz ER, Mieler WF. View 3: the case for pneumatic retinopexy. Br J Ophthalmol. 2003;87(6):787–9.
21. Tornambe PE, Hilton GF, The Retinal Detachment Study Group. Pneumatic retinopexy: a multicenter randomized controlled clinical trial comparing pneumatic retinopexy with scleral buckling. Ophthalmology. 1989;96:772–84.

22. Sinkar SN, Simon SJ, Gilhotra JS. Giant retinal tear after pneumatic retinopexy. Retin Cases Brief Rep. 2012;6(2):151–2.
23. Dhami A, Shah KK, Ratra D. Pneumatic retinopexy outcomes as primary or secondary surgical option for treating rhegmatogenous retinal detachment. Indian J Ophthalmol. 2018;66(3):420–5.
24. Tunc M, Lahey JM, Kearney JJ, Lewis JM, Francis R. Cystoid macular oedema following pneumatic retinopexy vs scleral buckling. Eye (Lond). 2007;21(6):831–4.
25. Taher RM, Haimovici R. Anterior chamber gas entrapment after phakic pneumatic retinopexy. Retina. 2001;21(1):681–2.
26. Feng H, Adelman RA. Cataract formation following vitreoretinal procedures. Clin Ophthalmol. 2014;8:1957–65.
27. Mougharbel M, Koch FH, Böker T, Spitznas M. No cataract two years after pneumatic retinopexy. Ophthalmology. 1994;101(7):1191–4.
28. Chan CK, Lin SG, Nuthi AS, Salib DM. Pneumatic retinopexy for the repair of retinal detachments: a comprehensive review (1986–2007). Surv Ophthalmol. 2008;53(5):443–78.
29. Ellakwa AF. Long term results of pneumatic retinopexy. Clin Ophthalmol. 2012;6:55–9.
30. Elhusseiny AM, Yannuzzi NA, Smiddy WE. Cost analysis of pneumatic retinopexy versus pars plana vitrectomy for rhegmatogenous retinal detachment. Ophthalmol Retina. 2019;3(11):956–61.

14 Primary Vitrectomy in Rhegmatogenous Retinal Detachment

Mahesh Shanmugam Palanivelu, Pradeep Sagar, and Divyansh K. C. Mishra

14.1 Introduction

Primary vitrectomy has largely replaced scleral buckling as the treatment of choice in rhegmatogenous retinal detachment (RRD) with proliferative vitreoretinopathy (PVR) [1, 2]. While most simple rhegmatogenous retinal detachments can be managed by scleral buckling, there are situations wherein vitrectomy is the treatment of choice.

14.2 Indications of Primary Vitrectomy in RRD

- Posterior breaks
- Multiple breaks at varying distance from the ora serrata
- RRD caused by/associated with macular hole [3, 4]
- Media haze significant enough to prevent visualization of break [5]
- Aphakic and Pseudophakic RRD [6–10]
- Cases in which primary break is not seen preoperatively [11]
- RRD associated with choroidal detachment (CD) [12, 13] and PVR more than C1

Rhegmatogenous retinal detachments associated with the above situations were managed with scleral buckling alone until a decade back. Improved anatomical results with vitrectomy in these situations and the lack of familiarity with the techniques of scleral buckling amidst younger generation surgeons has led to primary vitrectomy being the current treatment of choice.

14.3 Steps of Surgery

14.3.1 Conjunctival Peritomy

Conjunctival Peritomy would be necessary only if an encerclage is to be placed, which in itself is required only in select situations. Otherwise, a trans conjunctival entry is most often employed.

14.3.2 Encerclage

An encerclage is often not necessary in primary vitrectomy for RRD [14–16]. Select situations when one would feel safer to place an encerclage are:

(a) Phakic eye with multiple inferior breaks and/or lattices wherein a thorough vitreous base shaving would not be possible without lens touch [17].

M. Shanmugam Palanivelu (✉) · P. Sagar
D. K. C. Mishra
Sankara Eye Hospital, Bengaluru, India

A. Jain et al. (eds.), *Cutting-edge Vitreoretinal Surgery*,
https://doi.org/10.1007/978-981-33-4168-5_14

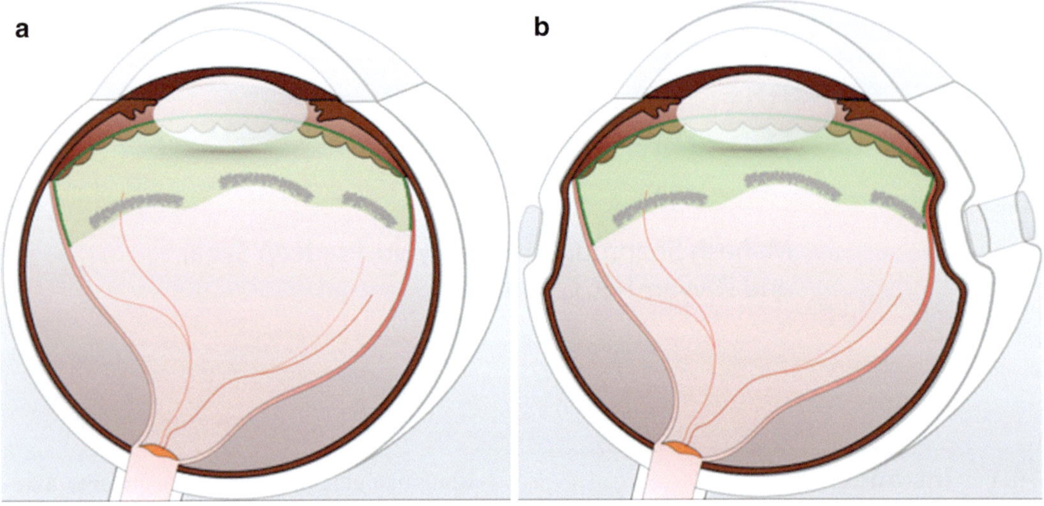

Fig. 14.1 (**a**) The vitreous attachment anterior to the lattice to the vitreous base is adherent and cannot be detached. (**b**) In such cases, an encerclage is used to indent the anterior retina

(b) RD associated with multiple rows of lattices in the detached retina at varying distances from the ora. In such cases, if the vitreous anterior to the lattice is detached, it would be possible to relieve this anterior traction satisfactorily. In such situations an encerclage is inessential. However, in most patients, the vitreous attachment would extend from the anterior lattice margin to the vitreous base. In such cases one may consider an encerclage (Fig. 14.1).

(c) Younger patients would have an adherent vitreous and one may consider an encerclage in them.

14.3.3 Sclerotomy

Trans conjunctival sclerotomies are placed 3.5–4 mm from the limbus in phakic eyes and 3–3.5 mm from the limbus in pseudophakic and aphakic eyes. The distance of sclerotomy from the limbus varies with age (Table 14.1). The temporal sclerotomies are placed in line with superior and inferior borders of the lateral rectus. The nasal sclerotomy is placed in line with superior border of the medial rectus. The infusion cannula is placed traditionally at the inferotemporal quadrant, but the use of a cannula system allows the flexibility of moving the infusion to the other sclerotomies as well.

Table 14.1 Distance of sclerotomy from the limbus [18]

Age	Distance of sclerotomy from limbus
0–6 months	1.5 mm
6–12 months	2.0 mm
1–2 years	2.5 mm
2–3 years	3.0 mm
Adult	3.5 mm

Trocar based systems of 23g, 25g, and 27g can be used to perform vitrectomy in RRD. These cannulas are usually 4 mm in length. The cannula is introduced into the vitreous cavity with the help of a trocar over which the cannula is loaded. The trocar is introduced in a biplanar direction in 23G and 25G to achieve a self-sealing wound [19]. The 27G trocar can be introduced perpendicular to the sclera and the sclerotomy is uniplanar [20, 21]. In eyes with RRD with CD, a 6-mm cannula is placed for infusion. A 6-mm cannula with the trocar cannula system is available for the 23g systems.

In rare situations, a 20g vitrectomy is performed. A limited peritomy of 1 clock hour superonasally and 3 clock hour temporally, straddling the lateral rectus is performed. A 20g micro vitreo retinal (MVR) blade is used to make the sclerotomy and it is placed circumferentially to the limbus. The infusion cannula is secured with polyglactin mattress suture with a slipknot that is placed away from the cornea to avoid disturbance in the visualization by the free ends of suture. A 20g entry may be required in the presence of RRD with choroidal detachment, wherein a 6-mm cannula is placed for infusion [22]. The 6-mm length of the cannula traverses the boggy choroid in eyes with choroidal detachment completely, thereby preventing inadvertent suprachoroidal infusion.

Special Situations:

(a) Sclerotomy in eyes with CD and RD:
In eyes with choroidal detachment, the choroidal detachment should be drained prior to placing the infusion cannula and the following modifications in the placement of sclerotomy are required:

1. Eyes with RD associated with CD are hypotonic: So an intravitreal injection of balanced salt solution is necessary to make the globe firm, prior to placement of the infusion cannula.
2. A simultaneous drainage of suprachoroidal fluid along with intravitreal injection would be required prior to placement of the cannula.
3. To drain the suprachoroidal fluid, the trocar of the trocar cannula system is used to make a partial entry into the globe. The trocar would reach the suprachoroidal space by penetrating the sclera until the broadest part of the tip of the trocar enters the eye (Fig. 14.2). It is indicated by drainage of the suprachoroidal fluid around the trocar. Twisting the trocar would enable the sclerotomy to remain open, allowing drainage of the suprachoroidal fluid. Simultaneous intravitreal injection through a superonasal site using a 30g needle aids replacement of the drained suprachoroidal fluid and pushes the choroid/ciliary body toward the sclera. With cessation of the suprachoroidal fluid drainage, the trocar is mounted with the cannula and re-entered with the trocar placed perpendicular to the sclera to allow the cannula to clear the boggy ciliary epithelium.

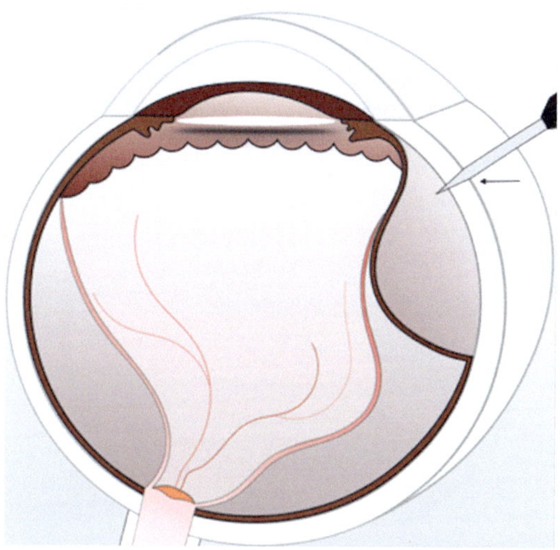

Fig. 14.2 The trocar is inserted until the broadest part (arrow) of the trocar enters the eye. The trocar reaches the suprachoroidal space and fluid starts draining

Once the sclerotomies are made or the cannulas are placed, the tip of the infusion cannula is inspected for its intravitreal location. It is particularly important in eyes with pre-existing CD. Failure to visualize the tip of the cannula within the vitreous cavity indicates that the cannula can be in the suprachoroidal space and the infusion should not be turned on. In such cases, a 24G needle or 23G MVR (in cases with 23G surgery) is introduced through the superonasal sclerotomy (in pseudophakic and aphakic eyes) to incise the ciliary epithelium overlying the infusion cannula to expose the cannula (Fig. 14.3). In 25G surgery, 26G needle can be used to achieve the same. In phakic eyes, trying to reach the inferotemporal infusion cannula from the superonasal port may result in iatrogenic lens damage. In such cases, one can try reaching it from the superotemporal port to incise the overlying ciliary epithelium (Fig. 14.4). It is preferable to switch to a 6-mm cannula if one is unsure of residual ciliary epithelium overlying the infusion cannula tip, rather than the risk of

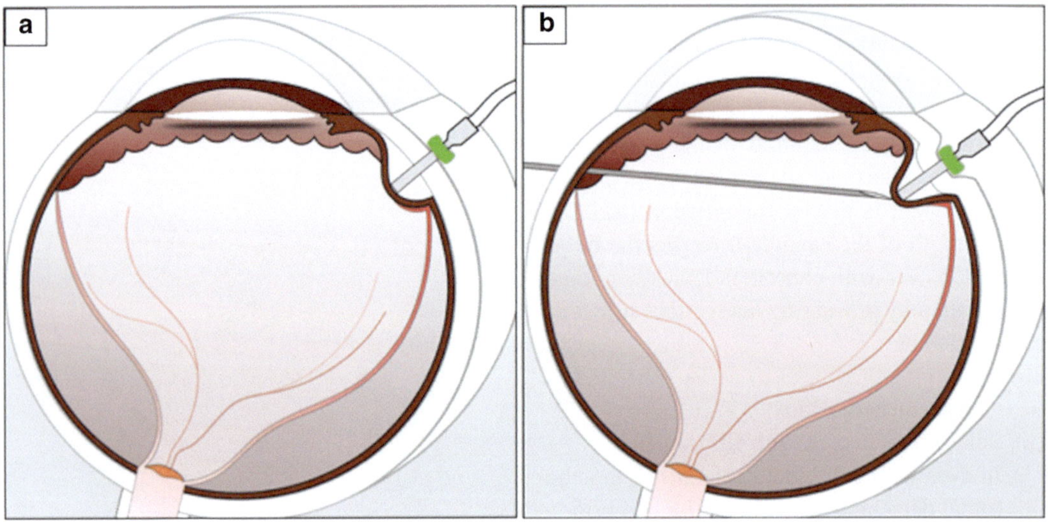

Fig. 14.3 (**a**) Suprachoroidal infusion cannula (**b**) 24G (or 26G) needle is introduced through the superonasal sclerotomy to incise the ciliary epithelium overlying the infusion cannula to expose the cannula

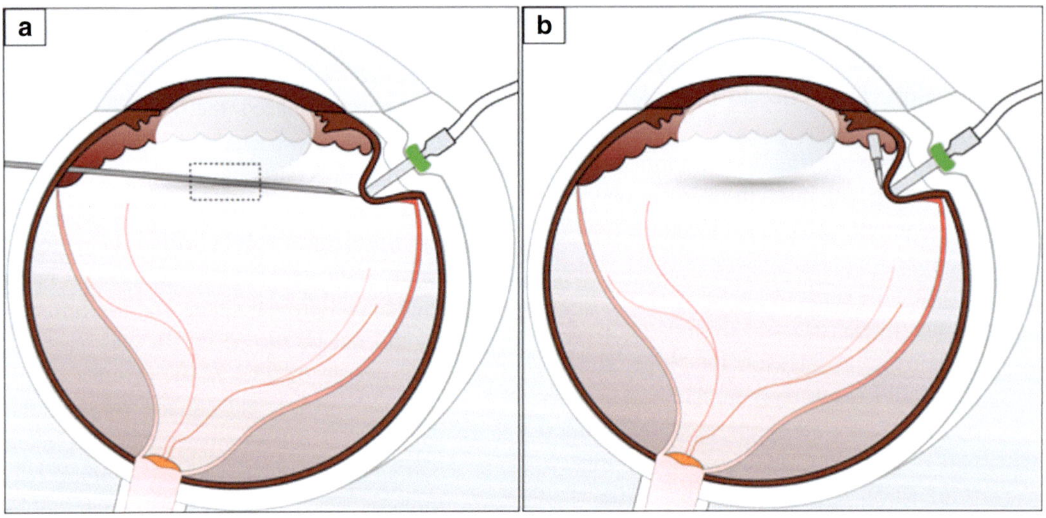

Fig. 14.4 (**a**) Using the opposite port to incise the ciliary epithelium in phakic eye can lead to lens touch (indicated by box). (**b**) The superotemporal port can be used to prevent lens touch

suprachoroidal infusion and its attendant complications.

(b) Placement of routine temporal sclerotomies using the trocar cannula system in an eye that has recently undergone a temporal small incision cataract surgery (SICS) can result in inadvertent gaping of the cataract wound, shallowing of the anterior chamber, hyphema, displacement of the lens, etc. In such eyes, it is preferable to expose the SICS wound and secure it with sutures prior to placing the sclerotomies. The inferotemporal and superotemporal sclerotomy placement needs to be modified, so that the sclerotomy does not go through the SICS wound.

14.3.4 Core Vitrectomy

Once the infusion is switched on, the vitreous gel at the port site and the anterior vitreous is removed with the cutter. Removal of the vitreous at the port sites at the beginning of the surgery decreases the risk of subsequent port site breaks. Mid and posterior vitrectomy is then performed with the aid of wide-angle viewing system. The highest cut-rate available with the vitrectomy console employed for the surgery is used to perform core vitrectomy to minimize vitreoretinal traction. A maximum vacuum of 300 mmHg (23g), 500–600 mmHg (25g and 27g) aids efficient removal of the vitreous.

Caution: A careful vitrectomy with a low vacuum is essential in eyes with bullous RD, as the mobile retina can get aspirated into the vitreous cutter and lead to iatrogenic retinal damage. Eyes with densely attached peripheral vitreous such as those with extensive lattices more often tend to get caught at the vitreous cutter port. Using perfluorocarbon liquid to stabilize the posterior retina, draining the subretinal fluid to flatten the retina, using the light pipe as a guard between the retina and the cutter are techniques one can employ to limit the risk of this complication.

14.3.5 Induction of Posterior Vitreous Detachment

Induction of Posterior Vitreous Detachment (PVD) is a crucial step in pars plana vitrectomy (PPV) for RRD. Posterior vitreous detachment extends up to the flap of the horse-shoe tear (HST) and over an operculated hole. Posterior vitreous detachment may not be present over atrophic holes and over patches of lattice degeneration. In myopic eyes, vitreoschisis and anomalous PVD is often seen.

Posterior vitreous detachment is induced in a posterior to anterior direction. Triamcinolone stain the posterior cortical vitreous and aids in its visualization and removal. Posterior hyaloid is densely adherent at the disc, macula, and along the retinal vessels. Grasping the hyaloid overlying the disc with the vitreous cutter in suction only mode and moving the cutter toward the mid vitreous cavity would aid separation of the hyaloid from the disc (Fig. 14.5). An aggressive core vitrectomy close to the posterior pole is better avoided, as there would be inadequate gel to be held by the cutter to aid PVD induction. Once hyaloid over the optic disc is detached, the detachment of hyaloid is advanced anteriorly by aspirating and lifting the posterior edge in all the directions up to the vitreous base.

In cases with difficulty in induction of PVD, a sharp needle (24G or 26G) or MVR blade can be used to make an opening in the posterior hyaloid by gently slicing it in a tangential motion. This is usually done over the papillomacular bundle or in the peripapillary region. Care is taken to prevent inadvertent damage to retina. Once an opening is created, the edge of the opening can be grasped with the active suction of the cutter and lifted to induce the PVD (Fig. 14.6). If there is a possibility of retinal incarceration in the vitreous cutter during this maneuver, forceps can be used to grasp and pull the edge of the hole created in the posterior hyaloid.

Injecting a bubble of perfluorocarbon liquid (PFCL) through the hole in the posterior hyaloid and slowly increasing the size of the bubble can help cleave the posterior hyaloid from the retina (Fig. 14.7). Alternatively, viscoelastic agents (hydoxypropyl methylcellulose) can be used for the same purpose.

Vitreoschisis is a fairly common occurrence in RRD particularly in young individuals and myopic eyes (Fig. 14.8). Repeated use of triamcinolone in these eyes will ensure identification and removal of all the layers of schitic vitreous. The residual adherent cortical vitreous in myopic eyes needs to be peeled with the aid of a micro forceps, needle or an instrument with a rough surface such as the Tano's diamond-dusted membrane scraper. Recently a technique of "vitreous wiping" has been described wherein a small piece of polyvinyl alcohol (PVA) sponge has been used to aid separation of the cortical vitreous [23]. The irregular surface of the PVA sponge entangles the vitreous fibrils enabling its removal. If the mobility of the retina is a hindrance to removal of the cortical vitreous, attaching the retinal using PFCL can aid removal of the same.

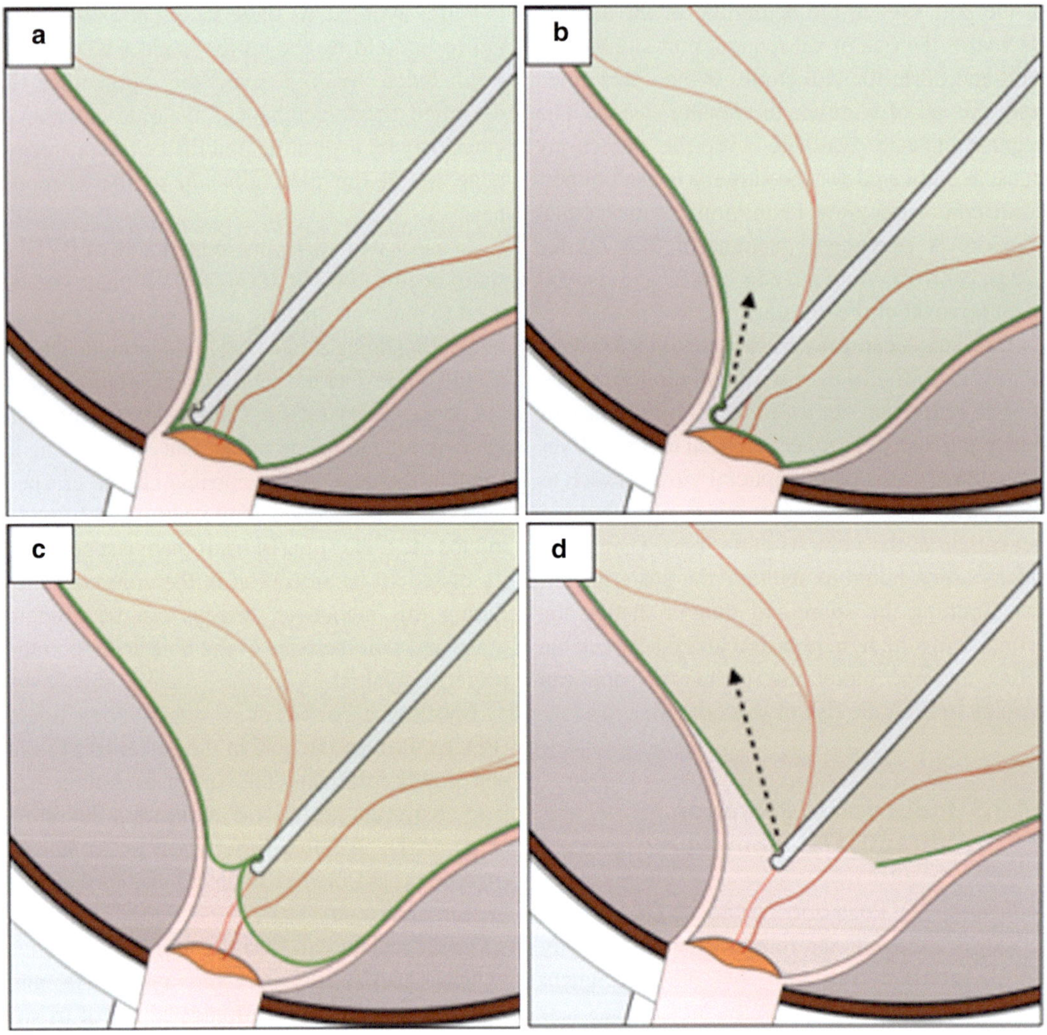

Fig. 14.5 (**a**) Suction is applied with the cutter in suction only mode over the optic disc. (**b**, **c**) Once the vitreous is grasped, the vitreous cutter is moved towards the mid-vitreous cavity. (**d**) Once the posterior hyaloid is detached from the disc, the PVD is extended anteriorly

14.3.5.1 Other Techniques of PVD Induction

A silicone tipped extrusion needle connected to an active aspiration port of the vitrectomy console is used to identify the cortical vitreous and aid PVD induction. The tip is gently swept over the retinal surface. In the presence of cortical vitreous, the tip of the silicone cannula bends down to attach itself to the residual cortical vitreous (Fish strike sign). Maintaining the aspiration and exerting anteroposterior traction aids PVD induction [24].

Non-aspiration technique of PVD induction is described by Takeuchi M et al. In this technique a hole is made in the posterior hyaloid with a diamond-dusted membrane scraper. The separation of posterior vitreous from the retina progresses due to the influx of irrigating fluid through the hole. The scraper is inserted under the posterior hyaloid through the hole and it is lifted to achieve PVD [25].

A hydro dissection technique is described by Dr. Paul Hahn. In this technique, the initial separation of posterior hyaloid is attempted along the

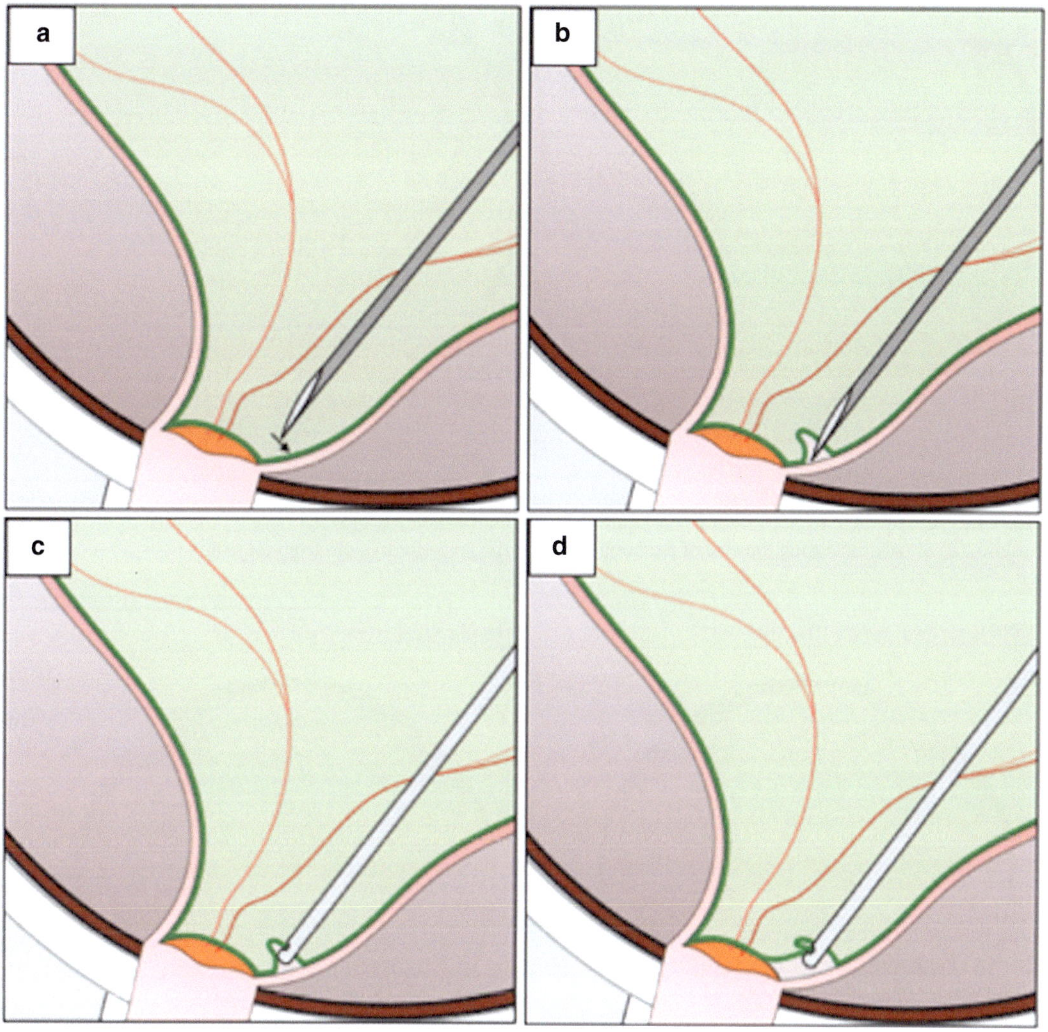

Fig. 14.6 (**a**) A sharp needle (24G or 26G) is used to slice the posterior hyaloid in a tangential motion. (**b**) A hole is created in the posterior hyaloid. (**c**, **d**) The edge of the opening is grasped with the active suction of the cutter and lifted to induce the PVD

temporal vascular arcade using a cutter with its port facing toward the retina. Then the cutter is used to achieve the separation circumferentially. The vitreous is aspirated anteriorly and the infusion fluid is forced posteriorly. This results in hydro dissection of posterior vitreous from the retina. This technique is claimed to have a lesser risk of iatrogenic break. But this would not be feasible in cases with detached mobile retina.

Combined sharp dissection of posterior hyaloid and active aspiration is described by Ellabban AA et al. In this technique, a micropick (25-gauge needle with bent tip) connected to active aspiration tubing of vitrectomy machine is used to induce PVD. Active aspiration is applied so as to engage the posterior hyaloid adjacent to optic disc. Then the tip of the micropick is used to penetrate the posterior hyaloid by tangential movement. Once the tip is in the subhyaloid space, the micropick is lifted toward the center of vitreous cavity to achieve separation of posterior hyaloid mechanically [26].

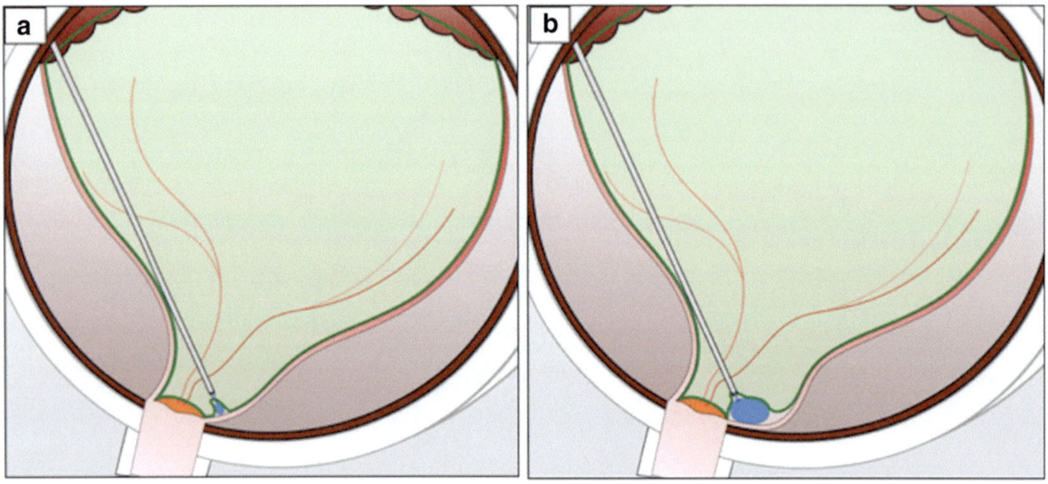

Fig. 14.7 (**a**) A bubble of perfluorocarbon liquid (PFCL) (blue bubble) is injected through the hole in the posterior hyaloid. (**b**) Slowly increasing the size of the bubble cleaves the posterior hyaloid from the retina

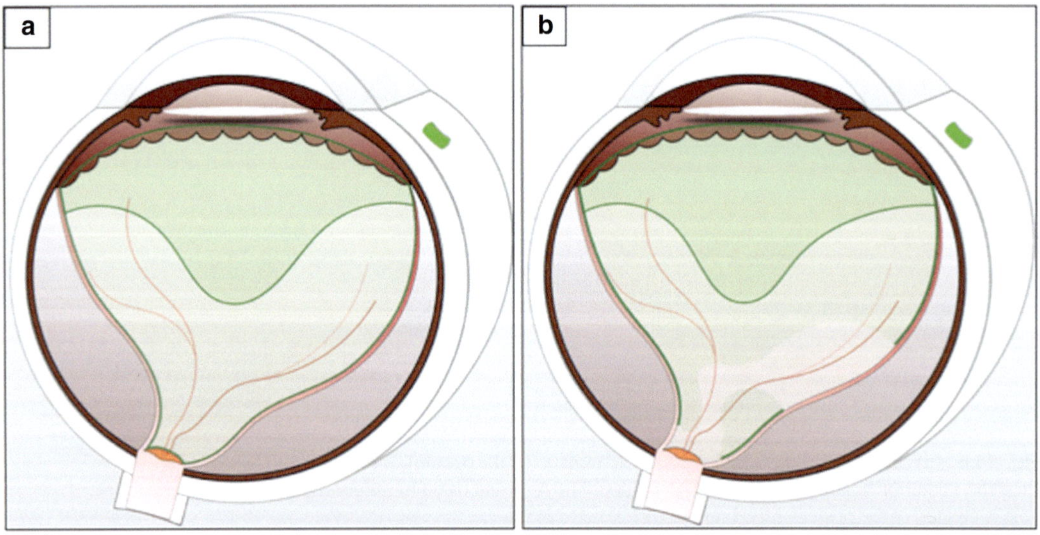

Fig. 14.8 Vitreoschisis. (**a**) During PVD, the cortical vitreous is split and a layer of remnant hyaloid is adherent to the retina as a continuous sheet (indicated by green line). (**b**) The remnant hyaloid is adherent to retina in multiple patches

14.3.6 Peripheral Vitrectomy

The induction of PVD is advanced anteriorly up to the point where vitreous is firmly adherent to retina and peeling beyond it may result in a retinal tear (Fig. 14.9). This point can be vitreous base, peripheral retinal degeneration, or in some myopic eyes anomalous posterior vitreous attachment. In cases with lattice degeneration or focal areas of vitreoretinal adhesion, an attempt can be made to induce the PVD anterior to the attachment, thereby isolating the island of the adherent vitreous from the rest of the posterior hyaloid (Figs. 14.10 and 14.11). Accomplishing this obviates the need for an encerclage and also minimizes the risk of recurrent RD.

The remnant vitreous adherent to the vitreous base or areas of abnormal vitreoretinal adhesion is shaved using high cut rates and low vacuum. Cutters with smaller/double ports and consoles

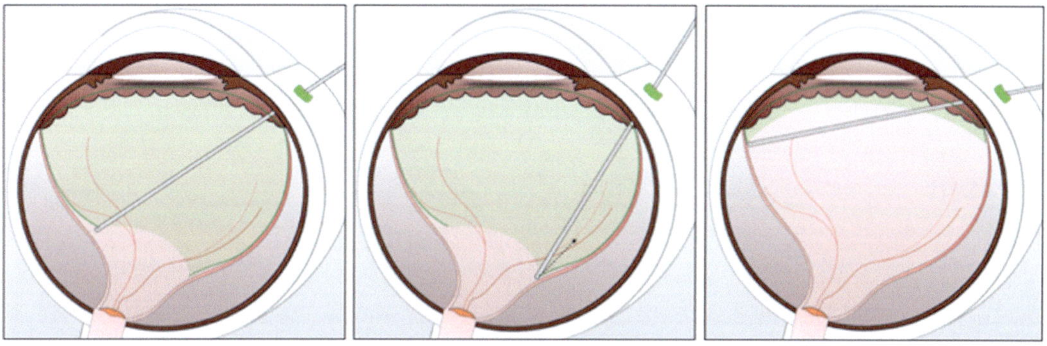

Fig. 14.9 PVD is advanced anteriorly in all directions up to the vitreous base

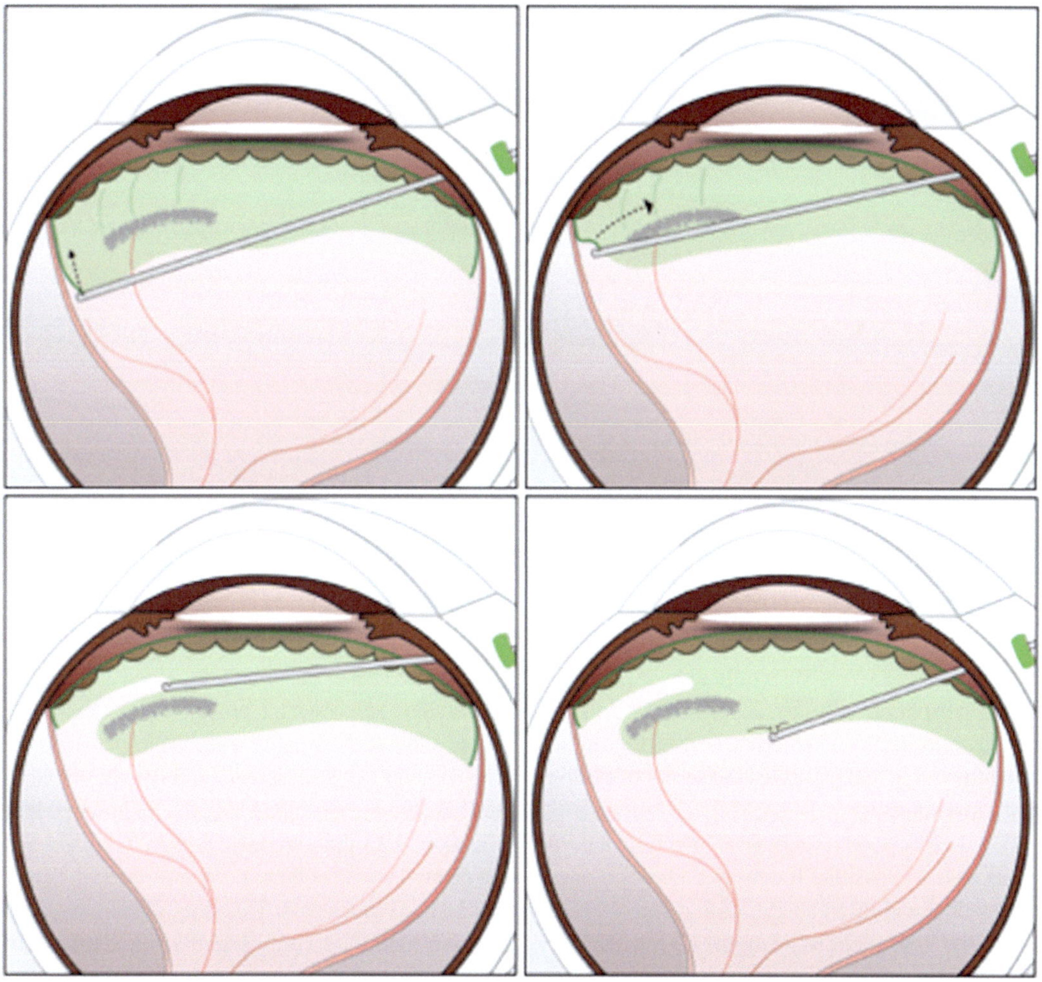

Fig. 14.10 Step-by-step illustration of peripheral vitrectomy in case with lattice degeneration. Posterior hyaloid is detached anterior to the lattice

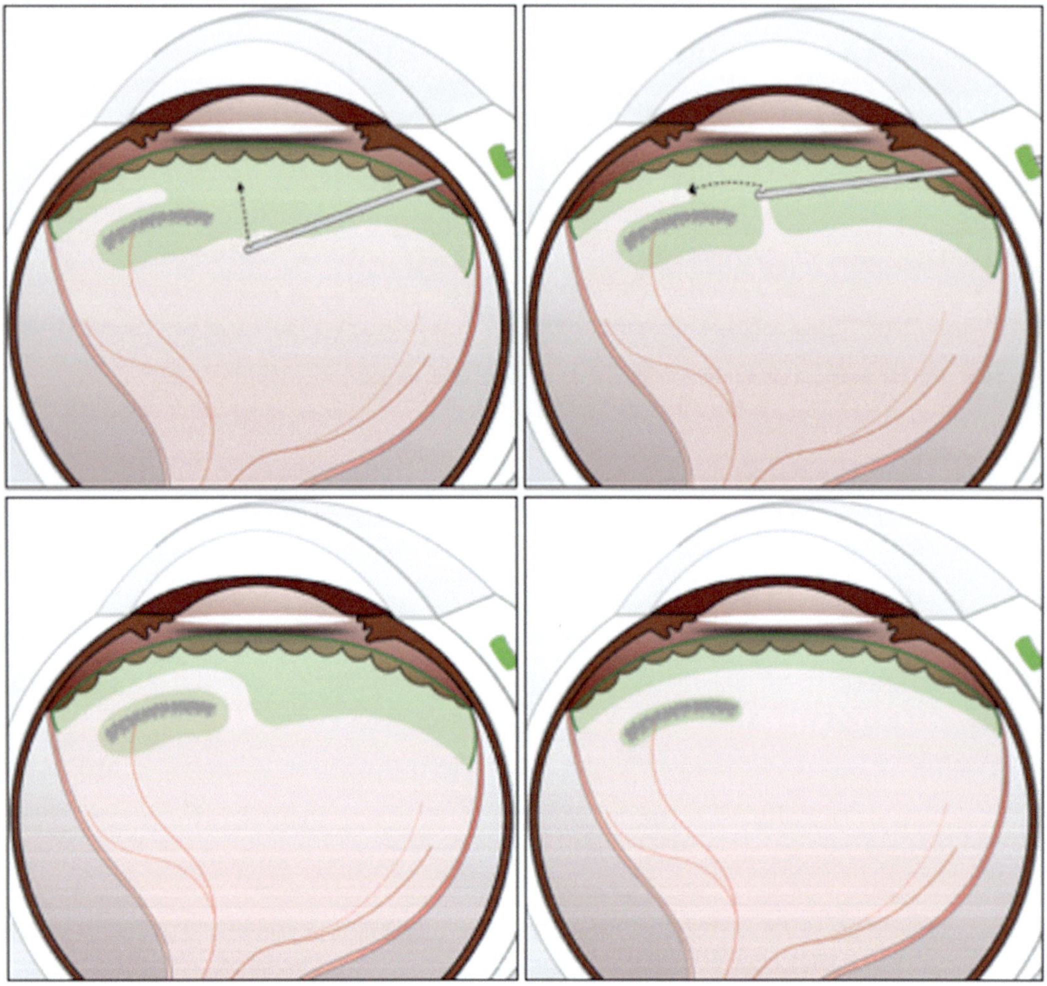

Fig. 14.11 Step-by-step illustration of peripheral vitrectomy in case with lattice degeneration (continued). Vitreous around the lattice is detached and cut to leave an island of vitreous adherent to lattice

with vitreous shave mode would aid safe removal of the peripheral vitreous. Using PFCL to keep the posterior retina attached decreases the mobility of the retina and increases the safety of peripheral vitrectomy.

While it is good to debulk as much of the vitreous base as possible, it may not always be necessary or possible. In an eye with a single break, it may be imprudent to be aggressive with vitreous base dissection. In contrast, in eyes with multiple breaks and peripheral retinal degeneration, it is preferable to do as complete vitrectomy as possible.

Vitreous base debulking is aided by scleral depression. An assistant aided scleral depression would allow surgery under wide-angle visualization. The surgeon can also depress and debulk the vitreous base by visualization using the microscope illumination, with the vitreous cutter in one hand and the depressor in the other. A cotton-tipped applicator can be used to depress. This does not slip over the sclera in contrast to a muscle hook. The advantage of the muscle hook is wider area of scleral depression.

Ease and completeness of vitreous base debulking would depend on the lens status of the patient. It is easiest and most complete in an apha-

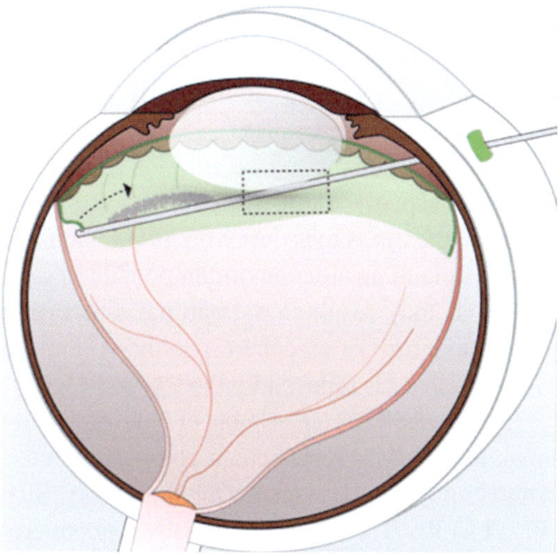

Fig. 14.12 Reaching the vitreous across the lens can lead to lens touch (indicated by the box) in cases with thicker lenses

kic eyes. In pseudophakic eyes, while one can attempt removal of the anterior vitreous base, there is a risk of iatrogenic zonular damage. This can result in migration of the tamponade agent (gas or silicone oil) into the anterior chamber resulting in elevated intraocular pressure and other complications. In young phakic eyes, the lens is thin and it is possible to debulk the vitreous base adequately with careful depression. Reaching an area across the lens should be avoided (Fig. 14.12). The sclerotomy on the side of area of interest is to be used preferably. In eyes wherein a good vitreous base dissection is preferred but not possible, an encerclage can be placed.

14.3.7 Internal Limiting Membrane Removal

Internal Limiting Membrane (ILM) need not be removed in every eye undergoing primary vitrectomy for RRD.

- ILM needs to be removed in RRD with a peripheral break and macular hole, to attempt macular hole closure.
- In eyes with residual cortical vitreous over the macular region, staining the ILM and removing it will aid removal of the irregular islands of cortical vitreous as well.
- In eyes with immature PVR wherein one is suspicious of subsequent PVR progression and re-detachment, ILM peeling can be done.
- ILM peeling in RRD is preferably performed under PFCL. Staining the ILM using BBG can be performed under air to ensure adequate staining. An initial nick in the stained ILM can be made using a forceps or needle. PFCL is injected to flatten the posterior pole. ILM can then be peeled from the site of initiation, peeling it under the PFCL in a tangential manner. Some would prefer ILM peeling without done PFCL.

14.3.8 Identification of Breaks

All retinal breaks need to be identified during vitrectomy to enable subsequent retinopexy. Intravitreal stream of yellow-colored fluid called schlieren, noticed during the process of PVD induction and peripheral vitrectomy guides one to the retinal break [27]. It is preferable to mark the breaks with cautery to aid in visualization of the breaks after retinal reattachment under air. This is particularly important in myopic eyes with chorioretinal atrophy wherein the break may "disappear" indistinctly after retinal reattachment following fluid gas exchange. Rolled edges of a retinal tear are rolled because of the PVR membranes, which may result in late failure of the surgery by reopening of the break. Diathermy to the edge of the tear results in necrosis of this PVR, decreasing the risk of re-detachment.

At times it may not be possible to identify the causative retinal break despite an extensive and careful inspection. Transretinal injection of a small quantity of a dye (trypan blue) with a narrow-gauge needle and injecting PFCL over the posterior pole will result in the expression of the subretinal dye into the vitreous cavity through the retinal break, allowing one to identify the break [28]. Our modification (unpublished data) is to inject the dye transclerally, using a 26g or 30g needle into the subretinal space, so that retinotomy can be avoided. The dye is injected transclerally by the dominant hand of the surgeon. The needle entry and the injection can be performed under direct visualization using wide-angle viewing system.

14.3.9 Fluid Air Exchange

A soft tip cannula or flute cannula or active suction is placed at the posterior most break and air is injected via the infusion cannula by the air pump of the vitrectomy console at 30–40 mm of Hg pressure. As the air flattens the peripheral retina, the subretinal fluid is driven towards the break and out of the eye through the flute needle.

An anterior break can also be used effectively to drain the subretinal fluid (SRF). It can be aided by rotating the eye toward the break so that the SRF gravitates toward the break (Fig. 14.13a). A fluid–fluid exchange wherein most of the SRF is removed under fluid infusion before turning on the air infusion when the retina is nearly flat, would also aid near complete drainage of the fluid. Once the intravitreal fluid level crosses the posterior edge of the retinal break, then the flute needle is moved to the optic disc to drain the residual intravitreal fluid. If the flow of the SRF through the break is impeded while performing FAE by moving the flute needle away from the break before complete drainage, it results in incomplete drainage of SRF.

When draining through an anterior break, SRF can get trapped posteriorly. This can be left to absorb if the eye is to be left with gas tamponade. If one is planning silicone oil tamponade in such a case, it may result in suboptimal tamponade due to under fill of silicone oil as the volume of vitreous cavity is reduced by the trapped SRF.

If residual SRF is undesirable or if the peripheral break is not easily accessible, a posterior drainage retinotomy may be made to drain the SRF (Fig. 14.13b). The drainage retinotomy is preferably placed in the superior half of the retina (if possible nasal half), in line with one of the sclerotomies to enable easy access and complete drainage. It is preferable to place it in an area with copious SRF. The area of the retinotomy is marked with cautery. Placing the flute at the area where retina was cauterized will result in the retinotomy and initiation of the drainage. Alternatively, PFCL can be injected to flatten the posterior retina up to the break. Then SRF is drained up to the break and then PFCL is drained completely (Fig. 14.14). In myopic eyes, longer cannulas can be used to perform FAE.

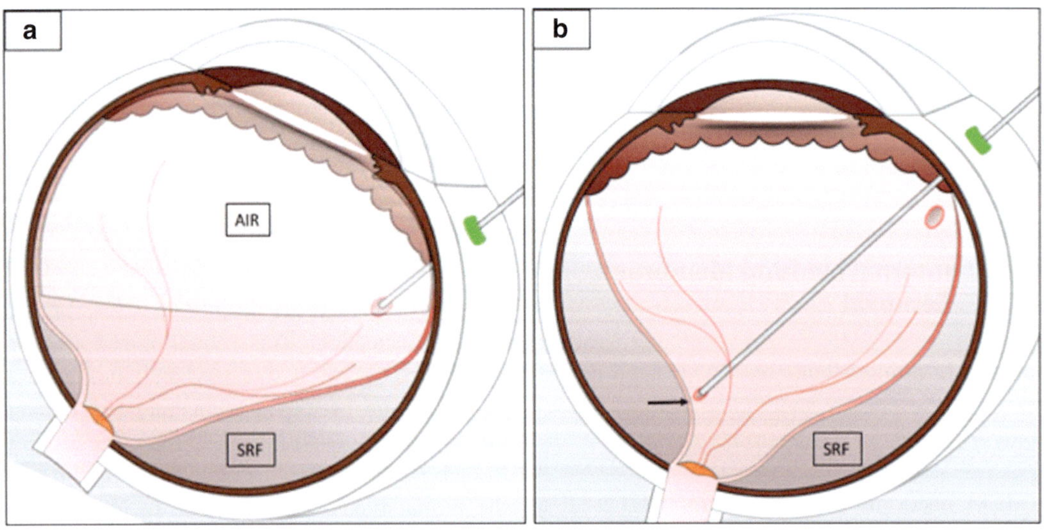

Fig. 14.13 (**a**) While draining the SRF through the anterior break, the eye is rotated toward the break so that the SRF gravitates toward the break. (**b**) A posterior drainage retinotomy (arrow) is used to drain SRF

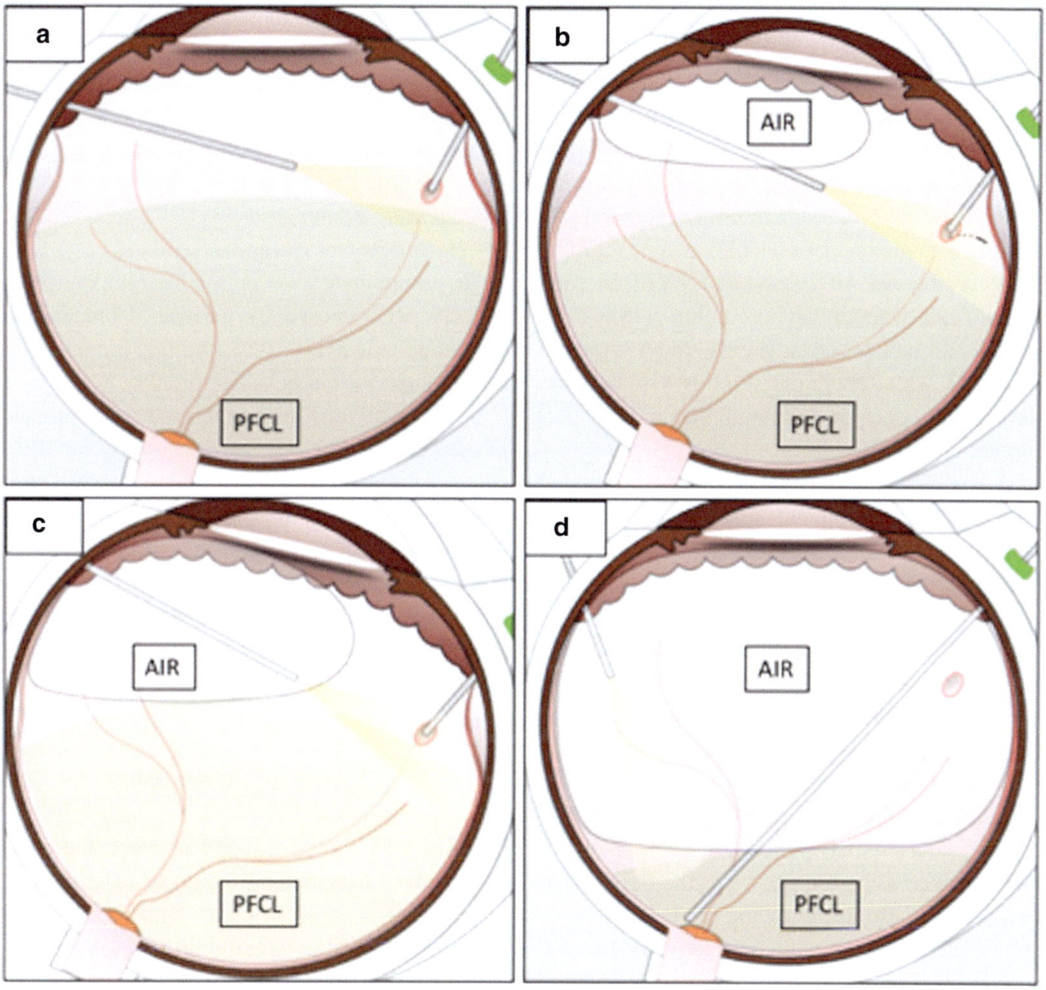

Fig. 14.14 Step-by-step illustration of PFCL assisted SRF drainage. (**a**) PFCL is filled up to the level of break. (**b**, **c**) The eye is rotated towards the break and the air infusion is started. (**d**) Once the fluid air exchange reaches the break, PFCL is exchanged with air

14.3.9.1 Difficulties during FAE

1. If the break is small, the retinal edges can block the cannula resulting in poor drainage of SRF. Keeping the tip of the cannula through the break close to the RPE will aid drainage. Alternately the break can be made larger with cautery.
2. Condensation of water vapor on the exposed posterior surface of intraocular lenses can result in poor visualization during FAE. Coating this surface with a small quantity of viscoelastic will clear the view.
3. Vanishing break—in an eye with an encerclage, the break may fall on the posterior slope of the indent making it invisible. Tightening the buckle after FAE or loosening it prior to FAE can prevent this issue.

14.3.10 Retinopexy

Once the retina is attached, 2–3 rows of contiguous laser burns are placed around each of the breaks. In HSTs, it is preferable to extend the laser up to the ora to prevent delayed opening of the anterior edge of the break due to contraction of the attached residue of the vitreous base. If laser photocoagulation is not possible due to anterior location, cryotherapy can be performed under visualization through the wide-angle viewing system. It is preferable to limit cryotherapy to treating a single break or a small area of retina to decrease the risk of subsequent PVR. In high myopic eyes wherein the poor contrast may limit identification of posterior breaks under air, or in situations with suboptimal fundus visualization through air, laser photocoagulation can be performed under PFCL.

Areas of lattice degeneration are surrounded by 2–3 rows of contiguous laser burns, extending them to the ora in lattices with associated HSTs. Laser photocoagulation to the vitreous base region (~5 rows) may be placed 360° in eyes wherein the causative break cannot be identified, in eyes with extensive peripheral retinal degeneration or in eyes wherein aggressive vitreous base dissection was performed, raising concerns of missing tiny breaks.

In high myopic eyes with breaks within pre-existing chorioretinal atrophy, laser uptake may be poor. Increasing the power or the duration of the laser can help surmount the issue; in rare situations, an endocryo may be necessary to treat such breaks.

14.3.11 Tamponade

The choice of tamponade depends on the location of break.

Short-acting or long-acting gases can be used. Air, sulfur hexafluoride, and perfluoro propane are the commonly used gases. The longevity of gases is listed in Table 14.2. In silicone study, short-acting gas was found to be inferior to long-acting gas in terms of anatomical success [29, 30]. However, completeness of vitrectomy and relief of traction is more important than choice of tamponade.

Table 14.2 Properties of gases used as tamponade

Gas	Percent of gas	Longevity
Air	–	5–7 days
Sulfur hexafluoride	18%	1–2 weeks
Perfluoropropane	14%	6–8 weeks

Exclusive use of air as tamponade is reported to have similar primary reattachment rate compared to long-acting gases [31]. It is reported that re-detachment was recognized early in cases with air as tamponade. We prefer air tamponade in superior RDs caused by peripheral breaks and gas tamponade in eyes with multiple breaks, inferior, or superior but posterior breaks.

Silicone oil may not be required as tamponade in eyes undergoing primary vitrectomy for RRD except in one-eyed patients wherein early visual rehabilitation is required, in patients who cannot maintain position, eyes with multiple inferior breaks at varying distances from the ora. A 1000 centistokes oil is adequate as tamponade with the silicone oil removal planned 3 months later.

14.3.12 Closure of Sclerotomy

In cases with trans conjunctival ports, the ports are removed by grasping the collar. The sclerotomy is self sealing. In cases with trans scleral ports, the sclerotomy is sutured with an absorbable polyglactin suture once the ports are removed. 20G sclerotomies need suturing. Intraocular pressure should be monitored during closure of sclerotomy. If peritomy is performed, it is closed with an absorbable suture or by electrocautery.

14.4 Results of Primary Vitrectomy for RRD

The single procedure retinal reattachment rate varies from 82% to 96.1% [32–35]. The final reattachment rate is close to 100%. In recent studies no statistically significant difference in the rate of anatomical success is seen in cases with established PVR and no PVR [34]. Similarly, no such difference is seen in cases with superior and inferior breaks [35].

References

1. Schwartz SG, Flynn HW. Primary retinal detachment: scleral buckle or pars plana vitrectomy? Curr Opin Ophthalmol. 2006;17:245–50.
2. Falkner-Radler CI, Myung JS, Moussa S, Chan RV, Smretschnig E, Kiss S, et al. Trends in primary retinal detachment surgery: results of a bicenter study. Retina. 2011;31:928–36.
3. Sasaki H, Shiono A, Kogo J, Yomoda R, Munemasa Y, Syoda M, et al. Inverted internal limiting membrane flap technique as a useful procedure for macular hole-associated retinal detachment in highly myopic eyes. Eye (Lond). 2017;31:545–50.
4. Takahashi H, Inoue M, Koto T, Itoh Y, Hirota K, Hirakata A. Inverted internal limiting membrane flap technique for treatment of macular hole retinal detachment in highly myopic eyes. Retina. 2018;38:2317–26.
5. Oshima Y, Emi K, Motokura M, Yamanishi S. Survey of surgical indications and results of primary pars plana vitrectomy for rhegmatogenous retinal detachments. Jpn J Ophthalmol. 1999;43:120–6.
6. Heimann H, Bartz-Schmidt KU, Bornfeld N, Weiss C, Hilgers RD, Foerster MH. Scleral buckling versus primary vitrectomy in rhegmatogenous retinal detachment study group. Scleral buckling versus primary vitrectomy in rhegmatogenous retinal detachment. Ophthalmology. 2007;114:2142–54.
7. Newman DK, Burton RL. Primary vitrectomy for pseudophakic and aphakic retinal detachments. Eye (Lond). 1999;13:635–9.
8. Brazitikos PD, Androudi S, Christen WG, Stangos NT. Primary pars plana vitrectomy versus scleral buckle surgery for the treatment of pseudophakic retinal detachment: a randomized clinical trial. Retina. 2005;25:957–64.
9. Sun Q, Sun T, Xu Y, Yang XL, Xu X, Wang BS, et al. Primary vitrectomy versus scleral buckling for the treatment of rhegmatogenous retinal detachment: a meta-analysis of randomized controlled clinical trials. Curr Eye Res. 2012;37:492–9.
10. Sharma YR, Karunanithi S, Azad RV, Vohra R, Pal N, Singh DV, et al. Functional and anatomic outcome of scleral buckling versus primary vitrectomy in pseudophakic retinal detachment. Acta Ophthalmol Scand. 2005;83:293–7.
11. Desai UR, Strassman IB. Combined pars plana vitrectomy and scleral buckling for pseudophakic and aphakic retinal detachments in which a break is not seen preoperatively. Ophthalmic Surg Lasers. 1997;28:718–22.
12. Sharma T, Gopal L, Badrinath SS. Primary vitrectomy for rhegmatogenous retinal detachment associated with choroidal detachment. Ophthalmology. 1998;105:2282–5.
13. Yang CM. Pars plana vitrectomy in the treatment of combined rhegmatogenous retinal detachment and choroidal detachment in aphakic or pseudophakic patients. Ophthalmic Surg Lasers. 1997;28:288–93.
14. Kinori M, Moisseiev E, Shoshany N, Fabian ID, Skaat A, Barak A, et al. Comparison of pars plana vitrectomy with and without scleral buckle for the repair of primary rhegmatogenous retinal detachment. Am J Ophthalmol. 2011;152:291–7.
15. Weichel ED, Martidis A, Fineman MS, McNamara JA, Park CH, Vander JF, et al. Pars plana vitrectomy versus combined pars plana vitrectomy-scleral buckle for primary repair of pseudophakic retinal detachment. Ophthalmology. 2006;113:2033–40.
16. Lindsell LB, Sisk RA, Miller DM, Foster RE, Petersen MR, Riemann CD, et al. Comparison of outcomes: scleral buckling and pars plana vitrectomy versus vitrectomy alone for primary repair of rhegmatogenous retinal detachment. Clin Ophthalmol. 2016;11:47–54.
17. Mehta S, Blinder KJ, Shah GK, Grand MG. Pars plana vitrectomy versus combined pars plana vitrectomy and scleral buckle for primary repair of rhegmatogenous retinal detachment. Can J Ophthalmol. 2011;46:237–41.
18. Lemley CA, Han DP. An age based method for planning sclerotomy placement during pediatric vitrectomy: a 12-year experience. Trans Am Ophthalmol Soc. 2007;105:86–9.
19. Chen JC. Sutureless pars plana vitrectomy through self-sealing sclerotomies. Arch Ophthalmol. 1996;114:1273–5.
20. Shah PK, Prabhu V, Narendran V. Outcomes of transconjuctival sutureless 27-gauge vitrectomy for stage 4 retinopathy of prematurity. World J Clin Pediatr. 2018;7:62–6.
21. Oshima Y, Wakabayashi T, Sato T, Ohji M, Tano Y. A 27-gauge instrument system for transconjunctival sutureless microincision vitrectomy surgery. Ophthalmology. 2010;117(1):93–102.
22. Ghoraba HH. Primary vitrectomy for the management of rhegmatogenous retinal detachment associated with choroidal detachment. Graefes Arch Clin Exp Ophthalmol. 2001;239:733–6.
23. van Overdam KA, van Etten PG, van Meurs JC, Manning SS. Vitreous wiping, a new technique for removal of vitreous cortex remnants during vitrectomy. Acta Ophthalmol. 2019;97(5):e747–52.
24. Kelly NE, Wendel RT. Vitreous surgery for idiopathic macular holes. Results of a pilot study. Arch Ophthalmol. 1991;109:654–9.
25. Takeuchi M, Takayama K, Sato T, Ishikawa S, Fujii S, Sakurai Y. Non-aspiration technique to induce posterior vitreous detachment in minimum incision vitrectomy system. Br J Ophthalmol. 2012;96:1378–9.
26. Ellabban AA, Barry R, Sallam AA. Surgical induction of posterior vitreous detachment using combined sharp dissection and active aspiration. Acta Ophthalmol. 2016;94:524–5.

27. Friberg TR, Tano Y, Machemer R. Streaks (schlieren) as a sign of rhegmatogenous detachment in vitreous surgery. Am J Ophthalmol. 1979;88:943–4.
28. Jackson TL, Kwan AS, Laidlaw AH, Aylward W. Identification of retinal breaks using subretinal trypan blue injection. Ophthalmology. 2007;114:587–90.
29. Silicone Study Group. Vitrectomy with silicone oil or sulfur hexafluoride gas in eyes with severe proliferative vitreoretinopathy: results of a randomized clinical trial. Silicone Study Report 1. Arch Ophthalmol. 1992;110:770–9.
30. Silicone Study Group. Vitrectomy with silicone oil or perfluoropropane gas in eyes with severe proliferative vitreoretinopathy: results of a randomized clinical trial. Silicone Study Report 2. Arch Ophthalmol. 1992;110:780–92.
31. Pak KY, Lee SJ, Kwon HJ, Park SW, Byon IS, Lee JE. Exclusive use of air as gas tamponade in rhegmatogenous retinal detachment. J Ophthalmol. 2017;2017:1341948.
32. Mohamed YH, Ono K, Kinoshita H, Uematsu M, Tsuiki E, Fujikawa A, et al. Success rates of vitrectomy in treatment of rhegmatogenous retinal detachment. J Ophthalmol. 2016;2016:2193518.
33. Romano MR, Das R, Groenwald C, Stappler T, Marticorena J, Valldeperas X, et al. Primary 23 gauge sutureless vitrectomy for rhegmatogenous retinal detachment. Indian J Ophthalmol. 2012;60:29–33.
34. Lumi X, Lužnik Z, Petrovski G, Petrovski BÉ, Hawlina M. Anatomical success rate of pars plana vitrectomy for treatment of complex rhegmatogenous retinal detachment. BMC Ophthalmol. 2016;16:216.
35. Stavrakas P, Tranos P, Androu A, Xanthopoulou P, Tsoukanas D, Stamatiou P, et al. Anatomical and functional results following 23-gauge primary pars plana vitrectomy for rhegmatogenous retinal detachment: superior versus inferior breaks. J Ophthalmol. 2017;2017:2565249.

Principles in the Management of Proliferative Vitreoretinopathy

15

Manish Nagpal, Shachi Wachasundar, Gayathri Mohan, and Ahmed Eltayib

15.1 Introduction

Proliferative vitreoretinopathy (PVR) formerly known by terms like “massive vitreous traction” or “massive periretinal proliferation” is the most common cause of failed repair of rhegmatogenous retinal detachment (RD). Surgical management of RD and PVR are pneumatic retinopexy, scleral buckling, and pars plana vitrectomy (PPV) alone or in combination. Newer techniques and instrumentation for vitrectomy have resulted in greatly improved outcomes of surgery. However, despite these advances, more than one-fourth of initially successful cases do land in re-detachment due to recurrent or persistent vitreoretinal traction [1]. As a result, PVR remains a challenge for the vitreoretinal surgeon and necessitates continuing efforts for development of other forms of therapy to inhibit the pathologic cascade causing traction. It is a well-known fact that retinal pigment epithelial (RPE) cells play a key role in triggering development of PVR [2]. The participation of soluble mediators and the extracellular matrix components is critical in cellular events like proliferation and tissue contraction, which result in PVR formation. Recent efforts have been directed toward the biochemical inhibition of cellular proliferation and membrane contraction in PVR. The need of the hour is a multimodal, combinatorial approach, involving inhibition of reactive oxygen species, blocking the direct and indirect pathway of platelet-derived growth factor receptor-α (PDGFRα) activation to halt the process of PVR. Furthermore, in the future, attention should be given to optimizing the correct dosing and administration of drugs, since some of the past failures may be due to the manner and time of administration rather than due to lack of true efficacy of the drugs tested [3].

M. Nagpal (✉) · S. Wachasundar · G. Mohan · A. Eltayib
Department of Retina and Vitreous, Retina Foundation, Ahmedabad, Gujarat, India

15.2 Risk Factors and Pathogenesis

Certain factors are associated with increased probability of PVR formation. These can be grouped as pre, intra, and post-operative. Preoperatively trauma, uveitis, giant tears, multiple breaks, large break, detachment involving more than two quadrants, vitreous hemorrhage with RD, aphakia, and multiple surgical interventions in the past contribute to the increased risk of PVR formation (Fig. 15.1). Presence of choroidal detachment with retinal detachment, pre- or postoperatively is a significant precursor to PVR formation [4–7]. In a recent study by Kunyong et al., association of cigarette smoking and macular involvement were identified as significant risk factors predictive of PVR formation

A. Jain et al. (eds.), *Cutting-edge Vitreoretinal Surgery*,
https://doi.org/10.1007/978-981-33-4168-5_15

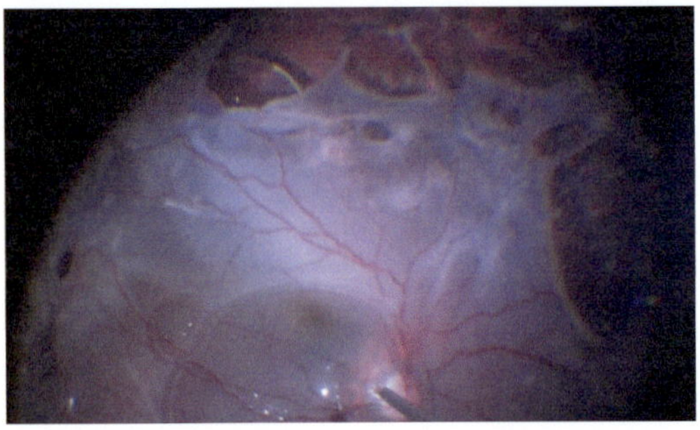

Fig. 15.1 Intraoperative photograph showing retinal detachment with advanced proliferative vitreoretinopathy. There is inferior retinal shortening along with multiple breaks noted inferiorly

after uncomplicated primary retinal detachment repair [8].

In giant retinal tears, the incidence of PVR varies from 16 to 41%, while in penetrating ocular traumas the mean incidence is 25%, range being from 10% to 45% [5]. In eyes with Rhegmatogenous retinal detachment (RRD) with grade B PVR, the incidence of severe PVR after surgery was reported to be 25.8% when using cryotherapy and 2.2% when using argon laser photocoagulation [6]. Intraoperatively, intraocular hemorrhage during or after surgery, use of air or sulfur hexafluoride, excessive cryotherapy, diathermy or photocoagulation, repeated surgical procedures, and loss of vitreous during subretinal fluid (SRF) drainage also lead to the increased incidence of PVR [7].

15.3 Pathogenesis of PVR

The pathological process of PVR is not completely understood but is thought to be analogous to the defective wound healing process leading to a keloid formation in the skin [9]. The retinal pigment epithelial cells play a key role by dedifferentiating and migrating through a retinal break and undergoing proliferation on the retinal surface. Retinal glial cells and macrophages may also play an important role, perhaps by providing the scaffold for membrane formation or by releasing trophic factors [3, 9].

Basically, PVR results from the growth and contraction of cellular membranes within the hyaloids, retina, and retinal surface owing to intraocular inflammation. These membranes exert traction, causing opening up of otherwise successfully treated retinal breaks, creating new retinal breaks, or promoting proliferation at the posterior vitreous base and anterior cortical vitreous resulting in re-detachment. This in turn causes antero-peripheral traction on the retina with a displacement of the peripheral retina toward the pars plana. Membrane contraction on the inner retina causes distortion and folding, resulting in star folds at the inferior quadrant [10].

Clinical and pathological changes occurring in eyes after posterior segment trauma and grade C PVR, was studied in a recent publication by Ying Zin et al. They documented PVR changes with intraoperative photographs during vitrectomy at serial intervals and observed that retinal fold formation occurred at around 30 days after injury. Within this time frame, they observed, that the retina was soft, easily flattened, thereafter, the retina was observed to become edematous, opaque and swollen, lost its elasticity subsequently to become stiff and undergo shortening [11].

15.4 Surgery in PVR

15.4.1 Scleral Buckling in PVR

Treatment of proliferative retinopathy, being essentially surgical, poses a challenging situation to the vitreoretinal surgeon. Although, vitrectomy with all its modern advances is the procedure of choice, some surgeons are still in favor of 360° scleral buckling for PVR. Scleral buckling acts as an adjunct in relieving the vitreoretinal traction, supporting the vitreous base and minimizing the chance of leakage from small postoperative retinal missed or de novo break. Inferiorly, the vitreous base continues to contract, as it is virtually impossible to remove the vitreous base completely. In eyes with focal or relatively inactive PVR, reattachment may be achieved by scleral buckling alone, with drainage of subretinal fluid and laser photocoagulation.

The width of the scleral buckle is decided based upon the contraction of the vitreous base and size of peripheral breaks if any. It may vary from a broad 7.0-mm, style 277 or 276 encircling tire and 40 band through a solid encircling 5.0-mm wide scleral band down to a 2.5-mm wide style 240 encircling band. The current trend is toward narrower bands. If larger, more posterior tears are present, an extra meridional explant can be placed under the tear, however, in most cases after complete relief of traction, internal tamponade and retinopexy may deem it unnecessary. The scleral sutures should be passed at two-third scleral thickness, at least 1 mm anterior and posterior to the encircling buckle, one or two in each quadrant. The sutures are tied and the buckle tightened at the end after completing vitrectomy.

15.4.2 Combined SB+ PPV Versus PPV Alone for PVR

The rate of successful reattachment of retina declines with increasing complexity of detachment. The anatomical success rate, i.e., retina remaining attached at the end 12 months after surgery for RRD with PVR is reported to be between 60 and 80%. In a study by Frank H et al., a comparison of the anatomical success of combined pars plana vitrectomy–scleral buckle (PPV–SB) and pars plana vitrectomy (PPV) for RRD with grade C PVR was done [12]. They achieved single surgery anatomical success rate of 70.1%, which was comparable to most studies. Even then, the utility of scleral buckle in addition to vitrectomy for PVR remains debatable. Storey et al. compared single surgery anatomical success rate in patients with retinal detachments at high-risk PVR, defined by the presence of preoperative PVR, vitreous hemorrhage, retinal tears >1 clock hour, or retinal detachment in two or more quadrants [13]. Single surgery attachment rate was 75.0% in the PPV and scleral buckle group versus 48.3% in the PPV alone group at 3 months follow-up. EVRS Retinal Detachment Study, on the other hand, postulated that combined vitrectomy and supplemental scleral buckling in Grades B and C1 PVR cases were associated with a higher failure rate of 8.9% versus 3.0%. Owing to the discrepancies in the above findings, determining the optimal management in PVR poses a challenge. Also, various confounding variables like the anatomical and pathological variables in patients with PVR add to the pre-existing dilemma [14].

With the advent of MIVS, most simple and moderate complexity RRD are best managed with PPV alone. Nonetheless, some surgeons may be inclined to add scleral buckle for more complicated retinal detachments. For noncomplex RRD, the addition of SB does not improve the anatomic success and is associated with slightly lower VA than with PPV alone. Current trend may be favoring the use of minimal and efficacious supplemental SB, as it inevitably causes a myopic shift and potentially extraocular movement dysfunction [15].

15.4.3 Vitrectomy in PVR

The vitreoretinal surgery for PVR is aimed at providing permanent support to the retina from any ongoing traction and to close any open retinal breaks. These can be successfully achieved by an encircling scleral buckle, meticulous relief of all retinal traction with vitrectomy, and temporary or long-term tamponade of the retina with long-acting agents. These steps must be achieved without causing prolonged ocular inflammation or further cellular access to the retinal surface or else recurrence is frequent. A comprehensive vitrectomy is essential in the management of PVR. Some surgeons rely on a meticulous vitrectomy and silicone oil (SO) tamponade without scleral buckling and report comparable results with a combined procedure. In any event, almost all eyes with retinal detachment and PVR also require a vitrectomy to remove all vitreous gel, cellular and inflammatory material, blood, and fibroblastic membranes. It is necessary to relieve all traction by division and peeling or delamination of fixed membranes and to remove as much as possible of the vitreous base.

15.5 Surgical Sequence and Techniques for Established PVR

15.5.1 Anesthesia

As with most vitreoretinal surgeries, either general or local peribulbar anesthesia is acceptable. The anesthetist must be informed if long-acting gas is to be used, so as to avoid nitrous oxide in general anesthesia cases. Most cases of PVR can be operated with local anesthesia. The block can be supplemented during the operation, if required, with further injection and by the attending anesthesiologist with intravenous sedation and analgesia.

15.5.2 Placement of Transconjunctival Cannulas

The three 23G, 25G entry ports are placed in the inferotemporal, superotemporal, and superonasal quadrants with an angled entry to diminish the risk of postoperative leakage of air or fluid. The first port is placed near the horizontal meridian in the inferotemporal quadrant, facilitating rotation of the eye downward during surgery while removing inferior vitreous base. The remaining two ports are for the fiberoptic and vitrector or other instruments such as endodiathermy, endolaser, vitreous scissors, vitreous forceps, and extrusion needle. A separate port has to be made if chandelier is to be used. The entry cannulas should be placed above the midline almost opposite each other, to facilitate peripheral visualization by superior and inferior globe rotation. Care must be taken to check that the position of indwelling ports inside the vitreous cavity and avoid subretinal or suprachoroidal infusion during vitrectomy.

15.5.3 Management of Lens in PVR

In cases of posterior PVR, the crystalline lens could be retained, however, presence of anterior PVR warrants its removal to facilitate adequate dissection of the anterior vitreous and prevent formation of cyclitic membrane. A planned cataract extraction with an intraocular lens (IOL) placed in the bag should be considered prior to starting vitrectomy. A posterior chamber IOL, if present, should be retained. Anterior chamber IOLs and iris plane lenses may have to be removed. Implant removal can occasionally result in an intraoperative hemorrhage or corneal and iris damage and compromise the surgical result. Clear lens always becomes cataractous with SO, for which phacoemulsification with or without IOL implantation at the time of SO removal can be done or when it hampers the view of the posterior segment. If the surgeon prefers pars plana lensectomy, there can be two situations, firstly when the capsule is removed completely, corneal decompensation can occur in the long term for which an inferior iridotomy can reduce risk. On the other hand, if capsule is left intact, then it almost always becomes opaque in the presence of SO. Subsequently, at the time of IOL implantation in the sulcus, YAG laser capsulotomy or formal capsulotomy can be done.

15.5.4 Core Vitrectomy and Removal of Vitreous Base

Complete removal of the central vitreous after induction of a posterior vitreous detachment is a critical step, although most patients with established PVR have a pre-existing PVD. Next step is the meticulous removal of the peripheral vitreous, with special care taken to completely remove inferior vitreous, as gravity causes pigment debris and inflammatory material to settle inferiorly.

Adherent vitreous membranes and the base can be visualized better by injecting intravitreal triamcinolone. With the advent of MIVS, the modern high-speed vitrectomy cutters having a port close to the tip facilitate shaving of the attached vitreous off the surface, without causing inadvertent retinal breaks. Scleral depression by an assistant can also help while removing the inferior vitreous base. In case of mobile detached retinas, filling of the vitreous cavity by heavy perfluorocarbon liquid can help to stabilize the retina while attempting removal of the peripheral vitreous. PFCL has a dual action, displacing subretinal fluid anteriorly by ironing the retina and breaking down invisible microscopic retinal bridges of scar tissue.

15.5.5 Epiretinal Membrane Removal and Use of Perfluorocarbon Liquid

After complete vitrectomy, any fixed folds or retinal contraction due to epiretinal membranes should be tackled. Peeling of the membranes is begun from the surface of the retina starting from the posterior pole and going outward. A blunt vitreous spatula or pick may help find a plane or elevate the membrane, if it is not pre-existing which can be peeled by vitreous forceps. Care must be taken to avoid creating iatrogenic retinal breaks. Fixed folds with the contracted membrane overlying tend to fold the retina in the crevices. Membrane spanning across the macula needs to be peeled (Figs. 15.2 and 15.3). An injection of vital dye such as methylene blue can be used to stain the internal limiting membrane and allow its peeling, especially if retinal surface at the posterior pole is stiff or shiny. The degree of adherence of epiretinal membranes to the retinal surface is variable, so that few may be peeled easily in a single sheet, while others have to be freed up in a piecemeal fashion or delaminated. In areas where retina is attached, peeling of surface retinal membranes and internal limiting membrane is easier. Next comes the drainage of the subretinal fluid, which can be done through an open retinal break or by creating a small retinotomy away from scar tissue. This process can be facilitated by the injection of the heavy liquid fluorocarbon.

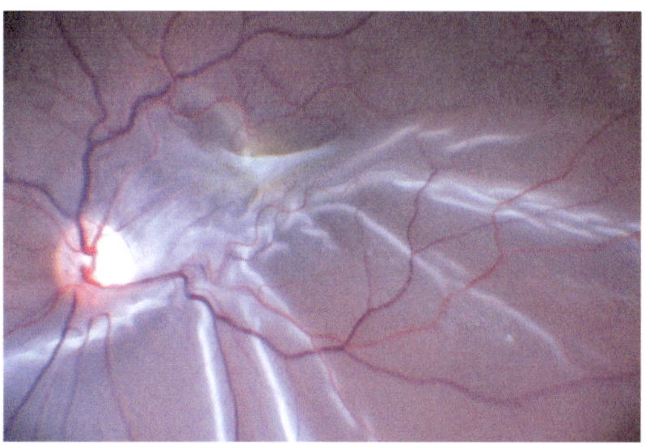

Fig. 15.2 Intraoperative photograph showing detached retina along with a star fold at macula and wrinkles on the retinal surface due to contraction of epiretinal membrane

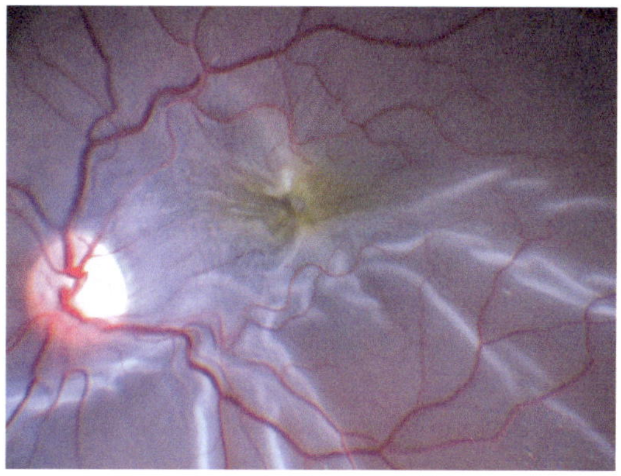

Fig. 15.3 Post-membrane peeling photograph of the eye in Fig. 15.2 showing the release of star-fold at macula

However, there is always a risk that the heavy fluid can pass through a retinal break to lie in the subretinal space which will make its removal difficult, apart from having unknown toxic effects. This risk escalates where tractional membranes are still elevating the retinal break. It is preferable to fill heavy liquid just short of any such retinal break until it is dissected, mobilized, and flattened.

15.5.6 Anterior PVR

By definition, anterior PVR occurs anterior to the posterior insertion of the vitreous base. Anterior PVR (A-PVR) is said to occur when proliferation extends over the ciliary body causing elevation of peripheral retina and anterior loop traction. It can also lead to hypotony, and the development of phthisis bulbi if left untreated, hence carries a poorer prognosis [16]. This makes complete dissection of the anterior loop traction extremely important. Ultrahigh speed cutters should be used to mobilize as much as peripheral retina as possible. Tatsuhiko et al. in their study concluded that

25G vitrectomy can be effective for A-PVR, although eyes with A-PVR in the study required more complex surgical procedures and longer surgical times. Wide-angle viewing system, bimanual surgery by using chandelier, and scleral depression are a value addition whose importance cannot be emphasized enough. Posterior pole can be kept stable during dissection of the anterior membranes by perfluorocarbon liquid. Although wide-angle viewing system facilitates complete anterior dissection, lens can be sacrificed, in case extensive anterior traction is noted preoperatively.

15.5.7 Testing Adequacy of Relief of Traction

Residual traction at the end of vitreous dissection prevents the retina from opposing to the pigment epithelial surface. This forms the major reason for poor anatomic results in PVR. The operating surgeon can test the adequacy of retinal mobilization by doing a complete fluid–air exchange. It can be performed by an extrusion needle aspirating all vitreous fluid, the injected heavy fluid and any residual subretinal fluid by positive suction. Residual subretinal fluid can also be aspirated by a silicone soft tubing extension on the needle. Incomplete relief of traction is evident when retina fails to flatten despite subretinal fluid drainage following fluid–air exchange, or subretinal passage of air over taut membranes. The cause being shortening of the retina by surface or intraretinal gliosis which will not permit adequate mobilization of the retina. At this stage, additional dissection around a retinal tear may help but more often than not, the surgeon will have to take a decision to perform a peripheral relaxing retinotomy or a circumferential or radial retinotomy and retinectomy in cases of badly fibrosed retina.

15.5.8 Relaxing Retinotomy and Retinectomy

The need for a relaxing retinotomy rarely arises in posterior PVR because the membranes can be removed surgically. The tractional vector forces contributing to anterior PVR are three, namely anteroposterior, circumferential, and perpendicular [17]. Relaxing retinotomy is the only savior when epiretinal membrane dissection and scleral buckling fail to relieve the preretinal traction and retinal foreshortening. Indeed, the retina can only be reattached by retinotomy in these very complicated cases [18].

In a study by Lim et al. [19], 30 cases having RRD and grade C PVR were subjected to combined large radial retinotomy and a circumferential retinectomy. The authors believed that although circumferential retinectomy can achieve a flat retina owing to release anteroposterior retinal shortening, more often to obtain adequate relief of circumferential intrinsic retinal shortening, large retinectomies are usually essential. As a result, patient is left to face potential complications such as large visual field defects, ocular hypotony causing phthisis bulbi, recurrent retinal detachment. To overcome this, the authors proposed making a large radial retinotomy with micro scissors, plus a radial retinotomy at 6-o'clock. The edges of radial retinotomy will be redistributed superiorly upon flattening. This salvages the retina from the PVR microenvironment inferiorly. In addition, the resultant loss of a superior visual field is usually better tolerated than an inferior one. The authors reported a 90% reattachment rate and a modest visual recovery with the above procedure.

In a study by the author [20], on 51 patients with RD complicated by grade D PVR who underwent retinectomy of 180° or more, 76.8% achieved improvement or stabilization of visual acuity with 35% achieved ambulatory vision. This finding stresses the importance of trial of surgical intervention in advanced PVR, more so in one-eyed patient. Literature suggests that in patients with PVR in one eye, 50–74.3% of fellow eyes can have a rhegmatogenous event resulting in profound visual loss, and often the eye that was initially thought to be worse, becomes the better-seeing eye with appropriate management. This study reported a 45.4% of one-eyed patients achieving ambulatory vision, supporting the work of some authors who suggested surgery of

PVR being cost effective as determined by the quality adjusted life year.

Even though retinotomy and retinectomies are done to salvage the eye in certain advanced PVR cases, its complications should be kept in mind. Contraction of the posterior free edge of the retina after a large circumferential retinotomy under SO tamponade can extend up to the disc and the macula, thereby compromising the visual outcome. To prevent this, a radial retinotomy sometimes helps. Hypotony is more prevalent in eyes that underwent retinectomy versus that did not, and silicone oil had a lower incidence of hypotony as compared to gas in the Silicone study. In a study by the author [20], size of retinectomy had no bearing on postoperative hypotony. Morse et al. found that hypotony was seen in 43% of attached retinas in a case series. In a study by Alturki et al., 40% hypotony was observed in patients in which 360° retinectomy was performed [21]. Diffuse anterior contraction is a significant predictor of postoperative hypotony. In a study by Federman et al., 78% of eyes having hypotony preoperatively became normotonic after surgery and it was attributed to removal of anterior PVR membranes which were covering ciliary epithelium of the pars plicata and resulting in ciliary body detachment [22]. To conclude, retinectomy aims to relieve all existing traction and should be minimum required to achieve retinal reattachment without causing significant hypotony [18].

15.5.9 Removal of Subretinal Membranes

In eyes with excessive inflammation, extensive PVR, subretinal bands may develop and contract to cause tenting of the retina [23]. Subretinal bands that prevent retinal reattachment should be removed prior to fluid–air exchange by creating a small retinotomy with scissors over the taut membrane, grasping the membrane through the retinotomy with 25G vitreous forceps, and pulling it through the retinotomy into the vitreous compartment [24, 25].

15.5.10 Technique of Stretching the Retina

In a study by Homayoun Tabandeh et al. [26], they described a surgical technique in seven patients with severe PVR in which they used two Tano diamond-dusted membrane scrapers to gently stretch the retina–PVR complex and facilitate partial relaxation of the pre-retinal membranes. The rationale behind this technique as described by the authors lies in the fact that the edges of the membranes are mostly indistinct and lifting the edge for peeling is limited by severe infolding of the retina. Using two membrane scrapers for bimanual gentle stretching of the PVR–retina complex results in partial relaxation of the contracted PVR membrane and loosening of its adhesion to the retina. They achieved complete reattachment in all patients at the end of follow-up period. The authors also suggested that this technique may be used in selected cases of diabetic tractional detachments with fibrovascular proliferation with caution, as the ischemic retina is often atrophic, thin, and predisposed to tearing, may also result in intraoperative bleeding and breaks.

15.5.11 Fluid–Air Exchange

After removal of all membranes and relaxing the retina, fluid–air exchange results in a flat retina. A 25G or 23G extrusion cannula is used to aspirate subretinal fluid, heavy fluid, vitreous fluid, and residual opacities such as blood maintaining continuous air infusion to maintain IOP. Subretinal fluid drainage may be completed via an open retinal break, or a small posterior retinotomy can be made after a diathermy mark on a spot chosen nasal to the disc, away from any fixed fold but over detached retina and avoiding retinal vessels. A suction cannula, 23G/25G, or a soft flexible silicone tip can then be used to make a small opening in the weakened spot, while keeping in mind the need to continuously aspirate the egressing subretinal fluid. Care should be taken to avoid spreading the mobilized pigment cells onto the retinal surface. Alternatively, it can also be passed under the pre-existing retinal break.

15.5.12 Retinopexy

Retinopexy is achieved most commonly by endolaser photocoagulation, although some surgeons prefer laser photocoagulation by indirect ophthalmoscope with scleral depression if required for 360°. All retinal breaks, along with retinotomies are surrounded by 2–3 rows of visible laser burns (Fig. 15.4). 360° laser burns are applied from the vitreous base extending posteriorly toward the equator. In case an extensive retinotomy or retinectomy has been carried out, endolaser is extended up to the arcades. The duration of laser should be longer than used for in office setting, but excessive increase in the power should be avoided for choroidal hemorrhage and rupture of Bruch's membrane can occur. Cryotherapy is generally avoided as it triggers more inflammation breakdown of the blood–vitreous barrier, cellular proliferation, and recurrence of PVR. In case there is persisting subretinal fluid or hazy view of the peripheral retina, cryotherapy may still be necessary.

15.5.13 Intraocular Tamponade

It was the Silicone Study Group, back in 1992 which established the superiority of longer acting tamponade agents, silicone oil, and perfluoro propane (C3F8), over sulfur hexafluoride (SF6) in PVR Grade C or worse. Long-term tamponade with silicone oil has many well-recognized advantages over long-acting gases like quicker visual rehabilitation and does not restrict air travel.

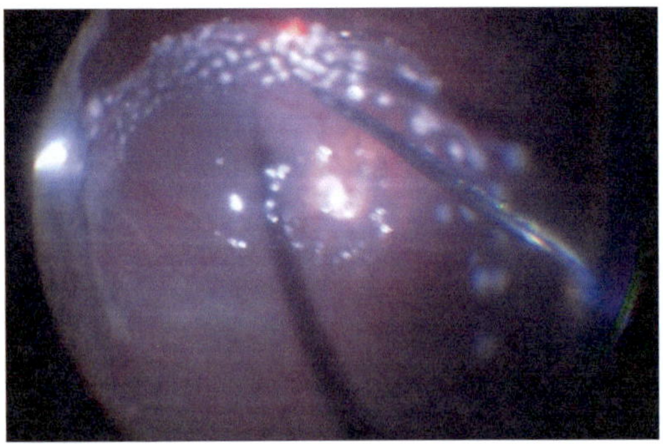

Fig. 15.4 Intraoperative photograph showing the margins of the retinectomy being treated extensively with 3–4 rows of endolaser photocoagulation

15.5.13.1 Silicone Oil

Silicone oil injection can be carried out after complete fluid air exchange, or if PFCL was injected, a direct PFCL–silicone oil exchange can also be done. Alternatively, some may prefer to do an intermediate step of PFCL–fluid exchange followed by fluid–air exchange. This step may be of particular importance to bring any fluid that may be trapped anteriorly under the heavy liquid to the posterior pole after air injection. The modern vitrectomy machines have a specially designed rigid syringe provided with SO injection driven by a pressurized air pump. The SO infusion is begun while air infusion is still connected to the eye, where air can pass out of the air infuser port, with continued infusion pressure is lowered to 10–15 mmHg as silicone enters the vitreous compartment from the superior site, thus maintaining IOP. As the oil reaches the sclerotomy port, air infusion stops, and IOP may rise exponentially. This is prevented by removing the air infusion cannula can allowing SO injection continued until the residual air is expelled. Alternatively, in case of valved cannulas, a vent can be placed to expel the air while injecting silicone oil. A complete fill of the vitreous cavity with SO, having IOP between 10 and 15 mmHg. 1000–1300 cSt silicone oil because is the choice of most surgeons owing to its relative ease of removal. Silicone oil with a higher viscosity is theoretically less prone to pass subretinal through breaks, however, incomplete relief of traction would be the primary reason for such an occurrence (Fig. 15.5).

15.5.13.2 Heavy Silicone Oil

Standard SO has the property of buoyancy resulting in inadequate tamponade to the inferior retina in upright position, which is the major cause of accumulation of inflammatory substrate for PVR occurrence. To tackle this problem, fluorinated SO or heavy SO can be used which effectively tamponades the inferior retina. It can be used in combination with conventional SO, but more

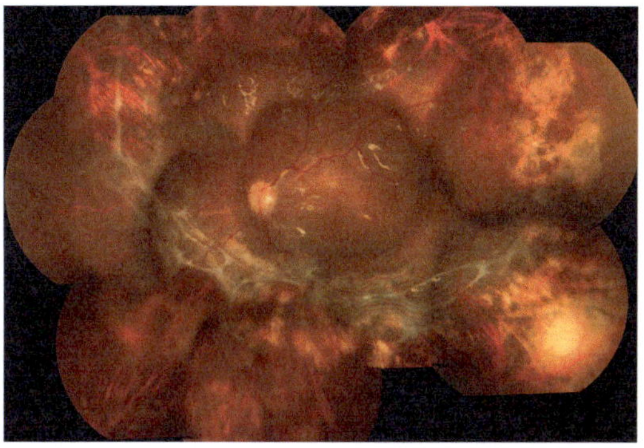

Fig. 15.5 Postoperative photograph showing a well-attached retina, after Pars Plana Vitrectomy for Proliferative vitreoretinopathy, with an inferior relaxing retinectomy andsilicone oil tamponade

often it is used as a substitute particularly after inferior relaxing retinotomy. Complications of these agents were frequent rise of IOP, inflammation, and earlier emulsification, with unknown long-term toxic effects warranting early removal. Multiple studies report excellent anatomical outcomes with the use of heavy silicone oils. Rizzo et al. [27] found out single surgery success rate of 84.6% and final anatomical attachment of 100%, improvement in visual acuity in 32 patients with inferior PVR heavy silicone oil. Other studies, however, failed to show any direct benefit of heavy silicone oils over standard silicone oil. In the Heavy Silicone Oil Study by Joussen et al. [28], visual acuity and anatomical success rates in patients with inferior PVR treated with standard silicone oil versus heavy silicone oil were compared and they found no statistically significant difference in visual acuity or reattachment rate.

15.5.13.3 PFCL as Medium-Term Tamponade

Sigler et al. [29] in their study on 44 eyes with recurrent inferior RD with grade C PVR, perfluoro octane was injected for 2–3 weeks, followed by its subsequent removal in a planned staged procedure. They found this technique to be effective management of recurrent inferior retinal detachments, achieving successful reattachment in 86%. However, it is associated with potential complications of transient inflammation and intraocular pressure elevation are potential complications associated with this technique.

15.6 Removal of Silicone Oil

Higher rate of retinal re-detachment after removal of silicone oil (ROSO) caused by PVR has been reported in the literature. Although, there is no consensus on an ideal time of silicone oil removal, most surgeons prefer removal after 3 months, as delayed removal has no benefits in terms of functional outcome. Retina should be screened at the time of SO removal for presence of missed breaks, ERM, tractional membranes which can be removed during surgery, in addition to laser. A retrospective study on 608 patients by Rizzo et al. [30], described adjunctive use of stains, which is mixture of trypan blue and brilliant blue G dyes re-detachment compared with standard care, which enabled achieving a higher probability of complete removal of ERM and PVR processes, perhaps including subclinical but active pathology.

In a study by Nagpal et al. [31], the presence of encirclage, laser retinopexy and presence of emulsified silicone oil were factors found to have a lower rate of re-detachment post SOR. However, the duration of tamponade had no bearing on the rate of re-detachment. In another study by the author [32], small hyper-reflective spherical bodies observed in sub-silicone oil-foveal depression (SSO-FD) space were studied using spectral domain optical coherence tomography (SD-OCT) in eyes undergoing silicone oil removal. The results were indicative of significantly improved visual outcomes after SOR, hyper-reflective bodies representing emulsified silicone oil globules.

Cataract occurs in 100% cases with silicone oil within 1 year, a combined phacoemulsification with implantation of an intraocular lens, and removal of the SO can be done in a single sitting. Occurrence of delayed glaucoma can occur with or without emulsified SO, and is an indication for removal, so is band keratopathy in young.

Newer generation vitrectomy machines are equipped with controlled active suction through a 23G or 25G, while maintaining IOP by continuous infusion. Heavy fluorinated silicone is more difficult to remove, automated equipment makes it relatively easy. Most surgeons prefer to have intraocular air at the end of surgery, while BSS in the remainder.

In a recently presented paper (publication underway) by the author, microperimetry was used to evaluate functional changes on the macula pre and post SOR. The results are indicative of improved retinal sensitivity in all patients even when best-corrected visual acuity remained the same, thus highlighting the importance of microperimetry in assessing functional status of the macula predicting visual prognosis post SOR.

15.7 Postoperative Care

Initial face down positioning in the first 24 h is deemed critical for the RPE to pump out residual SRF and retinopexy to develop initial adhesions. Strict face down positioning is advocated by some to be done for 7–10 days, more so for inferior breaks. In case of heavy SO tamponade, the patient needs to be supine for 24–48 h before being mobilized. Postoperative regime consists of corticosteroids, mydriatic/cycloplegic drops for 3–4 weeks, in addition, require antihypertensive drops and acetazolamide tablets for postoperative ocular hypertension. High IOP despite maximum tolerated medical therapy implies an overfill, and a small amount may need to be aspirated back from the vitreous cavity.

15.8 Complications of Surgery for PVR [33]

The surgery for PVR is not without complications. The patient of PVR posted for surgery should have realistic expectations, should understand that even after multiple procedures, visual gain may be moderate and that complications can occur during and after the surgery.

15.8.1 Intraoperative Complications

Intraoperative complications are creation of retinal breaks while membrane dissection, incidence of which depends on the degree of adherence of preretinal membrane to retina. It is acceptable to err on the side of creating a retinal break while peeling membranes to mobilize the retina. Hemorrhage while membrane dissection can be tackled by raising the infusion pressure, or the use of endodiathermy. Serous choroidal detachment can occur due to incorrect subretinal or suprachoroidal placement of the cannula, whereas hemorrhagic detachment can occur due to rupture of a choroidal vessel or prolonged hypotony. The former can be dealt with the placement of the infusion cannula at a different port, whereas the latter requires drainage during the same surgery or a later date.

15.8.2 Postoperative Complications

Early postoperative complications are a rise in IOP, inflammation which can most commonly be managed medically. IOP rise more than 25 mm Hg, not controlled by ocular hypotensive drops or oral acetazolamide can result from overfill of gas/SO, which may need to be removed partially. Endophthalmitis is very rare but is a possibility. The most frequent late complication of PVR is the recurrence of surface membranes or macular pucker. Under effective superior SO tamponade, there exists a vitreous pocket containing inflammatory substrate in between the silicone oil meniscus and inferior retina called "perisilicone oil proliferation." Progressive retinal shortening may be accompanied by the late development of large inferior retinal breaks and passage of the SO under the retina. Heavy SO formulations show promise of decreasing perisilicone proliferation. If the macula is not compromised, the membranes can be left alone or re-surgery can be considered. Prolonged intraocular silicone oil is associated with emulsification, cataract formation, glaucoma, corneal decompensation, more in aphakics. Late cystoid macular edema with or without preretinal membranes can be readily analyzed with spectral domain optical coherence tomography and treated with topical steroid and nonsteroidal drops, intravitreal triamcinolone injection, and peeling of the internal limiting membrane over the macula in selected can be tried.

15.9 Adjuncts to Surgery for PVR

15.9.1 Anti-VEGF Agents

Various adjunctive agents like 5-fluorouracil, heparin, daunomycin, corticosteroids, colchicine, and retinoids have been tried unsuccessfully to prevent the formation of PVR. As vascular endothelial growth factor (VEGF) is known to play a crucial role in proliferative diseases of the eye, the probability of anti-VEGF being effective for the treatment and prevention to have been investigated extensively. In a study by Ricker et al. [34] concluded the level of VEGF to be threefold higher in eyes with PVR-related RDs than RDs without PVR. Armstrong et al. [35] reported VEGF concentration in PVR-related membranes to be equivalent to proliferative diabetic retinopathy-related membranes. However, anti-VEGF drugs in PVR-related RDs have been of limited value. A meta-analysis on the effect of Bevacizumab on PVR by Xin-Yu Zhao et al. [36], found that bevacizumab neither enhanced the BCVA 6 months 6 nor reduced the rate of retinal re-detachment, disproving the role of bevacizumab in vitrectomy for PVR-related RD. As PVR is like healing process, the multifactorial pathways like cytokines have a role in its pathogenesis and should be targeted for its prevention. Also, it is believed by Hsu et al. [37] that once the inflammatory cascade begins, the application of anti-VEGF drugs is insufficient to stop the progression of the disease.

15.9.2 Steroids—Intra- and Post-operative

The rationale for including steroids in the prevention of PVR is obvious for their anti-inflammatory properties and by inhibition of cell proliferation by reducing histamine and prostaglandin levels. Agents, like prednisone, dexamethasone, and triamcinolone acetonide (TA), are routinely used during RRD surgery to reduce the risk of PVR. Intraoperative TA is used for delineating adherent posterior hyaloids and epiretinal membrane during vitrectomy, postoperatively it can suppress the intraocular inflammation reaction [38]. The meta-analysis by Hui Shi et al. documented that the use of steroids is an adjunct to RRD surgery to reduce incidence of PVR, more so grade B PVR [39].

Slow-release dexamethasone implant, Ozudex was evaluated in a recent study by Philip J. Banerjee for vitrectomy in PVR, did not show any difference in anatomical success rate compared to controls, but it suggested a greater reduction in CMO [40].

15.10 Pharmacotherapy

Preclinical research continues to throw light on the pathogenesis of PVR formation at a molecular level, aiding in the development of prophylactic and therapeutic agents. Drugs under investigation target one or more (combination therapy) of the involved pathologies, including anti-inflammatory agents, antiproliferative agents, antineoplastic agents, antigrowth factor agents, and antioxidant agents.

Low molecular weight heparin (LMWH, Fragmin) has also been used by adding it to the infusion fluid. It acts by binding to fibronectin which is the most potent stimulator for RPE cell migration, and prevents hypocellular gel contraction [41].

Antiproliferative agents aid by inhibiting the cell cycle and cellular proliferation, which follows the breakdown of blood–retinal barrier [42]. These include compounds like 5-fluorouracil (5-FU), daunorubicin, taxol, colchicine. But the optimal therapeutic dosage that does not cause ocular toxicity is yet to be determined.

Clinical research suggests the Anti-VEGF agents might have a role in the prevention of postoperative PVR. Vascular endothelial cell growth factor (VEGF) A has been reported to be able to activate the platelet-derived growth factor (PDGF) receptor α, a receptor tyrosine kinase that is key to the pathogenesis of PVR [43]. Intra-silicone oil injection of Bevacizumab has been tried [44].

TGF-β is another key player in the pathogenesis of this disease. It plays a role in extracellular matrix production, membrane contraction, and inflammation. Tranlisat, an inhibitor of TGF-β used as an antiallergy drug, showed promising results in terms of reducing the severity of PVR following intravitreal injection in a rabbit model in preclinical phase without apparent toxicity to the eye [45].

15.11 Future Scope

Future studies might further elucidate the real of Anti-VEGF in the prevention and management of PVR DNA–RNA chimeric ribozymes targeting proliferating cell nuclear antigen (*PCNA*), a cell cycle-controlling gene that inhibits cell division, have been tested [42].

Preclinical studies continue to throw light on different molecular pathologies, which leads to PVR development, thereby helping identify new targets for potential prophylactic or therapeutic agents in future.

References

1. Wickham L, Ho-Yen GO, Bunce C, Wong D, Charteris DG. Surgical failure following primary retinal detachment surgery by vitrectomy: risk factors and functional outcomes. Br J Ophthalmol. 2011;95:1234–8.
2. Casaroli Marano RP, Vilaro S. The role of fibronectin, laminin, vitronectin and their receptors on cellular adhesion in proliferative vitreoretinopathy. Invest Ophthalmol Vis Sci. 1994;35:2791–803.
3. Moysidis SN, Thanos A, Vavvas DG. Mechanisms of inflammation in proliferative vitreoretinopathy: from bench to bedside. Mediat Inflamm. 2012;2012:815937.
4. Nagasaki H, Shinagawa K, Mochizuki M. Risk factors for proliferative vitreoretinopathy. Prog Retin Eye Res. 1998;17:77–98.
5. Charteris DG, Sethi CS, Lewis GP, Fisher SK. Proliferative vitreoretinopathy – developments in adjunctive treatment and retinal pathology. Eye. 2002;16:369–74.
6. Bonnet M, Guenoun S. Surgical risk factors for severe postoperative proliferative vitreoretinopathy (PVR) in retinal detachment with grade B PVR. Graefes Arch Clin Exp Ophthalmol. 1995;233:789–91.
7. Jaccoma EH, Conway BP, Campochiaro PA. Cryotherapy causes extensive breakdown of the blood-retinal barrier. A comparison with argon laser photocoagulation. Arch Ophthalmol. 1985;103:1728–30.
8. Xu K, Chin EK, Bennett SR, et al. Predictive factors for proliferative vitreoretinopathy formation after uncomplicated primary retinal detachment repair. Retina. 2019;39(8):1488–95.
9. Garweg JG, Tappeiner C, Halberstadt M. Pathophysiology of proliferative vitreoretinopathy in retinal detachment. Surv Ophthalmol. 2013;58:321–9.
10. Khan MA, Brady CJ, Kaiser RS. Clinical management of proliferative vitreoretinopathy: an update. Retina. 2015;35(2):165–75.
11. Jin Y, Chen H, Xu X, Hu Y, Wang C, Ma Z. Traumatic proliferative vitreoretinopathy: clinical and histopathological observations. Retina. 2017;37(7):1236–45.
12. Lai FH, Lo EC, Chan VC, Brelen M, Lo WL, Young AL. Combined pars plana vitrectomy-scleral buckle versus pars plana vitrectomy for proliferative vitreoretinopathy. Int Ophthalmol. 2016;36(2):217–24.
13. Storey P, Alshareef R, Khuthaila M, et al. Pars plana vitrectomy and scleral buckle versus pars plana vitrectomy alone for patients with rhegmatogenous retinal detachment at high risk for proliferative vitreoretinopathy. Retina. 2014;34(10):1945–51.
14. Adelman RA, Parnes AJ, Sipperley JO, Ducournau D, European Vitreo-Retinal Society (EVRS) Retinal Detachment Study Group. Strategy for the management of complex retinal detachments: the European vitreo-retinal society retinal detachment study report 2. Ophthalmology. 2013;120(9):1809–13.
15. Totsuka K, Inui H, Roggia MF, Hirasawa K, Noda Y, Ueta T. Supplemental scleral buckle in vitrectomy for the repair of rhegmatogenous retinal detachment: a systematic review of literature and meta-analysis. Retina. 2015;35(11):2423–31.
16. Kim HC, Hayashi A, Shalash A, de E Jr. A model of chronic hypotony in the rabbit. Graefes Arch Clin Exp Ophthalmol. 1998;236:69–74.
17. Aaberg TM. Management of anterior and posterior proliferative vitreoretinopathy. XLV. Edward Jackson memorial lecture. Am J Ophthalmol. 1988;106:519–32.
18. Garnier S, Rahmi A, Grasswil C, Kodjikian L. Three hundred and sixty degree retinotomy for retinal detachments with severe proliferative vitreoretinopathy. Graefes Arch Clin Exp Ophthalmol. 2013;251(9):2081–5.
19. Lim AK, Alexander SM, Lim KS. Combined large radial retinotomy and circumferential retinectomy in

the management of advanced proliferative vitreoretinopathy. Retina. 2009;29(1):112–6.
20. Nagpal M, Jain P, Nagpal K. Outcomes of retinectomy of 180° or more in retinal detachment with advanced proliferative vitreoretinopathy. World J Retina Vitr. 2011;1(2):63–8.
21. Alturki WA, Peyman GA, Paris CL, Blinder KJ, Desai UR, Nelson NC Jr. Posterior relaxing retinotomies: analysis of anatomic and visual results. Ophthalmic Surg. 1992;23:685–8.
22. Federman JL, Eagle RC Jr. Extensive peripheral retinectomy combined with posterior 360 degrees retinotomy for retinal reattachment in advanced proliferative vitreoretinopathy cases. Ophthalmology. 1990;97:1305–20.
23. Wallyn RH, Hilton GF. Subretinal fbrosis in retinal detachment. Arch Ophthalmol. 1979;97:2128–9.
24. Machemer R. Surgical approaches to subretinal strands. Am J Ophthalmol. 1980;90:81–5.
25. Lewis H, Aaberg TM, Abrams GW, et al. Subretinal membranes in proliferative vitreoretinopathy. Ophthalmology. 1989;96:1403–14, discussion 1414–15.
26. Tabandeh H. A surgical technique for the management of retinal detachment associated with severe proliferative vitreoretinopathy. Retina. 2017;37(7):1407–10.
27. Rizzo S, Genovesi-Ebert F, Vento A, et al. A new heavy silicone oil (HWS 46-3000) used as a prolonged internal tamponade agent in complicated vitreoretinal surgery: a pilot study. Retina. 2007;27:613–20.
28. Joussen AM, Rizzo S, Kirchhof B, et al. Heavy silicone oil versus standard silicone oil in as vitreous tamponade in inferior PVR (HSO study): interim analysis. Acta Ophthalmol. 2011;89:483–9.
29. Sigler EJ, Randolph JC, Calzada JI, Charles S. Pars plana vitrectomy with medium-term postoperative perfluoro-N-octane for recurrent inferior retinal detachment complicated by advanced proliferative vitreoretinopathy. Retina. 2013;33(4):791–7.
30. Rizzo S, Barca F, Faraldi F, Caporossi T, Virgili G. Staining-assisted removal of silicone oil for the identification of subclinical proliferative vitreoretinopathy. Retina. 2017;37(11):2118–23.
31. Nagpal MP, Videkar RP, Nagpal KM. Factors having implications on re-retinal detachments after silicone oil removal. Indian J Ophthalmol. 2012;60(6):517–20.
32. Nagpal M, Bhatt KJ, Jain P, Taleb EA, Goswami S, Verma A. Correlation of spectral domain optical coherence tomography findings in sub-silicone oil foveal depression space and visual outcome in eyes undergoing silicone oil removal. Taiwan J Ophthalmol. 2016;6(1):21–5.
33. Constable I, Nagpal M. 111. Proliferative vitreoretinopathy. In: Retina. 6th ed. Cleveland: Elsevier; 2018. p. 2031–51.
34. Ricker LJ, Dieudonne SC, Kessels AG, et al. Antiangiogenic isoforms of vascular endothelial growth factor predominate in subretinal fluid of patients with rhegmatogenous retinal detachment and proliferative vitreoretinopathy. Retina. 2012;32:54–9.
35. Armstrong D, Augustin AJ, Spengler R, et al. Detection of vascular endothelial growth factor and tumor necrosis factor alpha in epiretinal membranes of proliferative diabetic retinopathy, proliferative vitreoretinopathy and macular pucker. Ophthalmologica. 1998;212:410–4.
36. Zhao XY, Xia S, Wang EQ, Chen YX. Efficacy of intravitreal injection of Bevacizumab in vitrectomy for patients with proliferative vitreoretinopathy retinal detachment: a meta-analysis of prospective studies. Retina. 2018;38(3):462–70.
37. Hsu J, Khan MA, Shieh WS, et al. Effect of serial intrasilicone oil bevacizumab injections in eyes with recurrent proliferative vitreoretinopathy retinal detachment. Am J Ophthalmol. 2016;161:65–70.
38. Furino C, Micelli Ferrari T, Boscia F, Cardascia N, Recchimurzo N, Sborgia C. Triamcinolone-assisted pars plana vitrectomy for proliferative vitreoretinopathy. Retina. 2003;23(6):771–6.
39. Shi H, Guo T, Liu PC, Wang QY, Du YR, Liu QY, He MM, Liu JL, Yu J. Steroids as an adjunct for reducing the incidence of proliferative vitreoretinopathy after rhegmatogenous retinal detachment surgery: a systematic review and meta-analysis. Drug Des Dev Ther. 2015;9:1393–400.
40. Banerjee PJ, Quartilho A, Bunce C, Xing W, Zvobgo TM, Harris N, Charteris DG. Slow-release dexamethasone in proliferative vitreoretinopathy: a prospective, randomized controlled clinical trial. Ophthalmology. 2017;124(6):757–67.
41. Kumar A, Nainiwal S, Sreenivas B. Intravitreal low molecular weight heparin in PVR surgery. Indian J Ophthalmol. 2003;51:67–70.
42. Sadaka A, Giuliari GP. Proliferative vitreoretinopathy: current and emerging treatments. Clin Ophthalmol. 2012;6:1325–33.
43. Pennock S, Haddock LJ, Eliott D, Mukai S, Kazlauskas A. Is neutralizing vitreal growth factors a viable strategy to prevent proliferative vitreoretinopathy? Prog Retin Eye Res. 2014;40:16–34.
44. Falavarjani KG, Hashemi M, Modarres M, Khani AH. Intrasilicone oil injection of bevacizumab at the end of retinal reattachment surgery for severe proliferative vitreoretinopathy. Eye. 2014;28(5):576–80. https://doi.org/10.1038/eye.2014.21.
45. Ito S, Sakamoto T, Tahara Y, et al. The effect of tranilast on experimental proliferative vitreoretinopathy. Graefes Arch Clin Exp Ophthalmol. 1999;237(8):691–6.

Giant Retinal Tear 16

Atul Kumar, Sandhya Gaur, and Divya Agarwal

16.1 Introduction

A Giant Retinal Tear (GRT) is a type of full-thickness retinal break located in the peripheral retina, which is extending equally to or more than 3 clock hours (>90°) in a circumferential pattern [1, 2], They are associated with posterior vitreous detachment. Vitreous is attached to the anterior flap of the break but the posterior flap is free from vitreous. Hence, it rolls back toward posterior pole. More retinal pigment epithelial (RPE) cells get released due to large size of the break, leading to more chances of proliferative vitreoretinopathy which makes its management challenging.

16.2 Epidemiology

GRTs comprise 1.5% out of all rhegmatogenous retinal detachments [3]. According to a British Giant Retinal Tear Epidemiology eye study, the incidence of GRT is between 0.094 and 0.114 per 100,000 persons in a year. Males constitute the majority of patients (65–91%) with a mean age of 42 years [4]. About 54% of GRTs are idiopathic, 12% are post traumatic, 25% in high myopic patients, 14% occur secondary to systemic conditions, i.e., Sticklers syndrome, Marfan syndrome, Ehlers Danlos syndrome, or Wagner Syndrome [4, 5]. Fellow eye has 6.6% GRT rate at presentation in a study by Freeman et al. [6]. In another study conducted on 128 eyes with GRT, 16.1% had detachment in the fellow eye of which 3.2% had GRT. Lattice degeneration was seen in 12.1% of eyes and 0.7% of eyes were treated for retinal tear by cryopexy or laser photocoagulation [7]. In another UK based study among the 50 nontraumatic non-iatrogenic GRT, 12% has previous or current GRT and 6% had previous or current non-GRT RD in the fellow eye [4].

16.3 Classification

Schepens et al. [2] have classified GRTs into three types based on etiology:

(a) Idiopathic (70% cases)
(b) Traumatic (15–20%)
(c) Along the posterior margin of chorioretinal degenerations (10%)

It is seen that idiopathic and traumatic GRTs are more common in males along with associated myopia.

Scott et al. [8] have classified GRTs on the basis of their location and pathophysiology into:

A. Kumar (✉) · S. Gaur · D. Agarwal
Dr. Rajendra Prasad Centre for Ophthalmic Sciences, All India Institute of Medical Sciences, New Delhi, India

A. Jain et al. (eds.), *Cutting-edge Vitreoretinal Surgery*,
https://doi.org/10.1007/978-981-33-4168-5_16

(a) Equatorial, located at the equator (most common)
(b) Equatorial with posterior extension (poor prognosis as posterior extension leads to more mobile posterior flap)
(c) Oral, located at the ora serrata (least common)

GRTs can also be classified on the basis of:

1. Extent: In degrees (90–360°) or clock hours [3–11]
2. Location: Superior, Temporal, Nasal, and Inferior
3. Configuration:
   (a) Giant tear without detachment
   (b) Giant tear with detachment with:
      - Flat or undisplaced posterior flap
      - Rolled posterior flap
      - Inverted posterior flap
      - Associated with posterior extensions, i.e., radial rips at or along the margin of the tear
4. Associated proliferative vitreoretinopathy changes (absent to severe)

16.4 Pathogenesis

Usually giant retinal tears occur due to abnormal vitreous traction around areas of peripheral vitreous condensation (white without pressure with central vitreous liquefaction). Subsequent contraction of the cortical vitreous causes focal vitreoretinal traction and neurosensory retinal tear in a circumferential manner. The vitreous is adherent to the anterior flap of the retinal break while the posterior flap remains free from vitreous. Hence, the posterior flap is freely mobile and has a tendency of rolling over posteriorly. Unlike GRT, the vitreous is adherent to the posterior margin of retinal tear in cases of retinal dialysis and hence the posterior flap is not very mobile.

Due to large area of retinal tear, RPE cells are released in greater numbers. They transdifferentiate into myofibroblasts and lead to severe proliferative vitreoretinopathy and intense inflammation.

16.5 Risk Factors

Trauma is one of the most important risk factors associated with GRT. Traumatic GRTs usually occur in young myopes. Open globe injuries can cause vitreous incarceration in the wound with subsequent traction and GRT. Closed globe injuries can also cause GRT due to shearing forces. Traumatic GRTs may not be associated with posterior vitreous detachment.

High myopia with large areas of white without pressure and posterior vitreous detachment, is also important risk factor for GRT. Complicated cataract surgery with vitreous loss, vitreous incarceration in wound or vitreous traction due to increased maneuvring increases the risk for GRT. Hereditary vitreoretinopathies such as Wagner syndrome, Stickler syndrome, Ehler Danlos syndrome, and Marfans syndrome pose an increased risk for GRT. Young age is a significant risk factor predisposing to giant retinal tears due to presence of tight vitreoretinal adhesions with greater predisposition to ocular trauma.

16.6 Clinical Features

Symptoms depend upon the status of macula and configuration of the flap with respect to macula. In cases of macula off retinal detachments and flaps covering macula, visual acuity is very poor.

Tobacco Dusting (Schaffer sign) is usually seen in anterior vitreous due to RPE pigment release in large numbers. It may be associated with vitreous hemorrhage if the tear involves a major retinal vessel. Examination of fellow eye may show WWOP areas and other retinal degenerations predisposing to detachments. Degenerations not usually leading to retinal detachments are sometimes treated in fellow eyes of GRTs due to increased risk of detachment.

16.7 Differential Diagnosis

GRTs should be differentiated from giant retinal dialysis, which is circumferential disinsertion of retina from the ora and is usually associated with blunt trauma. The main differentiating feature between the two is the presence of posterior vitreous detachment in case of GRT. In giant retinal dialysis, the break is located anteriorly at the vitreous base insertion. As the vitreous is usually attached to the posterior margin of the break, the flap does not invert or roll backward.

16.8 Management

We have come a long way in managing giant tears and complicated retinal breaks. The advent of wide-angle viewing system, microincision surgeries, and perfluorocarbon liquids (PFCL) have made vitrectomy the first choice in managing these patients. Complete vitrectomy up to or beyond the ora serrata is now possible under direct visualization. PFCL has unique properties like high specific gravity, low viscosity, and optical clarity. Due to its high interfacial tension than water, PFCL bubble has tendency to maintain its circular shape and helps in easy flap manipulation and helps in giving tamponade promoting apposition of detached retina with the RPE in complex vitreoretinal surgeries. This close apposition helps in laser or cryo retinopexy along the tear margins (Fig. 16.1). This has increased the primary attachment rate from 58% to 94% and also helped us to come out of some tedious procedures used before like retinal tacks, inverted surgical beds (Stryker Frame), transscleral suturing, retinal incarceration, etc. [9]. Final anatomical success rate of up to 98% has been reported in literature [10].

Scleral buckling is usually not the treatment of choice and can be tried in cases where the edge of the tear is not folded and there are no PVR changes or in children to salvage the lens and to get rid of postoperative positioning.

Complete vitrectomy along with the use of PFCL fluids with gas or oil tamponade is done to unfold the flap and settle the retina. After core vitrectomy, vitreous is freed from all of the edges of giant tear. PFCL bubble is then injected to unfold the retina. PFCL should be injected as a single bubble and fish eggs on dispersion should be avoided by keeping the PFCL level below the infusion. After stabilizing the posterior retina, anterior vitreous and anterior retinal flap should be removed. Any epiretinal membranes are removed under PFCL. Staining of the membrane with brilliant blue or ICG should be done prior to injecting PFCL. Edge of the tear should be managed well with removal of all vitreous traction as any residual vitreous traction in this area can lead to redetachment. Laser retinopexy is applied in two to three rows to the corners and edge of the tear up to the ora serrata (Fig. 16.2). Air–fluid exchange is a very crucial step as retinal slippage can occur if done incorrectly. All the fluid anterior to the PFCL edge should be removed prior to removing PFCL to prevent slippage of the retina. The residual PFCL can then be aspirated over the optic nerve. Direct PFCL silicone oil exchange is preferred over air–fluid exchange to prevent this

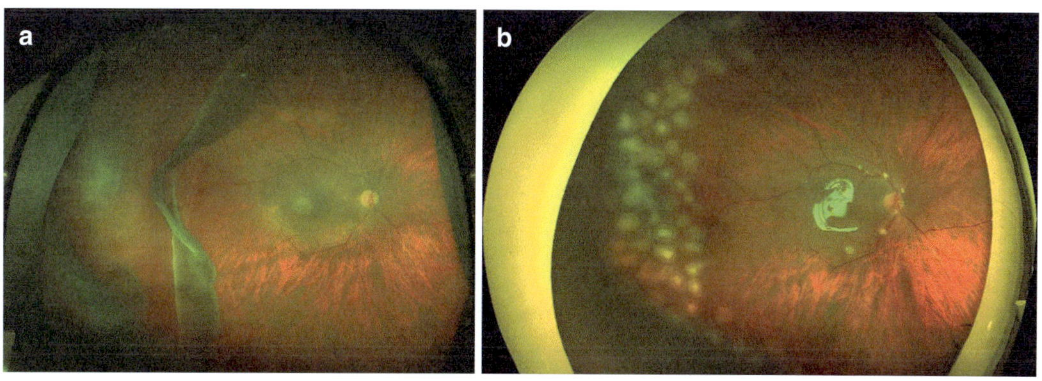

Fig. 16.1 (**a**) Preoperative ultrawidefield fundus photograph of a patient showing temporal GRT with macula on. (**b**) 6 weeks postoperative photograph showing well-attached retina with lasered flap

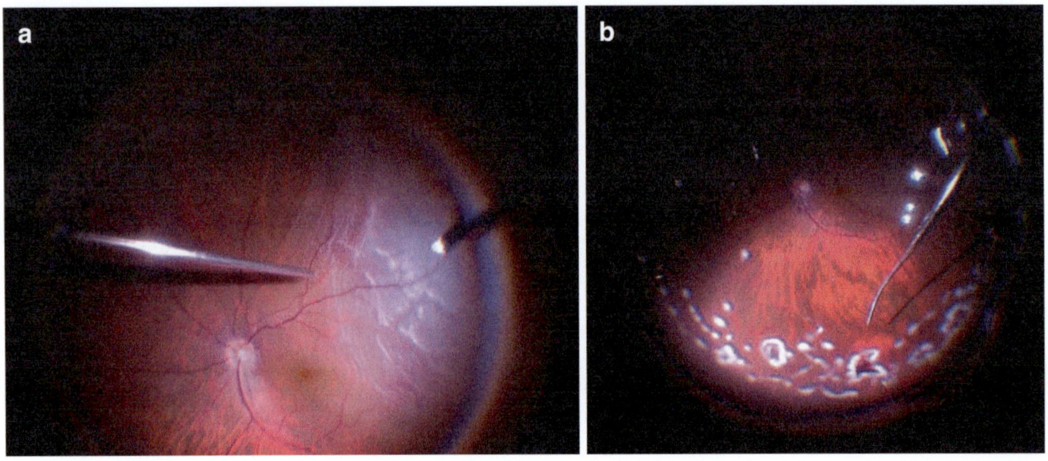

Fig. 16.2 (**a**) Important surgical steps showing complete release of vitreous traction. (**b**) Laser retinopexy of GRT flap in 2–3 rows

complication of retinal slippage. Phakic eyes may pose a problem in removing the anterior vitreous and anterior retinal flap due to risk of iatrogenic trauma to the lens. Scleral depression can be performed to prevent lenticular damage. Alternatively, lens can be removed by phacoemulsification or pars plan lensectomy. Use of encircling band in cases without PVR is not usually recommended as there are increased chances of tear fish mouthing, anterior retinal folds causing tear slippage and choroidal hemorrhage.

Proliferative vitreoretinopathy (PVR) is more commonly seen in GRTs in around 50% of cases due to large RPE dispersion and associated vitreous hemorrhage. It is more common in trauma-induced GRTs or long-standing GRTs. In these cases, encircling silicone band can be put to support the vitreous base and to counteract the axial shortening due to fibrous membranes. Fibrous proliferation on both the surfaces of the retina should be removed. Subretinal membranes if present should be removed prior to injection of PFCL.

There may be multiple factors responsible for surgical and visual outcomes in GRT surgery. Factors responsible for good postoperative visual acuities are no history of previous vitrectomies, no preoperative PVR changes, good preoperative vision, no need for retinotomies, etc. Factors found to be associated with poor visual outcome after surgery were poor preoperative vision, severe PVR changes, GRTs more than 180°, hypotony, concurrent choroidal detachment, pseudophakia, aphakia, etc.

16.9 Complications

The most common complication in vitrectomy for GRT repair is retinal slippage during air–PFCL exchange. It can be prevented by performing a direct PFCL–silicone oil exchange. Recurrent retinal detachment with PVR can occur due to residual traction and re-proliferation at the edges of the tear, missed breaks away from the tear, and the occurrence of PVR. Re-detachment due to PVR is more common in eyes with old detachments, associated vitreous hemorrhage, GRT extending more than 180° and pre-existing PVR. Other complications include progression of cataract, and PFCL remnants in subretinal space.

16.10 Treatment of Fellow Eyes

Due to high incidence of vitreoretinal pathologies and chances of RD in fellow eye of patients of GRT, proper screening of the fellow eye should be done. Incidence of bilateral nontraumatic GRT is between 0% and 21%. Freeman's 16-year observational study of fellow eyes of 226 nontraumatic GRTs found that bilateral GRTs occurred in 12.8% of patients [6]. In 3.7 years of follow up, 11% of eyes develop GRTs, among untreated 124 fellow eyes. Even 11.7% of patients had unrelated concurrent RDs not related to GRTs at initial visit. Overall incidence of RD was 15.9% in fellow eyes. Another study found 16.1% cases of bilateral RD of which 3.2% had GRT. 12.1% had lattice degeneration in the fellow eye and, 9.7% were treated by retinopaxy for a retinal tear in the fellow eye [7].

In the Freeman series, the most common predisposing lesion found to be in fellow eyes were WWOPs without any associated breaks (15.6%), lattices with or without retinal breaks (8%), and chorioretinal atrophy (5.3%).

There are no prospective randomized controlled trials regarding prophylactic treatment of fellow eyes in GRTs. Recommendations made by preferred practice panel of the American Academy of Ophthalmology are based on expert opinion but there is insufficient evidence to support prophylactic treatment in fellow eyes. A recent Cochrane review concluded that there was no supportive evidence of using 360° laser treatment of fellow eyes. Another study on 160 patients of GRT reported that prophylactic laser treatment reduced the occurrence of GRT in the fellow eye [11]. Peripheral vitreoretinal pathologies should be treated with laser retinopexy.

16.11 Conclusion

Modern-day vitrectomy practices like valved cannulas, chandelier illumination, PFCLs, and microincision surgeries have increased survival of retinal attachment. Final anatomical success has been reported in up to 98.4% of patients. Fellow eye of these cases should be examined thoroughly. Although prophylactic treatment is controversial, laser retinopexy is recommended in cases of retinal pathologies.

References

1. Kanski JJ. Giant retinal tears. Am J Ophthalmol. 1975;79(5):846–52.
2. Schepens CL, Dobble JG, McMeel JW. Retinal detachments with giant breaks: preliminary report. Trans Am Acad Ophthalmol Otolaryngol. 1962;66:471–9.
3. Shunmugam M, Ang GS, Lois N. Giant retinal tears. Surv Ophthalmol. 2014;59(2):192–216.
4. Ang GS, Townend J, Lois N. Epidemiology of giant retinal tears in the United Kingdom: the British giant retinal tear epidemiology eye study (BGEES). Invest Ophthalmol Vis Sci. 2010;51(9):4781–7.
5. Ghosh YK, Banerjee S, Savant V, Kotamarthi V, Benson MT, Scott RAH, et al. Surgical treatment and outcome of patients with giant retinal tears. Eye (Lond). 2004;18(10):996–1000.
6. Freeman HM. Fellow eyes of giant retinal breaks. Trans Am Ophthalmol Soc. 1978;76:343–82.
7. Lee S, Ong S, Wong D, et al. Giant retinal tear management: an Asian experience. Eye. 2009;23:601–5.
8. Scott JD. Giant tear of retina. Trans Ophthalmol Soc U K. 1975;95(1):142–4.10.
9. Berrocal MH, Chenworth ML, Acaba LA. Management of giant retinal tear detachments. J Ophthalmic Vis Res. 2017;12(1):93–7.
10. Falavarjani KG, Alemzadeh SA, Modarres M, Alemzadeh SA Parvarash MM, Naseripour M, Hashemi M, Robatmeili M. Outcome of surgery in patients with giant retinal tear: 10 years experience. Eye. 2017;31(9):1284–9.
11. Ripandelli G, Rossi T, Cacciamani A, Scarinci F, Piaggi P, Stirpe M. Laser prophylactic treatment of the fellow eye in giant retinal tears: long-term follow-up. Retina. 2016;36:962–26.

Management of Retinal Detachment in Eyes with Coloboma of Choroid

17

Lingam Gopal and Muna Bhende

17.1 Introduction

Ocular coloboma is a congenital disorder caused by defective closure of foetal fissure [1]. The spectrum of the disorder can include anterior segment structures such as iris, ciliary body and zonules as well as posterior segment structures such as choroid, retinal pigment epithelium (RPE), retina and optic disc. Retinal detachment is a complication of the fundus coloboma in a high percentage of cases and can occur at variable age [2].

17.2 Briefly on Embryology

The optic vesicle is an outpouching of the forebrain and hence of neuroectodermal origin. The optic vesicle next becomes the double-layered optic cup due to invagination. A ventral invagination then takes place in the optic cup and the optic stalk—called 'fetal fissure' [3]. This permits mesenchyme to enter the eye and supply vasculature. The outer layer of the optic cup is destined to become the retinal pigment epithelium, outer pigmented layer of ciliary body epithelium and the outer pigmented iris epithelium. The inner layer is destined to become the neurosensory retina, inner non-pigmented ciliary epithelium and inner pigmented iris epithelium. The foetal fissure closes by sixth week of gestation normally. Subsequently, the mesenchyme adds the choroid and scleral shell to complete the eye wall. Improper closure of the fissure is the cause of a spectrum of disorders affecting the eyeball—termed 'Fundus coloboma'. While the improper closure initially affects the development of retinal pigment epithelium and neurosensory retina, the development of the choroid and sclera are also influenced secondarily.

17.3 Structural Alterations Caused by Coloboma of Fundus

The effect of the improper closure can theoretically affect the entire length of the foetal fissure and hence be reflected in the iris, ciliary body, choroid, retina and the optic nerve. In addition, depending on the severity of the coloboma, the eyeball size can also be affected. Hence microphthalmos is a not uncommon association of the coloboma [4]. The visible coloboma of fundus is lacking in RPE, and choroid. The sclera very often is thinned out and could be

L. Gopal (✉)
Department of ophthalmology, National University Health System, Singapore, Singapore

M. Bhende
Sankara Nethralaya and Medical Research foundation, Chennai, India
e-mail: drmuna@snmail.org

A. Jain et al. (eds.), *Cutting-edge Vitreoretinal Surgery*,
https://doi.org/10.1007/978-981-33-4168-5_17

ectatic. The neurosensory retina is replaced by a nondescript membrane termed 'inter calary membrane (ICM)'.

17.4 Structural Changes at Junction of Coloboma with Normal Fundus

The junction between the normal fundus and the colobomatous area is the most important part of the anatomy that dictates the occurrence of coloboma-related retinal detachments. Several clinical and histopathological studies have elucidated these changes well. The inner layer of the neurosensory retina continues as the ICM, while the outer layer appears to bend backwards and merge with the RPE that is truncated at the margin of the coloboma. This junction is rather tenuous and aptly termed 'Zone of least resistance' [5].

17.5 Relationship of Structural Changes in Coloboma to Propensity for Occurrence of Retinal Detachment

For the purpose of the discussion that follows, the term 'retinal detachment' would refer to detachment of otherwise healthy retina from underlying RPE and the term 'intercalary membrane detachment' would indicate detachment of the ICM from underlying sclera (since there is no choroid or RPE under this area).

1. Non-rhegmatogenous retinal detachment: Shallow traction-related retinal detachments can occur at the edge of coloboma due to traction on the retina at the margin of the coloboma by the taut ICM. These are easily missed clinically since very often they remain asymptomatic, especially in the milieu of an already low visual acuity. The shallow detachment can be picked up on optical coherence tomography (OCT) [6]. The not uncommon occurrence of pigment degeneration at the margin of coloboma could be also due to spontaneous reattachment of such shallow detachments.
2. The ICM can become thin and give way at one or more places leading to breaks in ICM. These breaks can lead to detachment of the ICM from underlying sclera [7]. The sub ICM space is now communicating with the vitreous space but not necessarily with the sub-retinal space beyond the coloboma.
3. Breaks can occur in the healthy retina similar to what can happen in any other non-colobomatous eye. These can potentially lead to retinal detachment (again similar to an otherwise normal eye). This sub-retinal space is communicating with the vitreous cavity through the retinal break, but this does not necessarily communicate with the sub ICM space overlying the coloboma. For communication between sub-retinal and sub ICM space to exist, a break in continuity should occur at the 'zone of least resistance'.

17.6 Retinal Detachment and Coloboma of Fundus

Hence in a given eye with coloboma of fundus and retinal detachment, one has to decipher the contribution of each of these factors in the causation of the detachment. This enables the management to be appropriate. We will now discuss the various clinical presentations, the possible pathological mechanisms and appropriate management techniques.

1. *Detachment of ICM with no retinal detachment*:

   It is obvious that this does not cause any symptoms to the patient since the ICM is non-functional. Hence it is noted incidentally on routine examination—often in the fellow eye when one comes with issues in one eye. The risk of spread of the ICM detachment into healthy retina and causing clinical retinal detachment is very real. Hence one would offer prophylactic barrage laser (see below for techniques of treatment).

2. *Detachment of healthy retina with clearly no spillover into the colobomatous area, i.e. no ICM detachment*:

   In this situation, the cause of retinal detachment is unrelated to the coloboma and a peripheral break is usually fairly obvious. Technically it is possible to correct these detachments with techniques that one would adopt for retinal detachments in non-colobomatous eyes.

   Caveat: One should however be very certain that there is no spillover into the colobomatous area. Uncertainty can arise because of (1) nystagmus that makes it difficult to focus on one area for long enough time. (2) High frequency of coexisting microphthalmos that makes the ophthalmoscopy difficult (3) young age of the patient wherein the level of cooperation is variable. Even in cooperative children, the span of attention is very limited and they do not fixate steadily for a long enough time. A small rim of ICM detachment can thus be easily missed. Optical coherence tomography when possible can aid in the precision of diagnosis.

   When in doubt, it is best to treat the case as a coloboma-related retinal detachment.

3. *Detachment of healthy retina, which clearly has ICM detachment of variable extent in continuity*:

   There may or may not be visible breaks in the ICM, but a break in the Zone of least resistance can be assumed to be present in these cases (Fig. 17.1). In addition, a peripheral retinal break can coexist. These detachments are clearly due to the coloboma and the management is accordingly planned.

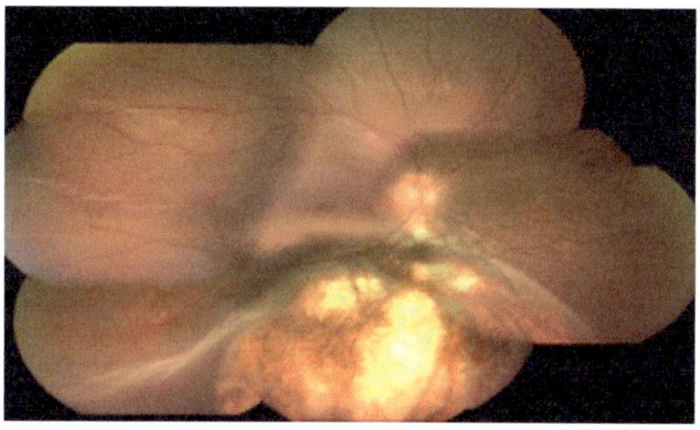

Fig. 17.1 Fundus photograph of a case of coloboma of choroid with partial retinal detachment sparing nasal quadrant. Note that the coloboma does not involve the disc and macula but disc is anomalous with an area of chorioretinal atrophy between inferior disc margin and coloboma margin. Note also the narrow rim of intercalary membrane detachment temporally along coloboma margin

17.7 Management

17.7.1 Barrage Laser

Laser when performed as a stand-alone procedure is done as a prophylaxis to prevent clinical detachment of the healthy retina beyond the coloboma.

In circumstances as described above with ICM detachment, it is definitely recommended. In an eye with coloboma but no evidence of ICM detachment, the role of prophylactic laser is more controversial. It is tempting to believe that laser to the coloboma margin will prevent retinal detachment. However, there are issues one should be aware of while performing laser.

(a) In eyes with fundus coloboma clearly away from optic disc and macula, there is no risk involved in the treatment and obviously should be offered.

(b) In eyes with fundus coloboma involving the optic disc, the treatment around the coloboma margin would involve treating the functional border of the optic disc with a risk to the nerve fibre layer. In the absence of any fluid under the retina, the neurosensory retina is not protected from accidental heavy burns that can potentially damage the nerve fibre layer.

(c) In the presence of nystagmus and in children, it may be difficult to treat with slit-lamp delivery. Treating them under general anaesthesia and with indirect delivery of laser has the risk of lack of precision in the intensity of burn.

(d) In eyes with coloboma just skirting the macula (a not uncommon presentation), treatment can potentially encroach on the foveal avascular zone (FAZ) or fovea itself. If one opts not to treat a segment of the border to avoid damage to fovea, the prophylactic value of such partial treatment becomes questionable.

17.7.2 Scleral Buckling

Scleral buckling may be possible only for eyes with retinal detachment unrelated to coloboma. Here the decision about scleral buckling or pars plana vitrectomy is based on other factors related to the retinal detachment and not the presence of coloboma.

17.7.3 Pars Plana Vitrectomy Approach

Considering the location of the pathology posterior to equator and mostly around the posterior pole of the eye, pars plana approach is the ideal way to manage the coloboma-related retinal detachments. Attempts at buckling the margin of the buckle with radial sponges were done in the pre vitrectomy era but have no place in the current day management [8]. Pars plana approach has several advantages including:

(a) Ability to identify precisely the extension of the retinal detachment into the ICM detachment.
(b) Ability to identify the ICM breaks.
(c) Permits surgery even in a microphthalmic eye unless the microphthalmos is extreme.
(d) Permits the understanding of the relative contribution of the factors discussed above based on the behaviour of the retina during fluid air exchange.
(e) Permits controlled laser photocoagulation to the margin of the coloboma.
(f) Permits long-term internal tamponade.

17.8 Specific Issues Related to Operating on an Eye with Coloboma of Fundus

17.8.1 Role of Additional Encirclage

Adding an encirclage perhaps has a limited role unless the peripheral vitreous debulking is not adequate and there is some unrelieved traction. In eyes that are aphakic/made aphakic/pseudophakic, there is probably no advantage of adding an encirclage. In phakic eyes, one may be excused for adding an encirclage in an attempt to reduce risk of recurrences. However, in eyes with significant microphthalmos, it is impractical to attempt an encirclage.

17.8.2 Location of Sclerotomies

The location of sclerotomies should appropriately be brought closer to limbus in eyes with microphthalmos. Thankfully the location of ora serrata does not correspond to the degree of microcornea and the limbus-ora serrata distance has been shown to be greater in eyes with microcornea compared to eyes with normal cornea [9].

17.8.3 Lens Management

In eyes with significant microphthalmos, a clear lens may sometimes need to be sacrificed. Eyes with pre-existing cataract would also need removal of the lens. In most cases, one can perform pars plana removal of the lens with the vitrector. However, dense nuclear sclerosis is not an uncommon association of coloboma of choroid and may necessitate the use of phaco fragmatome. In most cases with co-existing retinal detachment, one would not place an intraocular lens.

17.8.4 Inducing the Posterior Vitreous Detachment

The vitreous in most cases is not detached. Inducing Posterior Vitreous Detachment (PVD) could be tricky. The vitreous may be partly degenerated in the area of coloboma and may not give adequate purchase to peel the vitreous from the ICM. It is best to try and detach the vitreous from the healthy part of the retina first. The directionality of the peeling should be towards the coloboma so that one limits the possibility of inducing more ruptures of the zone of least resistance. If vitreous forceps is used to peel the vitreous collagen fibrils from the disc, it makes it easier to induce PVD with suction subsequently. Once a pocket of vitreous is detached, the rest of the separation is easy. A good debulking of the peripheral vitreous should be done, aided if necessary by peripheral indentation.

17.8.5 Inspection of the Coloboma Margin and ICM

Close inspection of the ICM should reveal the location of the breaks in the ICM. Where the ICM is extensively detached, the breaks in ICM are located usually away from the coloboma margin and can be multiple. Where the ICM detachment is restricted to just within the margin of the coloboma, the ICM break is usually at the margin of the ICM detachment, with only one edge lifted off the floor of the coloboma. The macula could be a site of break when it is involved in the coloboma.

One also estimates the extent of the coloboma margin that is involved in the ICM detachment, since the communication between the sub-retinal and sub ICM space is located only within this segment of the coloboma margin. However, the forcible induction of PVD can potentially induce additional areas of rupture in the zone of least resistance.

17.8.6 Mobilizing the Retina

When there is proliferative vitreoretinopathy, the steps of membrane peeling and obtaining relief of traction are similar to any other eye with retinal detachment.

17.8.7 Fluid–Air Exchange

If the retinal detachment is due to coloboma, and there is communication between sub-retinal and sub ICM space, air injection into vitreous cavity, will push the sub-retinal fluid into the floor of the coloboma. If there is a break in ICM, the fluid will find its way into the vitreous cavity. In most such cases, the retina can be flattened entirely without needing to suck the sub-retinal fluid through a peripheral break or through a drainage retinotomy.

However, in a few cases, the breaks in the zone of least resistance are small and do not permit rapid flattening of the retina. In such cases, a pre-existing peripheral break can be used to drain the sub-retinal fluid or one may have to create a mid-peripheral drainage retinotomy to facilitate this step.

17.8.8 Endolaser

Theoretically speaking, if there was no ICM detachment and there is a peripheral break to explain the retinal detachment, one can assume that the coloboma is not responsible for the detachment. However, the attempts at PVD induction can sometimes create breaks in the zone of least resistance even if there was none to start with. Hence it is best to assume that the margin of the coloboma is a threat for recurrent retinal detachment and treat the entire margin in all cases. Two to three rows of laser burns are applied.

Issues in performing laser along the coloboma margin:

(a) One can expect difficulty in producing burns in certain areas where the ICM is taut and the transition zone between retina and ICM is not pliable.
(b) Relationship of coloboma margin with the macula: Where the macula is clearly beyond the coloboma margin, it is easy to treat the entire coloboma margin with laser. Similarly, where the macula is totally involved in the coloboma of fundus, there is no issue with treating the coloboma margin with laser. There are, however, a group of cases where the macula is healthy but located just outside the coloboma margin. In some of these cases, there may not be enough space between macula and the coloboma margin to comfortably place 2–3 rows of laser burns. One may have to compromise by not treating a small extent of the margin of coloboma that is next to the macula.
(c) Treatment of the functional border of the optic disc in eyes wherein the disc is involved in the coloboma: It is always a cause for concern when laser is applied around the disc border due to fear of damaging the nerve fibre layer. This area should preferably be treated with a diode laser using light burns.
(d) After the margin of coloboma is treated, the treatment should be continued on to the ora serrata from the inferior limits of the coloboma margin. The necessity to treat the entire ora serrata is questionable. However, in cases with microphthalmos, the sclerotomies are closer to the ora serrata than in a normal-sized eyeball, hence there is a possibility of small, unidentified dialysis of the retina occurring in the meridians of the sclerotomies. Treating the ora serrata all round will reduce risk of recurrent retinal detachment. In phakic eyes, one may have to use cryopexy for this step.

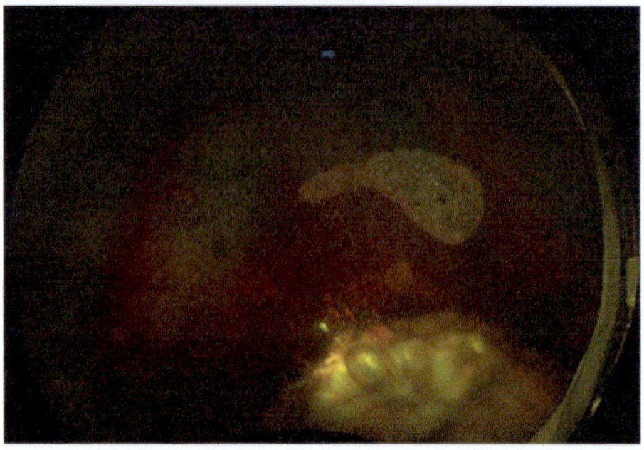

Fig. 17.2 Postoperative photograph of a case of coloboma of choroid following vitrectomy and silicone oil tamponade. Note choroidal coloboma involves the disc. The retina is attached with patches of emulsified oil bubbles made out

17.8.9 Internal Tamponade

The considerations for the choice of internal tamponade are as follows:

(a) The age group of patients and the possibility of compliance in prone positioning.
(b) The need to tamponade a long margin of the coloboma extending from the posterior pole towards infero nasal and infero temporal quadrants.

In the absence of PVR, both C_3F_8 and silicone oil should be adequate if compliance with prone positioning is not an issue (Fig. 17.2). However, considering the age group wherein the surgery is usually required, silicone oil has been the first choice [10].

Other than PVR, the causes for recurrent retinal detachment are:

(a) Peripheral retinal breaks—especially dialysis that has been missed.
(b) Inadequate vitrectomy leaving behind vitreous adherent to the coloboma margin—especially in the posterior pole.
(c) Inadequate retinopexy along the coloboma margin.

Sometimes the taut ICM can act as a membrane and keep the retina at the margin of coloboma relatively lifted. These situations can be corrected by measured excision or incision of the taut ICM-relaxing retinotomies. However, one should be cognizant of the fact that major blood vessels can transgress the ICM close to the coloboma margin and actually be supplying the healthy retina beyond. Any cutting of the ICM should strictly avoid these vessels.

17.9 Complications

17.9.1 Secondary Glaucoma

Raised intraocular pressure (IOP) can occur due to steroid use, gas tamponade (especially with C_3F_8) and silicone oil. Silicone oil can cause glaucoma due to emulsified material blocking the angles, or shallowing/flattening of anterior chamber in aphakic eyes. Inferior iris coloboma or a deliberately created peripheral iridectomy can be blocked by blood or fibrin and produce acute rise in IOP. Very often this is transient and the fibrin or blood can resolve and the anterior chamber reform while the acute rise of IOP is managed with medical therapy. It is only rare that surgical intervention is needed as emergency.

17.9.2 Emulsification of Silicone Oil

Emulsified silicone oil is natural sequelae of any eye with silicone oil present for a long enough time. In the milieu of a physically active child and some degree of inflammation, the emulsification occurs more rapidly.

17.9.3 Recurrent Retinal Detachment

Retinal re-detachment is either due to improper management at the time of primary surgery or due to proliferative vitreoretinopathy, new retinal breaks, or inability to induce posterior vitreous detachment during the first surgery.

17.10 Second Surgery

A second surgery is needed for (a) silicone oil removal, (b) recurrent retinal detachment and (c) secondary glaucoma that needs surgical intervention.

17.10.1 Silicone Oil Removal

This step is vital for the long-term health of the eye that underwent repair of coloboma-related retinal detachment. There is reluctance on the part of surgeons to take this step at the appropriate time and to allow complications to occur before the oil removal. In eyes with no preoperative proliferative vitreoretinopathy, oil can be removed safely after 3–4 weeks of time. After the oil is removed, one should inspect the peripheral retina as well as the border of the coloboma for any signs of sub-retinal fluid. Since these collections will be shallow, they can be easily missed and can result in recurrent retinal detachment post-oil removal.

17.11 Results

With the advanced techniques of vitreoretinal surgery, the success rates of reattaching the retina have improved tremendously. In a series of 85 eyes, 81.2% rate of anatomical success has been achieved. 10/200 or better visual acuity was achieved in 69.4% of these eyes [11]. The most important long-term complication was raised intraocular pressure, which needs medical and sometimes surgical management. Hocaoglu et al. had a 90% success with silicone oil tamponade in a small series of 10 eyes. They had 10% incidence of elevated IOP, band shaper keratopathy and PVR [12].

Pal et al. in a series of 42 eyes, reported a final anatomical success of 88.1% with 78.7% recovering 10/200 or better vision. Two out of the 21 eyes that had silicone oil removal had recurrent retinal detachment [13].

References

1. Pagon RA. Ocular coloboma. Surv Ophthalmol. 1981;25:223–36.
2. Jesberg DO, Schepens CL. Retinal detachment associated with coloboma of the choroid. Arch Ophthalmol. 1961;65:163–73.
3. Onwochei BC, Simon JW, Bateman JB, et al. Ocular colobomata. Surv Ophthalmol. 2000;45:175–94.
4. Gopal L, Badrinath SS, Kumar KS, Doshi G, Biswas N. Optic disc in fundus coloboma. Ophthalmology. 1996;103:2120–7.
5. Schubert HD. Schisis-like rhegmatogenous retinal detachment associated with choroidal colobomas. Graefes Arch Clin Exp Ophthalmol. 1995;233:74–9.
6. Gopal L, Khan B, Jain S, Prakash VS. A clinical and optical coherence tomography study of the margins of the choroidal colobomas. Ophthalmology. 2007;114:571–80.
7. Gopal L, Badrinath SS, Sharma T, Parikh T, Biswas J. Pattern of retinal breaks and retinal detachments in eyes with choroidal coloboma. Ophthalmology. 1995;102:1212–7.
8. Patnaik B, Kalsi R. Retinal detachment with coloboma of the choroid. Indian J Ophthalmol. 1981;29:345–9.
9. Liu T, Zhang M, Xu B, Wang W, Lee J, Gao Y, Zhang X. Evaluation of the safety of sclerotomy incision in patients with choroidal colobomas with/without associated microcornea. Retina. 2014;34:2300–5.
10. Gopal L, Kini MM, Badrinath SS, Sharma T. Management of retinal detachment with choroidal coloboma. Ophthalmology. 1991;98:1622–7.
11. Gopal L, Badrinath SS, Sharmat T, Parikh SN, Shanmugam MS, Bhende PS, Agarwal R, Deshpande D. Surgical management of retinal detachments related to coloboma of the choroid. Ophthalmology. 1998;105:804–9.
12. Hocaoglu M, Karacorlu M, Ersoz MG, Sayman Muslubas I, Arf S. Outcomes of vitrectomy with silicone oil tamponade for management of retinal detachment in eyes with chorioretinal coloboma. Retina. 2019;39(4):736–42.
13. Pal N, Azad RV, Sharma YR. Long-term anatomical and visual outcome of vitreous surgery for retinal detachment with choroidal coloboma. Indian J Ophthalmol. 2006;54:85–8.

Part V

Retinal Vascular Disorders

Surgical Management of High Risk Proliferative Diabetic Retinopathy: Vitreous Hemorrhage, Tractional Retinal Detachment, and Combined Tractional-Rhegmatogenous Retinal Detachment

18

Andrew X. Chen, Jessica Hsueh, Thais F. Conti, and Rishi P. Singh

18.1 Preoperative Management

18.1.1 Determining Surgical Candidates

Special considerations should be made for diabetic patients before surgery. Tight blood glucose control significantly reduces the risk of microvascular complications of diabetes, including progression of retinopathy [1, 2]. There is also evidence to suggest that preoperative glycemic control influences the risk of macular edema reduction in patients receiving vitrectomies for persistent diabetic macular edema. One study showed a 0.54 decreased probability of foveal thickness improvement for every 1% increase in HgbA1C 2 weeks before vitrectomy [3]. Furthermore, diabetic patients frequently have comorbidities such as hypertension, renal, and cardiac disease, which should be managed in conjunction with the patient's primary care physician or endocrinologist and reviewed by the anesthesiologist prior to surgery. One large, retrospective cohort study found that the occurrence of postoperative systemic adverse events after vitreoretinal surgery for all patients was 4%, and occurrence significantly increased in patients with coronary artery disease, asthma, chronic renal disease, and those requiring general anesthesia [4]. Optimal control of these conditions prior to surgery and anesthesia is ideal, and is thought to increase the likelihood of favorable outcomes and reduce the risk of complications.

In a retrospective, comparative study of 1267 eyes, 49.95% of patients had associated arterial hypertension [5]. A feared complication of uncontrolled hypertension during retinal surgery is suprachoroidal hemorrhage. The incidence of suprachoroidal hemorrhage in all patients under-

A. X. Chen · J. Hsueh
Case Western Reserve University School of Medicine, Cleveland, OH, USA
e-mail: axc701@case.edu; jxh889@case.edu

T. F. Conti
Cole Eye Institute, Cleveland Clinic Foundation, Cleveland, OH, USA

Center for Ophthalmic Bioinformatics, Cole Eye Institute, Cleveland Clinic Foundation, Cleveland, OH, USA

R. P. Singh (✉)
Case Western Reserve University School of Medicine, Cleveland, OH, USA

Cole Eye Institute, Cleveland Clinic Foundation, Cleveland, OH, USA

Center for Ophthalmic Bioinformatics, Cole Eye Institute, Cleveland Clinic Foundation, Cleveland, OH, USA
e-mail: SINGHR@ccf.org

A. Jain et al. (eds.), *Cutting-edge Vitreoretinal Surgery*,
https://doi.org/10.1007/978-981-33-4168-5_18

going victrectomy is 0.17% to 1.9% as reported in three case-control studies [6–8]. The rate in diabetic patients undergoing victrectomy is not well studied. Several studies have found that systemic hypertension at the time of pars plana vitrectomy was a significant risk factor for suprachoroidal hemorrhage [9, 10]. Furthermore, one case-controlled retrospective study has demonstrated that patients placed on antihypertensive medications 3 months before vitrectomy had 20% the risk of postoperative hemorrhage in comparison to patients without. Thus, control of hypertension with medications in diabetic patients should be achieved prior to retinal surgery.

Patients with diabetic end-stage renal disease were previously poor candidates for vitreoretinal surgery. However, recent improvements toward management of these patients have allowed patients with proliferative diabetic retinopathy on hemodialysis to receive vitreoretinal surgeries and improve visual outcomes [11]. Special postoperative care and education should be provided on maintaining head position during hemodialysis in order to prevent movement of any gas bubble tamponades.

In addition, patients with diabetes are often on antiplatelet or anticoagulant therapy, which is an important consideration before a procedure that may be complicated by intraoperative or postoperative hemorrhage. Multiple studies have found that the antiplatelet agent aspirin does not increase hemorrhage risk during retinal surgery. Thus, aspirin therapy is generally not discontinued for the procedure. On the other hand, anticoagulant medications have been demonstrated to increase risk of hemorrhage, but generally without serious consequences. A patient's anticoagulant may be held if there is low risk of an adverse cardiovascular event [12, 13].

Finally, the presence of cataracts or other opacities of the anterior media should be considered in order to ensure adequate visualization during the procedure. If cataracts are significant, a phacovitrectomy can be considered.

Preoperative testing accounts for billions of dollars in annual health care costs, and the volume of vitreoretinal surgeries has increased to over 225,000 in 2011 in the United States alone [14]. Although one retrospective cohort study using multivariate logistic regression analysis did not demonstrate any differences in rates of postoperative adverse events in patients who did or did not undergo preoperative testing prior to vitreoretinal surgery, it is still common practice to perform this preoperative testing [4]. Similarly, one randomized control study of cataract surgeries also demonstrated a nonsignificant increase in the safety of surgery when preoperative medical testing was performed [15].

18.1.2 Use of Preoperative Anti-VEGF

Vascular endothelial growth factor (VEGF) release by ischemic retinal tissue is thought to drive the development of PDR. Intravitreal injection of anti-VEGF medications, namely bevacizumab, aflibercept, and ranibizumab, have become an important component of long-term therapy for PDR, particularly in combination with prior pan-retinal photocoagulation (PRP) [16]. Anti-VEGF injections have also been used preoperatively prior to vitrectomy. It is presumed that the reduction of neovascularization prior to vitrectomy prevents hemorrhage during the intra and postoperative periods and thus produces more favorable outcomes. Use of preoperative anti-VEGF has also been associated with decreased surgical time, fewer retinal breaks, and facilitation of intraoperative fibroproliferative membrane dissection [17, 18].

One concern with the utilization of preoperative anti-VEGF is promotion of fibrovascular contraction, leading to worsening tractional retinal detachment and difficulty in identifying tissue planes, unfavorably termed "crunch syndrome." Generally, studies have demonstrated a low risk of complications and low incidence of TRD associated with preoperative anti-VEGF, especially if the dose and timing of the injections are well controlled. For instance, lower doses of bevacizumab (1.25 vs. 2.5 mg) were shown in one study to have an association with lower risk of TRD. Additionally, too short of a duration between anti-VEGF injection to surgery may not provide sufficient reduction of neovascularization, while too long of a duration may enhance fibrovascular contraction and likelihood of TRD. To date, there is little consensus in the literature on the exact timing of injections for maximal benefit. One report suggested surgery should ideally be performed within 4 days of injection. Another found that a group receiving intravitreal bevacizumab 5–10 days before vitrectomy had superior visual outcomes and fewer intraoperative complications compared with a group receiving it 1–3 days before [16, 19]. Further studies comparing anti-VEGFs treatments at various timeframes will better elucidate optimal timing for preoperative injections. Another drawback of preoperative anti-VEGF treatments is that patients may not return after treatment for re-evaluation prior to surgery.

18.1.3 Preoperative Pan-Retinal Photocoagulation

Argon laser pan-retinal photocoagulation is the gold standard for treatment of PDR, as established by the Diabetic Retinopathy Study (DRS), which showed that PRP decreased the rate of severe visual loss by 50% or more [20]. There is also a 50% reduction in risk of proliferative diabetic retinopathy progression and similar risk reduction of vitreous hemorrhage post-laser treatment according to a 2014 Cochrane Review [21]. Furthermore, the review found that laser treatments reduced the risk of severe visual loss by over 50% 12 months later. Laser-mediated destruction of ischemic retinal tissue reduces the production of VEGF and thereby causes regression of neovascularization [20, 23]. When possible, patients with PDR should receive laser treatment prior to surgical intervention, or during the procedure if not treated previously.

18.2 Intraoperative Approaches

18.2.1 PDR Pathophysiology

The pathophysiology of PDR involves microvascular damage secondary to diabetes mellitus secondary to diabetes mellitus [22]. Loss of capillary supply to the retina results in hypoxia and ultimately stimulates release of a variety of angiogenic growth factors and pro-inflammatory mediators, both of which are found at elevated levels within the vitreous humor. Neovascular buds then emerge from the retinal vasculature, accompanied by proliferation of fibrous tissue. The new, abnormal vessels tend to be friable and bleed easily, contributing to recurrent vitreous hemorrhage. Meanwhile, the posterior cortical surface of the vitreous acts as a scaffold upon which fibrovascular membranes grow. These membranes contract and exert progressive tractional forces on the retina and can eventually lead to retinal detachment [24].

Tractional retinal detachment (TRD) is less common than other types of retinal detachment and is caused by fibrovascular membranes exerting tractional forces on the retina. Rhegmatogenous detachments are more common and are caused by a break or tear in the retina which causes separation from the retinal pigment epithelium. As the name suggests, combined tractional-rhegmatogenous retinal detachment (CRD) involves features of both types of detachments described above.

18.2.2 Operative Principles in Sequential Order

PDR surgery involves removing the vitreous hemorrhage, releasing traction on the retina, dissection of fibrovascular proliferation, drainage of fluid through any retinal holes or breaks, pan-retinal photocoagulation, and retinal reattachment. Internal limiting membrane peeling may be performed during dissection of fibrovascular proliferation to help visualization and release tangential retinal traction, further flattening the posterior pole.

18.2.3 Pars Plana Vitrectomy

Pars plana vitrectomy (PPV) is one of the most common surgical approaches to management of complications secondary to PDR. It is most commonly indicated for recurrent vitreous hemorrhage. Tractional and combined retinal detachments are the second most common indication. The utility of PPV is multifaceted. Vitreous hemorrhage that has not been cleared spontaneously may be aspirated during the procedure. Epiretinal fibrovascular membranes can also be removed, relieving the retina of tractional forces promoting detachment. Furthermore, excision of the posterior vitreous cortex reduces the scaffold available for adherence of fibrovascular tissue, and helps to remove pro-angiogenic and pro-inflammatory factors present in the preretinal vitreous that are driving the disease process [25].

Timing of PPV for non-clearing vitreous hemorrhage is an important consideration. The Diabetic Retinopathy Vitrectomy Study continues to guide the decision of timing. This study assessed patients with severe vitreous hemorrhage that reduced visual acuity (VA) to 5/200 or less. Early PPV had improved long-term VA outcomes compared with delayed PPV in patients with type 1 diabetes. It is believed that a delay in surgery increases the risk of fibrovascular tissue growth leading to tractional or combined retinal detachment. For patients with type 2 diabetes, early PPV was not associated with improved long-term VA, but 80% still required PPV to resolve vitreous hemorrhage after 1 year. Based on these findings, patients with both type 1 and type 2 diabetes and vitreous hemorrhage are typically observed for 4 weeks. If the patient reports no spontaneous improvement at this point, PPV may be offered, particularly in type 1 diabetes. Those with type 2 diabetes could elect to wait 2–4 months for spontaneous clearance [26, 27].

PPV is normally performed as a 3-port transconjunctival, sutureless procedure with 23-gauge cannula entry. Use of smaller probes (25, 27-gauge) has recently become more common, with the presumed benefits of reduced postoperative inflammation, smaller sclerostomy wounds, and more controlled dissection of tissues. Instruments utilized in the three ports typically include a cutting/aspiration instrument such as a vitrector, intraocular light source, and an infusion system. Based on the surgeon's preference, additional instruments may be used temporarily in place of the cutting device, including a retinal pick, vertical or horizontal scissors, forceps, scraper, or spatula.

18.2.4 Removing Fibrovascular Membranes to Release Traction on the Retina

Removal of fibrovascular tissue from the retinal surface can be achieved through a number of methods, including delamination, viscodissection, en bloc, segmentation, and bimanual techniques. Typically, surgeons choose between (1) delamination and segmentation or (2) en bloc dissection. Various techniques are summarized in Table 18.1.

In delamination, all posterior hyaloid exerting anteroposterior traction on the retina is initially excised (Fig. 18.1). Using scissors, fibrovascular tissue is carefully severed from the surface of the retina. Segmentation may be performed when other methods are challenging, such as in the case of a highly mobile retina due to a retinal break. The fibrovascular membranes are cut vertically using scissors or a vitreous cutter, thereby relieving circumferential traction. Small localized pegs of fibrovascular tissue are left attached to the retina (Fig. 18.2). Segmentation has become a less common approach, as leaving membrane pegs may result in the recurrence of fibrovascular proliferation and postoperative bleeding. It may also prevent detection of small retinal breaks that would otherwise be seen.

Table 18.1 Techniques to remove fibrovascular membranes

Technique	Details
Delamination	Scissors or microvitrectomy instrument are used to remove fibrovascular tissue
Viscodissection	Creating potential space between posterior vitreous cortex and retina
En bloc	Initial preservation of posterior vitreous cortex until posterior hyaloid is cut so that membranes and vitreous are removed as one unit
Segmentation	Circumferential traction from fibrovascular membranes is released with scissors through vertical cuts
Bimanual removal	Performed using chandelier lighting systems that allow for forceps to be used along with vitrectomy probes or scissors

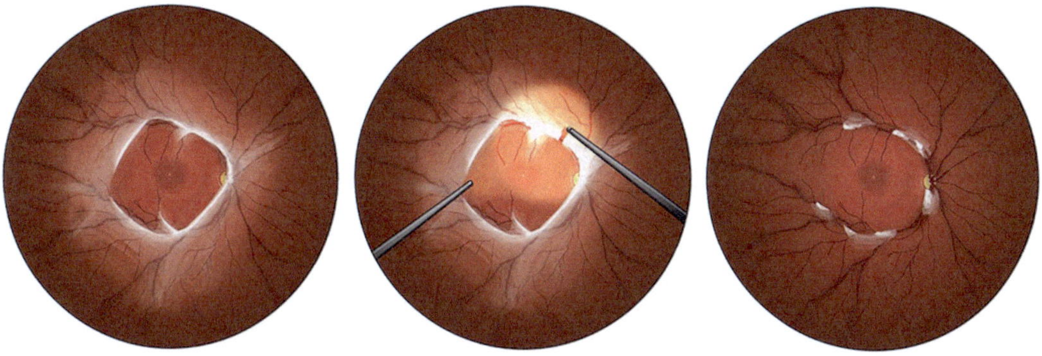

Fig. 18.1 Diagrammatic representation of en bloc dissection and delamination. All the posterior hyaloid exerting anteroposterior traction on the retina is excised

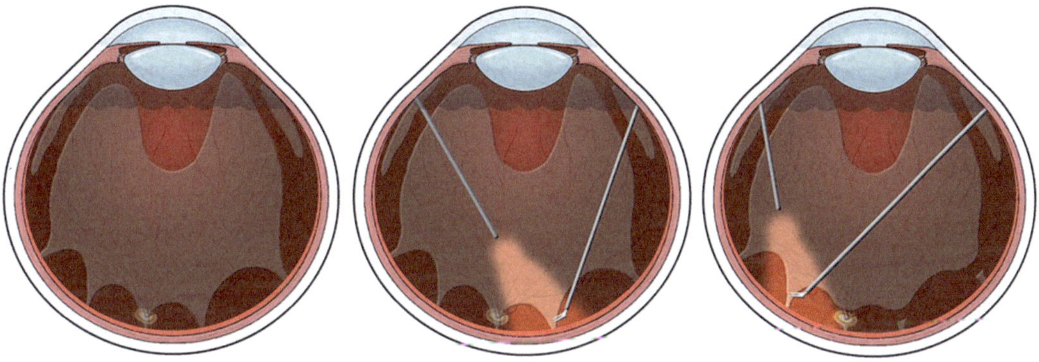

Fig. 18.2 Diagrammatic representation of segmentation. The fibrovascular membranes are cut vertically to relieve circumferential traction

In the en bloc technique, the posterior vitreous cortex is initially kept partially intact such that its anteroposterior traction aids in the dissection of fibrovascular material from the retinal surface. After dissecting the fibrovascular tissue as completely as possible, the remaining posterior hyaloid is cut so that the membranes and vitreous is removed together as one unit.

Viscodissection involves injection of viscoelastic material at the preretinal region to separate the posterior vitreous cortex from the retina and to create a potential space to aid in dissection of the fibrovascular tissue (Fig. 18.3).

Chandelier lighting systems or a lighted pick allow for bimanual removal of fibrovascular membranes that are tightly adhered. Combinations of forceps with vitrectomy probe or forceps and scissors can then be used to remove the membrane. One retrospective review indicated that bimanual microincision during vitreous surgery led to sustained visual improvement, anatomical restoration, and low complication rates, even in cases with complex tears [28]. Lenses that allow for wider angled views of the retina improve visualization and provide a three-dimensional view of the peripheral retina.

18.2.5 Retinal Tamponade

PPV is typically accompanied by use of intraocular tamponade to provide surface tension across retinal breaks. Various gases and silicone oils are used as tamponade agents. Common gases

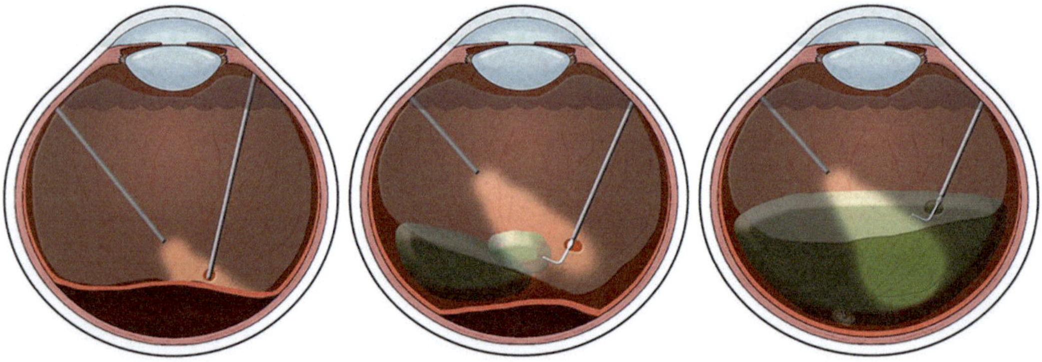

Fig. 18.3 Diagrammatic representation of viscodissection. Viscoelastic is used to create a potential space between the posterior vitreous cortex and the retina

include sulfur hexafluoride (SF6), perfluoroethane (C2F6) and perfluoropropane (C3F8), which take approximately 2, 4–5 weeks, and 8 weeks, respectively, to resorb spontaneously. During this period patients are advised to abstain from air travel. Silicone gas is a permanent tamponade agent, which has a lower specific gravity than the vitreous humor, thus will float. Silicone oil has a lower surface tension and lower buoyancy than gas tamponades has thus is thought to provide a less effective tamponade for inferior retinal breaks in comparison to gas bubbles [29]. Additionally, long term use of silicone oil is associated with microemulsification, band keratopathy, and increased intraocular pressure. Results from the Silicone Study, a randomized clinical trial, showed that there were significant differences at 1 year in anatomical and visual outcomes of patients with RD associated with proliferative retinopathy (PVR) who received silicone oil versus sulfur hexafluoride or perfluoropropane. However, no significant differences in anatomical and visual outcomes were found long term at 6 years [30].

Other tamponade agents include perfluorocarbon liquids (PFCs), can be used to flatten the retina transiently and are removed by the end of the procedure. They are especially useful in cases of combined retinal detachment as it stabilizes the retina when subretinal fluid is being drained through a break. Care must be taken with PFC use as the liquid can slip through posterior holes into the subretinal space.

18.2.6 Subretinal Fluid Drainage

Effective drainage of subretinal fluid brings retinal breaks in closer contact with the retinal pigment epithelium and may aid outcomes of scleral buckle procedures. This can be accomplished via various techniques. One method is to internally drain subretinal fluid through a preexisting retinal break or a retinotomy followed by using an extrusion cannula. This method requires adequate flattening of the posterior retina with PFCs up to the equator. Another method is to use an external needle (25–27 gauge). External needle drainage of subretinal fluid is performed by positioning the needle in the most bullous area of retinal detachment. The appearance of pigment granules in suspension in the draining subretinal fluid signifies adequate removal. Tension may be applied via a traction suture to assist in draining residual subretinal fluid out of the needle track [31]. Common complications of subretinal fluid drainage include subretinal hemorrhage, retinal incarceration, and retinal perforation.

18.2.7 Intraoperative Pan-Retinal Photocoagulation

Retinal breaks in cases of tractional or combined retinal detachments are repaired with photocoagulation endolaser. Subretinal fluid is removed through any breaks and a tamponade agent is used to readhere the retina against the pigment epithelium to permit for laser treatment. Complications of utilizing a gas bubble tamponade in an incompletely vitrectomized eye include additional traction on the peripheral retina. After, intraoperative 360° laser to the peripheral retina during vitrectomy can be performed to prevent the formation of new breaks and treat existing breaks. The effectiveness of laser treatment to the peripheral retina to prevent re-detachment is mixed. One randomized control study of patients with rhegmatogenous detachments found no significant reductions in retinal re-detachments between patients who received 360° laser versus those who did not [32]. Another randomized control study along with a retrospective study examined patients with rhegmatogenous detachments after silicone oil removal with and without laser and found that laser reduced the incidence of re-detachment [33, 34].

18.2.8 Additional Surgical Approaches and Considerations for Combined Retinal Detachments

A subset of tractional retinal detachments will progress to combined tractional-rhegmatogenous retinal detachment (CRD), which is associated with reduced surgical success rates and visual outcomes. CRD is characterized by existing retinal breaks along with fibrovascular membranes. Viscoelastics may be helpful in the dissection of preretinal or epiretinal membranes in CRD. Smaller gauged viscodissection instruments, such as a 25 gauge, will help minimize the considerable separation between retinal and fibrous tissue when performed using traditional 20 gauge instruments. Membrane delamination with viscodissection can allow for complete membrane removal and relief of traction. However, it is associated with increased bleeding. This can be controlled with PFCs during membrane removal. PFCs also aid in draining subretinal fluid through retinal breaks and help further flatten the retina. When removing fibrovascular membranes, peeling may be more effective than delamination with scissors. An indocyanine green (ICG) dye may be added for better visualization of the internal limiting membrane for peeling, though there have been some studies indicating possible toxicity with use [35]. Alternative dyes include trypan blue which has an affinity for the epiretinal membrane and can be mixed with glucose 5% or 10% to create a heavier dye. The double staining technique involves first staining the vitreous with triamcinolone acetonide and then a second injection with either ICG or trypan blue to stain and peel preretinal membranes.

For severe cases of CRD with anteriorposterior traction and rhegmatogenous etiology of detachment, particularly in phakic patients, a scleral buckle can be considered. Scleral buckles are not typically used unless anterior retinal breaks are present. Other indications for scleral buckling include rhegmatogenous detachments, younger patients with attached posterior hyaloid, and detachments due to dialysis without a retinal tear. The buckle helps to collapse the anatomic space between the sensory retina and the retinal pigment epithelium by indenting the sclera from the outside. This reduces the fluid underneath the retinal tear and re-apposes separated retinal layers.

18.2.9 Intraoperative OCT

For complex cases in which tissue planes are hard to identify, intraoperative OCT may be used. Real-time feedback may help improve surgical strategies and detect further residual membranes. In a prospective case series study of 81 eyes, surgeons reported that intraoperative OCT data provided valuable information for detection of dissection plans or retinal holes in 51% of cases and also altered decision making in 26% of cases [36].

18.3 Postoperative Management

The postoperative examination should assess for hemorrhage, proliferation of fibrovascular tissue, subretinal fluid reoccurrence, neovascularization in the anterior or posterior segments, and diabetic macular edema.

18.3.1 Prognostic Factors for VH, TRD, and CRD Post-vitrectomy

Prognostic factors of favorable visual outcomes for patients with VH include preoperative visual acuity of 5/200 or better absence of iris neovascularization, absence of neovascular glaucoma, clear lens or minimal cataract, and pan-retinal photocoagulation of least one-fourth of the fundus [37].

Prognostic factors of favorable visual outcomes for patients with TRD include patients <50 years of age, preoperative vision better than 20/400, and no macular ischemia [38]. Risk factors for poor visual outcome in patients with TRD include age >50, iris neovascularization, macular detachment >30 days, type 2 diabetics, and preoperative acuity worse than 20/200 [39]. According to a retrospective review study, poor prognostic factors for post vitrectomy procedures included: patients who required preoperative PRP, patients who had macula involving TRD, temporal TRD, and TRD complications such as neovascular glaucoma and proliferative retinopathy [40].

Prognostic factors of visual outcomes for patients with CRD is not well studied. However, they are likely to include or be similar to prognostic factors for TRD. A retrospective study found that preoperative BCVA, vitreoretinal adhesion, extent of retinal detachment, intraoperative retinectomy, and silicone oil use were significant prognostic factors in both CRD and TRD patients [41]. Another large, single-center retrospective study demonstrated that patients with advanced TRD and CRD who required silicone oil tamponade had lower single surgery reattachment rates and higher rates of vision loss. However, these patients were also more likely to have concurrent rhegmatogenous detachment and macular involving detachment [42].

18.3.2 General Complications Associated with Retinal Surgery

Cataract formation is the most common complication post vitrectomy. Increased ocular pressure is another complication of retinal surgeries, as much as 19–28% of cases. The cause is multifactorial and may be attributed to the surgery and co-morbid ocular diseases such as existing primary open-angle glaucoma [43]. Very rarely, rubeosis iridits can occur and severe pain and loss of vision due to intractable glaucoma can occur postoperatively. Patients with severe ischemia of the retina before surgery and new rhegmategenous breaks post-surgery are more at risk of this complication.

Additionally, recurrent vitreous hemorrhage (VH) can occur in up to 50% of cases due to leaking from residual hemorrhages that were not removed during surgery [43]. Postoperative VH can be early (within 2 months) or late. Early VHs are often related to surgical technique, and ensuring hemostasis of clots intraoperatively can prevent occurrence. Late VHs generally reduce with frequency and the initial management of postoperative VHs is observation if the retina is still attached. However, persistent hemorrhage may require laser therapy or even further vitrectomy. Prevention of VH includes anti-VEGFs treatments before surgery. Risk factors for postoperative VHs include iris neovascularization and history of lower extremity amputations. Antihypertensive treatments before vitrectomy may reduce the risk of hemorrhage [44].

Proliferative retinopathy (PVR) is the most common cause of retinal detachment repair failure. Risks for PVR include age, large retinal tears, more than two quadrants of involved retina, previous detachment repair, cryotherapy, vitreous hemorrhage, and choroidal detachment.

In complicated cases of diabetic retinal detachment, re-detachment may occur. Meticulous dissection of fibrovascular membranes can prevent new retinal tears and an examination of the peripheral retinal at the end of surgery for any remaining retinal tears may help prevent this complication.

18.3.3 PPV Postoperative Management

Intraoperative and postoperative VH are among the most common complications of PPV. Motoda and colleagues reported that a longer duration of surgery is a particularly strong predictor of postoperative bleeding within both 12 and 52 weeks following vitrectomy. Post-operative control of diabetes and blood pressure is important toward visual outcomes. High preoperative fasting blood glucose, use of antihypertensive drugs, and interestingly a lack of antiplatelet use, were associated with increased risk of postoperative hemorrhage within 1 year [45]. Conversely, evidence suggests that risk of postoperative VH may be reduced with intraocular perfluorocarbon gas tamponade and thorough removal of residual peripheral vitreous, but further study is needed [26].

18.3.4 Tamponade Agents and Postoperative Management

Certain precautions should be taken for patients with postoperative gas bubbles in the eye. Decompression of air pressure during air travel can result in massive IOP rise and even occlude the central retinal artery, thus air travel should be avoided entirely if the gas bubble is still present [46]. Additionally the risks of glaucoma and cataract are increased. Thus, patients should be followed for these complications postoperatively.

Complications of intravitreal silicone oil use include cataract, glaucoma, band keratopathy, and oil emulsification. These complications are related to the duration of silicone oil exposure and may or may not be reversible. It is recommended that silicone oil be removed as soon as retinal adherence has been stabilized.

PFC must be removed and replaced by another silicone oil if postoperative tamponade is needed because of a high risk for droplet formation and changes to retinal structures days or weeks after injection [47].

18.3.5 Scleral Buckling Postoperative Management

Patients should be seen the day following surgery to assess for complications such as choroidal detachment, high IOP, or persistent retinal detachment. Indentation of the globe from the silicone band can predispose the eye to secondary angle closure glaucoma. It is thought that the obstruction of venous draining from the buckle results in choroidal congestion, introducing transudates into the suprachoroidal space. Management with corticosteroids reduces inflammation of the ciliary body, which may take days to weeks [43]. Other complications include refractive change, intrusion or extrusion, and infection.

18.4 Conclusion

Advancements in surgical instrumentation and visualization of a wider retinal field have revolutionized diabetic eye surgery. These advancements in technology have improved surgical outcomes and allowed retinal specialists to address more difficult cases of diabetic retinopathy, the leading cause of blindness in the working population in the developed world. Along with improved understanding of disease pathophysiology and co-treatments with anti-VEGFs, diabetic patients can expect meaningful vision outcomes that will improve the quality of life measures after eye surgery.

Acknowledgment The authors would like to thank Mr. Michael M. Han, MD for creating the figures for this chapter.

References

1. Yau JWY, Rogers SL, Kawasaki R, Lamoureux EL, Kowalski JW, Bek T, et al. Global prevalence and major risk factors of diabetic retinopathy. Diabetes Care. 2012;35:556–64. https://doi.org/10.2337/dc11-1909.
2. UK Prospective Diabetes Study (UKPDS) Group. Intensive blood-glucose control with sulphonylureas or insulin compared with conventional treatment and risk of complications in patients with type 2 diabetes (UKPDS 33). Lancet (Lond). 1998;352:837–53.
3. Kojima T, Terasaki H, Nomura H, Suzuki T, Mori M, Ito Y, et al. Vitrectomy for diabetic macular edema: effect of glycemic control (HbA(1c)), renal function (creatinine) and other local factors. Ophthalmic Res. 2003;35:192–8. https://doi.org/10.1159/000071170.
4. Shalwala A, Hwang RY, Tabing A, Sternberg P, Kim SJ. The value of preoperative medical testing for vitreoretinal surgery. Retina. 2015;35:319–25. https://doi.org/10.1097/IAE.0000000000000306.

5. Brănişteanu DC, Bilha A, Moraru A. Vitrectomy surgery of diabetic retinopathy complications. Rom J Ophthalmol. 2016;60:31–6.
6. Speaker MG, Guerriero PN, Met JA, Coad CT, Berger A, Marmor M. A case-control study of risk factors for intraoperative suprachoroidal expulsive hemorrhage. Ophthalmology. 1991;98:202–9; discussion 210.
7. Piper JG, Han DP, Abrams GW, Mieler WF. Perioperative choroidal hemorrhage at pars plana vitrectomy. A case-control study. Ophthalmology. 1993;100:699–704.
8. Sharma T, Virdi DS, Parikh S, Gopal L, Badrinath SS, Mukesh BN. A case-control study of suprachoroidal hemorrhage during pars plana vitrectomy. Ophthalmic Surg Lasers. 1997;28:640–4.
9. Laube T, Brockmann C, Bornfeld N. Massive suprachoroidal hemorrhage: surgical management and outcome. GMS Ophthalmol Cases. 2015;5:Doc10. https://doi.org/10.3205/oc000032.
10. Tabandeh H, Sullivan PM, Smahliuk P, Flynn HW, Schiffman J. Suprachoroidal hemorrhage during pars plana vitrectomy. Risk factors and outcomes. Ophthalmology. 1999;106:236–42. https://doi.org/10.1016/S0161-6420(99)90062-3.
11. Su L, Huang G, Yin S, Hua X, Tang X. A clinical analysis of vitrectomy for severe vitreoretinopathy in patients with chronic renal. BMC Ophthalmol. 2018;18:34. https://doi.org/10.1186/s12886-018-0704-7.
12. Oh J, Smiddy WE, Kim SS. Antiplatelet and anticoagulation therapy in vitreoretinal surgery. Am J Ophthalmol. 2011;151:934–939.e3. https://doi.org/10.1016/j.ajo.2010.09.035.
13. Narendran N, Williamson TH. The effects of aspirin and warfarin therapy on haemorrhage in vitreoretinal surgery. Acta Ophthalmol Scand. 2003;81:38–40.
14. Lalezary M, Kim SJ, Jiramongkolchai K, Recchia FM, Agarwal A, Sternberg P. Long-term trends in intraocular pressure after pars plana vitrectomy. Retina. 2011;31:679–85. https://doi.org/10.1097/IAE.0b013e3181ff0d5a.
15. Schein OD, Katz J, Bass EB, Tielsch JM, Lubomski LH, Feldman MA, et al. The value of routine preoperative medical testing before cataract surgery. Study of medical testing for cataract surgery. N Engl J Med. 2000;342:168–75. https://doi.org/10.1056/NEJM200001203420304.
16. Arevalo JF, Liu TYA, Pan-American Collaborative Retina Study Group (PACORES). Intravitreal bevacizumab in diabetic retinopathy. Recommendations from the Pan-American collaborative retina study group (PACORES): the 2016 Knobloch lecture. Asia-Pac J Ophthalmol (Phila). 2018;7:36–9. https://doi.org/10.22608/APO.2017466.
17. Smith JM, Steel DHW. Anti-vascular endothelial growth factor for prevention of postoperative vitreous cavity haemorrhage after vitrectomy for proliferative diabetic retinopathy. Cochrane Database Syst Rev. 2015;8:CD008214. https://doi.org/10.1002/14651858.CD008214.pub3.
18. Simunovic MP, Maberley DAL. Anti-vascular endothelial growth factor therapy for proliferative diabetic retinopathy: a systematic review and meta-analysis. Retina. 2015;35:1931–42. https://doi.org/10.1097/IAE.0000000000000723.
19. Bahrami B, Hong T, Gilles MC, Chang A. Anti-VEGF therapy for diabetic eye diseases. Asia-Pac J Ophthalmol (Phila). 2017;6:535–45. https://doi.org/10.22608/APO.2017350.
20. The Diabetic Retinopathy Study Research Group. Photocoagulation treatment of proliferative diabetic retinopathy. Clinical application of diabetic retinopathy study (DRS) findings, DRS report number 8. Ophthalmology. 1981;88:583–600.
21. Evans JR, Michelessi M, Virgili G. Laser photocoagulation for proliferative diabetic retinopathy. Cochrane Database Syst Rev. 2014;11:CD011234. https://doi.org/10.1002/14651858.CD011234.pub2.
22. Wang W, Lo ACY. Diabetic retinopathy: pathophysiology and treatments. Int J Mol Sci. 2018;19:1816. https://doi.org/10.3390/ijms19061816.
23. Moutray T, Evans JR, Lois N, Armstrong DJ, Peto T, Azuara-Blanco A. Different lasers and techniques for proliferative diabetic retinopathy. Cochrane Database Syst Rev. 2018;3:CD012314. https://doi.org/10.1002/14651858.CD012314.pub2.
24. Abcouwer SF. Angiogenic factors and cytokines in diabetic retinopathy. J Clin Cell Immunol. 2013;S1:011. https://doi.org/10.4172/2155-9899.
25. Cury CE, Rodrigues EB, Meyer CH, Farah ME. VEGF inhibitors and vitrectomy for diabetic vitreoretinopathy. Dev Ophthalmol. 2009;44:69–81. https://doi.org/10.1159/000223947.
26. El Annan J, Carvounis PE. Current management of vitreous hemorrhage due to proliferative diabetic retinopathy. Int Ophthalmol Clin. 2014;54:141–53. https://doi.org/10.1097/IIO.0000000000000027.
27. Oellers P, Mahmoud TH. Surgery for proliferative diabetic retinopathy: new tips and tricks. J Ophthalmic Vis Res. 2016;11:93–9. https://doi.org/10.4103/2008-322X.180697.
28. Shroff CM, Gupta C, Shroff D, Atri N, Gupta P, Dutta R. Bimanual microincision vitreous surgery for severe proliferative diabetic retinopathy: outcome in more than 300 eyes. Retina. 2018;38(Suppl 1):S134–45. https://doi.org/10.1097/IAE.0000000000002093.
29. Vaziri K, Schwartz SG, Kishor KS, Flynn HW. Tamponade in the surgical management of retinal detachment. Clin Ophthalmol. 2016;10:471–6. https://doi.org/10.2147/OPTH.S98529.
30. Abrams GW, Azen SP, McCuen BW, Flynn HW, Lai MY, Ryan SJ. Vitrectomy with silicone oil or long-acting gas in eyes with severe proliferative vitreoretinopathy: results of additional and long-term follow-up. Silicone study report 11. Arch Ophthalmol. 1997;115:335–44.
31. Kitchens JW. Modified external needle drainage of subretinal fluid in the management of rhegmatogenous retinal detachment using a "guarded needle"

approach. Arch Ophthalmol. 2011;129:949. https://doi.org/10.1001/archophthalmol.2011.165.
32. Iwase T, Jo Y-J, Oveson BC. Effect of prophylactic 360° laser treatment for prevention of retinal detachment after phacovitrectomy: (prophylactic 360° laser treatment for prevention of retinal detachment). BMC Ophthalmol. 2013;13:77. https://doi.org/10.1186/1471-2415-13-77.
33. Avitabile T, Longo A, Lentini G, Reibaldi A. Retinal detachment after silicone oil removal is prevented by 360 degrees laser treatment. Br J Ophthalmol. 2008;92:1479–82. https://doi.org/10.1136/bjo.2008.140087.
34. Laidlaw DAH, Karia N, Bunce C, Aylward GW, Gregor ZJ. Is prophylactic 360-degree laser retinopexy protective? Risk factors for retinal redetachment after removal of silicone oil. Ophthalmology. 2002;109:153–8.
35. Wu Y, Zhu W, Xu D, Li Y-H, Ba J, Zhang X-L, et al. Indocyanine green-assisted internal limiting membrane peeling in macular hole surgery: a meta-analysis. PLoS One. 2012;7:e48405. https://doi.org/10.1371/journal.pone.0048405.
36. Khan M, Srivastava SK, Reese JL, Shwani Z, Ehlers JP. Intraoperative OCT-assisted surgery for proliferative diabetic retinopathy in the DISCOVER study. Ophthalmol Retin. 2018;2:411–7. https://doi.org/10.1016/j.oret.2017.08.020.
37. Thompson JT, de Bustros S, Michels RG, Rice TA. Results and prognostic factors in vitrectomy for diabetic traction-rhegmatogenous retinal detachment. Arch Ophthalmol. 1987;105:503–7.
38. Abunajma MA, Al-Dhibi H, Abboud EB, Al Zahrani Y, Alharthi E, Alkharashi A, et al. The outcomes and prognostic factors of vitrectomy in chronic diabetic traction macular detachment. Clin Ophthalmol. 2016;10:1653–61. https://doi.org/10.2147/OPTH.S98555.
39. La Heij EC, Tecim S, Kessels AGH, Liem ATA, Japing WJ, Hendrikse F. Clinical variables and their relation to visual outcome after vitrectomy in eyes with diabetic retinal traction detachment. Graefes Arch Clin Exp Ophthalmol. 2004;242:210–7. https://doi.org/10.1007/s00417-003-0815-5.
40. Usui A, Kiyokawa M, Kimura I, Sakuma T, Ito R, Hatano N, et al. Effects of vitrectomy as a treatment for proliferative diabetic retinopathy in young patients. Nihon Ganka Gakkai Zasshi. 2011;115:516–22.
41. Hsu Y-J, Hsieh Y-T, Yeh P-T, Huang J-Y, Yang C-M. Combined tractional and rhegmatogenous retinal detachment in proliferative diabetic retinopathy in the anti-VEGF era. J Ophthalmol. 2014;2014:917375. https://doi.org/10.1155/2014/917375.
42. Storey PP, Ter-Zakarian A, Philander SA, Olmos de Koo L, George M, Humayun MS, et al. Visual and anatomical outcomes after diabetic traction and traction-rhegmatogenous retinal detachment repair. Retina. 2018;38:1913–9. https://doi.org/10.1097/IAE.0000000000001793.
43. Sahoo NK, Balijepalli P, Singh SR, Jhingan M, Senthil S, Chhablani J. Retina and glaucoma: surgical complications. Int J Retin Vitr. 2018;4:29. https://doi.org/10.1186/s40942-018-0135-x.
44. Soto-Pedre E, Hernaez-Ortega MC, Vazquez JA. Risk factors for postoperative hemorrhage after vitrectomy for diabetic retinopathy. Ophthalmic Epidemiol. 2005;12:335–41. https://doi.org/10.1080/09286580500227068.
45. Motoda S, Shiraki N, Ishihara T, Sakaguchi H, Kabata D, Takahara M, et al. Predictors of postoperative bleeding after vitrectomy for vitreous hemorrhage in patients with diabetic retinopathy. J Diabetes Investig. 2018;9:940–5. https://doi.org/10.1111/jdi.12791.
46. Neffendorf JE, Gupta B, Williamson TH. The role of intraocular gas tamponade in rhegmatogenous retinal detachment. Retina. 2018;38:S65–72. https://doi.org/10.1097/IAE.0000000000002015.
47. Ghoraba HH, Zaky AG, Abd Al Fatah HM, El Gemai EEDM, Heikal MA. Sticky silicone oil. Retina. 2017;37:1599–606. https://doi.org/10.1097/IAE.0000000000001377.

19 Surgical Management of Diabetic Macular Edema

Mikel Mikhail and Tarek S. Hassan

19.1 Introduction

Macular edema is an important cause of vision loss in diabetic patients [1]. Diabetic macular edema (DME) develops in approximately 30% of patients who have had diabetes mellitus for more than 20 years and constitutes a major cause of visual impairment worldwide. Identifying treatments that can effectively treat DME is critical to managing this increasing number of patients.

Currently, the first line of treatment of DME is intravitreal pharmacotherapy. All phase III randomized clinical trials (RISE/RIDE, RESTORE, VIVID/VISTA) have demonstrated the superiority of anti-vascular endothelial growth factor (anti-VEGF) agents, such as ranibizumab and aflibercept, over laser photocoagulation and/or surgery. Nevertheless, anti-VEGF agents confer high direct and indirect costs to patients and payers that can exceed those of laser and vitrectomy. In addition, there is a subset of nonresponders who may benefit from alternative therapy.

In 1988, Nasrallah et al. demonstrated a lower prevalence of DME in eyes with a posterior vitreous detachment compared to eyes without [2]. Hikichi et al. similarly showed resolution of macular edema in almost half of the eyes which underwent a posterior vitreous separation [3]. Lewis et al. also reported the improvement of DME in eyes with posterior hyaloid traction who underwent vitrectomy [4]. In 1996, Tachi et al. reported good results after vitrectomy in patients with diffuse edema in the presence of an attached, albeit not thickened hyaloid [5]. In his series, macular edema resolved in 90% of these cases and vision improved in 50% of treated eyes.

19.2 Pathophysiology

We must appreciate the physiology of the diabetic vitreous and its interaction with the retina to understand the role of vitrectomy in the management of DME.

The vitreous cortex adheres tightly to the internal limiting membrane (ILM) through an extracellular matrix of laminin, opticin, fibronectin, and other constituents [6, 7]. In diabetic patients, there is an abnormal cross-linking of fibrils that results in stronger adhesions between

M. Mikhail
Associated Retinal Consultants, P.C., Royal Oak, MI, USA

Oakland University School of Medicine, Rochester, MI, USA

Lakeridge Health, Queen's University, Ontario, Canada
e-mail: mmikhail@lh.ca

T. S. Hassan (✉)
Associated Retinal Consultants, P.C., Royal Oak, MI, USA

Oakland University School of Medicine, Rochester, MI, USA

A. Jain et al. (eds.), *Cutting-edge Vitreoretinal Surgery*, https://doi.org/10.1007/978-981-33-4168-5_19

the posterior vitreous cortex and the ILM. This is the result of the deposition of advanced glycosylation end-products at the sites of vitreoretinal adhesion [7]. The ILM is noted to be pathologically thickened in diabetic patients due to this accumulation of extracellular matrix components (such as collagen type I, III, IV, V, proteoglycans, laminin, and fibronectin), as well as macrophages and fibroblasts [8].

There is sufficient clinicopathologic correlation to suggest that these changes are relevant in the diabetic eye. For example, Hagenau et al. examined specimens from eyes with DME that underwent vitrectomy. All eyes showed pathologic changes at the vitreomacular interface, regardless of the appearance of the retina on prior OCT or clinical examination. They reported trans-differentiation of hyalocytes into myofibroblasts, as well as thickening and remodeling of the vitreous cortex [9]. This thickened posterior hyaloid–ILM complex can impede the outflow of fluids accumulated in the retina and prevents proper diffusion of oxygen into the retina from the vitreous [10].

The vitreous is an important contributor to the development of DME in other ways. Intact vitreous causes traction on Muller cells, resulting in cellular proliferation and leakage [11]. Vascular permeability is increased as traction distorts the retinal vessels and results in disruption of the macular microcirculation [12–16].

19.3 Role of Vitrectomy

There are three main hypothesized methods by which a vitrectomy is thought to improve macular edema in diabetic, non-vitrectomized patients: (1) relief of vitreoretinal traction, (2) increase in retinal and vitreous oxygenation, and (3) reduction of intravitreal VEGF load.

A vitrectomy with detachment of the posterior hyaloid effectively relieves any traction that may contribute to anatomic thickening and/or increased vascular permeability. Independent of the relief of traction, vitrectomy has also been shown to effectively decrease certain growth factors, such as vascular endothelial growth factor (VEGF), interleukin-6 (IL-6), and platelet-derived growth factor (PDGF). These growth factors play an important role in the development and progression of macular edema in diabetic retinopathy and venous occlusive disease [17–20]. Vitrectomy also increases oxygen tension in the posterior segment and allows for increased retinal and, potentially, choroidal oxygenation [21–27].

19.4 Indications for Vitrectomy

19.4.1 Eyes with Clinically Visible Vitreomacular Traction

Vitreomacular interface abnormalities are common in patients with diabetic macular edema. Chang et al. showed that in patients treated with intravitreal anti-VEGF injections, vitreomacular interface abnormalities were present in 6.4% of eyes, and vitreomacular adhesion (VMA) was a predictor of poor baseline vision. Nevertheless, the presence of VMA did not affect response to treatment [28]. This was corroborated in other studies [29]. A spontaneous release of VMA seems to be associated with a positive anatomic response to anti-VEGF treatment with decreased DME.

There is evidence to suggest that in the presence of clinically identifiable vitreomacular traction (VMT), vitrectomy confers some anatomic and functional benefit, with a relatively favorable anatomic success rate and a low rate of complications [30]. Vitrectomy proves to be particularly useful in eyes with diffuse macular edema that present with a taut posterior hyaloid or clinical evidence of VMT by clinical examination and/or on optical coherence tomography (OCT). Whereas focal macular edema generally results from microaneurysmal leakage, diffuse macular edema is associated with widespread breakdown of the blood–retinal barrier and is often associated with a taut posterior hyaloid [31–34]. The posterior hyaloid tends to condense and cause tangential vitreomacular traction, with a subsequent increase in the permeability of the retinal vasculature [31]. All eyes showed pathologic changes at the vitreomacular interface, regardless of the appearance of the retina on prior OCT or clinical examination [35]. They reported trans-differentiation of hyalocytes into myofibroblasts, as well as thickening and remodeling of the vitreous cortex. This thickened posterior hyaloid–ILM complex is thought to impede the outflow of fluid accumulated in the retina and prevent diffusion of oxygen into the retina from the vitreous.

In the absence of macular ischemia, removing the posterior hyaloid in eyes with traction at the fovea improves macular edema and visual function in up to 90% of eyes, according to some studies [31]. Lewis et al. showed that in eyes with macular edema that did not adequately respond to laser photocoagulation and had biomicroscopic evidence of a taut posterior hyaloid, vitrectomy improves anatomic and functional outcomes. In their study, 9 of 10 vitrectomized eyes showed improvement in macular edema, and vision improved by two or more Snellen lines in 6 eyes [4]. Harbour et al. showed that eyes with a taut posterior hyaloid similarly benefitted from surgery, with vision improving in 4 out of 10 eyes, with the rest remaining stable [33]. Other studies have corroborated these findings [36]. Rosenblatt et al. similarly showed improvements in retinal thickness and vision in a series of 26 eyes with a taut posterior hyaloid [37]. Otani et al. also demonstrated improvement in foveal thickness and vision after vitrectomy [38]. Even in eyes with "massive" exudation, vitrectomy has been shown to be useful in obtaining some functional and/or anatomic improvement [39].

The Diabetic Retinopathy Clinical Research Network (DRCRnet) Vitrectomy Study evaluated the role of vitrectomy in DME in a prospective, data-gathering study of 87 eyes with clinical evidence of VMT, baseline vision of 20/63 to 20/400, and OCT subfield thickness of greater than 300 um [40]. After vitrectomy with or without epiretinal and/or ILM peeling, there was a statistically significant anatomic and functional improvement. Median OCT thickness decreased by 160 um. Vision improved in 38% of eyes, although 22% of eyes showed some loss of visual acuity. There were several pitfalls with this study that should be taken into account which can limit our ability to apply these findings to routine clinical practice. There was no assessment of the degree of macular ischemia in these eyes. Vitreomacular traction was also not universally defined. There was no control group. Surgical technique and indication was left up to the surgeon's discretion. Surgery was performed only if it was deemed that the eye would likely not improve after further sessions of macular laser photocoagulation, thereby selecting patients who were more than likely to present with a poorer functional and anatomic baseline. Despite any controlled and standardized approach to this condition with respect to preoperative macular status, preoperative imaging, timing of intervention, inclusion criteria, surgical technique, and follow-up, the study nevertheless outlined the potentially positive role vitrectomy can have on DME.

Even in the absence of a taut posterior hyaloid on examination or OCT, a clinically identifiable epiretinal membrane (ERM) can also cause underlying macular traction and contribute to DME. Although most studies evaluating the role of surgery in DME have examined eyes with a taut posterior hyaloid, some groups have examined the role of ERM peeling in DME. For example, Yamamoto et al. included a group of DME eyes with a posterior vitreous detachment and ERM that underwent vitrectomy and membrane peeling. Although mean foveal thickness decreased, the difference was not statistically significant. Nevertheless, vision improved in 60% of eyes [41].

19.4.2 Eyes Without Clinically Visible Vitreomacular Traction

As mentioned earlier, most of the earlier studies evaluating the role of vitrectomy for DME focused on eyes with a clinically visible taut posterior hyaloid, and these reports suggest a clear benefit. Nevertheless, this is a small subset of the overall population of eyes with DME. Thomas et al. demonstrated that only 4% of patients with DME had a taut thickened posterior hyaloid that could be definitively identified in the clinical setting [42].

Traction is a significant cause of diffuse retinal leakage in DME that can improve with vitrectomy. If the hyaloid is detached and there is no evidence of VMT, there is less evidence to suggest surgery is beneficial. Despite some evidence suggesting the efficacy of vitrectomy in these cases, there is still controversy over the criteria used for selecting surgical cases if the clinical examination and/or OCT does not reveal a tractional component.

There is a body of literature that suggests that vitrectomy is only useful in eyes with clinical evidence of traction. In a comparative, prospective case series, Shah et al. demonstrated that vitrectomy was only useful in eyes with OCT signs suggestive of macular traction. Vision only improved in eyes with tractional signs preoperatively [43]. A randomized controlled trial by the same group demonstrated that in eyes previously treated with macular laser, there was no significant improvement in macular thickness in eyes with no macular traction [44]. This result was replicated by Patel et al. [45]. Massin et al. similarly showed that vitrectomy was only beneficial in eyes with prior evidence of vitreomacular traction [46]. Ikeda et al. examined five DME eyes with a posterior vitreous detachment on exam. After vitrectomy, four eyes showed improved macular thickening, and all exhibited some improvement in vision. The authors attributed this to a reduction in pro-inflammatory cytokines in the vitrectomized eye and an increase in oxygen tension [47]. Kumagai et al. followed eyes with non-tractional DME that underwent vitrectomy and reported long-term visual acuity gains in 52.7% of eyes [48]. Le Heij et al. similarly demonstrated visual acuity improvement in eyes without evident VMT. Eyes that had prior macular laser photocoagulation showed a 14% improvement in vision, whereas eyes with no prior macular laser showed a 77% improvement in vision [49]. Michalewska et al. examined a cohort of treatment-naïve eyes that underwent vitrectomy for diabetic macular edema. These eyes tended to have a poorer visual acuity at presentation [50]. Nevertheless, the authors noted a significant improvement in central retinal thickness from a mean of 595 um to 266 um which was sustained for a period of 6 months. Vision also improved in all but 1 of 44 eyes. These patients were not followed for more than 6 months.

Figure 19.1 demonstrates the resolution of macular edema in a patient with no OCT evidence of hyaloid traction who underwent vitrectomy for treatment-resistant DME.

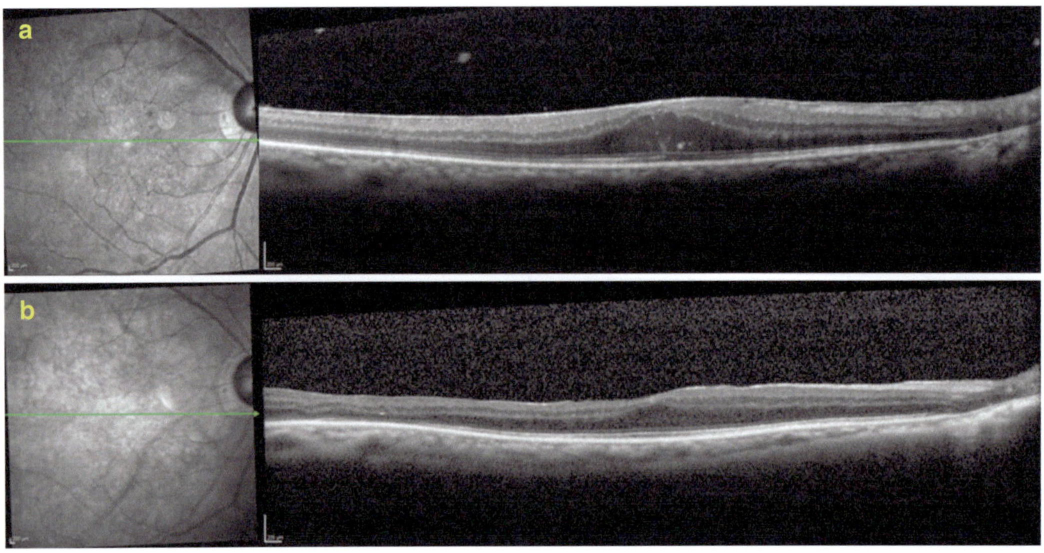

Fig. 19.1 Pre- (**a**) and postoperative (**b**) OCT examination demonstrating resolution of macular edema after vitrectomy, right eye in a 64-year-old male. The patient had no OCT evidence of hyaloid traction and was resistant to anti-VEGF treatment. Six months after surgery, the patient demonstrated anatomic resolution of macular edema. There was also significant improvement in subfoveal ellipsoid zone disruption with the reconstitution of this layer postoperatively. The patient's best-corrected visual acuity improved from 20/80 to 20/60

19.5 Surgical Procedure

The choice of anesthesia remains largely surgeon-, anesthesia-, and institution-dependent. However, special consideration should be given to the general health status of the patient and his or her suitability for general and/or local anesthesia. The patient's systemic health, particularly in the context of possible cardiovascular and renal complications secondary to diabetes, should be considered by the anesthesia team.

The standard surgical technique involves a thorough posterior vitrectomy using a standard three-port pars plana technique, using a separate infusion cannula, a fiberoptic endoilluminator, and an automatic vitrectomy probe. In order to prevent lens opacification in phakic patients, dextrose should be instilled into the Balanced Salt Solution (BSS) Plus infusion solution. This is not necessary in pseudophakic or aphakic patients. Epinephrine can also be added to reduce intraoperative bleeding, although the increased risk of vasoconstriction and decreased vascular perfusion should also be evaluated by the surgeon.

The choice of gauge is surgeon-dependent, and a diabetic vitrectomy can be successfully performed using 23-G, 25-G, or 27-G vitrectomy systems. The authors routinely perform 25-G diabetic vitrectomies due to the ability of the vitrector to effectively engage and cut membranes obviating the need for scissors. The 25-G probe has a sufficiently small sphere of influence to allow efficient and safe dissection and is now complemented with a wide range of instruments that are available in this gauge size [51]. Smaller gauge instrumentation has also been successfully used, although the surgeon should be aware of their increased flexibility and the lack of a full range of instrumentation at the time of writing.

A detachment of the posterior hyaloid is critical for the success of a diabetic vitrectomy, regardless of indication. Intravitreal triamcinolone can be used to stain the hyaloid and provide improved visualization. Posterior vitreous detachment may be difficult to achieve particularly in cases where there is a component of a tractional retinal detachment. The hyaloid can be engaged with active suction. Care must be taken to ensure that excessive aspiration does not result in the worsening of a focal tractional detachment or the creation of a rhegmatogenous component. A sharp edge dissection may be needed with the help of a myringotomy blade or a micro-vitreoretinal forceps. Once an opening in the hyaloid is achieved, this can be lifted carefully with the aid of suction using a small-gauge vitrector. Alternatively, end-grasping forceps or diamond-dusted forceps can also be used to engage the posterior hyaloid and extend the hyaloidal detachment peripherally. The surgeon should ensure that the posterior hyaloid is elevated off the macula as well. This may require additional attempts to elevate other hyaloidal remnants particularly given that there is a reasonably high chance that vitreoschisis (or splitting of the hyaloid) may be encountered. The posterior hyaloid detachment should be extended as far out to the periphery as can be safely achieved without causing iatrogenic breaks. The internal limiting membrane may be peeled, and the role of ILM peeling will be further explored in this chapter. Peripheral shaving of the vitreous is recommended to ensure that traction is adequately relieved. Scleral depression is important to identify any peripheral breaks, which should be treated with endolaser or cryotherapy, although the former is preferred by the authors, due to a reduced risk of postoperative inflammation. A fluid–air exchange can be performed to ensure adequate closure of sclerotomies. Gas or silicone oil can be used as a long-term tamponade agent, the choice of which depends on the status of the retina and the presence of any concomitant breaks or detachment at the conclusion of the surgery. The surgeon should ensure that the incisions are water-tight and suture the sclerotomies if there is any leak. Sutureless diabetic vitrectomies with small-gauge instrumentation is effective and safe, as demonstrated by Mikhail et al. [30]. This is contingent on creating well-constructed sclerotomies and ensuring no immediate postoperative leak. If there is any doubt, leaking sclerotomies must be sutured.

19.6 Adjunctive Techniques

19.6.1 Internal Limiting Membrane Peeling

The ILM may contribute to DME because of its rigidity, and removing it may allow for the release of tangentially oriented tractional forces. Some have advocated routine ILM peeling in DME cases, although the literature is still unclear as to the benefits of this approach. Similar to a taut posterior hyaloid or vitreomacular traction, tangential traction caused by an ILM is relieved once it is peeled. A thickened ILM also acts as a barrier to the diffusion of oxygen from the vitreous and its removal may improve retinal oxygenation [22, 52]. More importantly, these patients often have an attached cortical vitreous, and peeling ILM ensures complete detachment of the posterior hyaloid, particularly in cases where vitreoschisis is suspected. Removing the ILM scaffold may help prevent the formation of epiretinal membranes postoperatively. Figures 19.2 and 19.3 demonstrate a representative case.

In practice, the results of ILM peeling for diabetic DME remain mixed, as in the DRCR.net Vitrectomy Study which showed that 54% of surgeons elected to routinely peel ILM [40]. As techniques have been refined in recent years, greater numbers of surgeons peel ILM in macular surgery.

The actual contribution of the ILM to tractional DME was explored by Abe et al. [53]. The authors performed 3-D OCT imaging on preoperative DME eyes and only peeled ILM on eyes that demonstrated fine folds or a frank epiretinal membrane. They demonstrated an improvement in retinal thickness in these eyes and suggested that folds on 3-D imaging can help stratify patients who may benefit from ILM peeling [53].

This subject has been explored extensively in the literature and the results have been conflicting. Kamura et al. examined 34 eyes with DME that underwent vitrectomy with or without ILM peeling and reported no significant functional difference between the two groups [54]. This was replicated by Yamamoto et al. who looked at 15 eyes undergoing vitrectomy with or without ILM peeling and determined that no significant difference in vision or anatomy [55]. These results were corroborated by Bahadir et al. who again found no difference between patients who under-

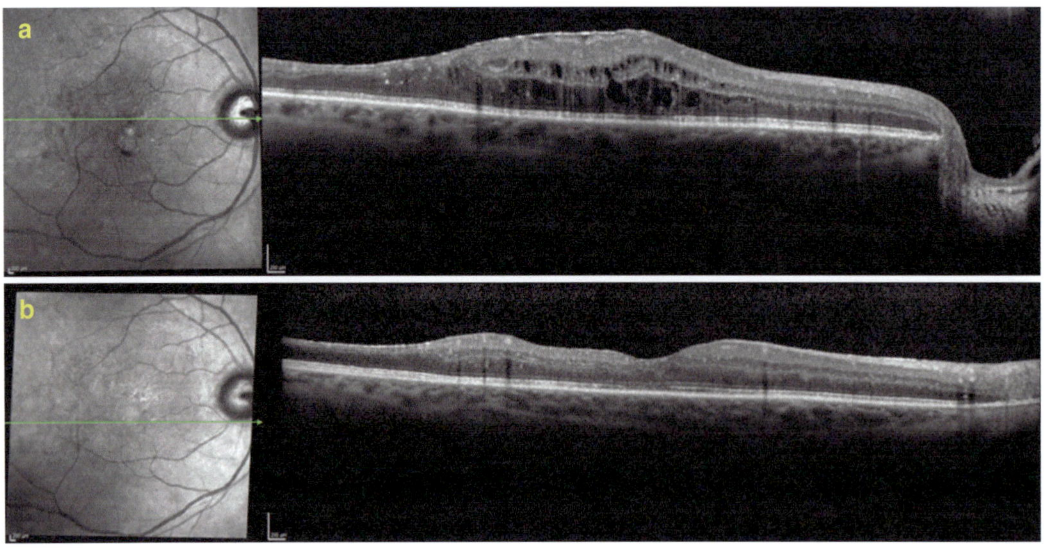

Fig. 19.2 Pre- (**a**) and postoperative (**b**) OCT examination demonstrating resolution of macular edema after vitrectomy, right eye in a 62-year-old male. Epiretinal and internal limiting membrane peeling was performed. There is significant improvement in cystoid macular edema and these results were maintained over a period of 4 years. Vision improved from 20/100 to 20/60

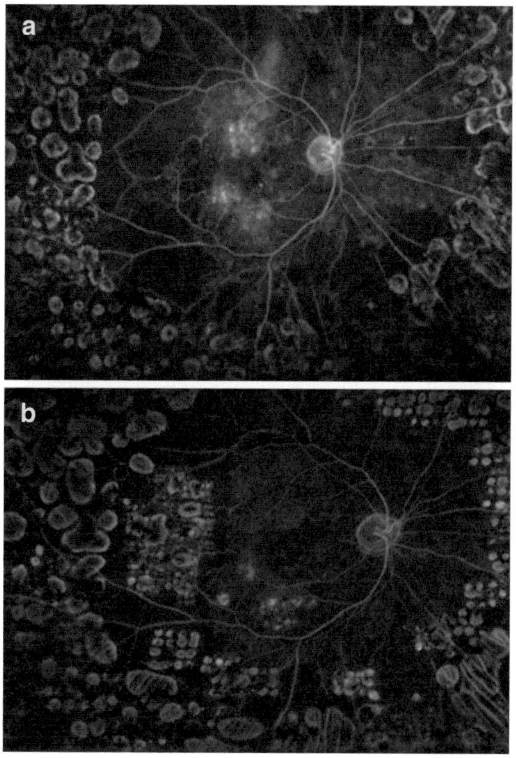

Fig. 19.3 Pre- (**a**) and postoperative (**b**) fluorescein angiography of the patient noted in this figure, demonstrating interval improvement in late leakage consistent with macular edema. There is no significant improvement in vascular perfusion

went vitrectomy alone, compared to those who had their ILMs peeled [56]. Rinaldi et al. examined this topic in detail in a meta-analysis, looking solely at eyes who underwent vitrectomy and ILM peeling vs eyes that underwent vitrectomy alone. The authors included eyes with no clinical evidence of traction [10]. They concluded that ILM peeling as an adjunct to vitrectomy did not significantly improve visual or anatomic outcomes.

Others have suggested a beneficial role for ILM peeling. Patel et al. assessed 10 eyes with refractory DME after vitrectomy and ILM peeling and found significant anatomical improvement, but no gains in visual acuity [45]. Rosenblatt et al. reviewed 26 of their eyes with refractory DME without evidence of clinical traction and reported significant gains in vision and reduction of mean foveal thickness after vitrectomy and ILM peeling [37]. Recchia et al. studied 10 patients who underwent vitrectomy and ILM peeling for refractory DME previously treated with laser and reported improvements in macular edema and vision [57]. Yanyali et al. compared eyes undergoing vitrectomy and ILM peeling vs. focal laser alone, and reported gains in the former group, with no significant improvement in the latter [58]. Similarly, in this cohort, 27 eyes that underwent vitrectomy with ILM peeling reported significant gains in vision and anatomy [59]. Most recently, a meta-analysis by Hu et al. examined 14 studies and concluded that a vitrectomy with ILM peeling demonstrated a higher rate of reduction of central macular thickness and improved vision compared to vitrectomy alone [60].

In summary, the majority of these studies reported some additional benefit to ILM peeling. It is often impossible for the surgeon to determine with certainty whether there is evidence of clinically silent posterior hyaloidal traction, for which an ILM peel may prove beneficial. OCT examination may not adequately address this, and it remains difficult to ascertain whether refractory DME is secondary to subclinical traction by the ILM itself. As the primary goal in such surgeries is to separate the posterior hyaloid from the macula, at a minimum, peeling ILM ensures that all hyaloidal elements are removed. For a number of such reasons, the authors prefer to perform ILM peeling in all cases of vitrectomy for DME.

If a decision is made to peel ILM, the surgeon should use adjunctive staining techniques to identify any residual cortical vitreous, as well as ILM. In the attached retina, ILM peeling is not technically challenging and may provide for a reduction in traction or, at the very least, a reduced risk of epiretinal proliferation in those eyes. In detached retina, the decision is less clear, and it remains up to the surgeon's discretion whether ILM can be safely peeled without causing further damage. At the very least, while several studies have shown that ILM peeling may not provide an additional benefit, none have suggested additional harm. These studies may lack long-term follow-up and the implications of an

ILM peel on the macula's anatomic status remains unclear. An ILM peel is likely to improve a patient's anatomic status but vision may not necessarily improve, which may be a reflection of a diseased retinal microcirculation.

19.6.2 Removal of Hard Exudates

Recently, Imai et al. reported en bloc removal of cystoid lesions during vitrectomy. En block removal resulted in improvement in central retinal thickness, with no significant change in vision. The authors hypothesized that a cystoid lesion is an aggregate of fibrinogen, a provasogenic factor that contributes to further worsening of DME [61]. Subretinal forceps have also been introduced through paramacular retinotomies and used to manually extract hard exudates [62]. There are no large-scale studies to evaluate the efficacy of these techniques, and in the age of widespread intravitreal anti-VEGF injections, they are likely not commonly used.

19.6.3 Iatrogenic Subfoveal Detachment

Subfoveal detachment has been described as a technique to remove subretinal inflammatory mediators and flush out chronic subretinal fluid. For example, Takagi et al. described a procedure by which they detached the fovea and flushed out hard exudates with subretinally injected BSS. Their patients included those with massive foveal exudation with largely end-stage eyes [63]. Nevertheless, they observed some, albeit minimal, improvement in postoperative visual acuity [63]. This technique has been popularized by other authors as a means to rapidly induce resolution of macular thickening. Morizane et al. evaluated a similar technique using 41-G focal subretinal BSS injections in treatment-naïve eyes, as well as those which had been previously treated with anti-VEGF agents [64]. In their series of 20 eyes, mean central retinal thickness decreased significantly, and vision improved in 13 eyes. Subretinal BSS is thought to change the oncotic pressure of subretinal fluid, and may allow for its drainage into the underlying choroid [65]. The authors also hypothesized that BSS flushes out inflammatory mediators, thereby allowing for an improved microenvironment and a potentially more active RPE pump. It is notable that in their eyes, the effect of their surgery lasted for greater than 6 months without further treatment.

This technique has been previously described in the treatment of macular holes, macular translocation in age-related macular degeneration, displacement of submacular hemorrhages, and gene therapy [66]. Extrapolating from our experience in these cases, the authors recommend that if a subfoveal detachment is attempted, the surgeon should use a controlled viscous fluid injection system that is widely available on most vitrectomy machines. The surgeon should test the most optimal injection pressure that would allow a safe, steady, and controlled injection of fluid in the subretinal space prior to entering the eye. This allows for more controlled subretinal injection and reduces the risk of macular hole induction with forceful injection or choroidal injury. If the surgeon experiences difficulty with the initial retinotomy puncture, consideration should also be given to peeling the overlying ILM.

19.7 Prognosis

There are multiple prognostic predictors for the improvement of DME after vitrectomy. These include the duration of macular edema, the extent of previous laser treatment, the degree of macular ischemia, and the amount of exudation. Dysfunction of the photoreceptor layer due to chronic edema, damage induced by laser photocoagulation, and loss of macular perfusion are known to limit visual recovery, despite anatomic improvement.

In a study by Iglicki et al., the timing of surgery was significantly correlated with functional results. For every day vitrectomy was postponed, the patient's chances of gaining greater than five letters at 24 months decreased by 1.8% [67]. Chronic edema can result in outer retinal damage and more permanent vision loss [50]. The preoperative length of photoreceptor outer segment length was shown to positively predict a positive response in these patients [68]. The presence of submacular fluid was also shown to predict a more positive visual prognosis after 24 months for patients undergoing vitrectomy [69].

It is important to closely follow these patients. While vitrectomy is often thought to be a "permanent" solution to recalcitrant diabetic macular edema, this has not been validated extensively. Yamamoto showed that in treated eyes, a reduction in macular thickness is only seen 4 months after the procedure [70]. Yang showed that resolution occurred 3 months after surgery [39]. Results may be sustained up to 24 months after surgery [70]. Regardless, these patients require lifelong follow-up and adjuvant pharmacotherapy may be required.

19.8 Conclusion

Despite the advent of intravitreal pharmacology for the treatment of DME, pars plana vitrectomy, with or without adjunctive techniques, remains an important tool in the vitreoretinal surgeon's armamentarium, particularly in cases of recalcitrant and treatment-naïve DME, with or without clinically identifiable vitreomacular traction. The current literature is replete with multiple, retrospective, noncontrolled studies with limited evidence, but the general trend seen by most is for anatomic and/or functional improvement in those eyes. While there is clear evidence to suggest the role of vitrectomy in eyes with a clinically visible taut, thickened hyaloid, the absence of OCT or clinical evidence of vitreomacular traction should not be used as an exclusion criterion. The decision to pursue surgery should be based on a mutual discussion between surgeon and patient, with an assessment of other factors, such as visual acuity, response to prior intravitreal anti-VEGF treatment, duration and extent of macular edema, presence and degree of macular ischemia, systemic comorbidities as well as an assessment of the direct and indirect costs of alternative therapy. Regardless, further prospective, controlled clinical, long-term trials are sorely needed to address the usefulness of this powerful tool for the management of DME, particularly in this age of widespread intravitreal injection therapy with anti-VEGF agents and steroids.

References

1. Moss SE, Klein R, Klein BE. The 14-year incidence of visual loss in a diabetic population. Ophthalmology. 1998;105:998–1003.
2. Nasrallah FP, Jalkh AE, Van Coppenolle F, et al. The role of the vitreous in diabetic macular edema. Ophthalmology. 1988;95:1335–9.
3. Hikichi T, Fujio N, Akiba J, Azuma Y, Takahashi M, Yoshida A. Association between the short-term natural history of diabetic macular edema and the vitreomacular relationship in type II diabetes mellitus. Ophthalmology. 1997;104:473–8.
4. Lewis H, Abrams GW, Blumenkranz MS, Campo RV. Vitrectomy for diabetic macular traction and edema associated with posterior hyaloidal traction. Ophthalmology. 1992;99:753–9.
5. Tachi N, Ogino N. Vitrectomy for diffuse macular edema in cases of diabetic retinopathy. Am J Ophthalmol. 1996;122:258–60.
6. Sebag J. Structure, function, and age-related changes of the human vitreous. Bull Soc Belge Ophtalmol. 1987;223(Pt 1):37–57.
7. Sebag J. Ageing of the vitreous. Eye. 1987;1(Pt 2):254–62.
8. Abari E, Kociok N, Hartmann U, et al. Alterations in basement membrane immunoreactivity of the diabetic retina in three diabetic mouse models. Graefes Arch Clin Exp Ophthalmol. 2013,251:763–75.
9. Hagenau F, Vogt D, Ziada J, et al. Vitrectomy for diabetic macular edema: optical coherence tomography criteria and pathology of the vitreomacular interface. Am J Ophthalmol. 2018;200:34–46.
10. Rinaldi M, dell'Omo R, Morescalchi F, et al. ILM peeling in nontractional diabetic macular edema: review and metanalysis. Int Ophthalmol. 2018;38:2709–14.
11. Bringmann A, Grosche A, Pannicke T, Reichenbach A. GABA and glutamate uptake and metabolism in retinal glial (Muller) cells. Front Endocrinol. 2013;4:48.
12. Scholl S, Kirchhof J, Augustin AJ. Pathophysiology of macular edema. Ophthalmologica. 2010;224(Suppl 1):8–15.
13. Augustin AJ. Oxidative tissue damage. Klin Monatsbl Augenheilkund. 2010;227:90–8.
14. Augustin A, Loewenstein A, Kuppermann BD. Macular edema. General pathophysiology. Dev Ophthalmol. 2010;47:10–26.

15. Lindqvist N, Liu Q, Zajadacz J, Franze K, Reichenbach A. Retinal glial (Muller) cells: sensing and responding to tissue stretch. Invest Ophthalmol Vis Sci. 2010;51:1683–90.
16. Wolfensberger TJ, Gregor ZJ. Macular edema--rationale for therapy. Dev Ophthalmol. 2010;47:49–58.
17. Yamasaki M, Noma H, Funatsu H, et al. Changes in foveal thickness after vitrectomy for macular edema with branch retinal vein occlusion and intravitreal vascular endothelial growth factor. Int Ophthalmol. 2009;29:161–7.
18. Noma H, Funatsu H, Sakata K, Harino S, Mimura T, Hori S. Macular microcirculation in hypertensive patients with and without branch retinal vein occlusion. Acta Ophthalmol. 2009;87:638–42.
19. Praidou A, Papakonstantinou E, Androudi S, Georgiadis N, Karakiulakis G, Dimitrakos S. Vitreous and serum levels of vascular endothelial growth factor and platelet-derived growth factor and their correlation in patients with non-proliferative diabetic retinopathy and clinically significant macula oedema. Acta Ophthalmol. 2011;89:248–54.
20. Praidou A, Klangas I, Papakonstantinou E, et al. Vitreous and serum levels of platelet-derived growth factor and their correlation in patients with proliferative diabetic retinopathy. Curr Eye Res. 2009;34:152–61.
21. Williamson TH, Grewal J, Gupta B, Mokete B, Lim M, Fry CH. Measurement of PO2 during vitrectomy for central retinal vein occlusion, a pilot study. Graefes Arch Clin Exp Ophthalmol. 2009;247:1019–23.
22. Stefansson E. Diabetic maculopathy. Acta Ophthalmol Scand. 1999;77:612–3.
23. Holekamp NM, Shui YB, Beebe DC. Vitrectomy surgery increases oxygen exposure to the lens: a possible mechanism for nuclear cataract formation. Am J Ophthalmol. 2005;139:302–10.
24. Siegfried CJ, Shui YB, Holekamp NM, Bai F, Beebe DC. Oxygen distribution in the human eye: relevance to the etiology of open-angle glaucoma after vitrectomy. Invest Ophthalmol Vis Sci. 2010;51:5731–8.
25. Giblin FJ, Quiram PA, Leverenz VR, Baker RM, Dang L, Trese MT. Enzyme-induced posterior vitreous detachment in the rat produces increased lens nuclear pO2 levels. Exp Eye Res. 2009;88:286–92.
26. Quiram PA, Leverenz VR, Baker RM, Dang L, Giblin FJ, Trese MT. Microplasmin-induced posterior vitreous detachment affects vitreous oxygen levels. Retina. 2007;27:1090–6.
27. Gamulescu MA, Herrmann WA, Helbig H. Surgical treatment of diabetic macular oedema. Klin Monatsbl Augenheilkund. 2009;226:910–3.
28. Chang CK, Cheng CK, Peng CH. The incidence and risk factors for the development of vitreomacular interface abnormality in diabetic macular edema treated with intravitreal injection of anti-VEGF. Eye. 2017;31:762–70.
29. Mikhail M, Stewart S, Seow F, Hogg R, Lois N. Vitreomacular interface abnormalities in patients with diabetic macular oedema and their implications on the response to anti-VEGF therapy. Graefes Arch Clin Exp Ophthalmol. 2018;256:1411–8.
30. Mikhail M, Ali-Ridha A, Chorfi S, Kapusta MA. Long-term outcomes of sutureless 25-G+ pars-plana vitrectomy for the management of diabetic tractional retinal detachment. Graefes Arch Clin Exp Ophthalmol. 2017;255:255–61.
31. Pendergast SD, Hassan TS, Williams GA, et al. Vitrectomy for diffuse diabetic macular edema associated with a taut premacular posterior hyaloid. Am J Ophthalmol. 2000;130:178–86.
32. Pendergast SD. Vitrectomy for diabetic macular edema associated with a taut premacular posterior hyaloid. Curr Opin Ophthalmol. 1998;9:71–5.
33. Harbour JW, Smiddy WE, Flynn HW Jr, Rubsamen PE. Vitrectomy for diabetic macular edema associated with a thickened and taut posterior hyaloid membrane. Am J Ophthalmol. 1996;121:405–13.
34. Kirber WM, Nichols CW, Grimes PA, Winegrad AI, Laties AM. A permeability defect of the retinal pigment epithelium. Occurrence in early streptozocin diabetes. Arch Ophthalmol. 1980;98:725–8.
35. Kaiser PK, Riemann CD, Sears JE, Lewis H. Macular traction detachment and diabetic macular edema associated with posterior hyaloidal traction. Am J Ophthalmol. 2001;131:44–9.
36. Kalvodova B, Zahlava J. Results of vitrectomy in cystoid diabetic macular edema detected by optical coherence tomography. Cesk Slov Oftalmol. 2002;58:224–32.
37. Rosenblatt BJ, Shah GK, Sharma S, Bakal J. Pars plana vitrectomy with internal limiting membranectomy for refractory diabetic macular edema without a taut posterior hyaloid. Graefes Arch Clin Exp Ophthalmol. 2005;243:20–5.
38. Otani T, Kishi S. Tomographic assessment of vitreous surgery for diabetic macular edema. Am J Ophthalmol. 2000;129:487–94.
39. Yang CM. Surgical treatment for severe diabetic macular edema with massive hard exudates. Retina. 2000;20:121–5.
40. Haller JA, Qin H, Apte RS, et al. Vitrectomy outcomes in eyes with diabetic macular edema and vitreomacular traction. Ophthalmology. 2010;117:1087–93.
41. Yamamoto T, Akabane N, Takeuchi S. Vitrectomy for diabetic macular edema: the role of posterior vitreous detachment and epimacular membrane. Am J Ophthalmol. 2001;132:369–77.
42. Thomas D, Bunce C, Moorman C, Laidlaw AH. Frequency and associations of a taut thickened posterior hyaloid, partial vitreomacular separation, and subretinal fluid in patients with diabetic macular edema. Retina. 2005;25:883–8.
43. Shah SP, Patel M, Thomas D, Aldington S, Laidlaw DA. Factors predicting outcome of vitrectomy for diabetic macular oedema: results of a prospective study. Br J Ophthalmol. 2006;90:33–6.
44. Thomas D, Bunce C, Moorman C, Laidlaw DA. A randomised controlled feasibility trial of vitrec-

tomy versus laser for diabetic macular oedema. Br J Ophthalmol. 2005;89:81–6.
45. Patel JI, Hykin PG, Schadt M, et al. Diabetic macular oedema: pilot randomised trial of pars plana vitrectomy vs macular argon photocoagulation. Eye. 2006;20:873–81.
46. Massin P, Duguid G, Erginay A, Haouchine B, Gaudric A. Optical coherence tomography for evaluating diabetic macular edema before and after vitrectomy. Am J Ophthalmol. 2003;135:169–77.
47. Ikeda T, Sato K, Katano T, Hayashi Y. Vitrectomy for cystoid macular oedema with attached posterior hyaloid membrane in patients with diabetes. Br J Ophthalmol. 1999;83:12–4.
48. Kumagai K, Furukawa M, Ogino N, Larson E, Iwaki M, Tachi N. Long-term follow-up of vitrectomy for diffuse nontractional diabetic macular edema. Retina. 2009;29:464–72.
49. La Heij EC, Hendrikse F, Kessels AG, Derhaag PJ. Vitrectomy results in diabetic macular oedema without evident vitreomacular traction. Graefes Arch Clin Exp Ophthalmol. 2001;239:264–70.
50. Michalewska Z, Stewart MW, Landers MB 3rd, Bednarski M, Adelman RA, Nawrocki J. Vitrectomy in the management of diabetic macular edema in treatment-naive patients. Can J Ophthalmol. 2018;53:402–7.
51. Dugel PU, Zhou J, Abulon DJ, Buboltz DC. Tissue attraction associated with 20-gauge, 23-gauge, and enhanced 25-gauge dual-pneumatic vitrectomy probes. Retina. 2012;32:1761–6.
52. Stefansson E. Physiology of vitreous surgery. Graefes Arch Clin Exp Ophthalmol. 2009;247:147–63.
53. Abe S, Yamamoto T, Kashiwagi Y, Kirii E, Goto S, Yamashita H. Three-dimensional imaging of the inner limiting membrane folding on the vitreomacular interface in diabetic macular edema. Jpn J Ophthalmol. 2013;57:553–62.
54. Kamura Y, Sato Y, Isomae T, Shimada H. Effects of internal limiting membrane peeling in vitrectomy on diabetic cystoid macular edema patients. Jpn J Ophthalmol. 2005;49:297–300.
55. Yamamoto T, Hitani K, Sato Y, Yamashita H, Takeuchi S. Vitrectomy for diabetic macular edema with and without internal limiting membrane removal. Ophthalmologica. 2005;219:206–13.
56. Bahadir M, Ertan A, Mertoglu O. Visual acuity comparison of vitrectomy with and without internal limiting membrane removal in the treatment of diabetic macular edema. Int Ophthalmol. 2005;26:3–8.
57. Recchia FM, Ruby AJ, Carvalho Recchia CA. Pars plana vitrectomy with removal of the internal limiting membrane in the treatment of persistent diabetic macular edema. Am J Ophthalmol. 2005;139:447–54.
58. Yanyali A, Nohutcu AF, Horozoglu F, Celik E. Modified grid laser photocoagulation versus pars plana vitrectomy with internal limiting membrane removal in diabetic macular edema. Am J Ophthalmol. 2005;139:795–801.
59. Yanyali A, Horozoglu F, Celik E, Nohutcu AF. Long-term outcomes of pars plana vitrectomy with internal limiting membrane removal in diabetic macular edema. Retina. 2007;27:557–66.
60. Hu XY, Liu H, Wang LN, Ding YZ, Luan J. Efficacy and safety of vitrectomy with internal limiting membrane peeling for diabetic macular edema: a meta-analysis. Int J Ophthalmol. 2018;11:1848–55.
61. Imai H, Otsuka K, Tetsumoto A, Miki A, Nakamura M. Effectiveness of en bloc removal of fibrinogen-rich component of cystoid lesion for the treatment of cystoid macular edema. Retina. 2018;40(1):154–9.
62. Takaya K, Suzuki Y, Mizutani H, Sakuraba T, Nakazawa M. Long-term results of vitrectomy for removal of submacular hard exudates in patients with diabetic maculopathy. Retina. 2004;24:23–9.
63. Takagi H, Otani A, Kiryu J, Ogura Y. New surgical approach for removing massive foveal hard exudates in diabetic macular edema. Ophthalmology. 1999;106:249–56.
64. Morizane Y, Kimura S, Hosokawa M, et al. Planned foveal detachment technique for the resolution of diffuse diabetic macular edema. Jpn J Ophthalmol. 2015;59:279–87.
65. Abdel Hadi AM. Evaluation of Vitrectomy with planned Foveal detachment as surgical treatment for refractory diabetic macular edema with or without Vitreomacular Interface abnormality. J Ophthalmol. 2018;2018:9246384.
66. Kimura S, Morizane Y, Hosokawa M, et al. Submacular hemorrhage in polypoidal choroidal vasculopathy treated by vitrectomy and subretinal tissue plasminogen activator. Am J Ophthalmol. 2015;159:683–9.
67. Iglicki M, Lavaque A, Ozimek M, et al. Biomarkers and predictors for functional and anatomic outcomes for small gauge pars plana vitrectomy and peeling of the internal limiting membrane in naive diabetic macular edema: the VITAL study. PLoS One. 2018;13:e0200365.
68. Kogo J, Shiono A, Sasaki H, et al. Foveal microstructure analysis in eyes with diabetic macular edema treated with Vitrectomy. Adv Ther. 2017;34:2139–49.
69. Iglicki M, Loewenstein A, Barak A, Schwartz S, Zur D. Outer retinal hyperreflective deposits (ORYD): a new OCT feature in naive diabetic macular oedema after PPV with ILM peeling. Br J Ophthalmol. 2019;104(5):666–71.
70. Yamamoto T, Takeuchi S, Sato Y, Yamashita H. Long-term follow-up results of pars plana vitrectomy for diabetic macular edema. Jpn J Ophthalmol. 2007;51:285–91.

20 Vitreoretinal Surgery in Eales' Disease

Sandeep Saxena, Somnath De, and Astha Jain

20.1 Introduction

Eales' disease was first described by Henry Eales, a British ophthalmologist, in 1880 and 1882 [1, 2]. Eales' disease is an idiopathic retinal periphlebitis that primarily affects the peripheral retina in young adults. Elliot first recognized the inflammation of the retinal vein and described it as periphlebitis retinae. Several investigators have documented both venular and arteriolar inflammation in this disease [3–8].

Eales' disease commonly affects healthy young adult males. It is an important cause of preventable blindness in young adults. The predominant age of onset of symptoms is 20–30 years. Eales' disease is more commonly seen in the Indian subcontinent. However, it has been reported from the UK, the USA, Canada, Germany, Greece, and Turkey.

Eales' disease is characterized by retinal periphlebitis, peripheral retinal ischemia, and neovascularization (Figs. 20.1 and 20.2). Visual loss is characteristically caused by recurrent vitreous hemorrhage [9].

S. Saxena (✉) · S. De
Department of Ophthalmology, King George's Medical University, Lucknow, Uttar Pradesh, India

A. Jain
Aditya Jyot Foundation for Twinkling Little Eyes, Mumbai, India

Aditya Jyot Eye Hospital, Mumbai, India

A. Jain et al. (eds.), *Cutting-edge Vitreoretinal Surgery*,
https://doi.org/10.1007/978-981-33-4168-5_20

Eales' disease appears to be an immunologic reaction that may be triggered by an exogenous exposure. Retinal S-antigen and Inter photoreceptor Retinoid Binding Protein play a role in the etiopathogenesis. An extraneous agent results in the exposure of normally sequestered uveito pathogenic antigens of the immune system, leading to an immune response in the eye that initiates the disease process [10].

Oxidative stress has been found to play an important role in etiopathogenesis [11–18].

Elevated lipid peroxides have been found in the proliferative stage, which induce the synthesis of cytokines and growth factors in the retina during neovascularization [13]. Cytokines have been found to play a significant role in the pathogenesis of intraocular inflammation and neovascularization. During the inflammatory and proliferative stages of the disease, a significant increase in IL-1β, IL-6, IL-10, and TNF-α expression has been observed, highlighting the role of pro- and anti-inflammatory cytokines in pathogenesis. Thus, the IL-1 system and TNF-α represents a novel target for controlling inflammatory activity and/or the associated long-term sequelae related to angiogenesis in Eales' disease [19–21].

A close relationship between the prominent neovascular proliferation in Eales' disease and the intense expression of VEGF has been found. The increased expression of VEGF, when compared to other conditions inducing neovascularization, might explain the severity of neovascular

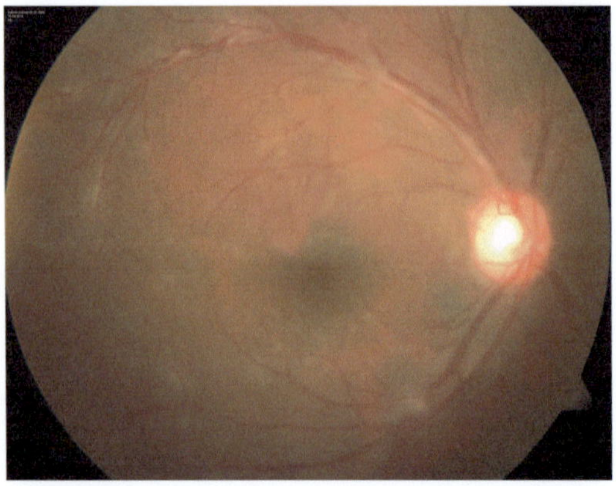

Fig. 20.1 Color fundus photograph showing retinal periphlebitis

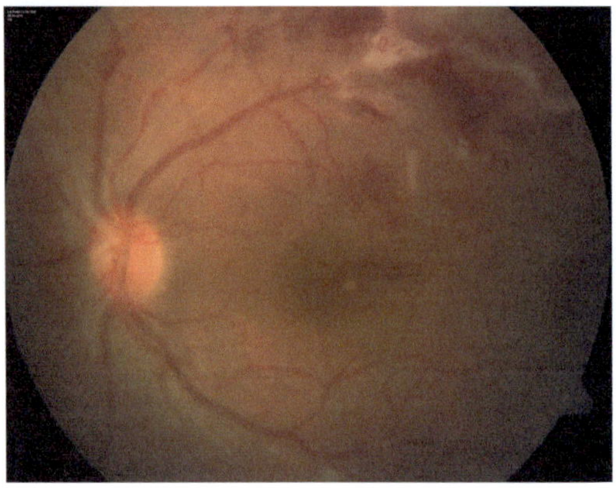

Fig. 20.2 Color fundus photograph shows vascular sheathing along with superficial retinal hemorrhages and neovascularization elsewhere

growth and the propensity of repeated vitreous hemorrhage in Eales' disease [22].

Retinal photoreceptors and platelets have been shown to be an easy target of oxidants because of the high proportion of polyunsaturated fatty acids. The decreased membrane fluidity in platelets suggests alterations in the physiological events, which may result in alterations in the functioning of retinal photoreceptors [18].

20.2 Clinical Features

Eales' disease with a characteristic clinical picture, fluorescein angiographic findings, and natural course is considered a specific disease entity.

Table 20.1 Classification system for Eales' disease

Stages	Features
A. Peripheral Eales disease	
Stage 1a	Periphlebitis of small caliber vessels with superficial retinal hemorrhages
Stage 1b	Periphlebitis of large caliber vessels with superficial retinal hemorrhages
Stage 2a	Peripheral capillary non-perfusion
Stage 2b	Neovascularization elsewhere/ neovascularization of the disc
Stage 3a	Fibrovascular proliferation
Stage 3b	Vitreous hemorrhage
Stage 4a	Traction/combined rhegmatogenous detachment
Stage 4b	Rubeosisiridis, neovascular glaucoma, complicated cataract, and optic atrophy
B. Central Eales' disease	

Recurrent vitreous hemorrhage is the hallmark of this disease. A novel classification system has been proposed by the author [23]. This staging system, based on standard terminology and features, provides a simple method to categorize, according to the severity of the disease. This staging system takes into consideration the fundoscopic and fluorescein angiographic variables that have been shown to be prognostic of visual outcome (Table 20.1). Macular involvement is uncommon. Macular ischemia and traction macular detachment are associated with poor visual outcome [24]. This classification system is consistent, simple, and easy to recall. It can also be used to monitor the effect of medical, laser, and/or surgical treatment.

Areas of capillary non-perfusion and retinal neovascularization can be easily delineated by fluorescein angiography. Capillary non-perfusion of more than 20 disc area and 60 disc area are associated with neovascularization elsewhere (NVE) and neovascularization of the disc (NVD) [25]. Retinal neovascularization sites have been found to cluster around specific anatomic foci. The quadrantic distribution of the sites of NVE in Eales' disease is: superotemporal, 46%; inferotemporal, 24%; superonasal, 16%; and inferonasal, 14% [26].

20.3 Management

The management of Eales' disease depends on the severity of the disease. Management strategies can also be defined according to the stage of the disease. *Stage 1*, the stage of inflammation, is amenable to medical therapy. *Stage 2*, the stage of ischemia and neovascularization, requires observation/laser photocoagulation. *Stage 3*, the stage of proliferation, requires laser/pars plana vitrectomy and laser. *Stage 4*, the stage of complications, requires sophisticated surgical management strategies [23].

20.3.1 Medical Therapy

Corticosteroids: Anti-inflammatory corticosteroid drugs are potent therapeutic agents for a wide range of ocular and systemic disorders and remain the mainstay of therapy in retinal periphlebitis in Eales' disease (1 mg/kg/day).

Methotrexate: Predominantly T cell involvement has been demonstrated in the lymphocytic infiltration of epiretinal and subretinal membranes in Eales' disease, indicating that treatment should be directed to the downregulation of the activated T cells. As opposed to the more "cytostatic" effects of corticosteroids, the "cytotoxic" immunosuppressives exert their beneficial effects by actually killing the rapidly dividing clones of lymphocytes that are responsible for inflammation.

Methotrexate, a folic acid antagonist, has anti-inflammatory and immunomodulatory actions. The drug reduces the synthesis of DNA by acting on the enzyme dihydrofolate reductase. Methotrexate is used as a weekly "pulsed" therapy. A "pulse" differs from chronic moderate dose therapy in its ability to "reset" an aberrant immune response. Inhibition of the proliferating lymphocyte clones, the temporary removal of recirculating T lymphocytes from the blood and eye, and the profound suppression of peripheral inflammation, all occur simultaneously. Antigens exposed by viral, bacterial, or autoimmune injury are normally perpetuated by the inflammatory response but in such a system a pulse may abolish the source of antigen at the same time as it suppresses the immune response. When memory T cells recirculate, the disease falters in the absence of the antigen [27, 28].

20.3.2 Photocoagulation

Photocoagulation is the mainstay of therapy in the proliferative stage of the disease. In cases of gross capillary, non-perfusion photocoagulation is suggested. For NVE and NVD, sectoral scatter photocoagulation and panretinal photocoagulation, respectively, are suggested.

20.3.3 Vitreoretinal Surgery

Vitreous hemorrhage is the primary cause for diminution of vision (Fig. 20.3). The episodes of vitreous hemorrhage do not necessarily correlate with the retinal changes. Vitrectomy is often not required in the first episode of vitreous hemorrhage. The first episode of vitreous hemorrhage usually clears within 6–8 weeks. However, recurrent vitreous hemorrhages may lead to the formation of traction bands and membranes in the vitreous and resulting complications (Figs. 20.4, 20.5, 20.6, 20.7). Ultrasonography

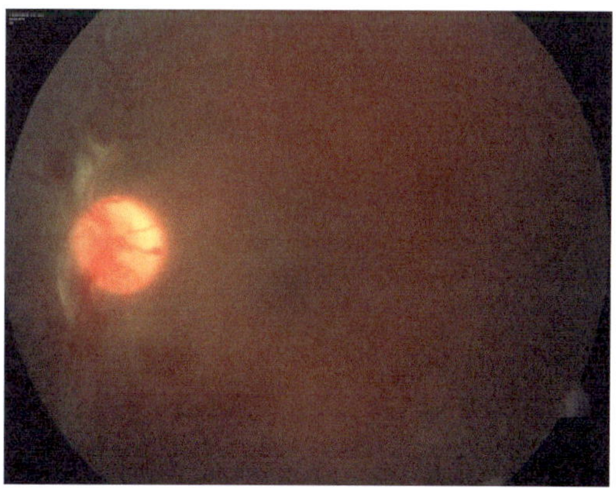

Fig. 20.3 Color fundus photograph showing neovascularisation at disc and vitreous hemorrhage

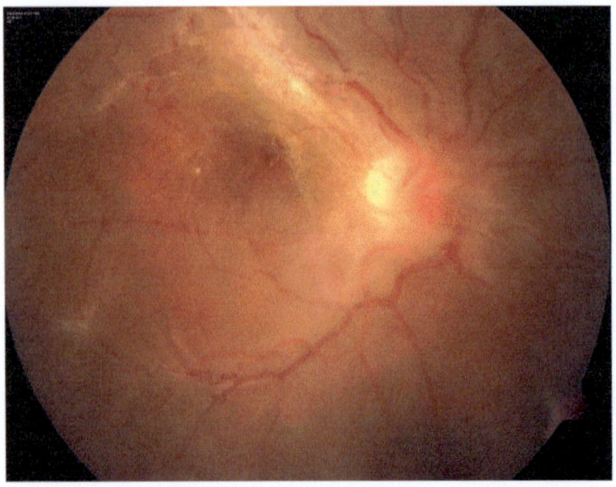

Fig. 20.4 Color fundus photograph showing retinal vasculitis, fibrovascular proliferation along the superotemporal vascular arcade and epiretinal membrane at macula

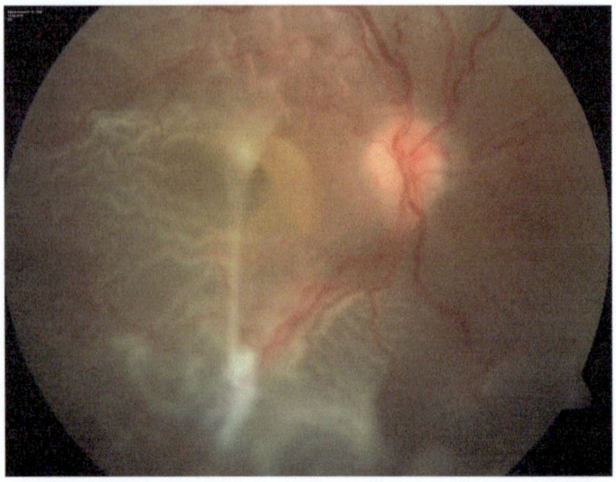

Fig. 20.6 Color fundus photograph showing retinal detachment along with fibroproliferative membrane across macula

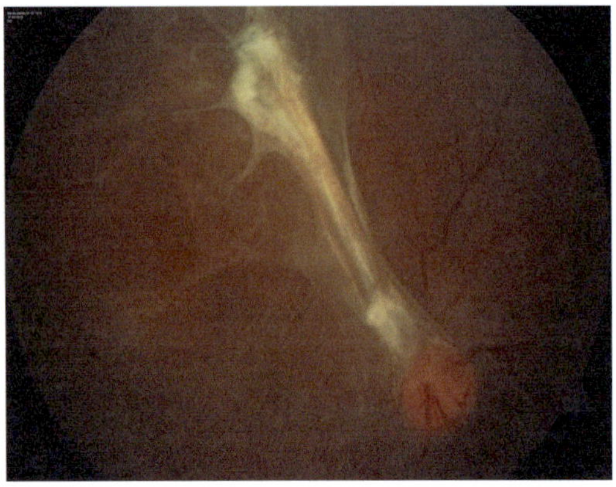

Fig. 20.5 Color fundus photograph showing residual fibrous proliferation from the disc and epiretinal membrane

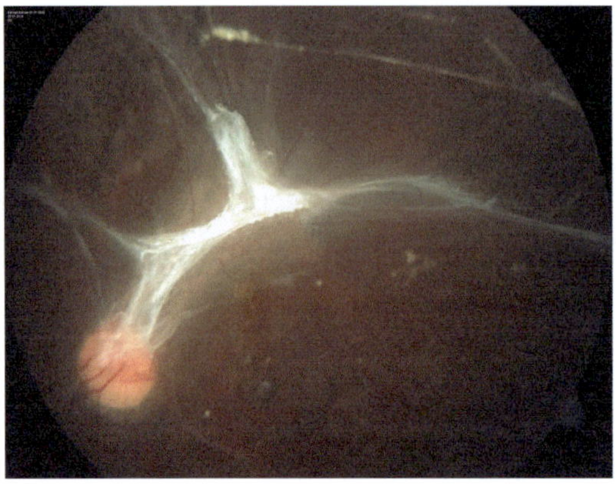

Fig. 20.7 Color fundus showing optic disc pallor, residual fibrous proliferation, and ischemic macula

should always be performed to exclude the presence of an associated retinal detachment.

Vitrectomy alone or combined with other vitreoretinal surgical procedures is often required. Surgical results have been variable in the published literature [29–36]. The reported outcomes differ considerably with the surgical indication (vitreous hemorrhage versus tractional complications), the extent of posterior vitreous detachment (PVD), and the surgical techniques employed [30–35].

The main indications for vitrectomy include non-resolving vitreous hemorrhage, tractional retinal detachment involving the posterior pole, multiple vitreous membranes with or without tractional retinal detachment, and combined tractional and rhegmatogenous retinal detachment.

The aim of vitreoretinal surgery is to clear the vitreous opacities and also to critically evaluate the fundus for any retinal neovascularization. In the presence of tractional retinal detachment, extensive vitreous membranes and epiretinal membranes early vitrectomy may be considered. A standard three-port pars plana 23- or 25-gauge vitrectomy may be employed for vitreous hemorrhage removal. Excision of posterior hyaloid face and clearing of any subhyaloid hemorrhage is performed. Epimacular membranes are peeled off. Posterior vitreous usually detaches from the retinal surface early except the attachment at the optic disc, and unlike diabetic retinopathy, there are less often multiple retinal attachments and vitreous schisis. The latter helps the surgeon in getting into the correct plane for a safe vitreous surgery. Endolaser application is mandatory at the conclusion of vitreous surgery. Additional procedures, such as belt buckling and lensectomy, are occasionally required.

Visual improvement is better with fewer episodes and shorter duration of vitreous hemorrhage. It has also been shown that the patients who had photocoagulation before vitreous surgery had a better prognosis. The indication for surgery, status of PVD, and complexity of the surgical procedure performed affect the final outcome. Results of vitrectomy in Eales' disease have been reported for nearly three decades. Vitrectomy was generally performed after long waiting periods. Excellent results have been obtained in the presence of total PVD. Poor outcomes had been reported with preoperative or intraoperative detachments. The overall surgical results had been satisfactory because a majority of cases were operated on for vitreous hemorrhage and had complete PVD [29–39].

Posterior vitreous detachment is not necessarily common in Eales' disease. Incomplete PVD may be detected in eyes operated for Eales' disease [40]. Fibrous and fibrovascular proliferation have multiple areas of adhesions to the posterior vitreous cortex. The presence of type II collagen in the epiretinal membrane indicated a possible vitreous collagen component to the double-layered membranes (vitreoschisis). Recognition of the double-layered membranes aids in the relief of traction during surgery by delamination [15].

The major postoperative complications are recurrent vitreous hemorrhage, rubeosis iridis, neovascular glaucoma, and early development of cataract.

20.3.4 Role of Bevacizumab

Intravitreal bevacizumab has been found to be effective as an adjunctive treatment of retinal neovascularization in patients with Eales' disease [41]. However, repeated intravitreal bevacizumab in patients with Eales' disease with dense vitreous hemorrhage may not hasten the resolution of vitreous hemorrhage or reduce the need for vitrectomy. Moreover, tractional retinal detachment may be a serious complication of therapy and hence should be closely monitored because it entails a poor visual prognosis [42]. Intravitreal bevacizumab, 5–7 days before surgery, is a useful adjunct. It reduces intraoperative bleeding thereby decreasing the surgical time and improving the visual outcome.

20.4 Outcome

Kumar et al. [31] reported excellent visual outcome in Eales' disease (≥6/18 in 92%; PVD: 70–100%) [6], whereas El-Asrar and Al-Kharashi [30] reported acuity ≥6/12 in a modest 26% (incidence of PVD not reported; preoperative RD in 27%). Majji et al. [34] had a final acuity ≥20/50 in 30% of cases. Membrane peeling was performed in all, suggesting incomplete PVD. Smiddy et al. [35] reported dismal results with vitrectomy in Eales' disease (functional improvement in only 26.5%). Triester and Machemer [36] reported final acuity of ≥20/50 in 51%; but 42% presented with the same vision preoperatively. Shukla et al. [41] obtained a final BCVA ≥ 6/12 in 60% eyes, notwithstanding an incomplete PVD in 60% eyes; only three (4%) of their cases had BCVA ≥ 6/12 preoperatively. The presence of preoperative RD in only a third of eyes probably improved the prognosis. But the absence of RD did not necessarily mean a simple surgery. Adjunctive procedures such as sclera buckling/C_3F_8/silicone oil were required in 43% of cases.

Preoperative panretinal photocoagulation does affect the surgical outcome [29–32]. Additional surgical procedures (sclera buckling/C_3F_8/silicone oil) have a relatively high incidence of postoperative cataract formation.

Surgical failure rate is mostly related to the difficulty of peeling tractional membranes in the peripheral retina. Peripheral tears or retinotomies may be observed in all the persistent/inoperable detachments [43]. Encirclage helps in neutralizing the peripheral traction from fibrovascular membranes.

20.5 Conclusion

Vitrectomy with removal of persistent vitreous hemorrhage and focal neovascular membranes and endolaser photocoagulation may lead to improved visual acuity in the majority of eyes with Eales' disease. However, extensive fibrovascular membranes and long-standing retinal detachment result in poor visual outcome. Earlier surgery can be considered to prevent visual loss in patients [44]. Although surgical outcomes in Eales' disease depend on preoperative PVD/RD to some extent, good results are possible in the presence of incomplete PVD and tractional sequelae.

References

1. Eales H. Retinal hemorrhage associated with epistaxis and constipation. Brim Med Rev. 1880;9:262.
2. Eales H. Primary retinal hemorrhage in young men. Ophthalmic Rev. 1882;1:41.
3. Duke-Elder S, Dobree JH. Primary perivasculitis of the retina: Eales disease. In: Elder D, Perkins EJ, editors. System of ophthalmology, vol. X. London: Henry Kimpton; 1967. p. 222–36.
4. Elliot AJ. 30-year observation of patients with Eales disease. Am J Ophthalmol. 1975;80:404–8.
5. Kimura SJ, Carriker FR, Hogen MJ. Retinal vasculitis with intraocular hemorrhage. Classification and results of special studies. Arch Ophthalmol. 1956;56:361–5.
6. Cross AG. Vasculitis retinae. Trans Ophthalmol Soc UK. 1963;83:133.
7. Keith-Lyle T, Wybark A. Retinal vasculitis. Br J Ophthalmol. 1961;45:77–8.
8. Gilbert TW. Periphlebitis and endovasculitis of retinal vessels. Klin Monatsbl Augenheilkd. 1935;94:335–49.
9. Kumar D, Saxena RC, Saxena S. Vitreous hemorrhage in Eales' disease. Afro-Asian J Ophthalmol. 1995;13:109–12.
10. Saxena S, Rajasingh J, Biswas S, et al. Cellular response to retinal S-antigen and Interphotoreceptor retinoid binding protein fragments in patients with Eales' disease. Pathobiology. 1999;67:37–44.
11. Saxena S, Khanna VK, Kumar D, et al. Enhanced oxidative stress in Eales' disease. Ann Ophthalmol. 2001;33:40–2.
12. Saxena S, Kumar D, Srivastava P, et al. Low levels of platelet glutathione in Eales' disease. Med Sci Res. 1999;42:125–6.
13. Srivastava P, Saxena S, Khanna VK, et al. Raised platelet thiobarbituric acid reacting substances in proliferative Eales disease. Indian J Ophthalmol. 2000;48:307–10.
14. Saxena S, Khanna VK, Kumar D, et al. Impaired antioxidant defense mechanism in centralEales' disease. Ann Ophthalmol. 2004;36:29–31.
15. Bhooma V, Sulochana KN, Biswas J, Ramakrishnan S. Eales' disease: accumulation of reactive oxygen intermediates and lipid peroxides and decrease of antioxidants causing inflammation, neovascularization and retinal damage. Curr Eye Res. 1997;16:91–5.
16. Sulochana KN, Biswas J, Ramakrishnan S. Eales' disease: increased oxidation and peroxidation products of membrane constituents chiefly lipids and antioxidant enzymes and reduced glutathione in vitreous. Curr Eye Res. 1999;19:254–9.
17. Swamy-Mruthinti S, Miriam KC, Kumar SK, et al. Immunolocalization and quantification of advanced glycation end products in retinal neovascular membranes and serum: a possible role in ocular neovascularization. Curr Eye Res. 2002;25:139–45.
18. Saxena S, Srivastava P, Kumar D, et al. Decreased platelet membrane fluidity in retinal periphlebitis in Eales' disease. Ocul Immunol Inflamm. 2006;14:113–6.
19. Saxena S, Pant AB, Khanna VK, et al. Interleukin-1 and tumor necrosis factor- alpha: novel targets for immunotherapy in Eales' disease. Ocul Immunol Inflamm. 2009;17:201–6.
20. Saxena S, Pant AB, Khanna VK, et al. Tumor necrosis factor-α-mediated severity of idiopathic retinal periphlebitis in young adults (Eales' disease): implication for anti-TNF-α therapy. J Ocul Biol Dis Inform. 2010;3:35–8.
21. Saxena S, Khanna VK, Pant AB, et al. Elevated tumor necrosis factor-α in serum is associated with increased retinal ischemia in proliferative Eales'disease. Pathobiology. 78:261–5.
22. Perentes Y, Chan CC, Bovey E, et al. Massive vascular endothelium growth factor (VEGF) expression in Eales' disease. Klin Monatsbl Augenheilkd. 2002;219:311–4.
23. Saxena S, Kumar D. A new staging system of idiopathic retinal periphlebitis. Eur J Ophthalmol. 2004;14:236–9.
24. Saxena S, Kumar D. Macular involvement in Eales' disease. Ann Ophthalmol. 2000;32:98–100.
25. Saxena S, Kumar D, Maitreya A, et al. Retinal neovascularization in Eales' disease. Ann Ophthalmol. 2003;35:25–7.
26. Saxena S, Kumar D. Topographic distribution of retinal neovascularisation in Eales' disease. Ann Opthamol. 2005;37:273–5.
27. Saxena S, Kumar D, Kapoor S. The efficacy of oral methotrexate pulsed therapy in Eales' disease. Ann Ophthalmol. 2000;32:60–2.

28. Bali T, Saxena S, Kumar D, Nath R. Response time and efficacy of oral methotrexate pulsed therapy in idiopathic retinal periphlebitis. Eur J Ophthalmol. 2005;15:374–8.
29. Biswas J, Sharma T, Gopal L, et al. Eales disease—an update. Surv Ophthalmol. 2002;47:197–214.
30. El-Asrar AM, Al-Kharashi SA. Full panretinal photocoagulation and early vitrectomy improve prognosis of retinal vasculitis associated with tuberculoprotein hypersensitivity (Eales' disease). Br J Opthalmol. 2002;86:1248–51.
31. Kumar A, Tiwari HK, Singh RP, et al. Comparative evaluation of early vs deferred vitrectomy in Eales' disease. Acta Ophthalmol Scand. 2000;78:77–8.
32. Shanmugam MP, Badrinath SS, Gopal L, et al. Long term visual results of vitrectomy for Eales disease complications. Int Ophthalmol. 1998;22:61–4.
33. Atmaca LS, Nagpal PN. Eales' disease: medical, laser, and surgical treatments. Ophthalmol Clin N Am. 1998;11:619–6.
34. Majji AB, Vemuganti GK, Shah VA, et al. A comparative study of epiretinal membranes associated with Eales' disease: a clinicopathologic evaluation. Eye. 2006;20:46–54.
35. Smiddy WE, Isernhagen RD, Michels RG, et al. Vitrectomy for nondiabetic vitreous hemorrhage: retinal and choroidal vascular disorders. Retina. 1988;8:88–95.
36. Treister G, Machemer R. Results of vitrectomy for rare proliferative and hemorrhagic disease. Am J Ophthalmol. 1977;84:394–412.
37. Mason JO III, Colagross CT, Haleman T, et al. Visual outcome and risk factors for light perception and no light perception vision after vitrectomy for diabetic retinopathy. Am J Ophthalmol. 2005;140:231–5.
38. Atmaca LS, Batioglu F, Sonmez PA. A long-term follow-up of Eales' disease. Ocul Immunol Inflam. 2002;10:213–21.
39. Dehghan MH, Ahmadieh H, Soheilian M. Therapeutic effects of laser photocoagulation and/or vitrectomy in Eales' disease. Eur J Ophthalmol. 2005;15:379–83.
40. Badrinath SS, Gopal L, Sharma T, et al. Vitreoschisis in Eales' disease: pathogenic role and significance in surgery. Retina. 1999;19:51–4.
41. Küçüerdönez C, Akova YA, Yilmaz G. Intravitreal injection of bevacizumab in Eales disease. Ocul Immunol Inflamm. 2008;16:63–5.
42. Patwardhan SD, Azad R, Shah BM, Sharma Y. Role of intravitreal bevacizumab in Eales disease with dense vitreous hemorrhage: a prospective randomized control study. Retina. 2011;31:866–70.
43. Shukla D, Kanungo S, Prasad NM, Kim R. Surgical outcomes for vitrectomy in Eales' disease. Eye. 2008;22:900–4.
44. Hui Y, Wang L, Cao X. Vitrectomy for complicated Eales disease. Yan Ke Xue Bao. 1997;13:25–8.

Management of Coats' Disease

21

Ramesh Venkatesh, Bharathi Bavaharan, K. Bhujang Shetty, and Naresh Kumar Yadav

21.1 Introduction

Coats' disease was first described in 1908 by George Coats as a retinal vascular disorder characterized by the presence of abnormal retinal telangiectasias along with massive exudation and fluid within and/or underneath the retina [1]. The condition occurs commonly unilaterally in young males, usually within the first decade of life, can be congenital with no familial predilection, and is not associated with systemic diseases [2]. In childhood, the disease presents with decreased vision, leukocoria, or strabismus. The spectrum of clinical findings in Coats' disease is broad, ranging from asymptomatic perifoveal telangiectasias, such as that seen in type 1 idiopathic macular telangiectasia [2–5], to exudation in mid-peripheral/peripherally to total exudative retinal detachment with poor visual prognosis [2, 6–8] and may progress to neovascular glaucoma with eventual painful blind eye [2, 7]. In adults, the clinical symptoms may either be identical to that seen in children, or a milder variant of the disease with predominantly macular findings may be seen [9]. On the basis of findings of enucleated specimens, Coats' early description showed many characteristic features: subretinal exudation, mononuclear cellular infiltrate, and prominent cholesterol crystals [1, 10]. Histologically, Coats' disease frequently displays foam or "ghost cells" (histiocytes) in the inner retinal layers and glial proliferation [11, 12]. Although considerable progress has been made in understanding patient characteristics and treatment, the true underlying mechanism of Coats' disease remains unclear.

21.2 Classification of Coats' Disease

During its early description, Coats classified the disease into three groups based on clinical findings: Group I with massive subretinal exudate alone, group II with massive subretinal exudate, intra- and subretinal hemorrhage, and retinal vascular dilatations, and group III included eyes with subretinal exudate and retinal arteriovenous malformations. Later, Von Hippel identified group III as a separate entity, angiomatosis retinae [13, 14], which led to the exclusion of this group from the spectrum of Coats' disease. In 1912, Theodor Leber described a disorder similar to Coats' disease, but without massive subretinal exudate, hemorrhage, and serous retinal detachment. This became known as Leber multiple miliary aneurysms, and Leber concluded that this entity was probably an earlier

R. Venkatesh (✉) · B. Bavaharan · K. B. Shetty
N. K. Yadav
Narayana Nethralaya, Bengaluru, India
e-mail: chairman@narayananethralaya.com

A. Jain et al. (eds.), *Cutting-edge Vitreoretinal Surgery*,
https://doi.org/10.1007/978-981-33-4168-5_21

or less severe form of the disease previously described by Coats [15, 16]. In 2000, based on the methods and management of a large series of patients with Coats' disease, Shields et al. [2] proposed a new practical classification system. One-hundred and fifty consecutive patients with Coats' disease were retrospectively reviewed. In 117 patients (124 eyes) with a mean follow-up of 55 months, primary management was observation in 22 eyes (18%), cryotherapy in 52 (42%), laser photocoagulation in 16 (13%), various methods of retinal detachment surgery in 20 (17%), and enucleation in 14 (11%). Anatomic improvement or stability was achieved in 76% of eyes, and final visual acuity was 20/50 or better in 17 eyes (14%), 20/60 to 20/100 in eight (6%), 20/200 to finger counting in 30 (24%), and hand motion to no light perception in 49 (40%) Enucleation was ultimately necessary in 20 eyes (16%). Coats' disease was classified into stage 1, telangiectasia only; stage 2, telangiectasia and exudation (2A, extrafoveal exudation; 2B, foveal exudation); stage 3, exudative retinal detachment (3A, subtotal; 3B, total); stage 4, total detachment and secondary glaucoma; and stage 5, advanced end-stage disease (Table 21.1). Poor visual outcome (20/200 or worse) was found in 0% of eyes with stage 1, 53% with stage 2, 74% with stage 3, and 100% of stages 4 and 5 Coats' disease. Enucleation was ultimately necessary in 0% of stages 1 and 2, 7% of stage 3, 78% of stage 4, and 0% of stage 5 disease.

Table 21.1 Shields' staging of Coats' disease

Stage	Clinical findings
I	Retinal telangiectasia alone
II	Telangiectasia and exudation IIA: Extrafoveal location IIB: Foveal location
III	Exudative retinal detachment IIIA: Subtotal detachment IIIA1: Extrafoveal detachment IIIA2: Foveal detachment IIIB: Total retinal detachment
IV	Total retinal detachment and glaucoma
V	Advanced end-stage disease

Table 21.2 Differential diagnosis of Coats' disease

(A) Tumors	(1) Retinoblastoma (2) Hamartomas and vasoproliferative tumors
(B) Inherited congenital and vitreoretinal disorders	(1) Retinitis pigmentosa (2) Norrie' disease (3) Familial exudative vitreoretinopathy (4) Persistent fetal vasculature
(C) Idiopathic retinal vascular diseases and inflammation	(1) Uveitis and retinal vasculitis (2) Macular telangiectasias type 1
(D) Other retinal vascular diseases	(1) Diabetic retinopathy (2) Hypertensive retinopathy

21.3 Differential Diagnosis of Coats' Disease

The more common differential diagnosis of Coats' disease in adults and children are mentioned in Table 21.2. Coats' disease is seen usually in children before the first decade of life. In such cases, retinoblastoma needs to be ruled out as it is a life-threatening condition. Identification of calcification on ultrasonography or CT helps to rule out the diagnosis of Coats' disease. Other retinal vascular and inflammatory conditions routinely confused with Coats' disease include MacTel Type 1, retinal vasculitis, IRVAN syndrome, diabetic and hypertensive retinopathy.

21.4 Investigations

The role and findings of various investigative modalities in Coats' disease are described in Table 21.3. Posterior segment imaging in Coats' disease is done with the intention of diagnosing the condition, planning the management, and differentiating cases of advanced Coats' disease from malignant lesions producing a similar clinical picture. Ocular B-scan ultrasonography is useful, especially in clinical situations where the posterior segment examination is limited by media opacity or poor patient cooperation. Ultrasonography can

Table 21.3 Imaging findings in Coats' disease

(A) Ultrasonography	– To assess the disease extent – To identify choroidal mass in advanced disease – To rule out calcification and potential malignancy	– Relatively immobile, serous retinal detachment contiguous with the optic nerve head – Hyperreflective masses of exudate, or clear subretinal space without significant choroidal thickening – Vitreoretinal traction – Absence of calcification
(B) Angiography	– For early and peripheral detection of vascular abnormalities	– Areas of nonperfusion – Telangiectatic capillaries most prominent in the temporal macula, and "light bulb" aneurysms – Vascular leakage, tortuosity, and blockage from overlying exudate
(C) Optical coherence tomography (OCT)	– To identify subtle macular edema or cystic changes – To monitor response to treatment	– Identification of SRF, exudate, and hemorrhage – Assessment of the integrity of specific retinal layers
(D) Computerized tomography	– To differentiate cases of advanced Coats' disease from malignant lesions producing a similar clinical picture	– Demonstrates calcifications that are common in retinoblastoma but not in Coats – Vascularity – Presence of subretinal lesions, and extraocular orbital or intracranial lesions such as metastases from an underlying malignancy – Globe volumes may be significantly lower than for normal eyes or retinoblastoma
(E) Magnetic resonance imaging (MRI)	– To differentiate cases of advanced Coats' disease from malignant lesions producing a similar clinical picture	– Hyperintense T1- and T2-weighted signal converging on the optic nerve head corresponding to an exudative retinal detachment – In retinoblastoma, the lesion is relatively hypointense on T2-weighted images – Mass-like enhancement noted in RB after contrast administration

confirm the disease extent and absence of a choroidal mass lesion in Coats' disease and helps to rule out retinoblastoma. Fluorescein angiography facilitates early or peripheral detection of vascular abnormalities in stage 1 disease (Fig. 21.1). Optical coherence tomography (OCT) is useful in identifying subtle macular edema or cystic changes and to monitor response to treatment. OCT's role in Coats' disease parallels those for other retinal disorders in the era of anti-VEGF therapy. Radiologic imaging of the globe and orbit may be obtained with computed tomography (CT) and magnetic resonance imaging (MRI). CT and MRI are particularly useful in identifying malignant cases and to differentiate cases of advanced Coats' disease, producing a similar clinical picture.

21.5 Management

The existing treatment modalities for Coats' disease include nonsurgical options, surgical options, or a combination of both. Nonsurgical options include ablative therapy with laser, cryotherapy, and intravitreal anti-vascular endothelial growth factor (VEGF) therapy while surgical options include external subretinal (SRF) drainage with or without scleral buckling and vitrectomy. This can be combined either with laser therapy, cryotherapy, or anti-VEGF therapy. The choice of treatment to be performed and decisions are usually made based by the retinal specialists depending on their preferences, stage, and severity of the disease.

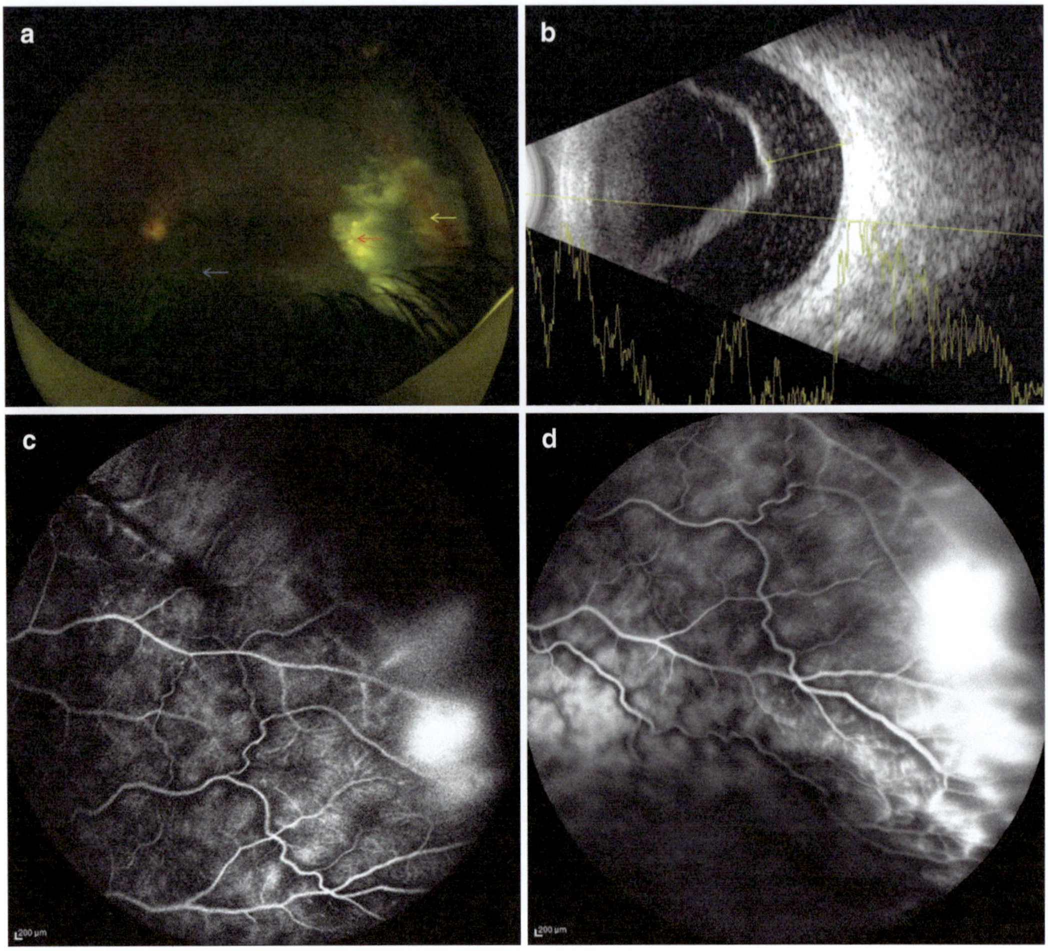

Fig. 21.1 A 4-year-old boy with Coats' Disease (Stage 3A2). (**a**) Fundus photo showing exudative retinal detachment (blue arrow), extensive subretinal exudation (red arrow), and telangiectatic vessels (yellow arrow) in the temporal periphery. (**b**) Ultrasound B-scan showing retinal detachment with plenty of subretinal dot echoes suggestive of subretinal exudates. (**c**) and (**d**) Early and late stages of fluorescein angiogram showing increasing leakage and characteristic "light bulb appearance" suggestive of Coats' disease

21.5.1 Ablative Therapy

21.5.1.1 Laser Photocoagulation

Laser therapy for Coats' disease has been the standard of care for treatment since the 1960s when Meyer-Schwickerath et al. [17] had described the procedure. The basic aim of laser therapy is to cause the obliteration of abnormal and aneurysmal retinal vessels by the heat produced by the monochromatic, coherent light. Fluorescein angiography is a useful guide in identifying and treating all the abnormal leaking vessels. The absorptive property of the abnormal retinal vessels to 532 nm (green) [18] or 577 nm (yellow) [19] laser light with a relatively longer duration is adequate for vascular absorption of laser energy, and to produce direct photocoagulation of vascular abnormalities even in the presence of SRF. Infrared light laser therapy seems to be ineffective due to poor absorption of the laser energy by the intravascular anomalies. However, Namba et al. [20] showed complete resolution of SRF in a 15-year-old boy with photodynamic therapy when the aneurysms and telangiectasias are located closer to the posterior pole. Following the reattachment of the retina, laser therapy is required to the areas of capillary nonperfusion which acts as a source of VEGF. The disadvantages with therapy include the need for multiple sessions and ineffective treatment in the presence of vascular anomalies in more than two quadrants and the presence of SRF [2, 18]. Complications include an increase in exudation, inflammation, choroidal detachment, ERM formation, and hemorrhage. An interval of 4–6 weeks is required to assess the therapeutic effect of laser therapy.

21.5.1.2 Cryotherapy

Triple freeze–thaw cryotherapy under indirect ophthalmoscopy has been advocated when the retinal telangiectasias are located far in the periphery and massive SRF is present preventing adequate treatment with laser [7]. Similar to laser treatment, an interval of 4–6 weeks is required to gauge the treatment effect and decide on retreatment if needed. Cryotherapy induces more inflammation than laser therapy and can cause epiretinal membrane formation and retinal traction [21, 22]. Therefore, we prefer to avoid cryotherapy in Coats' disease, because adequate ablation of retinal telangiectasias can be achieved with laser photocoagulation, even in the setting of SRF, as described. Even then, cryotherapy is a known effective solution to achieve resolution of exudates, telangiectasias, and vascular ablation in Coats' retinopathy.

21.5.2 Intravitreal Pharmacotherapy

21.5.2.1 Anti-VEGF Therapy

Increased levels of VEGF have been identified in the vitreous and SRF obtained during the external drainage procedure [23, 24]. VEGF causes increased vascular permeability from the retinal vessels leading to exudation and edema into the adjacent tissues. VEGF levels are also elevated secondary to retinal ischemia due to abnormal vasculature. Therefore, anti-VEGF agents have been tried either in monotherapy or in combination with intraocular steroids or ablation to improve the disease conditions in Coats' disease. Recently, newer VEGF antagonists like conbercept or ranibizumab have been used successfully in the treatment of Coats' disease [25]. A possible limiting factor for anti-VEGF therapy use is that it may induce vitreoretinal fibrosis leading to tractional retinal detachment [26, 27]. However, it is not clear if such findings are solely due to anti-VEGF therapy because similar phenomena are also seen after ablation therapy alone. There is overwhelming evidence available in literature supporting the use of anti-VEGF therapy for Coats' disease with retinal edema or exudate involving the macula or when adequate ablative therapy cannot be used.

21.5.2.2 Intravitreal Steroids

Intravitreal steroids are usually used as adjuvants to laser or cryopexy. Intravitreal triamcinolone acetonide (IVTA) is effective in reducing macular edema and subretinal exudation [28, 29]. Othman and colleagues used 4 mg of IVTA with ablative therapy in 15 eyes. All patients experienced an improvement in visual acuity. Cataract progression requiring cataract surgery was seen in 40% of the eyes, and one patient required intraocular pressure-lowering drops. In recent times, intravitreal dexamethasone implant (Ozurdex) has been used in the resolution of macular edema, hard exudates, and SRF in Coats' disease [30, 31].

21.5.3 Surgery

The SRF in Coats' disease contains high concentrations of VEGF which the VEGF antagonists are not able to reach the subretinal space due to its high molecular weight. Also, the presence of large cholesterol clumps in the subretinal space and extensive exudative retinal detachment prevent the adequate cryo or laser uptake of the telangiectatic vessels and are unable to cause the resolution of the SRF.

Hence, surgery for Coats' disease is usually reserved for: (1) severe cases (stage 4 and 5); (2) refractory cases of Coats' disease with no improvement (i.e., retinal reattachment) following ablation or anti-VEGF therapy; (3) secondary glaucoma due to the forward push of the iris–lens diaphragm by the extensive exudative retinal detachment; (4) in cases where immediate reattachment of the retina is required to facilitate treatment with laser or cryotherapy; and (5) in cases with epiretinal membrane, proliferative vitreoretinopathy and tractional retinal detachment.

Surgical techniques include external drainage of SRF or vitrectomy with internal drainage with endotamponade.

21.5.3.1 External Drainage

The most preferred surgical technique for Coats' disease is the external drainage of SRF in the previous several decades [2, 23, 32–35]. In this technique, a full-thickness scleral cut-down is made in the quadrant with maximum SRF and choroidal puncture is done with either needle or laser probe. The SRF gets drained through the choroidal opening (Fig. 21.2). Sometimes, the choroidal opening may get blocked by large choroidal crystals present in the subretinal space preventing the drainage of SRF. To normalize intraocular pressure, BSS Plus may be injected either into the anterior chamber or into the vitreous space through the pars plana. Injection into the anterior chamber is safer because it has no possibility of retinal damage.

21.5.3.2 Vitrectomy

The vitreous in eyes with Coats' disease contain high concentrations of VEGF. Vitrectomy is beneficial in reducing the VEGF load; however, this could be achieved with anti-VEGF injections as well [23, 24]. Vitrectomy is indicated in eyes with the presence of epiretinal membrane or traction over the retina. Disadvantages of vitrectomy include technical difficulty and a higher risk of complications. The most common difficulty encountered by surgeons is the visualization of the infusion cannula tip in the vitreous space due to the bullous exudative retinal detachment. In such a scenario, a combined approach of initial external drainage creating sufficient space for the placement of infusion cannula followed by vitrectomy can be considered. The most serious complication is probably the creation of an iatrogenic retinal break. If such a break occurs in an eye with minimal disease with surrounding exudate, the retinal break can be sealed and the retina reattached without much difficulty. However, if it is created on a retina with large amounts of surrounding exudates in an eye with a high disease burden, retinal reattachment can be very challenging. This is because laser burn cannot be created on a retina with underlying exudate, high risk of developing proliferative vitreoretinopathy in an eye with high concentrations of VEGF, and higher chances of recurrence of exudative/rhegmatogenous retinal detachment. In eyes with peripheral retinal traction, scleral buckling can be considered as a viable treatment option along with anti-VEGF therapy or ablation to avoid the risks of vitrectomy [41].

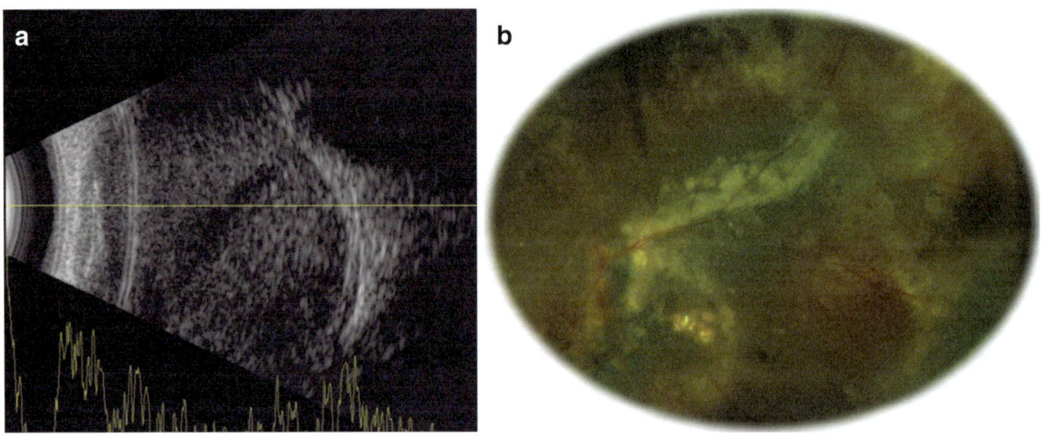

Fig. 21.2 A 3-year-old boy diagnosed with Coats' disease (Stage IV). (**a**) Ultrasound showing total retinal detachment with plenty of subretinal echoes suggestive of subretinal exudation. The child underwent external drainage of SRF with cryotherapy to the telangiectatic vessels. (**b**) Postoperatively, the retina was reattached with residual exudation at the posterior pole and retinal periphery

After retinal reattachment, laser or cryotherapy is done to the retinal telangiectasias and aneurysms depending upon the surgeons' preferences. Surgical results with or without vitrectomy are relatively successful, with success rates ranging from 50% to 100% [33–40].

21.6 Clinical Approach to Coats' Disease management

A step-wise approach in the treatment of Coats' disease is depicted in Table 21.4.

21.7 Prognosis

Prognosis in Coats' disease depends upon the stage of the disease at presentation, involvement of macula, and timing of treatment. Early stages of the disease such as stages I, II, and III have a favorable visual outcome [2]. However, the involvement of macula due to deposition of the intra- and subretinal hard exudates/cholesterol deposits can lead to a permanent decrease in visual acuity. Development of retinal neovascularisation, iris neovascularization, and neovascular glaucoma are associated with poor visual prognosis. Compromise of the optic nerve head function due to a rise in the intraocular pressure following the forward displacement of iris–lens diaphragm and neovascularization can lead to a permanent decrease in the visual acuity.

Table 21.4 Step-wise approach in the treatment of Coats' disease

Disease stage	Treatment
Stage I	(a) Observation
	(b) Laser photocoagulation
Stage II	(a) Anti-VEGF therapy
	(b) Laser photocoagulation
	(c) Cryotherapy
Stage III a	(a) Anti-VEGF therapy
	(b) Laser photocoagulation
	(c) Cryotherapy
Stage III b	Without high IOP
	(a) Anti-VEGF therapy
	(b) Laser photocoagulation
	(c) Cryotherapy
	With high IOP
	(a) Surgery
Stage IV	With peripheral traction
	(a) External drainage
	(b) Scleral buckling
	(c) Vitrectomy
	With posterior pole traction
	(a) Vitrectomy
Stage V	Asymptomatic
	(a) Observation
	Painful blind eye
	(a) Enucleation

21.8 Conclusion

In spite of significant progress being made in understanding the pathogenesis of Coats' disease and its clinical spectrum, the etiology still remains unclear. With the development of VEGF antagonists, retinal specialists have found a new and effective adjunct in the treatment of Coats' disease. For milder forms of the disease, ablation and/or anti-VEGF therapy seems to be effective while in severe forms of the disease, surgery seems to be preferred. Overall, surgery needs to be considered as a last resort, especially in eyes with severe disease that have a higher risk of developing proliferative vitreoretinopathy.

References

1. Coats G. Forms of retinal diseases with massive exudation. R Lond Ophthalmol Hosp Rep. 1908;17:440–525.
2. Shields JA, Shields CL, Honavar SG, Demirci H, Cater J. Classification and management of Coats disease: the 2000 proctor lecture. Am J Ophthalmol. 2001;131:572–83.
3. Campbell FP. Coats' disease and congenital vascular retinopathy. Trans Am Ophthalmol Soc. 1976;74:365–424.
4. Gass JD, Oyakawa RT. Idiopathic juxtafoveolar retinal telangiectasis. Arch Ophthalmol. 1982;100:769–80.
5. Yannuzzi LA, Bardal AM, Freund KB, Chen KJ, Eandi CM, Blodi B. Idiopathic macular telangiectasia. Arch Ophthalmol. 2006;124:450–60.
6. Budning AS, Heon E, Gallie BL. Visual prognosis of Coats' disease. J AAPOS. 1998;2:356–9.
7. Haik BG. Advanced Coats' disease. Trans Am Ophthalmol Soc. 1991;89:371–476.

8. Mrejen S, Metge F, Denion E, Dureau P, Edelson C, Caputo G. Management of retinal detachment in Coats disease. Study of 15 cases. Retina. 2008;28:S26–32.
9. Beselga D, Campos A, Mendes S, Carvalheira F, Castro M, Castanheira D. Refractory Coats' disease of adult onset. Case Report Ophthalmol. 2012;3:118–22.
10. Duke JR. The role of cholesterol in the pathogenesis of Coats' disease. Trans Am Ophthalmol Soc. 1963;61:492–544.
11. Takei Y. Origin of ghost cell in Coats' disease. Investig Ophthalmol. 1976;15:677–81.
12. Tripathi R, Ashton N. Electron microscopical study of Coat's disease. Br J Ophthalmol. 1971;55:289–301.
13. Lindau A. Zur frage der angiomatosis retinae und ihrer hirnkomplikationen. Acta Ophthalmol. 1927;4:193.
14. Von Hippel E. Ueber eine seltene erkrankung der netzhaut. Arch f Augenh. 1904;59:83.
15. Leber T. Die aneurysmen der zentralarterie und ihrer verzweigungen. Retinaldegeneration bei multiplen miliaraneurysmen. In: Saemisch T, editor. Handbuch der Gesamten Augenheilkunde. 2nd ed. Leipzig: Wilhelm Engelmann; 1915. p. 20–35.
16. Leber T. Verber ein durch yorkommen miltipler miliaraneurisi men characterisierte form von retinaldegeneration. Graefes Arch Clin Exp Ophthalmol. 1912;81:1–14.
17. Pesch KJ, Meyer-Schwickerath G. Light coagulation in morbus Coats and Leber's retinitis. Klin Monatsbl Augenheilkd. 1967;151:846–53.
18. Nucci P, Bandello F, Serafino M, et al. Selective photocoagulation in coats' disease: ten-year follow-up. Eur J Ophthalmol. 2002;12:501–5.
19. Levinson JD, Hubbard GB 3rd. 577-nm yellow laser photocoagulation for coats disease. Retina 2016 Jul;36(7):1388–1394.
20. Namba M, Shiode Y, Morizane Y, Kimura S, Hosokawa M, Doi S, et al. Successful resolution of coats disease by photodynamic therapy: a case report. BMC Ophthalmol. 2018;18(1):264.
21. Glaser BM, Vidaurri-Leal J, Michels RG, Campochiaro PA. Cryotherapy during surgery for giant retinal tears and intravitreal dispersion of viable retinal pigment epithelial cells. Ophthalmology. 1993;100:466–70.
22. Yadav NK, Vasudha K, Gupta K, Shetty KB. Vitrectomy for epiretinal membrane secondary to treatment for juvenile Coats' disease. Eye. 2013;27(2):278–80.
23. He YG, Wang H, Zhao B, Lee J, Bahl D, McCluskey J. Elevated vascular endothelial growth factor level in coats' disease and possible therapeutic role of bevacizumab. Graefes Arch Clin Exp Ophthalmol. 2010;248:1519–21.
24. Sun Y, Jain A, Moshfeghi DM. Elevated vascular endothelial growth factor levels in coats disease: rapid response to pegaptanib sodium. Graefes Arch Clin Exp Ophthalmol. 2007;245:1387–8.
25. Zhang L, Ke Y, Wang W, Shi X, Hei K, Li X. The efficacy of conbercept or ranibizumab intravitreal injection combined with laser therapy for Coats' disease. Graefes Arch Clin Exp Ophthalmol. 2018;256(7):1339–46. https://doi.org/10.1007/s00417-018-3949-1.
26. Ramasubramanian A, Shields CL. Bevacizumab for Coats' disease with exudative retinal detachment and risk of vitreoretinal traction. Br J Ophthalmol. 2012;96:356–9.
27. Bhat V, D'Souza P, Shah PK, et al. Risk of tractional retinal detachment following intravitreal bevacizumab along with SRF drainage and cryotherapy for stage 3B Coats' disease. Middle East Afr J Ophthalmol. 2016;23:208–11.
28. Othman IS, Moussa M, Bouhaimed M. Management of lipid exudates in Coats disease by adjuvant intravitreal triamcinolone: effects and complications. Br J Ophthalmol. 2010;94:606–10.
29. Jarin RR, Teoh SC, Lim TH. Resolution of severe macular oedema in adult Coat's syndrome with high-dose IVTA. Eye. 2006:20, 163–125.
30. Kumar K, Raj P, Chandnani N, Agarwal A. Intravitreal dexamethasone implant with retinal photocoagulation for adult-onset Coats' disease. Int Ophthalmol. 2018;39(2):465–70. https://doi.org/10.1007/s10792-018-0827-0.
31. Saatci AO, Doruk HC, Yaman A. Intravitreal dexamethasone implant (Ozurdex) in coats' disease. Case Rep Ophthalmol. 2013;4(3):122–8.
32. Ridley ME, Shields JA, Brown GC, Tasman W. Coats' disease. Evaluation of management. Ophthalmology. 1982;89:1381–7.
33. Adam RS, Kertes PJ, Lam WC. Observations on the management of Coats' disease: less is more. Br J Ophthalmol. 2007;91:303–6.
34. Stanga PE, Jaberansari H, Bindra MS, Gil-Martinez M, Biswas S. Transscleral drainage of SRF, anti-vascular endothelial growth factor, and wide field-imaging-guided laser in Coats exudative retinal detachment. Retina. 2016;36:156–62.
35. Peng J, Zhang Q, Jin H, Fei P, Zhao P. A modified technique for the transconjunctival and sutureless external drainage of SRF in bullous exudative retinal detachment using a 24-G i.v. catheter. Ophthalmologica. 2017;238:179–85.
36. Cai X, Zhao P, Zhang Q, Jin H. Treatment of stage 3 Coats' disease by endolaser photocoagulation via a two-port pars plana nonvitrectomy approach. Graefes Arch Clin Exp Ophthalmol. 2015;253:999–1004.
37. Li AS, Capone A Jr, Trese MT, Sears JE, Kychenthal A, De la Huerta I, et al. Long-term outcomes of total exudative retinal detachments in stage 3B Coats disease. Ophthalmology. 2018;125(6):887–93.
38. Mrejen S, Metge F, Denion E, et al. Management of retinal detachment in Coats disease. Study of 15 cases. Retina. 2008;28(Suppl 3):S26–32.

39. Suesskind D, Altpeter E, Schrader M, et al. Pars plana vitrectomy for treatment of advanced Coats' disease--presentation of a modified surgical technique and long-term follow-up. Graefes Arch Clin Exp Ophthalmol. 2014;252:873–9.
40. Karacorlu M, Hocaoglu M, Sayman M, Arf S. Long-term anatomical and functional outcomes following vitrectomy for advanced Coats disease. Retina. 2017;37:1757–64.
41. Huang YC, Lai CC, Wu WC. Integrating scleral buckling, Transscleral drainage of SRF, Intravitreal anti-vascular endothelial growth factor, and laser photocoagulation in stage 3B Coats' Total retinal detachment. Ophthalmic Surg Lasers Imaging Retina. 2016;47(9):865–8.

Part VI

Macular Surgery

Surgical Techniques of Macular Hole Repair

22

Rene Alfredo Cano-Hidalgo
and Tatiana Urrea-Victoria

22.1 Introduction

A macular hole (MH) is a round full- or partial-thickness defect in the macular region, specifically in the foveal center [1, 2].

The majority occur as an age-related primary idiopathic condition with a female predominance in the seventh decade of life [3]. They are bilateral in 12–13% in 2 years after presentation in one eye [4].

Macular holes were first described in 1869 by Knapp in a traumatic case [1, 3], in a patient who had sustained a severe contusion and in whom an initial diagnosis of macular hemorrhage was made [5].

Later, Noyes in 1871 gave a detailed ophthalmoscopic description of a traumatic case, and in 1900 Ogilvie was the first to use the term "hole at the macula" [1].

The modern history of MH started in 1988 when Gass introduced the concept of tangential vitreous traction on the posterior pole in macular holes and proposed, on the basis of his biomicroscopic observations, a staging system ranging from impending to full-thickness MH [1, 5].

R. A. Cano-Hidalgo (✉) · T. Urrea-Victoria
Department of Retina and Vitreous, Institute of Ophthalmology Foundation Conde de Valenciana, National Autonomous University of Mexico, Mexico City, Mexico
e-mail: canoh@unam.mx

Kelly and Wendel performed the first successful surgery of MH [1], developing the concept of using vitrectomy and fluid–gas exchange to treat these patients [6].

22.2 Epidemiology

The prevalence of MH reported in the literature varies greatly [1]. Few population-based studies have reported on the prevalence of full-thickness macular holes (FTMH). The Beaver Dam Eye Study used fundus photography to evaluate fundus morphology in 4926 individuals aged 63–102 years [1, 7] found FTMHs to be prevalent in 0.3% of the population [7].

A follow-up to the Beaver Dam Eye Study found a 10-year incidence of MHs in 0.7% of the population [7].

The relatively frequent occurrence of MHs was confirmed by the Blue Mountains Eye Study in Australia with 0.2 per 1000 and 3.3 per 1000 in the Baltimore Eye Study [1, 7].

MHs affect women three times more often than men [7]. The data on the incidence of bilateral MH vary considerably from 5% to 16% [1]. Age 65 years or older and female gender are the only two relevant systemic risk factors yet identified [1].

A. Jain et al. (eds.), *Cutting-edge Vitreoretinal Surgery*,
https://doi.org/10.1007/978-981-33-4168-5_22

22.3 Pathogenesis

There are three basic historical theories regarding the etiology of MHs: Traumatic theory, cystoid degeneration theory, and vascular theory [3].

Lister in 1924 was the first of many to implicate anteroposterior vitreous forces in the pathogenesis of MHs [5]. Following this traumatic theory, the hole formation was explained by rupture of fovea from mechanical energy created by vitreous fluid waves [5]. Two main tractions were described: anteroposterior traction may be a result of dynamic tractional forces on an abnormally persistent vitreofoveal attachment following perifoveal vitreous separation that slowly tears the macula in a circumferential fashion [6, 8] and tangential traction may result from contraction of prefoveal vitreous cortex following invasion and proliferation of Muller cells [8].

Coats was among the first to recognize that macular cystoid degeneration was often not related to trauma [5], suggesting that cystoid degeneration could be involved in part of the physiopathogenesis of MH development.

It was also believed that aging and other changes of the retinal vasculature led to cystoid retinal degeneration and subsequent MH formation [5].

Later, Morgan and Schatz in 1986 proposed a mechanism of MH formation that they describe as involutional macular thinning, which incorporates vitreous, vascular, and cystic degeneration theories [5].

In recent decades the etiology of MH has been debated along two general lines: vitreomacular traction and some form of degenerative dissolution of inner retinal layers in the fovea [9, 10].

Even though in 1952 Grignolo provided histologic evidence of strong vitreomacular adherence to the fovea [1], the routine visualization of the vitreofoveal interface has been possible since the advent of ocular coherence tomography (OCT) allowing the differentiation of lamellar from pseudo- and FTMHs and permitting the vitreomacular traction syndrome diagnosis.

Recent innovations in macular imaging and surgery have provided relevant new information concerning the pathogenesis and treatment of idiopathic MH. New imaging data suggest that localized perifoveal vitreous detachment (an early stage of age-related posterior vitreous detachment, PDV) is the primary pathogenic event in idiopathic MH formation [11].

22.4 Grading

Gass proposed a system of MH staging, from impending to FTMH [1]. In this grading system, he described the evolution of the MH and defined the clinical appearance of the different stages of its development [7]. The process of MH formation was divided into four stages that are still used today [1].

Stage 1

The earliest stage, according to Gass, is an impending hole, characterized by a yellow spot (foveal intraretinal cyst) [4] [stage 1a] or a yellow ring (ring of cysts) [4] [stage 1b] in the fovea [7]. At this point, the patient may be asymptomatic or have mild blur or distortion [4].

Since the advent of OCT the diagnosis of stage 1 has been easier to identify, evidencing the hole like a cystic lesion in the inner retinal layers [7].

Stage 2

In stage 2 MH, there is a foveal full-thickness defect less than 400 μm in diameter; these holes can be round, ovoid, or slit-like in shape.

Stage 3

The fully developed, stage 3 MH appears as a round, full-thickness defect larger than 400 μm in diameter [7].

In the majority of patients, a small vitreous opacity, or operculum, can be seen suspended in front of the lesion (Fig. 22.1). In more chronic lesions yellow dots can be seen on the surface of the pigment epithelium at the bottom of the lesion [7].

Stage 4

A hole with a complete posterior vitreous detachment associated, frequently evidenced by a visible Weiss's ring [4, 7].

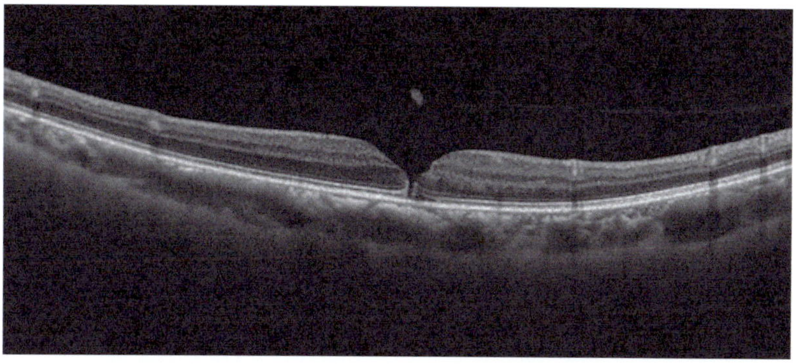

Fig. 22.1 Full-thickness macular hole with an operculum

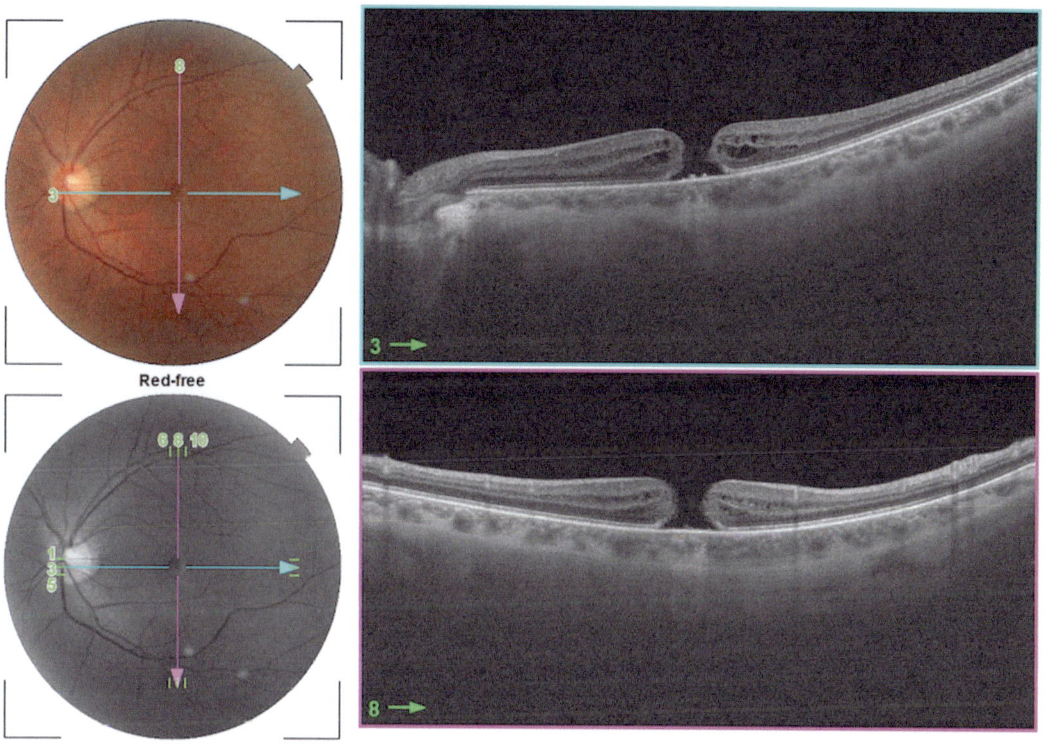

Fig. 22.2 Fundus photo and OCT of a full-thickness macular hole

22.5 Clinical Features

In the early stages, patients could present blurred vision, distortion or notices a small central gray patch without distortion of the image. Distortion becomes a feature as the fovea dehisces and the photoreceptors are moved outward onto the rim of the hole [4].

The receptors are on the perimeter of the hole and spread out by the dehiscence. The brain, therefore, receives fewer signals than it should in the center of the macula and interprets this as a falsely small image centrally. Eventually, the receptors at the edge of the hole will stop functioning (stages 3 and 4) and the patient will only perceive a central scotoma [4].

Biomicroscopically, a fully developed MH appears as a punched out, full-thickness defect in the fovea (Fig. 22.2) [7].

The phenomena of distortion and loss of vision are exploited in the Watzke–Allen test, described in 1969. This involves shining a thin line of light (usually vertically) via the slit lamp biomicroscope over the macular hole, while asking the patient to describe whether the line of light is straight or has a narrowing (waist) or gap (break) centrally [4]. The test is considered positive if the patient reports a gap in the slit. A positive Watzke–Allen test result represented an inclusion criterion in the Vitrectomy for Macular Hole Trial [7].

Most stage 1 and some stage 2 lesions are asymptomatic. In later stages, patients complain of metamorphopsia and loss of central vision [7].

22.6 OCT Classification of Macular Hole

OCT has been recognized as an extremely useful tool for making or confirming diagnoses of MH, as well as for defining the stage of the lesion and postoperative monitoring [7].

A new classification has been proposed based on both the MH diameter and the status of the vitreous attachment at the hole edge. It has indeed been shown that the hole size was correlated with the need for internal limiting membrane (ILM) peeling, face-down positioning, or the indications of enzymatic vitreolysis [1].

The aperture size is measured using the caliper function on OCT devices. The minimum hole width is measured at the narrowest hole point in the mid retina, using the OCT caliper function, as a line parallel to the retinal pigment epithelium (RPE) [1].

22.7 International Vitreomacular Traction Study Group Classification

FTMH is an anatomic defect in the fovea featuring interruption of all neural retinal layers from the ILM to the RPE [12]. FTMH was further classified based on the hole size, the presence or the absence of a vitreomacular traction (VMT), and the cause of the hole [1, 12].

The VMT was defined as present or absent [1]. The hole size (diameter) was defined as small, medium, or large [1]. Small holes have an aperture size of less than 250 μm. These holes usually represent less than 10% of operated MH [1, 12]. The cutoff for small FTMHs at 250 μm is derived from studies showing that these holes are associated with a small rate of spontaneous closure, have a very high closure rate with vitrectomy (approaching 100%) [12]. A medium hole is defined by an aperture size ranging between 250 and 400 μm [1, 12].

Studies exploring postsurgical FTMH closure rates by aperture size consistently show a very high anatomic closure rate (>90% in all recent series) with complete removal of residual hyaloid, with or without ILM peeling [12]. Pharmacologic therapy can be successful as well, but at a lower rate than for small macular holes [12].

Almost half of FTMHs are large (diameter > 400 μm) at the time of diagnosis [1, 12]. Vitrectomy with ILM peel is associated with high closure rates (90–95%), even for these large holes. Without an ILM peel, the vitrectomy success rate is closer to 75%. In the few eyes with large FTMH that have undergone pharmacologic vitreolysis, no anatomic success has been recorded [12].

This classification does not take into account the possible presence of an epiretinal membrane (ERM) around the hole, which is more frequent in large MH [1] and are found in approximately two-thirds of eyes with MHs [7].

FTMHs are categorized secondarily according to the absence or presence of vitreous attachment. Only MHs with concurrent VMT should be considered for pharmacologic vitreolysis [12].

FTMHs can also be subdivided into primary and secondary forms. Primary FTMH (formerly referred to as idiopathic) results from vitreous traction on the fovea from anomalous PVD. A secondary FTMH is caused directly by other pathologic features and does not have preexisting or concurrent VMT [12].

Abortive macular holes may result in lamellar holes, in which only the inner part of the fovea is torn away from the retina [7].

A special circumstance exists when an individual develops FTMH in one eye and OCT reveals VMA or VMT in the fellow eye. Studies show that these fellow eyes are at increased risk for the development of FTMH. In the past, the finding of VMA in a fellow eye has been referred to as a stage 0 macular hole, but the term *impending macular hole* should be used instead to describe a case in which FTMH is observed in one eye and VMT is observed on OCT in the fellow eye [12].

22.8 Natural History

Impending macular holes can resolve, remain stable, or progress to FTMH. If complete PVD develops, the fovea can return to normal, or a lamellar hole can develop if some part of the Müller cell cone is torn off the retinal surface [7].

For a patient with a newly diagnosed FTMH, an important consideration in deciding whether or not to proceed with surgery concerns the risk of developing a macular hole in the fellow eye. There are two important factors to consider when determining this risk. The first concerns the presence of a stage 1 MH in the fellow eye, which implies a high risk (40%) of FTMH formation in this eye within 1 year and the second concerns the state of the posterior vitreous. If the posterior vitreous is detached in the fellow eye, then this eye has a very low risk (<2%) of progression to an FTMH [7].

22.9 Management of Macular Hole

Previously, surgeons focused their attention on the MH only if retinal detachments were associated [5].

Vitrectomy with gas tamponade to achieve retinal reattachment in eyes with large retinal detachment and macular holes was reported in 1982 [5]. Since then, this procedure has become one of the most successful vitreoretinal surgeries [1].

The first article reporting on the results of vitrectomy for hole closure was published in 1991 [13], this first pilot study of idiopathic MH surgery was presented at the Annual Meeting of the American Academy of Ophthalmology where two important surgical techniques emerged from it: the identification and removal of the ILM and the identification and removal of the cortical vitreous [14].

Kelly and Wendel are to be credited for the introduction and developments of vitreous surgery for FTMH [10], they hypothesized that vision might stabilize or improve if it were possible to surgically relieve the tangential traction, reduce the cystic changes, and reattach the cuff of detached retina surrounding an MH using traditional vitrectomy techniques [5].

After the pilot surgical series published by Kelly and Wendel, which showed remarkable success in improving vision by sealing FTMHs, there was a quick acceptance of the technique reported by many vitreous surgeons and results have been duplicated by other investigators around the world. Since then, surgical techniques have been gradually improving along with the visual results [5]; the concept of core vitrectomy, the induction of PVD, the ILM and any ERM peeling off the macula, followed by fluid–gas or an exchange using an isoexpansive mixture of air and SF_6 or C_3F_8 gas tamponade, and face-down positioning for up to 14 days postoperatively have become standardized techniques [6, 11].

The surgical objectives are to relieve vitreomacular tractions, anteroposterior traction or tangential traction, and to provide retina tamponade [5, 15]. Likewise, surgical success should be defined as the clinical disappearance of the hole, reconstitution of the foveal anatomy on OCT, and marked improvement in vision (Fig. 22.3a, b) [6].

Freeman et al. have shown that the size of the MH is the only preoperative factor that has been proven to predict surgical closure rates; however, MH duration has an important influence on final visual outcomes [6, 16].

Surgical strategies for the repair of MHs are designed to relieve vitreofoveal traction and to promote flattening and reapposition of the MH edges [8, 17]. The removal of the attached cortical

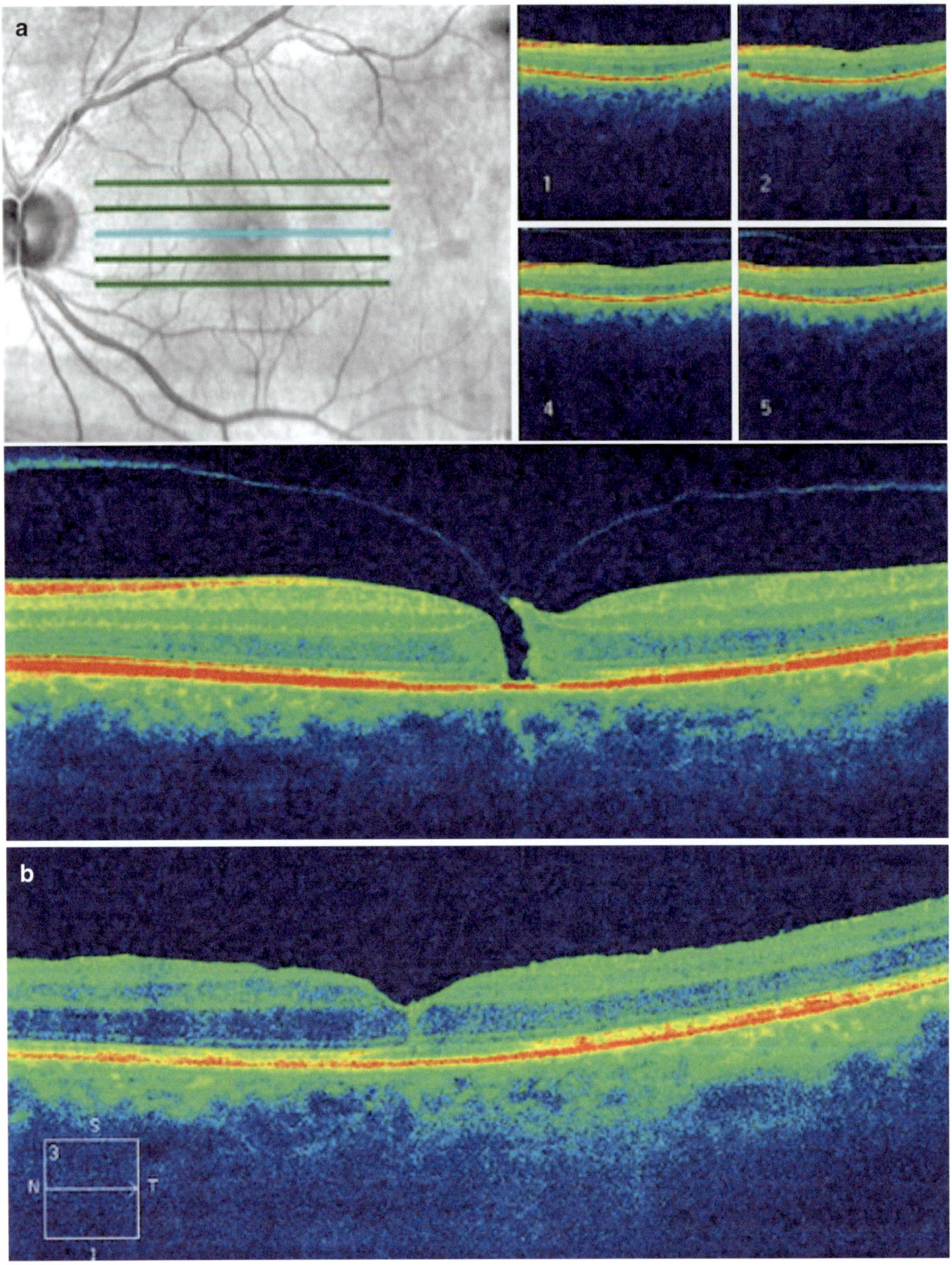

Fig. 22.3 (**a**, **b**) Pre- and postoperative OCT of vitreomacular traction and macular hole showing macular hole closure and complete resolution of the vitreomacular adhesion

vitreous had been previously described by numerous authors, including Han et al.; however, it was not until MH surgery that the technique became widely used [14].

The indications for surgery also depend on the stage of the MH, it is known that in the case of stage 1 holes should be managed conservatively while the outcomes are particularly favorable for stage 2 holes and holes of less than 6 months duration [8].

Two large randomized controlled trials have been done to compare the effects of surgery with the natural history of MHs. The Vitrectomy for Macular Hole Study (VMHS) was a multicenter, randomized clinical trial set up to evaluate the newly developed MH surgery [7]. The VMHS is still the only randomized clinical trial to have compared MH surgery with observation [7]. In the Moorfields Macular Hole Study (MMHS), the overall anatomical closure rate for stages 2, 3, and 4 macular holes was 81% at 24 months following surgery compared to 11% in the observation group, and surgery was associated with a significant reduction in MH dimensions [8].

In particular cases like traumatic MHs, where they can spontaneously close in the first 4–6 weeks, a period of observation should precede the determination of operability [6].

Visual acuity improvements are known to differ depending on the stage of MH, mean visual acuity has been reported to improve to 20/50 for stage 2 holes, 20/110 for stage 3 holes, and 20/145 for stage 4 holes [18].

An understanding of anatomical changes and the physiopathology occurring at the vitreomacular interface has led to the development of an adequate surgical approach [8].

22.9.1 Healing

Suggested mechanisms by which the edges of the orifice approximate include the formation of a fibrin membrane or plug and the resolution of intraretinal hydration by blocking the passage of vitreous fluid through the orifice [8].

22.9.2 Posterior Hyaloid Detachment

A group headed by Dr. Ron Michels introduced the concept of detaching the posterior vitreous cortex after completing core vitrectomy in the late 1980s, which is still considered a crucial step in MH with VMT [1].

Some of the tools used to separate the vitreous cortex from the retinal surface, included an aspirating cannula with a rigid or soft tip, a microvitreoretinal blade or an aspirating forceps, and the vitreous probe. The most effective way of lifting the vitreous cortex en bloc, appears to be direct aspiration of the vitreous fibers attached to the Weiss ring and gradually extending its detachment to the equator in all the quadrants of the fundus [1].

The 23- and even 25- or 27-G vitreous probes are very effective for firm aspiration and detachment of the posterior hyaloid (their aspirating port is narrower and closer to the tip of the probe). Before starting posterior hyaloid (PH) detachment, it is also possible to inject diluted triamcinolone or brilliant blue G in front of the posterior pole for clearer visualization of the vitreous cortex [1].

22.9.3 Extensive Vitrectomy

Extensive vitrectomy refers to the detachment of the PH up to the equator, followed by shaving of the vitreous base. There are several arguments that favor the most extensive vitrectomy possible since it allows more gas mixture to be injected into the eye, consequently prolonging the effect of the gas tamponade. Shaving the vitreous base, especially in the lower periphery, also reduces the risk of postoperative lower retinal breaks and detachment by preventing the gas bubble from exerting traction on the remaining vitreous fibers [1].

22.9.4 Epiretinal Membrane Peeling

ERMs are usually soft and friable around the hole and when present, they should be peeled off [1]. Since these ERMs adhere firmly to the thickness of the hole edge [1], removal of the cortical vitreous and the ERMs surrounding the hole allows tangential traction release. While the anteroposterior traction is relieved by the removal of vitreous and its attachments to the fovea [5, 15]. These ERM adhere firmly to the thickness of the hole edge [1].

22.9.5 Internal Limiting Membrane Peeling

The internal limiting membrane (ILM), dubbed membrana limitante by the Italian anatomist Filippo Pacini in 1845, represents the structural interface between the retina and the vitreous, which acts as a scaffold for cellular proliferation such as myofibroblasts, fibrocytes, and retinal pigment epithelium cells, and those glial cells might migrate onto the surface of the ILM generating a tangential contractile force [14].

ILM peeling as a method of improving the MH closure rate was first described by Eckardt et al. in 1997 [1]. The ILM received virtually no clinical attention until vitrectomy removal of ERM became routine in the 1980s [14]. Although there was a debate on ILM peeling in the past, ILM peeling with or without the aid of a vital dye has been established to improve surgical success rates [19], becoming one of the preferred steps in contemporary MH surgical technique [9].

Surgical removal of ILM is advocated to ensure thorough removal of any tangential tractional components including any residual cortical vitreous [8] and to guarantee successful removal of ERMs that are occasionally present [6].

ILM peeling increases retinal elasticity by over 50%, which enables lateral surface tension forces to close the hole as soon as the air–gas bubble makes contact with the hole. It is also likely that ILM peeling also initiates mechanical signaling to the astrocytes to heal the hole margins days after the hole is closed by lateral surface tension [6, 11].

Several meta-analyses have indicated that ILM peeling can significantly improve initial postoperative closure rate and visual recovery and reduce the chance of a second operation [2]. Current evidence suggests that ILM peeling can improve anatomical outcomes but the effect on visual function is less predictable; unsuccessful attempts to peel the ILM can be associated with poor visual outcome [8].

Mester and Kuhn reported a meta-analysis of 1654 eyes from published reports of idiopathic MHs from 1992 to 1999. They found 96% hole closure rates in eyes that had ILM peeling versus only 77% of eyes without ILM peeling [13, 14]. The study also showed an increased rate of visual acuity improvement from 55% to 81% in those eyes with ILM peeling [13].

Although Zhao Peng et al. informed that there is no difference between peeling and nonpeeling for stages 1 and 2 MHs according to studies analyzed, there is a significant difference for stages 3 and 4 between peeling and nonpeeling, regarding the closure rate [2, 18].

End-gripping forceps are used to pinch and tear a flap of ILM without touching the optic nerve fibers. The ILM is then peeled off in a circular movement, thus creating a "maculorrhexis." The use of a diamond-dusted scraper has also been proposed to initiate and complete ILM peeling, but this instrument could be more dangerous for the optic nerve fibers than a forceps [1].

Vitreoschisis, or splitting of the posterior hyaloid face, is a common occurrence during vitrectomy in diabetic eyes and may give the false impression of hyaloid separation when in reality vitreomacular adhesion persists. Therefore, removal of the ILM guarantees complete separation of the posterior hyaloid from the macular surface [14].

Kunho Bae et al. concluded that larger extent of ILM peeling during MH surgery is beneficial with respect to reduction of metamorphopsia, alleviating asymmetric elongation of foveal tissue [19].

Several studies using OCT have reported the dynamic sealing process after MH surgery [19]. OCT demonstrated restoration of near-normal or normal foveal anatomy in successfully operated cases [6]. Foveal tissue elongation and macular migration have been noted following ILM peeling after surgery for MH and diabetic macular edema. In addition, there is a significant correlation between these morphologic changes and visual function such as metamorphopsia [19].

However, visual acuity outcomes differ by the MH type, the postoperative visual outcomes for high myopic MH are limited compared with the idiopathic MH. For idiopathic MHs, Tewari et al. reported a final visual acuity of 20/50 following ILM peeling. Wuand Kung reported that the

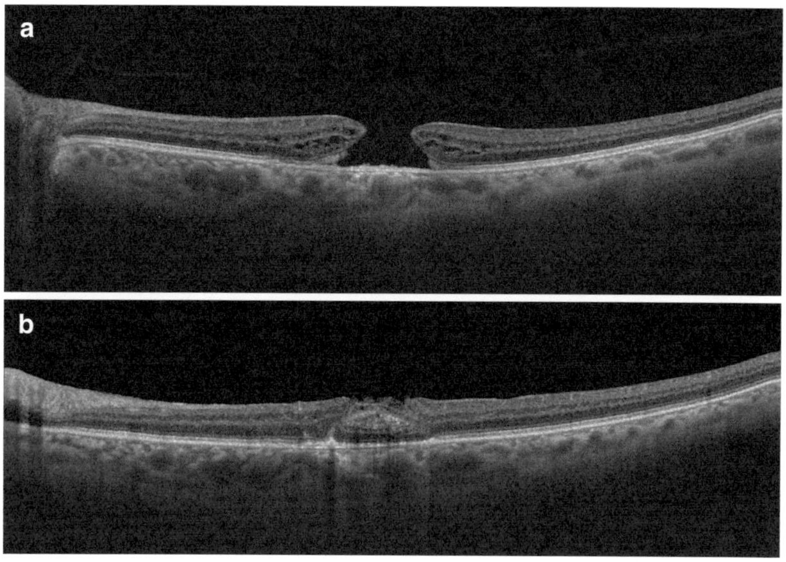

Fig. 22.4 (a, b) Preoperative and 8 weeks postoperative OCT images for large macular hole treated with autologous retinal graft. Courtesy of Dr. Antonio López Bolaños

mean logMAR visual acuity improved in a group with high myopia from 0.92 to 0.63, while a group without high myopia showed an improvement from 1.02 to 0.48. Thus, visual outcomes were less successful in highly myopic eyes [18]. Due to the relatively less favorable outcomes of ILM peeling techniques for myopic eyes and for large and refractory MHs, the inverted flap technique was proposed in 2010.

Michalewska et al. have proposed not to remove the dissected ILM from the eye but to cover the hole with an ILM flap, especially in myopic eyes and large or refractory MH [1]. In 2010, the authors reported an inverted ILM flap technique, which resulted in an improvement of the postoperative closure rates and visual functions for large MHs with a minimum diameter > 400 μm [18, 20].

After Michalewska et al. first report, there have been many studies on the inverted ILM flap technique with or without some modification, including temporal inverted ILM flap, pedicle ILM flap, autologous and pedicle ILM flap with perfluoro-n-octane, autologous ILM flap, and double ILM insertion [16, 18, 20].

Guber et al. reported that most patients with large MHs (diameter > 400 μm) showed best-corrected visual acuity (BCVA) improvements of 1–2 lines following surgery using the inverted flap technique [18]. A meta-analysis by Yuan et al. in 2017 reported that the ILM flap technique was significantly better than the previous non-flap technique for MH-induced retinal detachment [20].

Chen and Yang reported a technique that uses the autologous anterior or posterior lens capsule flap as a scaffold to plug the MH and, finally, Grewal and Mahmoud introduced a new technique involving the use of the autologous neurosensory retinal free flap for closure of refractory myopic MHs (Fig. 22.4a, b) [18].

22.9.6 Type of Tamponade in Macular Hole Surgery

Two kinds of tamponades can be used in the vitreous cavity: gas and silicone oil. Gas plays a very important role in MH surgery because air not only can provide scaffolds for cellular proliferation but also can cause the extrusion of subretinal fluid from surface tension [18].

Standard MH surgery typically includes a long-acting v gas bubble with a period of postoperative face-down positioning lasting 7–14 days [11].

Randomized controlled trials have shown that surgical intervention, using pars plana vitrectomy

(PPV) and intraocular gas tamponade, is effective in allowing for closure of the MH [14]. The role of gas in MH closure has been extensively debated. The more likely role is that the gas bubble acts first by dehydrating the hole edge and then by preventing fluid currents from hampering the healing process [1].

Various gases have been used for MH surgery, including C3F8, C2F6, SF6, and air. The rationale for preferring one gas to another is based on the expected duration of the gas bubble [1]. The degree of gas fill also affects MH closure, as a gas fill above at least 65% on postoperative day 4 has been shown to reduce the risk of poor gas–macula contact and surgical failure [18].

Steve Charles et al. have determined in recent years that surface tension management using air or SF6 combined with ILM peeling is required to restore normal or near-normal foveal anatomy and improve or eliminate symptoms when operating on symptomatic partial-thickness holes [6].

Silicone oil, which is also used as a tamponade, is available in heavy and light varieties [18]. It has been used to avoid the need for positioning in patients unable to maintain the face-down position, to allow air travel after surgery, or to ensure prolonged tamponade in case of failure of the initial surgery [1].

Heavy silicone oil can also cause complications such as intraocular inflammation reaction, media opacification, and secondary glaucoma. Face-down posturing is not strictly necessary when using silicone oil, and heavy silicone oil only requires that the patient be lied flat. Silicone oil is mainly used for patients who cannot tolerate face-down posturing for large MHs, for MHs that remain open after the first operation, for highly myopic MHs with retinal detachment, and for cases involving posterior staphyloma [18].

The time for which a tamponade is needed depends on the duration of the healing process, which is certainly related to hole diameter [1].

22.9.7 Vital Dyes

The use of dyes to stain the ERM and ILM, also known as chromovitrectomy, has made the peeling of the retinal surface more precise, more complete, reduce the duration of surgery, and decrease the risk of mechanical trauma to the retina and less traumatic [1, 18].

Commonly used dyes include indocyanine green (ICG), trypan blue (TB), brilliant blue G (BBG), and adjuvants include triamcinolone acetonide (TA) and blood [18].

Indocyanine green dye has been used to facilitate ILM removal, however, because of some potential toxicity concerns, their routine usage has decreased considerably [9].

TB stains the ERM well but the ILM poorly. To improve TB staining of the ILM, it must be used after fluid–gas exchange or mixing the dye isovolumetrically in 10% glucose to create heavy TB, which falls onto the posterior pole and results in an acceptable staining after a 2-min contact. However, it has been suggested that this may also increase its osmolarity to toxic levels. TB showed no signs of toxicity to the RPE or neuronal tissue [1].

BBG, also known as Coomassie or acid blue, is a synthetic dye [15], has a selective affinity for the ILM and gives a good staining in an iso-osmolar solution of 0.25 mg/ml (0.025%) [1]. The staining occurs after a brief contact with the dye injected onto the retinal surface [1]. No clinical signs of toxicity have been observed in the long term [15].

If a dye that stains the ILM, such as BBG, is used before removing the ERM, the ERM is not stained and appears as a "negative" at the surface at the ILM. The ERM can also be removed en bloc together with the ILM [1].

22.9.8 Postoperative Positioning

The aim of positioning is to keep the MH insulated from liquid currents until the healing process has started to close the hole [1].

The Face-down position (FDP) has become a standard treatment for MH, since Kelly and Wendel used air to fill the vitreous cavity after vitrectomy and required patients to remain face down for a week. However, there is still debate about the need and duration of the face-down posturing [18].

A period of face-down positioning postoperatively is conventionally advised. However, the evidence to support this recommendation is weak and practice varies considerably [8].

In addition, posturing was recommended for MHs with a diameter of ≥400 μm, while posturing was not so effective for MHs with a diameter of <500 μm [20].

A meta-analysis of the closure rates of MH with and without posturing reported that the borderline diameter of posturing should be between 500 and 600 μm [20].

As a result of meta-analysis, Zizhong Hu et al. found substantial evidence that post-operative no FDP treatment is as effective as FDP treatment when MH is smaller than 400 μm. However, the conclusion seems not valid in condition of MH larger than 400 μm [17].

The duration of face-down posturing is strongly related to the type of tamponade that is used in MH surgery [18].

Face-down posturing is accompanied by great inconvenience, and some patients, especially children and the elderly, cannot tolerate it [18].

22.9.9 Type of Macular Hole Closure

The closure of macular holes is usually defined as a flattened and reattached hole rim along the whole circumference of macular hole [21], and is usually associated with a decrease in size of the hole with the edges appearing to have slide together and becoming imperceptible in some cases [5].

The anatomical status of the macula after macular hole surgery was classified in 1998 by Tornambe et al. into three types [22]. In one, the hole remains elevated, its circular edges are visible, and there is fluid beneath the hole. In the second, the hole is flat against the retinal pigment epithelium (RPE), but the edges of the hole are visible and separated; and, in the third, the hole is flat against the RPE, but the edges of the hole are not visible and sometimes a pinpoint defect is noted [22], these findings suggested that flat and closed outcomes have a better visual prognosis than flat and open outcomes.

Imai et al. categorized the successfully repaired macular hole into three patterns with OCT; U-type (normal foveal contour), V-type (steep foveal contour), and W-type (foveal defect of neurosensory retina). The authors reported that postoperative visual acuity was well correlated with these patterns (U > V > W) [21].

22.10 Outcome

Although the surgical technique of macular hole has been improved and the hole closure rate after the operation has recently been reported to be about 90%, with vitrectomy and adjuvant therapy, the postoperative visual outcome is not always satisfactory even in eyes with anatomical success [21].

A number of possible prognostic factors such as the duration of symptoms, preoperative macular hole size, preoperative visual acuity, axial length, age, and sex have been reported [21]. Long-lasting and large size are MH characteristics that are considered poor prognostic factors for MH surgery [1]. Nevertheless, the introduction of ILM peeling has improved the closure rate dramatically and the anatomic prognosis for large holes, which is nearly the same as for smaller ones, and even long-standing MH may benefit from surgery [1, 23].

In 2010, Michalewska et al., as previously mentioned, described a novel technique of inverted internal limiting membrane (ILM) flap [24] for the treatment of large macular holes and found that this technique achieved better anatomical and visual outcomes compared to conventional ILM peeling (ILMP). It has also been reported that this technique increased the rate of complete MH closure to 98% for large idiopathic MHs (diameter exceeding 400 μm), whereas in conventional vitrectomy with ILM peeling, 88% closure rate was achieved [24].

Grewal and Mahmoud described a technique involving the use of an autologous neurosensory retinal free flap for closure of refractory myopic MH. This technique involves using an autologous neurosensory retinal free flap and positioning it over the MH to provide a scaffold and plug for hole closure [25]. The limitations of this procedure include limited follow-up to date on a limited number of cases and unknown potential long-term complications. Likewise, the success rate of long-term closure, as well as recovery of visual acuity, is still unknown [25].

Reported closure rates, therefore, vary depending on the cases included in each series. In 2013, National Ophthalmology Database study of Vitreoretinal Surgery was performed in the United Kingdom [26], the reported results showed that all operations undertaken for primary MH included a PPV; 1014 (94.1%) also included ILM peel, 437 (40.5%) included cataract surgery, 1008 (93.5%) included gas tamponade, four included silicone oil tamponade, and in 66 (6.1%) the tamponade used was not recorded. The most commonly selected intravitreal gas was C2F6, with approximately equal numbers of eyes receiving SF6 and C3F8, finding that the choice of gas did not significantly alter the visual outcome [26].

Kang et al. performed a meta-analysis of the recent literature to examine what factors were important with regards to improving the results of surgery [27]. The authors considered for the analysis of 389 macular holes. There were 88 stage 2, 124 stage 3 and 67 stage 4 holes. The parameters examined included staging and duration of the MH, VA before and after surgery, use of adjuvants and postoperative anatomical closure. They found that over 80% of the macular holes reported in the literature were successfully closed, although the definition of anatomical success varied [27]. The visual outcome of the macular hole surgery in the literature was not as favorable as the anatomical results and the stage of the macular hole had a significant association with both the preoperative VA and duration of the hole.

The meta-analysis showed that the anatomical success rates do not differ greatly between the stages but in the more long-standing cases, adjuvants may improve the chance of anatomical closure of the hole, but it is not clear whether this will translate to a better visual outcome [27].

According to the authors' knowledge, a multivariate analysis has not been established between the findings in OCT of post-surgical closure and the type of technique used.

22.11 Conclusions

The standard surgical procedure for idiopathic macular hole repair consists of a three-port PPV, removal of the posterior cortical vitreous, peeling of obvious ERM, and gas tamponade with postoperative face-down positioning for 7–14 days [11]. PPV is performed for stages 2–4 MH [10]. The most important factor for MH closure is internal tamponade [10]. OCT monitoring of the outer layers of the retina after MH surgery may play an important prognostic role [10].

References

1. Gaudric A, Tadayoni R. Macular hole. In: Ryan retina. 6th ed. Elsevier: Amsterdam; 2004. p. 2280–2302.
2. Zhao P, Wang S, Liu N, Shu Z, Zhao J. A review of surgical outcomes and advances for macular holes. J Ophthalmol. 2018;2018:7389412.
3. Corcostegui B, Pimentel LP. Macular hole. In: Quiroz-Mercado H, Kerrison JB, editors. Macular surgery. 2nd ed. Philadelphia, PA: Lippincott Williams & Wilkins. p. 271–82.
4. Williamson TH. Macular hole. In: Vitreoretinal surgery. 2nd ed. Heidelberg: Springer; 2013. p. 209–18.
5. Sharma YR, Pal N. Management of macular hole. In: Retinal detachment surgery: a practical guide. 1st ed. Noida: Jaypee Publishers; 2006. p. 107–31.
6. Charles S, Calzada J, Wood B. Macular holes. In: Charles S, Calzada J, Wood B, editors. Vitreous microsurgery. 5th ed. Philadelphia, PA: Lippincott Williamns and Wilkins; 2001. p. 164–70.
7. la Cour M, Friis J. Macular holes: Classification, epidemiology, natural history and treatment. Acta Ophthalmol Scand. 2002;80(6):579–87.
8. Bainbridge J, Herbert E, Gregor Z. Macular holes: vitreoretinal relationships and surgical approaches. Eye. 2008;22:1301–9.
9. Smiddy WE, Flynn HW. JR. M. Pathogenesis of macular holes and therapeutic implications. Am J Ophthalmol. 2004;137(3):525–37.
10. Pieczynski J, Kuklo P, Grzybowski A. Pars plana vitrectomy with silicone oil tamponade for primary and secondary macular hole closure: Is it still a useful procedure? Eur J Ophtalmol. 2018;28(5):1–12.
11. Johnson MW. Improvements in the understanding and treatment of macular hole. Curr Opin Ophthalmol. 2002;13(3):152–60.

12. Duker JS, Kaiser PK, Binder S, De Smet MD, Gaudric A, Reichel E, et al. The international vitreomacular traction study group classification of vitreomacular adhesion, traction, and macular hole. Ophthalmology. 2013;120(12):2611–9. https://doi.org/10.1016/j.ophtha.2013.07.042.
13. MESTER V, KUHN F. Internal limiting membrane removal in the Management of Full-Thickness Macular Holes. Am J Ophthalmol. 2000;129(6):769–77.
14. Almony A, Nudleman E, Shah GK, Blinder KJ, Eliott DB, Mittra RA, et al. Techniques, rationale, and outcomes of internal limiting membrane peeling. Retina. 2012;32(5):877–91.
15. Natarajan S, Hussain N, Dabir S. Textbook of vitreoretinal diseases and surgery. Noida: Jaypee Brothers, Medical Publishers; 2009.
16. De Novelli FJ, Preti RC, Ribeiro Monteiro ML, Pelayes DE, Junqueira Nóbrega M, Takahashi WY. Autologous internal limiting membrane fragment transplantation for large, chronic, and refractory macular holes. Ophthalmic Res. 2015;55(1):45–52.
17. Hu Z, Xie P, Ding Y, Zheng X, Yuan D, Liu Q, et al. Face-down or no face-down posturing following macular hole surgery: a meta-analysis. Acta Ophthalmol. 2016;94:326–34.
18. Zhao P, Wang S, Liu N, Shu Z, Zhao J. A review of surgical outcomes and advances for macular holes. J Opt. 2018;2018:7389412.
19. Bae K, Kang SW, Kim JH, Kim SJ, Kim JM, Yoon JM. Extent of internal limiting membrane peeling and its impact on macular hole surgery outcomes: a randomized trial. Am J Ophthalmol. 2016;169:179–88. https://doi.org/10.1016/j.ajo.2016.06.041.
20. Yamashita T, Sakamoto T, Terasaki H, Iwasaki M, Ogushi Y, Okamoto F, et al. Best surgical technique and outcomes for large macular holes: retrospective multicentre study in Japan. Acta Ophthalmol. 2018;96(8):1–7.
21. Kang SW, Ahn K, Ham DI. Types of macular hole closure and their clinical implications. Br J Ophthalmol. 2003;87(8):1015–9.
22. Tornambe P, Poliner LS, Cohen RG. Definition of macular hole surgery end points. Retina. 1998;18(3):286–7.
23. Kusuhara S, Negi A. Predicting visual outcome following surgery for idiopathic macular holes. Ophthalmologica. 2013;231(3):125–32.
24. Shroff D, Gupt P, Atri N, Gupta C, Shroff C. Inverted internal limiting membrane (ILM) flap technique for macular hole closure: patient selection and special considerations. Clin Ophthalmol. 2019;13:671–8.
25. Grewal DS, Mahmoud TH. Autologous neurosensory retinal free flap for closure of refractory myopic macular holess. JAMA Ophthalmol. 2016;134(2):229–30.
26. Jackson TL, Donachie PHJ, Sallam A, Sparrow JM, Johnston RL. United Kingdom national ophthalmology database study of vitreoretinal surgery: report 3, retinal detachment. Ophthalmology. 2014;121(3):643–8. https://doi.org/10.1016/j.ophtha.2012.09.003.
27. Kang HK, Chang AA, Beaumont PE. The macular hole: report of an Australian surgical series and meta-analysis of the literature. Clin Exp Ophthalmol. 2000;28(4):298–308.

Management of Vitreo-macular Traction and Epiretinal Membrane 23

Purva Date, Matteo Forlini,
and Maria Rosaria Carbotti

23.1 Vitreo-macular Traction Syndrome

23.1.1 Natural History

The vitreous is a gel-like structure that occupies about 4 ml of intraocular space. It is composed mostly (98%) of water, and two major macromolecules-collagen (type II, hybrid of types V/XI and type IX collagen in a molar ratio of 75:10:15) and hyaluronan [1].

With advancing age, the vitreous gel undergoes initial phase of liquefaction. The attachment between vitreous and internal limiting membrane (ILM) weakens and it gets completely separated called posterior vitreous detachment (PVD). PVD begins in the perifoveal macula and occurs in 4 stages: [2, 3] Stage 1: separation of the vitreous perifoveally with adhesion to fovea, optic disc, and mid-peripheral retina; Stage 2: Vitreofoveal separation with adhesion to optic disc and mid-peripheral retina; Stage 3: Vitreous attached only to optic disc; Stage 4: Complete PVD where the vitreous is detached from the optic disc also. PVD is considered as an acute event precipitated by the abrupt development of a break in the thin posterior cortical vitreous layer overlying the macular region [2]. Weiss ring is the sign of completion of vitreo–papillary separation. It is usually an acute and symptomatic event. Inadequate or incomplete vitreo–retinal interface separation result in anomalous PVD with vitreo-macular interface (VMI) anomalies.

23.1.2 Definition and Classification of Vitreo-macular Adhesion

Vitreo-macular adhesion (VMA) denotes residual strong adhesion between vitreous and macula when PVD is incomplete.

Vitreo-macular Traction (VMT), as described by Jaffe in 1967, is a well-recognized complication of PVD [3] where vitreous separates from the retina throughout the peripheral fundus but remains adherent posteriorly, resulting in anteroposterior traction on a broad, dumbbell-shaped area encompassing the macula and optic nerve. Johnson et al. [4] described complications of PVD with respect to the area of adhesion. VMT is characterized by macular adhesions of the hyaloid

Electronic Supplementary Material The online version of this chapter (https://doi.org/10.1007/978-981-33-4168-5_23) contains supplementary material, which is available to authorized users.

P. Date (✉)
Pramukh Swami Eye Hospital, Mumbai, India

M. Forlini
Domus Nova' Private Hospital, Ravenna, Italy

M. R. Carbotti
Institute of Ophthalmology, University of Modena and Reggio Emilia, Modena, Italy

A. Jain et al. (eds.), *Cutting-edge Vitreoretinal Surgery*,
https://doi.org/10.1007/978-981-33-4168-5_23

of about 1500 μm, whereas vitreofoveolar traction is when the macular adhesion is less than 500 μm.

With the evolution of Optical Coherence Tomography (OCT) visualization and understanding of the vitreo–retinal interface has improved [5]. OCT is central for diagnosis and detection of VMT. Focal VMA is usually asymptomatic [6]. If traction is enough to cause disturbance in macular architecture VMA can lead to VMT, which is always pathologic and symptomatic.

International Vitreo-macular Traction Study (IVTS) Group in 2013 has proposed evidence-based clinically applicable classification system to identify, monitor, and manage vitreo-macular interface disorders. This is based on multiple OCT B-line scans images and classified by the size of attachment or lesion and presence of retinal or vitreo–retinal conditions [7] (Table 23.1).

23.1.3 Clinical Features of Vitreo-macular Traction Syndrome

There is a wide spectrum of severity and clinical findings. Visual symptoms such as blurring of vision, metamorphopsia and difficulty in reading, central scotoma, alteration in image size and decreased visual acuity may arise due to antero-posterior traction exerted on the macula leading to cystoid macular edema, epiretinal membrane. Progressive traction can lead to the development of a hole in the macula and worsening visual function [8].

23.1.4 Treatment of Vitreo-macular Adhesion

23.1.4.1 Observation

During the process of PVD, the vitreous remains attached to the foveal region in the last stages. Therefore, VMA can be considered as a normal stage in the natural history of PVD associated with vitreous aging. Patients with VMA who are asymptomatic can be safely observed and reexamined for a period of 3 months. Cases becoming symptomatic or showing foveal anatomical changes needs intervention.

23.1.4.2 Pharmacological Vitreolysis

Agents break down the peptide bonds in laminin and fibronectin molecules which keeps the adhesion between ILM and vitreous. Collagenase,

Table 23.1 International Vitreo-macular Traction Study (IVTS) Group classifications [9]

Anatomical state	IVTS classification system Definition	Based on the extent of foveal attachment	Associated retinal condition
VMA	Perifoveal vitreous detachment from retinal surface with vitreous cortex attached to macula within a radius of 3 mm. There is no change in foveal anatomy	*focal* < 1500 μm, *Broad* > 1500 μm	*Isolated*-no retinal anomaly *Concurrent*: With retinal anomaly
VMT	Perifoveal vitreous detachment from retinal surface vitreous cortex attached to macula within a radius of 3 mm. It is associated with distortion of foveal surface, intraretinal structures	*focal* < 1500 μm, *Broad* > 1500 μm	*Isolated*-no retinal anomaly *Concurrent*: With retinal anomaly
FTMH	Full-thickness macular lesion, interrupting all layers from ILM to RPE	Small ≤ 250 μm Medium—250–400 μm Large ≥ 400 μm	Etiology Primary-initiated by VMT Secondary: Due to trauma or associated retinal pathology
LMH	Loss of foveal contour, with defect in the inner foveal layers causing splitting, but photoreceptor layer is intact		
Macular pseudohole	Concomitant ERM with central opening with invaginated or heaped foveal edges No loss of retinal tissue Near normal central foveal thickness		

plasmin, chondroitinase, hyaluronidase, plasminogen activator are the agents that are used for vitreolysis. Ocriplasmin is a recombinant truncated form of human plasmin with a molecular weight of 27.8 kDa. This DNA molecule is more stable than plasmin and has emerged as a new vitreolytic agent. It is a recombinant protease with activity against fibronectin and laminin.

Ocriplasmin was approved for treatment of VMT, including macular hole with a diameter < 400 μ. Around 29.8% VMT patients had resolution by 28 days after single injection of 0.125 mg/0.1 ml ocriplasmin compared to placebo injection where resolution was seen in 7.7% only [9].

Side Effects of Ocriplasmin

Ocular adverse effects of Ocriplasmin injection are vitreous floaters, photopsia, blurred vision, potential for lens subluxation, retinal breaks, retinal detachments, and dyschromatopsia (yellow vision). ERG changes in the form of reduced "a" and "b" wave amplitude are reported in patients experiencing dyschromatopsia. Patients can experience transient loss of vision, which is attributed to the disruption in the ellipsoid layer which is reversible. Widespread retinal dysfunction can develop in patients due to its effect on laminin, which is present in outer layers of retina including bruch membrane, inter-photoreceptor matrix, and external limiting membrane. Though the effect on photoreceptor outer segment is transient, the action on rods is more prolonged.

23.1.4.3 Surgical Treatment

Pars Plana Vitrectomy (PPV) with ILM peeling is the standard treatment advocated for VMT (Fig. 23.1). The success of relieving VMT ranges from 80 to 90%. The surgery helps to improve blurred and distorted vision. But this can be associated with various complications of vitrectomy like retinal breaks, macular hole formation, retinal detachment, endophthalmitis, and development of cataract.

23.1.4.4 Non-vitrectomizing Vitreous Surgery (NVS)

Surgical procedure aiming to remove VMT and ERM without removing the vitreous has been described for the first time by Charles [10]. Saito et al. [11] showed this technique is safe and efficient to remove ERM and prevent the development or progression of nuclear sclerosis. In our modified technique by Dr. Cesare Forlini, 27G

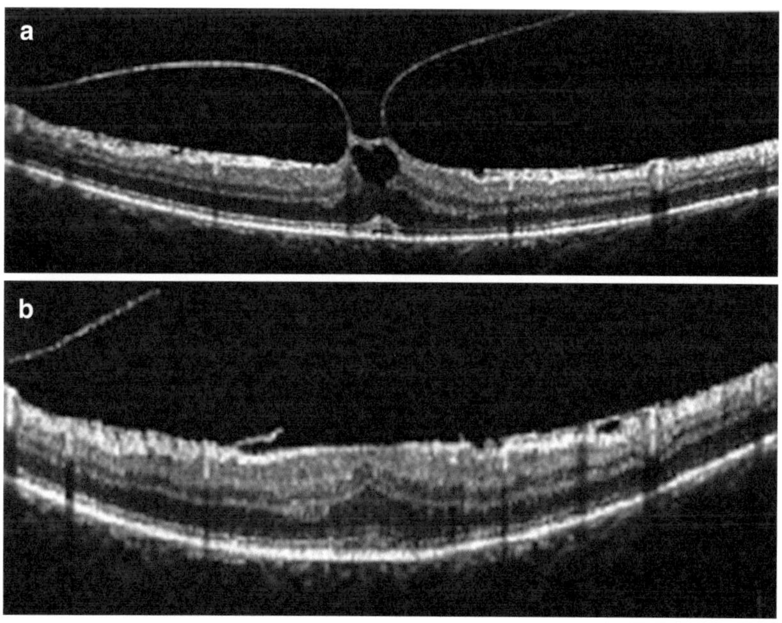

Fig. 23.1 (**a**) Oct scan of symptomatic vitreo-macular traction in a 51-year-old male, (**b**) OCT scan showing complete resolution VMT post vitrectomy 1 month

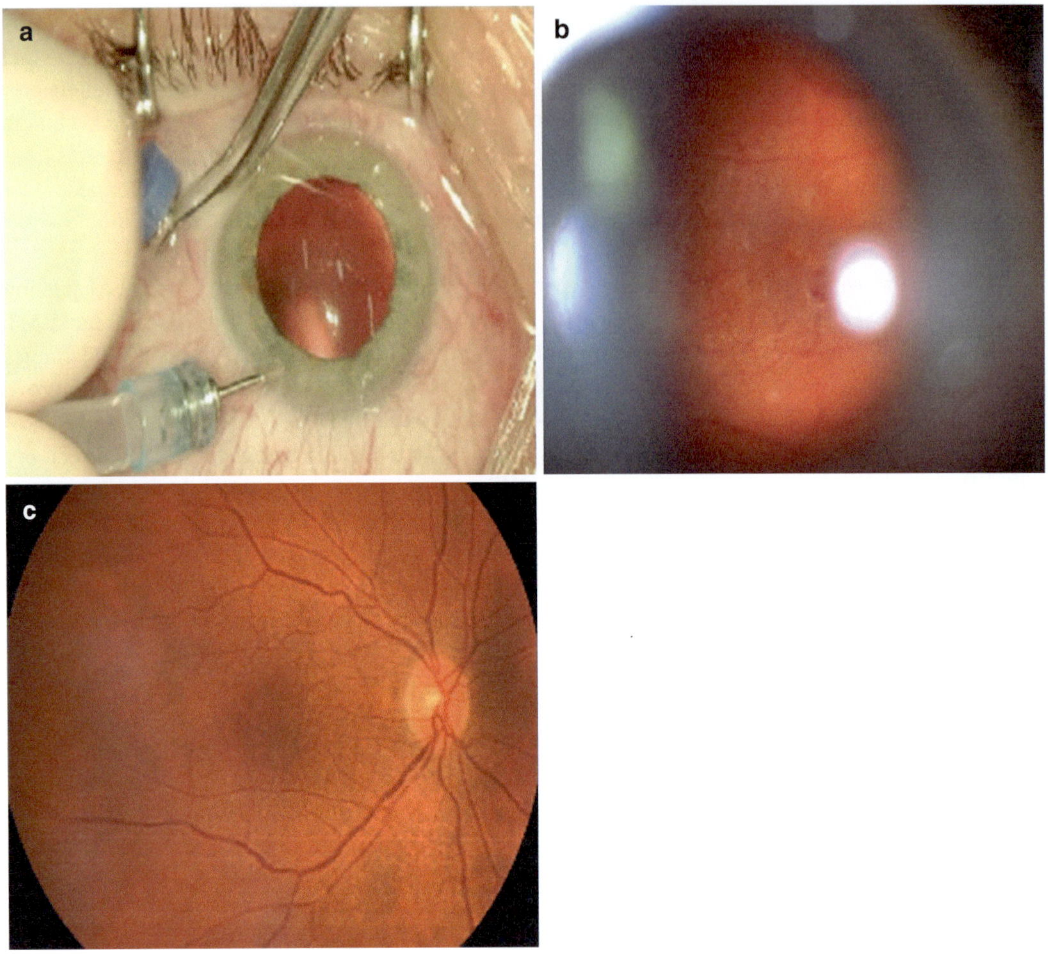

Fig. 23.2 Non-vitrectomizing vitreous surgery (NVS) in the left eye of a 55-year-old phakic patient. (**a**) Inferotemporal single port with superior anterior chamber maintainer, (**b**) Intraoperative Fundus view through slit-lamp illumination system, (**c**) 1 month postoperative fundus view

single port is used for removal of VMT and anterior chamber maintainer for maintaining the intraocular pressure. Fundus is viewed by a slit-lamp illumination system installed on a surgical microscope (Visulux, Carl Zeiss, Oberkochen, Germany) (Figs. 23.2 and 23.3)

23.2 Epiretinal Membrane

23.2.1 Natural History

Epiretinal membrane (ERM) was first described by Iwanoff in 1865 as an avascular, fibrocellular membrane that proliferates on the inner surface of the retina. The prevalence of macular ERMs is 2% under the age of 60 years and 12% in those over 70 years [12].

23.2.2 Etiology and Pathogenesis

Epiretinal membranes can be idiopathic, which are found in otherwise healthy eyes with no specific cause. Idiopathic ERMs are associated with anomalous posterior vitreous detachment (PVD) [13], which occurs when vitreous liquefaction occurs without sufficient vitreo–retinal adhesion weakening resulting in vitreoschisis and vitreo-macular traction. The retained corti-

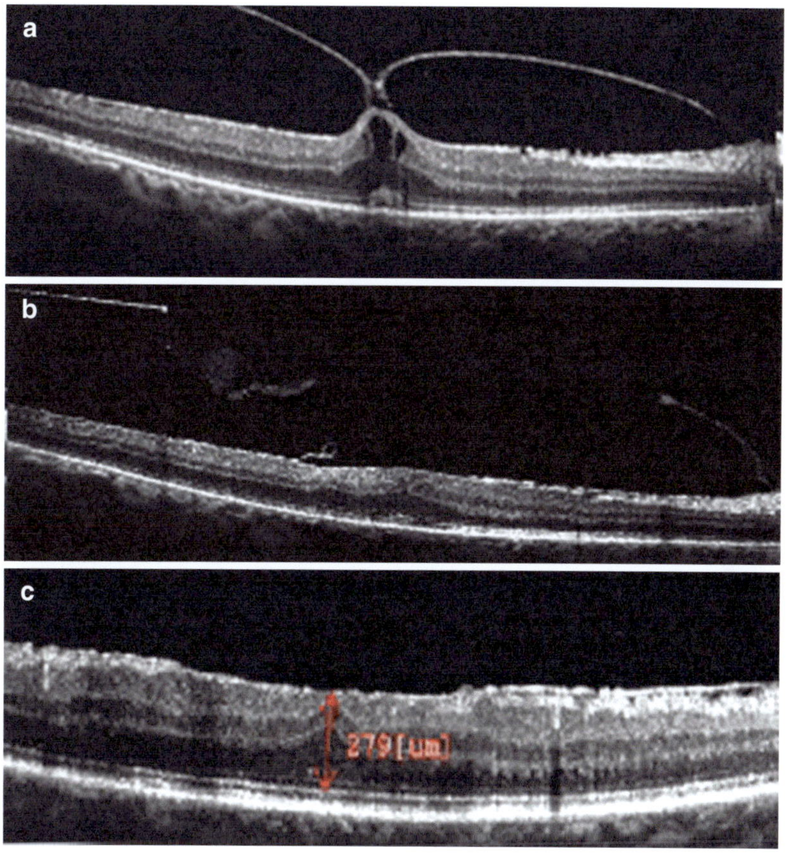

Fig. 23.3 (**a**) OCT scan of the above patient showing vitreo-macular traction, (**b**) postoperative 1 week OCT with resolution of traction, (**c**) OCT showing restoration of macular anatomy with thin ERM and CMT measuring 279 microns

cal vitreous induces the production of cytokines such as basic fibroblast growth factor and nerve growth factor, which stimulate cellular proliferation over ILM [14–16]. Alternatively, PVD can cause a dehiscence in the internal limiting membrane, which allows microglial cells to interact with hyalocytes and laminocytes in the vitreous leading to the formation of ERM [17, 18]. These cells transdifferentiate into myofibroblasts like cells, which can contract and create a macular pucker [19].

Secondary ERMs are associated with other ocular conditions, such as posterior uveitis, retinal detachment, retinal vascular diseases such as diabetic retinopathy or venous occlusive disease, trauma, intraocular surgery, post-vitrectomy, retinal laser, and cryotherapy. Secondary ERM can be considered as an abnormal wound healing triggered by inflammation.

23.2.3 Diagnosis and Classification of ERM

Clinical classification of ERM was given by Gass [20] as Grade 0—Cellophane maculopathy: fine membrane over macula with glistening light reflex and no retinal distortion. Patient is usually asymptomatic; Grade 1—Crinkled cellophane maculopathy: there is distortion of retinal vasculature with inner retinal folds. Metamorphopsia is the main symptom; Grade 2—Macular pucker: opaque ERM with obscuration of the underlying retina, marked distortion, and puckering of macula. Visual acuity is less than 20/200 with metamorphopsia. Foos [21] also has classified ERM based on clinical appearance and etiology into simple: no feature of contraction or any associated ocular disease; intermediate: thicker ERM with pigments and features of contraction; com-

Table 23.2 OCT-based ERM classification according to foveal involvement modified from Hwang et al. study [22]

Group 1: fovea-involving ERM	
1A	Outer retinal thickening and minimal inner retinal change
1B	Exaggerated tenting of outer retinal layer in the foveal area with slight thickening and distorted configuration of inner retinal layer
1C	Prominent thickening of the inner retinal layer
Group 2: fovea-sparing ERM	
2A	Formation of a macular pseudohole
2B	Macular pseudohole with marked intraretinal splitting

plex: ERM secondary to retinal detachment, surgery or trauma. Contraction of these membranes can lead to tractional retinal detachment.

OCT provides noninvasive high-resolution cross-sectional images of retina and is therefore considered as a gold-standard in ERM diagnosis and staging. Hwang et al. has classified ERM as fovea involving and non-involving based on OCT (Table 23.2).

23.2.4 Treatment of ERM

The treatment options for ERM consists of either observation or surgical intervention. Asymptomatic ERM diagnosed on routine evaluation can well be observed. Most of the ERMs do not progress and may even regress. Hence conservative management is advised if the patient is asymptomatic. Regular follow up with SD-OCT and clinical examination for recording visual acuity and metamorphopsia should be advised. Surgical intervention is considered for patients who have visual symptoms of metamorphopsia or decreased visual acuity below 20/40. Optimal surgical time has not yet been well standardized, it varies case to case basis. Surgical removal of ERM may be more beneficial for patients with progressive, secondary ERM than patients with stable idiopathic ERM.

Surgery involves a three-port pars plana vitrectomy and removal of ERM, with or without peeling of the internal limiting membrane (ILM). Different methods of staining, and peeling of ERM, have been described below.

23.2.4.1 Vitrectomy

A small guage three-port pars plana vitrectomy is performed. PVD can be induced actively by the cutter or passively by the flute needle. Triamcinolone acetonide can be used to stain the vitreous to ensure complete PVD.

23.2.4.2 Membrane Removal

Once the vitrectomy is completed, ERM is visualized for existing edges. Preoperative 3D OCT can also help in planning the optimal area of initiating the peel. If a preexisting edge is not found, it can be created using an MVR blade. On rare occasions where the ERM is highly adherent to the underlying retina, scissors can be used to delaminate the membrane.

The edge is then grasped with an end gripping forceps and a circumscribed flap is created. When the edge of the membrane is not easily grasped by the forceps, a Tano diamond-dusted membrane scraper (DDMS) can be used. The dissection can be carried out from periphery to the center (outside in technique) or the membrane can be grasped centrally and peeled toward the periphery (inside out technique). An alternative is the pinch and peel technique where the forceps are used to pinch the membrane without creating an edge, and then peeled circumferentially. Retinal contact is avoided in this method and so is the risk of retinal damage [23].

23.2.4.3 Role of ILM Peeling

Role of ILM peeling in cases of ERM is controversial. ILM serves as a platform for cellular proliferation and may cause residual glial cells and myofibroblasts to proliferate and reform the ERM. Peeling of ILM also ensures complete removal of ERM and hence reduced risk of recurrence. Few studies have compared the results of removing the ERM alone by removing both the ERM and the ILM. Few studies found that peeling the ILM with the ERM led to a lower incidence of recurrent ERM. whereas others showed no difference between peeling or no peeling the ILM. No article reported better results for peeling the ERM alone [24–30]. However, ILM peeling can cause damage to the nerve fiber layer, retinal edema, retinal hemorrhage, electrophysiological, and visual field changes [31].

23.2.4.4 Staining of Membrane

To enhance the visualization of these transparent or semitransparent membranes and to prevent ERM recurrence, various staining methods have been used, including indocyanine green, trypan blue, and brilliant blue G. Indocyanine green stains acellular collagen of the ILM. In contrast, cellular ERM is stained negatively. It provides a "negative staining" of ERM. Trypan blue at a concentration of 0.2%, gives a bluish discoloration of ERMs that facilitates surgery. The area of ERM is usually larger than that estimated ophthalmoscopically. With the stain, a larger area of the membrane can be identified and enables a more complete removal. Brilliant Blue G mostly stains the ILM, but the ERM is also stained to some degree. It is preferred for simultaneous removal, when dual staining is necessary [32].

23.2.5 Complications

ERM peeling is usually a safe procedure. Intraoperative complications include retinal petechiae, vitreous hemorrhage, retinal hemorrhage, peripheral iatrogenic retinal breaks, posterior retinal breaks, and retinal surface damage. Focal retinal petechiae and retinal hemorrhage usually resolve on their own. Peripheral retinal breaks can occur due to vitreous traction at the sclerotomy site or at the time of PVD induction. Careful examination of the periphery toward the end of surgery should be done to look for any peripheral break which can later cause a retinal detachment. Eccentric full-thickness macular hole has been reported with an incidence of 0.6% [33]. They usually occur at the site where ILM peeling is initiated or completed. Muller cell damage during ILM peeling can cause weakening of the retina and lead to hole formation. Contraction of the edge of the ERM can also lead to continued traction and secondary hole formation [34].

The most common postoperative complication of ILM peeling is cataract progression. Retinal detachment can occur due to a missed peripheral retinal break. Visual field defects can occur as a result of damage to the nerve fiber layer [35]. Recurrence has been reported from 1 to 16% more on cases of secondary ERMs. Other less common complications include cystoid macular edema, macular phototoxicity, and endophthalmitis.

23.2.6 Outcome

Improved visual acuity and reduced metamorphopsia have been reported after ERM removal surgery. After surgery, vision improves in 60–87% of by 2 Snellen lines. The improvement continues for more than 6 months and the meantime to achieve the best final vision is about 1 year [36] (Fig. 23.4).

The prognostic factors for improvement in visual acuity include better baseline visual acuity, preoperative degree of metamorphopsia, shorter duration of symptoms, intact inner segment–outer segment photoreceptor junction, less ganglion, and inner plexiform layer thickness [37]. The parafoveal inner nuclear layer (INL) is the only retinal structural parameter that was found to be associated with VA and metamorphopsia [38]. Ectopic inner fovea layer has been described in idiopathic ERM and its presence is considered a negative prognostic factor for anatomical and functional recovery [39].

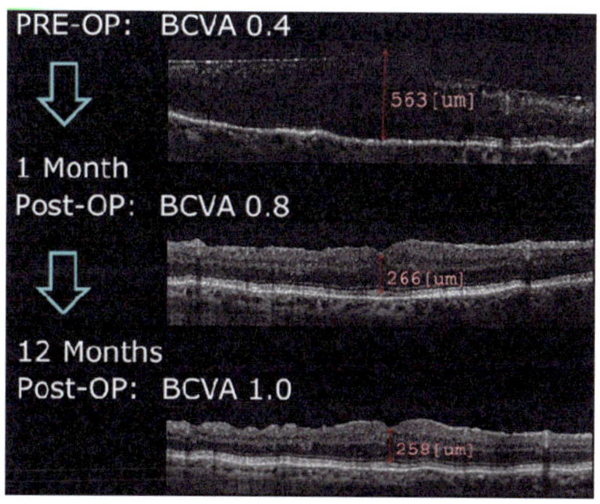

Fig. 23.4 OCT scans of a 62-year male with ERM showing preoperative, postoperative, and follow-up scans

23.3 Conclusion

Despite the favorable results of surgery for the treatment of ERM, debate remains regarding a preferable treatment strategy. Decision for surgery and selection of the proper method depends on the surgeon's preference and on the patients' characteristics. Early intervention may prevent the evolvement of nonreversible damage to the outer retina; however, ERM progression concerns only a small percentage of patients. Follow-up with SDOCT and clinical examination for recording visual acuity and metamorphopsia is imposed in early cases prior to decision-making.

References

1. Balazs EA. Molecular morphology of the vitreous body. In: Smelser GK, editor. The structure of the eye. New York: Academic; 1961. p. 293–310.
2. Eisner G. Posterior vitreous detachment. KlinMBlAugenheilk. 1989;194:389–92.
3. Jaffe NS. Vitreous traction at the posterior pole of the fundus due to alterations in the vitreous posterior. Trans Am Acad Ophthalmol Otolaryngol. 1967;71:642–52.
4. Johnson MW. Posterior vitreous detachment: evolution and complications of its early stages. Am J Ophthalmol. 2010;149:371–82.
5. Koizumi H, Spaide RF, Fisher YL, et al. Three dimensional evaluation of vitreo-macular traction and epiretinal membrane using spectral domain optical coherence tomography. Am J Ophthalmol. 2008;145:509–17.
6. Kroll P, Wiegand W, Schmidt J. Vitreopapillary traction in proliferative diabetic vitreoretinopathy. Br J Ophthalmol. 1999;83:261–4.
7. Duker JS, Kaiser PK, Binder S, et al. The international Vitreomacular Traction Study Group classification of Vitreomacular adhesion, traction, and macular hole. Ophthalmology. 2013;120:2611.
8. Jackson TL, Nicod E, Simpson A, Angelis A, Grimaccia F, Kanavos P. Symptomatic vitreomacular adhesion. Retina. 2013;33(8):1503–11.
9. Stalmans P, Benz MS, Gandorfer A, et al. Enzymatic vitreolysis with ocriplasmin for vitreomacular traction and macular holes. N Engl J Med. 2012;367:606–15.
10. Charles S. Vitreous microsurgery. 2nd ed. Baltimore: Williams & Wilkins; 1987. p. 153–7.
11. Saito Y, Lewis JM, Park I, et al. Nonvitrectomizing vitreous surgery: a strategy to prevent postoperative nuclear sclerosis. Ophthalmology. 1999;106:1541–5.
12. Mitchell P, Smith W, Chey T, Wang JJ, Chang A. Prevalence and associations of epiretinal membranes. The Blue Mountains Eye Study, Australia. Ophthalmology. 1997;104:1033–40.
13. Sebag J. Anomalous posterior vitreous detachment: a unifying concept in vitreo-retinal disease. Graefes Arch Clin Exp Ophthalmol. 2004;242(8):690–8.
14. Hikichi T, et al. Relationship between premacular cortical vitreous defects and idiopathic premacular fibrosis. Retina. 1995;15(5):413–6.
15. Joshi M, et al. Inflammatory mechanisms of idiopathic epiretinal membrane formation. Mediators Inflamm. 2013;2013:192582.
16. Lindqvist N, et al. Retinal glial (Muller) cells: sensing and responding to tissue stretch. Investig Ophthalmol Vis Sci. 2010;51(3):1683–90.
17. Bringmann A, et al. Involvement of Muller glial cells in epiretinal membrane formation. Graefes Arch Clin Exp Ophthalmol. 2009;247(7):865–83.
18. Kohno RI, et al. Possible contribution of hyalocytes to idiopathic epiretinal membrane formation and its contraction. Br J Ophthalmol. 2009;93(8):1020–6.
19. Parapuram SK, et al. Differential effects of TGFbeta and vitreous on the transformation of retinal pigment epithelial cells. Investig Ophthalmol Vis Sci. 2009;50(12):5965–74.
20. Gass JDM. Macular dysfunction caused by epiretinal membrane contraction. In: Stereoscopic atlas of macular diseases: diagnosis and treatment, vol. 2. 4th ed. St. Louis: Mosby; 1997. p. 938–50.
21. Foos RY. Vitreoretinal juncture—simple epiretinal membranes. Graefes Arch Clin Exp Ophthalmol. 1974;189:231–50.
22. Hwang JU, et al. Assessment of macular function for idiopathic epiretinal membranes classified by spectral-domain optical coherence tomography. Invest Ophthalmol Vis Sci. 2012;53(7):3562–9.
23. Charles S. Techniques and tools for dissection of epiretinal membranes. Graefes Arch Clin Exp Ophthalmol. 2003;241:347–52.
24. Bovey EH, Uffer S, Achache F. Surgery for epimacular membrane: impact of retinal internal limiting membrane removal on functional outcome. Retina. 2004;24:728–35.
25. Kwok A, Lai TY, Yuen KS. Epiretinal membrane surgery with or without internal limiting membrane peeling. Clin Exp Ophthalmol. 2005;33:379–85.
26. Oh HN, Lee JE, Kim HW, Yun IH. Clinical outcomes of double staining and additional ILM peeling during ERM surgery. Korean J Ophthalmol. 2013;27:256–60.
27. Park DW, Dugel PU, Garda J, et al. Macular pucker removal with and without internal limiting membrane peeling: pilot study. Ophthalmology. 2003;110:62–4.
28. Sandali O, El Sanharawi M, Basli E, et al. Epiretinal membrane recurrence: incidence, characteristics, evolution, and preventive and risk factors. Retina. 2013;33:2032–8.

29. Shimada H, Nakashizuka H, Hattori T, et al. Double staining with brilliant blue G and double peeling for epiretinal membranes. Ophthalmology. 2009;116:1370–6.
30. Koestinger A, Bovey EH. Visual acuity after vitrectomy and epiretinal membrane peeling with or without premacular indocyanine green injection. Eur J Ophthalmol. 2005;15:795–9.
31. Andrea DV, Wu L. To peel or not to peel the internal limiting membrane in idiopathic epiretinal membranes. Retina. 2018;38:S5–S11.
32. Totan Y, Guler E, Dervisogullari MS. Brilliant Blue G assisted epiretinal membrane surgery. Sci Rep. 2014;4:3956.
33. Sandali O, El Sanharawi M, Basli E, et al. Paracentral retinal holes occurring after macular surgery: incidence, clinical features, and evolution. Graefes Arch Clin Exp Ophthalmol. 2012;250:1137–42.
34. Steven P, Laqua H, Wong D, Hoerauf H. Secondary paracentral retinal holes following internal limiting membrane removal. Br J Ophthalmol. 2006;90:293–5.
35. Pichi F, Lembo A, Morara M, et al. Early and late inner retinal changes after inner limiting membrane peeling. Int Ophthalmol. 2014;34(2):437–46.
36. Pesin SR, Olk RJ, Grand MG, et al. Vitrectomy for premacular fibroplasia. Prognostic factors, long-term follow-up, and time course of visual improvement. Ophthalmology. 1991;98:1109–14.
37. Miguel AI, Legris A. Prognostic factors of epiretinal membranes: a systematic review. J Fr Ophtalmol. 2017;40(1):61–79.
38. Okamoto F, Sugiura Y, Okamoto Y, Hiraoka T, Oshika T. Inner nuclear layer thickness as a prognostic factor for metamorphopsia after epiretinal membrane surgery. Retina. 2015;35(10):2107–14.
39. Govetto A, Virgili G, Rodriguez FJ, Figueroa MS, Sarraf D, Hubschman JP. Functional and anatomical significance of the ectopic inner foveal layers in eyes with idiopathic epiretinal membranes: surgical results at 12 months. Retina. 2019;39(2):347–57.

Management of Submacular Hemorrhage

24

Grazia Pertile and Emilia Maggio

24.1 Introduction

Submacular hemorrhage (SMH) is a severe and relatively common complication of choroidal neovascularization (CNV). Its visual prognosis is dramatically poor when left untreated [1, 2] as a consequence of blood component toxicity, such as hemosiderin, fibrin, and iron [3, 4], the physical separation of photoreceptors from the retinal pigment epithelium (RPE), and the traumatic insult to the outer photoreceptor segments secondary to hemorrhage contraction [5]. Moreover, large, thick SMH prevents an examination of the underlying macular features. This may raise diagnostic issues, as it can become difficult to distinguish whether the SMH is due to neovascular age-related macular degeneration (AMD), or secondary to other causes, such as retinal macroaneurysm or myopic CNV.

The optimal treatment for SMH still remains uncertain. In fact, all the major clinical trials for neovascular AMD with anti-vascular endothelial growth factor (VEGF) agents and photodynamic therapy (PDT) have excluded eyes with significant SMH [6, 7]. Previous evidence has shown that the most severe and irreversible retinal damage occurs between 7 and 14 days after hemorrhage [3], and has suggested removing SMH within 7 days to preserve retinal morphology [8]. Therefore, different techniques have been proposed to displace the blood away from the macular region, thus allowing extrafoveal resorption and preventing macular photoreceptor damage [9–12].

Previous literature has reported several techniques for SMH management, including pneumatic displacement with intravitreal injection of recombinant tissue plasminogen activator (rtPA) and gas; vitrectomy followed by a subretinal rtPA injection and gas or air tamponade [10–13]; anti-VEGF injections as a monotherapy; and submacular surgery, such as full macular translocation (FMT) and autologous RPE–choroid patch graft. Several studies have focused on evaluating the functional outcomes, complete SMH displacement rates, and major post-procedural complications, while literature reviews and meta-analyses have focused on comparing these data. Besides the treatment modality, several variables may affect the treatment outcome, including the initial visual acuity (VA), the thickness, the duration and the size of the hemorrhage, and the neuroretinal damage secondary to CNV activity.

Electronic Supplementary Material The online version of this chapter (https://doi.org/10.1007/978-981-33-4168-5_24) contains supplementary material, which is available to authorized users.

G. Pertile (✉) · E. Maggio
IRCCS – Istituto di Ricovero e Cura a Carattere Scientifico, Sacro Cuore – Don Calabria, Ospedale Classificato e Presidio Ospedaliero Accreditato – Regione Veneto, Verona, Italy
e-mail: emilia.maggio@sacrocuore.it

A. Jain et al. (eds.), *Cutting-edge Vitreoretinal Surgery*,
https://doi.org/10.1007/978-981-33-4168-5_24

24.2 Pneumatic Displacement with rtPA and Gas

Recombinant tissue plasminogen activator (rtPA) is a thrombolytic agent that activates plasminogen into plasmin, which enzymatically liquefies hemorrhages by lysing fibrin. In SMH treatment, this allows a subsequent gas tamponade to displace the liquefied blood from the macula to a site where it potentially causes less functional damage to central visual acuity. Moreover, since fibrin is located between the photoreceptors in the context of SMH, SMH liquefaction also allows for detaching the fibrin from the outer retina, thereby minimizing shearing damage to the outer photoreceptor segments.

Among the gases commonly used in vitreoretinal surgery, sulfur hexafluoride gas (SF6) is the most frequently used for SMH displacement because of its short temporal permanence in the vitreous cavity, which allows for early verification of treatment effectiveness. Other gases used for this purpose include C3F8 and C2F6 [14].

Intravitreal rtPA and gas injection is performed in the operating room, after topical anesthesia and preoperative antisepsis with povidone iodine using sterile gloves, a drape, and a lid speculum. The treatment consists of injecting the eye via the pars plana, using a 27-gauge needle with 50 μg of alteplase diluted with a balanced salt solution of up to 0.05 mL, followed by an intravitreal injection of 100% SF6 up to 0.3 mL. Before the procedure, an anterior chamber paracentesis to reduce intraocular pressure is recommended. Patients need to be instructed to maintain a face-down position overnight and as much as possible during the ensuing week. The day after the procedure, IOP evaluation and dilated fundus examination are also recommended. The efficacy of blood displacement is evaluated 1 week after the procedure (Fig. 24.1). Blood displacement by intravitreal rtPA and gas injection also allows for postoperative diagnostic testing, the evaluation of macular features, and the identification of CNV type and location, and thus guide further treatment opportunities.

Other previously described techniques have included either only intravitreal gas [15–17] or only rtPA [18] injection, either combined or not combined with anti-VEGF agents, and applied either preoperatively or postoperatively [19, 20].

In the previous literature, intravitreal rtPA and gas injection treatment, either combined with anti-VEGF agents or not, has reported a 50–100% complete displacement rate. The reported range of SMH recurrence is 0–27%, and the range of vitreous hemorrhages 0–45% [14]. Previous studies have also shown that rtPA and gas injection has a better visual outcome when compared with the natural history of SMH. A recent literature review has reported a mean BCVA improvement from 20/726 at baseline to 20/324 upon the final visit [21].

Pneumatic displacement with rtPA and SF6 is a fast, minimally invasive, and quite feasible procedure. Additional advantages include the lack of need for trained personnel or dedicated equipment, and considerably lower costs compared to other procedures. Moreover, this strategy is unlikely to interfere with subsequent AMD treatments, whereas in eyes requiring further treatments for CNV, previous vitrectomy could reduce the effect of anti-VEGF therapy by shortening the drug's temporal permanence in the vitreous cavity.

Some concerns have been raised regarding the opportunity to use rtPA in association with gas for hemorrhage displacement. In fact, certain previous studies have found a high displacement rate in eyes treated with gas only [15–17]. Moreover, because of its molecular weight, doubts remain whether rtPA penetrates the retina. However, Kamei et al. [22] discovered a rtPA signal in the neural retina of some rabbit eyes after injection into the vitreous cavity. The authors suggested that its diffusion into the subretinal space occurred through microscopic retinal tears secondary to the subretinal hemorrhage. In addition, a recent experimental study demonstrated that rtPA administered into the vitreous cavity is capable of penetrating the intact retina and reaching the subretinal space in

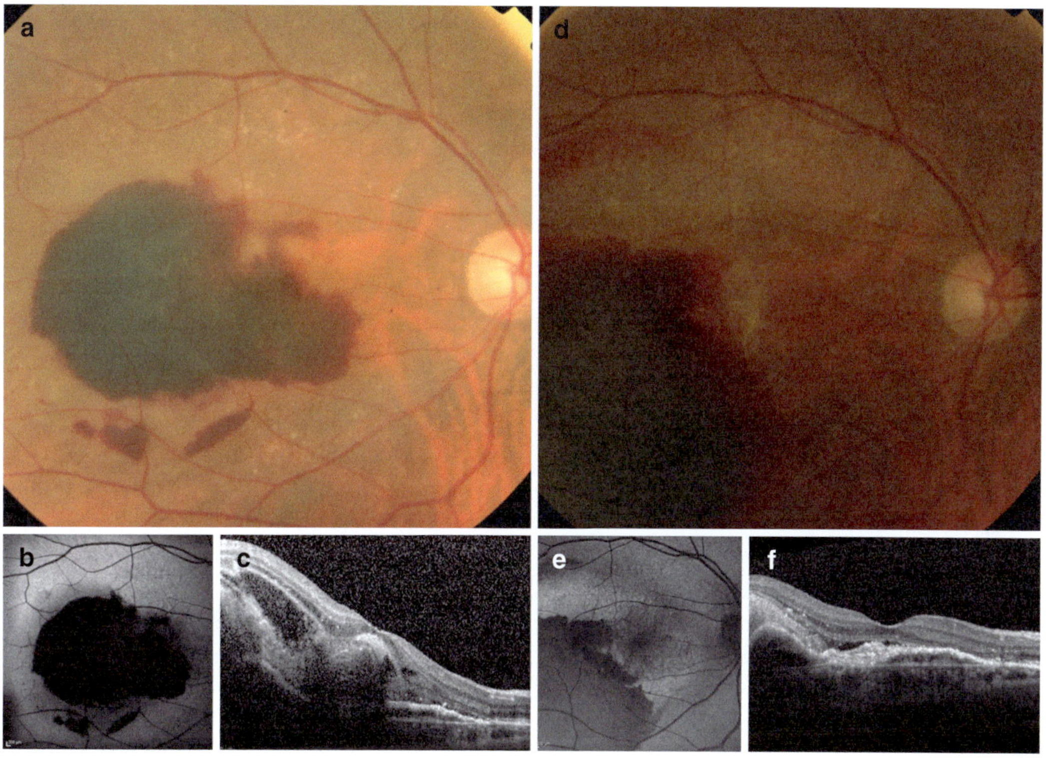

Fig. 24.1 Example of submacular hemorrhage displacement with intravitreal rTPA and SF6. (**a**) Color fundus photography showing submacular hemorrhage involving the fovea. Female patient, aged 82 years, BCVA 1.5 logMar. (**b**, **c**) Autofluorescence and OCT at the presentation: the blood blockage prevents an examination of the underlying macular features. The hemorrhage hides essential information from the diagnostic tools, precluding the determination of the type, size, and location of CNV, as well as the evaluation of anatomic factors that potentially predict improvement in visual acuity. (**d**) Color fundus photography 1-week after the treatment with intravitreal rTPA and SF6. SMH is displaced away from the foveal area. BCVA: 0.2 logMar. (**e**, **f**) Autofluorescence and OCT 1-week after the treatment: the hemorrhage displacement allows the evaluation of macular features, lesion type and location identification, and outer retinal layer integrity

rats [23]. The use of rtPA in association with gas seems to provide additional therapeutic advantages, since rtPA has been found to effectively liquefy hemorrhages by lysing fibrin [24]. SMH liquefaction may facilitate its separation from the retina and RPE, and thus prevent a possible traumatic insult to the outer photoreceptor segments due to pneumatic SMH displacement [14]. Moreover, rtPA is not toxic to the retina at a specific concentration when administrated either subretinally and intravitreally [25, 26]. Therefore, the use of rtPA in association with gas might be a safe and effective way to improve blood displacement.

24.3 Vitrectomy Followed by Subretinal rtPA Injection

More invasive procedures for SMH displacement have included vitrectomy followed by a subretinal rtPA injection and gas or air tamponade [10–13], either combined or not combined with internal limiting membrane peeling (ILM), and/or anti-VEGF agent administration [14].

After a complete pars plana vitrectomy, subretinal rtPA is injected into the subretinal space through a self-sealing retinotomy, using a 41-gauge needle connected to a tuberculin syringe by tubing, and filled with the rtPA solution at a 12.5-μg in 0.1 mL concentration. Once the 41-G tip is inserted through the retina, the fluid is injected into the subretinal space (injected volumes range from 0.05 to 0.15 mL) creating a local retinal detachment that encompasses the blood clot. Then, the vitreous cavity is filled with an SF6 gas/air mixture (18–20%) and the patient is instructed to maintain a facedown position. In some studies, ILM peeling at the posterior pole was performed to prevent the formation of a macular pucker or proliferative vitreoretinopathy (PVR) after surgery. Moreover, the co-application of subretinal rtPA and anti-VEGF was described. No cleavage or functional inactivation of bevacizumab by rtPA was found in vitro.

Postoperative complications include recurrent submacular hemorrhage, retinal detachment (RD), or vitreous hemorrhages. The complete displacement rates for these techniques are reported at 53–100%. The range of submacular hemorrhage recurrence is 0–27%. The range of RD is 0–11%, and the percentage of vitreous hemorrhages reaches from 0 to 67% [14]. No toxicity was reported after subretinal TPA.

Previous studies have also reported a high percentage of eyes with improved VA [14]. Researchers have highlighted a possible relief of any vitreomacular traction that could affect visual function [21], a likely increase in vitreous oxygenation, and potentially more complete and certain SMH removal [21] as possible advantages of these procedures. The disadvantages include vitrectomy reducing the effect of anti-VEGF therapy by shortening the temporal permanence of the drug in the vitreous cavity, and a higher rate of complications as RD when compared with intravitreal injections [21]. Vitrectomy also requires vitreoretinal expertise, an operating room, and dedicated equipment that may delay treatment, while also having much higher costs [21].

24.4 Intravitreal Anti-VEGF Injections

Some studies [27–30] have investigated the efficacy of intravitreal anti-VEGF injections as a monotherapy for SMH treatment in AMD-affected eyes, reporting improvements in or stabilization of VA in most patients. However, a recent, large, retrospective study [30] has found limited efficacy in eyes with extensive hemorrhage or severe subfoveal hemorrhage. Moreover, in some cases, patients were offered the treatment when the SMH was located primarily outside of the foveola [27]. Although intravitreal anti-VEGF agents are the standard of care for CNV, anti-VEGF alone—without SMH displacement away from the macular region—might not prevent the retinotoxic effect caused by the presence of blood in the subfoveal area, which is a fundamental, causative factor for permanent retinal damage. In addition, a thick SMH might limit anti-VEGF penetration into the neovascular lesion [30].

Therefore, the majority of patients affected by AMD with acute SMH are most likely to benefit from an early displacement by rtPA and gas injection, followed by continued anti-VEGF treatment.

24.5 Submacular Surgery

Another possible approach to SMH management is submacular surgery as a first therapeutic option, without any prior gas/rtPA blood displacement. Although the Submacular Surgery Trial [31] was unable to demonstrate any benefit from simply removing CNV and blood in eyes with predominantly hemorrhagic CNV secondary to AMD, diverse surgical approaches such as FMT or autologous RPE–choroid patch graft, which are able to restore the RPE–choroid complex underneath the macula, have been found to preserve macular function and improve vision in selected cases [32–37]. The rationale for submacular surgery is to relocate functioning foveal neuroretina from the compromised RPE area below the SMH to an undamaged RPE–choroid complex.

Full macular translocation is preferable in case of low visual acuity in the fellow eye to prevent postoperative diplopia due to the compensatory and contextually performed muscular surgery. Only when the angle of rotation cannot be predicted because of massive subretinal hemorrhage are the muscles adjusted after retinal rotation. In phakic eyes, phacoemulsification with intraocular lens implantation is undertaken. After a pars plana vitrectomy, the posterior hyaloid is detached and the vitreous base is shaved carefully with a vitreous cutter. Retinal detachment is induced by injecting a balanced salt solution with a 41-gauge cannula into the subretinal space, and complete detachment is accomplished through fluid–air exchange. After the retina is detached, a 340° retinotomy is performed at the ora serrata. While lifting the retina, the SMH and the CNV are removed and the afferent vessel is cauterized. Thereafter, the 360° retinotomy is completed and the retina is stabilized with perfluorocarbon liquid (PFCL). The retina is rotated carefully approximately 45°, preferably upward. After the translocation is completed, PFCL is injected up to the ora serrata to reattach the retina, and laser photocoagulation is performed at the edge of the retinotomy. Finally, PFCL is exchanged with silicone oil. The silicone is removed after 2–3 months.

Autologous RPE–choroid patch graft permits replacing the CNV-damaged choroidal tissue by positioning a healthy RPE transplant from the mid-periphery of the same eye under the macula. Phacoemulsification and IOL implantation are performed in phakic eyes. After the induction of a posterior vitreous detachment, a complete vitrectomy is performed. Then, the temporal retina is detached with the injection of a balanced salt solution (BSS) into the subretinal space through a 41-gauge cannula, followed by fluid–air exchanges to complete the detachment. A 180° temporal retinotomy is performed as close as possible to the ora serrata. The SNH and the CNV are removed after exposing the subretinal space with the temporal retina overlying the nasal retina. Before harvesting the graft, a laser is utilized to delineate the shape and size of the graft, which may reduce hemorrhage risk. Then, a full-thickness patch of choroid, choriocapillaries, Bruch's membrane, and RPE is isolated from the mid-periphery. Perfluorocarbon liquid (PFCL) is injected into the subretinal space to prevent shrinkage of the graft and facilitate its positioning in the sub-foveal area. The PFCL is aspirated from the subretinal space, the temporal retina is flipped over from its position, and the PFCL is reinjected into the preretinal space to reattach the retina. Peripheral laser endophotocoagulation is performed at the edge of the retinotomy. A PFCL–silicone oil 1000 exchange completes the surgery (Video 24.1). The silicone oil is removed about 2 months later. Postoperative complications for submacular surgery include RD, PVR, CNV recurrence, choroidal hemorrhage, epiretinal membrane, cystic macular edema, and diplopia.

Significant long-term visual gains are reported for SMH submacular surgery, and there are interesting, although complex, therapeutic alternatives for the management of the disease. Consequently, these alternatives should be reserved for selected cases, including patients with very thick and extensive SMH and/or association with extensive vitreous hemorrhage. Moreover, these techniques may be applied as second treatments after rtPA and gas displacement in cases where displacing the blood reveals severe subretinal damage, such as subfoveal RPE tearing or RPE atrophy. In these cases, therapeutic strategies targeting the lack of RPE are more likely to obtain a visual improvement when compared to anti-VEGF treatment as a monotherapy, or to vitectomy with a subretinal rtPA injection.

24.6 Submacular Hemorrhage Due to Causes Other than AMD

Submacular hemorrhage (SMH) occurs most commonly in association with exudative age-related macular degeneration (AMD). However, it may arise from several other conditions, such as high myopia, angioid streaks, ocular histoplasmosis syndrome, ruptured retinal arterial macroaneurysm (RAM), trauma, Valsalva retinopathy, Terson's syndrome, and coagulopathies.

In eyes affected by high myopia, SMH may be a consequence of myopic choroidal neovascularization (CNV) or related to the formation of new lacquer cracks (LCs). In the process of new

LC formation, the mechanical rupture of Bruch's membrane and the choriocapillaris complex may result in subretinal bleeding. Moreover, SMH may also be subsequent to the progression of a preexisting LC. In these cases, SMHs are commonly small and may not require any treatment. After SMH absorption, the visual prognosis may be fair, above all when LCs do not occur across the central fovea. SMH associated with LC is not considered a risk factor for the development of myopic CNV [38–40]. On the contrary, subretinal bleeding from a myopic CNV may be more detrimental to visual function and require treatment with anti-vascular endothelial growth factor (anti-VEGF) therapy.

Angioid streaks result from breaks in a degenerated Bruch's membrane, due to the degradation and mineralization of collagen and elastic lamina [41]. SMH may occur with no evidence of CNV, resulting from spontaneous rupture at the area of the angioid streak, or as a consequence of mild ocular trauma or even indirect trauma. These hemorrhages usually resolve spontaneously and, in case of small SMH, the course may be favorable over the short follow-up period. However, angioid streaks may be associated with CNV, which may cause subretinal bleeding with a more severe prognosis.

Also, ocular histoplasmosis syndrome may be associated with SMH as a result of a CNV and/or a disruption of the choriocapillaris and Bruch's membrane [42].

The rupture of a RAM causes extravasation of blood, which may spread into the vitreous, under the hyaloid, under the internal limiting membrane (ILM), within the retina or under the retina [43]. The treatment modalities differ depending on the SMH site and on the involved ocular structures. Intravitreal rtPA and gas injection is suitable for the displacement of hemorrhages limited to the macular area involving the subretinal space. Pre-macular hemorrhages usually occur at the interface between the posterior hyaloid and the ILM. They may be treated with an Nd:YAG laser. The laser treatment aims at the photodisruption of the posterior hyaloid and ILM to drain the entrapped hemorrhage underneath. After the Nd:YAG laser photodisruption, the blood drainage through the cleft into the vitreous cavity may become visible [44]. Vitrectomy with subretinal injection of rtPA and air or gas tamponade has been described for the treatment of massive submacular hemorrhages or multilevel macular hemorrhages, with or without vitreous hemorrhage, caused by a ruptured RAM [43, 45]. The visual prognosis of pre-macular hemorrhages is usually favorable. On the contrary, hemorrhages involving the subretinal space may be more detrimental to visual function.

Blunt ocular trauma may be associated with macular hemorrhages. They may be combined with other ocular alterations, such as vitreous hemorrhage, Berlin's edema, and choroidal rupture. The occurrence of a choroidal rupture may be complicated by the subsequent development of CNV.

Macular hemorrhages occurring in Terson's syndrome and Valsalva retinopathy are mostly sub-ILM. In Terson's syndrome, intraocular hemorrhage is associated with subarachnoid hemorrhaging, resulting from a spike in intracranial pressure that may occur as a consequence of multiple conditions, including carotid artery occlusion, cortical venous sinus thrombosis, and lumbosacral myelomeningocele. It may be present in the vitreous, sub-hyaloid, or intraretina/sub-ILM. Unilateral or bilateral hemorrhages in Valsalva retinopathy result from the rupture of small superficial capillaries in the macula due to a sudden increase in intrathoracic or intraabdominal pressure. It may be subsequent to activities such as coughing, vomiting, labor, and straining for a bowel movement. The extravasation of blood usually spreads below the ILM, but may also involve the vitreous cavity or subhyaloid space.

Several coagolopathies may be associated with macular and/or ocular hemorrhages, including disseminated intravascular coagulation, Von Willebrand Disease, sickle cell disease, thrombotic thrombocytopenic purpura, and idiopathic thrombocytopenic purpura. Manifestations and management may differ depending on the underlying etiology.

24.7 Conclusion

The natural history of submacular hemorrhage secondary to AMD is potentially devastating when left untreated, mainly as a consequence of blood persisting in the subfoveal area. Many procedures have been described for SMH management, most of which displaces the blood away from the macular region. All these procedures—both the invasive and the less invasive—have shown a high rate of complete displacement and demonstrated significant visual improvement. Nevertheless, invasive procedures have generated a higher rate of complications [14, 21]. In a recent literature review, the authors concluded that intravitreal rtPA and gas injection might be as effective as vitrectomy followed by submacular rtPA, while most likely being associated with fewer complications [21].

Intravitreal rtPA and gas injection have the advantage of being prompt and readily available. Moreover, it does not preclude the subsequent application of other therapeutic strategies. In fact, blood displacement also allows the identification of the lesion responsible for the bleeding, which can then be treated with a diverse approach, such as intravitreal injections of anti-VEGF or submacular surgery. Therefore, in the management of SMH, it may be reasonable to attempt rtPA and gas displacement as first-line treatment, and afterward consider the need for further, more invasive procedures.

References

1. Avery RL, et al. Natural history of subfoveal subretinal hemorrhage in age-related macular degeneration. Retina. 1996;16(3):183–9.
2. Bennett SR, et al. Factors prognostic of visual outcome in patients with subretinal hemorrhage. Am J Ophthalmol. 1990;109(1):33–7.
3. Toth CA, et al. Fibrin directs early retinal damage after experimental subretinal hemorrhage. Arch Ophthalmol. 1991;109(5):723–9.
4. Gillies A, Lahav M. Absorption of retinal and subretinal hemorrhages. Ann Ophthalmol. 1983;15(11):1068–74.
5. Glatt H, Machemer R. Experimental subretinal hemorrhage in rabbits. Am J Ophthalmol. 1982;94(6):762–73.
6. Rosenfeld PJ, et al. Ranibizumab for neovascular age-related macular degeneration. N Engl J Med. 2006;355(14):1419–31.
7. Brown DM, et al. Ranibizumab versus verteporfin for neovascular age-related macular degeneration. N Engl J Med. 2006;355(14):1432–44.
8. Benner JD, et al. Fibrinolytic-assisted removal of experimental subretinal hemorrhage within seven days reduces outer retinal degeneration. Ophthalmology. 1994;101(4):672–81.
9. Chen CY, et al. Management of submacular hemorrhage with intravitreal injection of tissue plasminogen activator and expansile gas. Retina. 2007;27(3):321–8.
10. Haupert CL, et al. Pars plana vitrectomy, subretinal injection of tissue plasminogen activator, and fluid-gas exchange for displacement of thick submacular hemorrhage in age-related macular degeneration. Am J Ophthalmol. 2001;131(2):208–15.
11. Olivier S, et al. Subretinal recombinant tissue plasminogen activator injection and pneumatic displacement of thick submacular hemorrhage in age-related macular degeneration. Ophthalmology. 2004;111(6):1201–8.
12. Chang W, et al. Management of thick submacular hemorrhage with subretinal tissue plasminogen activator and pneumatic displacement for age-related macular degeneration. Am J Ophthalmol. 2014;157(6):1250–7.
13. Hillenkamp J, et al. Management of submacular hemorrhage with intravitreal versus subretinal injection of recombinant tissue plasminogen activator. Graefes Arch Clin Exp Ophthalmol. 2010;248(1):5–11.
14. van Zeeburg EJ, van Meurs JC. Literature review of recombinant tissue plasminogen activator used for recent-onset submacular hemorrhage displacement in age-related macular degeneration. Ophthalmologica. 2013;229(1):1–14.
15. Ron Y, et al. Pneumatic displacement of submacular hemorrhage due to age-related macular degeneration. Ophthalmologica. 2007;221(1):57–61.
16. Gopalakrishan M, et al. Pneumatic displacement of submacular hemorrhage: safety, efficacy, and patient selection. Retina. 2007;27(3):329–34.
17. Fujikawa M, et al. Comparison of pneumatic displacement for submacular hemorrhages with gas alone and gas plus tissue plasminogen activator. Retina. 2013;33(9):1908–14.
18. Tsymanava A, Uhlig CE. Intravitreal recombinant tissue plasminogen activator without and with additional gas injection in patients with submacular hemorrhage associated with age-related macular degeneration. Acta Ophthalmol. 2012;90(7):633–8.
19. Cakir M, Cekic O, Yilmaz OF. Pneumatic displacement of acute submacular hemorrhage with and without the use of tissue plasminogen activator. Eur J Ophthalmol. 2010;20(3):565–71.
20. Mizutani T, et al. Pneumatic displacement of submacular hemorrhage with or without tissue plasminogen activator. Graefes Arch Clin Exp Ophthalmol. 2011;249(8):1153–7.

21. Stanescu-Segall D, Balta F, Jackson TL. Submacular hemorrhage in neovascular age-related macular degeneration: a synthesis of the literature. Surv Ophthalmol. 2016;61(1):18–32.
22. Kamei M, Misono K, Lewis H. A study of the ability of tissue plasminogen activator to diffuse into the subretinal space after intravitreal injection in rabbits. Am J Ophthalmol. 1999;128(6):739–46.
23. Tal K, et al. Retinal penetration of intravitreally injected tissue plasminogen activator: a rat model study. Ophthalmic Res. 2018;59(4):235–40.
24. Kamei M, Estafanous M, Lewis H. Tissue plasminogen activator in the treatment of vitreoretinal diseases. Semin Ophthalmol. 2000;15(1):44–50.
25. Luke M, et al. The retinal tolerance to bevacizumab in co-application with a recombinant tissue plasminogen activator. Br J Ophthalmol. 2007;91(8):1077–82.
26. Hesse L, Schmidt J, Kroll P. Management of acute submacular hemorrhage using recombinant tissue plasminogen activator and gas. Graefes Arch Clin Exp Ophthalmol. 1999;237(4):273–7.
27. Stifter E, et al. Intravitreal bevacizumab therapy for neovascular age-related macular degeneration with large submacular hemorrhage. Am J Ophthalmol. 2007;144(6):886–92.
28. Chang MA, et al. Prospective one-year study of ranibizumab for predominantly hemorrhagic choroidal neovascular lesions in age-related macular degeneration. Retina. 2010;30(8):1171–6.
29. Shienbaum G, et al. Management of submacular hemorrhage secondary to neovascular age-related macular degeneration with anti-vascular endothelial growth factor monotherapy. Am J Ophthalmol. 2013;155(6):1009–13.
30. Kim JH, et al. Intravitreal anti-vascular endothelial growth factor for submacular hemorrhage from choroidal neovascularization. Ophthalmology. 2014;121(4):926–35.
31. Bressler NM, et al. Surgery for hemorrhagic choroidal neovascular lesions of age-related macular degeneration: ophthalmic findings: SST report no. 13. Ophthalmology. 2004;111(11):1993–2006.
32. van Zeeburg EJ, et al. A free retinal pigment epithelium-choroid graft in patients with exudative age-related macular degeneration: results up to 7 years. Am J Ophthalmol. 2012;153(1):120–7 e2.
33. Skaf AR, Mahmoud T. Surgical treatment of age-related macular degeneration. Semin Ophthalmol. 2011;26(3):181–91.
34. van Romunde SH, et al. Long-term results of full macular translocation for choroidal neovascularization in age-related macular degeneration. Ophthalmology. 2015;122(7):1366–74.
35. van Romunde SHM, et al. Retinal pigment epithelium-choroid graft with a peripheral retinotomy for exudative age-related macular degeneration: long-term outcome. Retina. 2019;39(2):288–95.
36. Cereda MG, et al. Surgery for CNV and autologous choroidal RPE patch transplantation: exposing the submacular space. Graefes Arch Clin Exp Ophthalmol. 2010;248(1):37–47.
37. Polito A, et al. Macular translocation with 360 degrees retinotomy for management of retinal pigment epithelial tear: long-term results. Br J Ophthalmol. 2011;95(1):74–8.
38. Ohno-Matsui K, Ito M, Tokoro T. Subretinal bleeding without choroidal neovascularization in pathologic myopia. A sign of new lacquer crack formation. Retina. 1996;16(3):196–202.
39. Liu B, Zhang X, Mi L, Chen L, Wen F. Long-term natural outcomes of simple hemorrhage associated with lacquer crack in high myopia: a risk factor for myopic CNV? J Ophthalmol. 2018;2018:3150923.
40. Klein RM, Green S. The development of lacquer cracks in pathologic myopia. Am J Ophthalmol. 1988;106(3):282–5.
41. Tripathy K, Quint JM. Angioid Streaks (Knapp Streaks). StatPearls [Internet]. Treasure Island (FL): StatPearls Publishing; 2019.
42. Diaz RI, Sigler EJ, Rafieetary MR, Calzada JI. Ocular histoplasmosis syndrome. Surv Ophthalmol. 2015;60(4):279–95.
43. van Zeeburg EJ, Cereda MG, van Meurs JC. Recombinant tissue plasminogen activator, vitrectomy, and gas for recent submacular hemorrhage displacement due to retinal macroaneurysm. Graefes Arch Clin Exp Ophthalmol. 2013;251(3):733–40.
44. Sonmez K, Ozcan PY. Nd:YAG laser photodisruption for multilevel premacular hemorrhage due to isolated retinal venous macroaneurysm. Case Rep Ophthalmol Med. 2017;2017:4630187.
45. Inoue M, Shiraga F, Shirakata Y, Morizane Y, Kimura S, Hirakata A. Subretinal injection of recombinant tissue plasminogen activator for submacular hemorrhage associated with ruptured retinal arterial macroaneurysm. Graefes Arch Clin Exp Ophthalmol. 2015;253(10):1663–9.

Management of Foveoschisis

25

Tamer Ahmed Macky,
Mohamad Amr Salah Eddin Abdelhakim,
and Hassan Aly Mortada

25.1 Introduction

Foveoschisis, foveal retinoschisis or foveomacular retinoschisis, is splitting of retinal layers in the foveal area. It can be classified as:

1. Juvenile X-linked Retinoschisis [1]
2. Myopic Foveoschisis [2]
3. Vitreomacular Traction Syndrome [3]
4. Optic Disc Pit Maculopathy [4]
5. Idiopathic Foveomacular Retinoschisis [5]

25.2 Juvenile X-Linked Retinoschisis

JXLRS is one of the most common juvenile macular degenerations with an estimated prevalence of 1 in 5000 to 1 in 20,000 [6]. It is a progressive disorder with predominately ocular manifestations and minimal systemic associations affecting almost exclusively males. Female carriers do not demonstrate fundus changes, but there have been reports of heterozygotes with clinical signs [7]. General characteristics are mild to severe loss in central vision, radial streaks arising from foveal schisis, peripheral retinoschisis, and a negative electroretinogram (ERG) due to marked reduction in b-wave amplitude. It was first described in 1898 in two brothers by the Austrian ophthalmologist Josef Haas [1], and later Jager was the first to use the term "retinoschisis" in 1953 [8]. Today, both terms X-linked and congenital retinoschisis are synonymous with JXLRS.

25.2.1 Pathogenesis and Genetic Background

JXLRS is an X-linked recessive disorder due to numerous mutations, predominantly missense, in the retinoschisin 1 (RS1) gene, which encodes for the protein retinoschisin [9] important for the adhesive properties of different cell types [7]. Retinoschisin is expressed in the retina during early development and maintained throughout life, which explains the progressive nature of this disorder, and allows gene replacement to be a potential target for therapeutic intervention [10].

Electronic Supplementary Material The online version of this chapter (https://doi.org/10.1007/978-981-33-4168-5_25) contains supplementary material, which is available to authorized users.

T. A. Macky (✉) · M. A. S. E. Abdelhakim
H. A. Mortada
Department of Ophthalmology, Cairo University, Cairo, Egypt

A. Jain et al. (eds.), *Cutting-edge Vitreoretinal Surgery*,
https://doi.org/10.1007/978-981-33-4168-5_25

25.2.2 Clinical Features

The consistent clinical feature of JXLRS is the presence of foveal schisis appearing distinctly as a small cyst centered in the fovea and arranged in a stellate pattern or with radial striae as a spoke-wheel pattern. In some cases, it might not be initially apparent by clinical examination and may require optical coherence tomography (OCT). Peripheral retinoschisis is found in 50% of patients, most commonly in the inferotemporal quadrant [6].

JXLRS has been classified into four phenotypes (Figs. 25.1, 25.2, 25.3 and 25.4) based on examination and characteristics: type 1, foveal (without peripheral); type 2, foveo-lamellar (without peripheral); type 3, complex (foveal, lamellar, and peripheral); and type 4, foveo-peripheral [11]. Foveal schisis is appreciated on clinical examination whereas; lamellar schisis is recognized on OCT in areas that appear normal on clinical examination. Type 3 appears to be the predominant phenotype in 70% of patients [11]. The presence of retinoschisin in the inner and outer retina may account for the presence of lamellar schisis, deep to the nerve fiber layer (NFL). Currently, no studies have evaluated the prognostic significance of the various phenotypes of JXLRS.

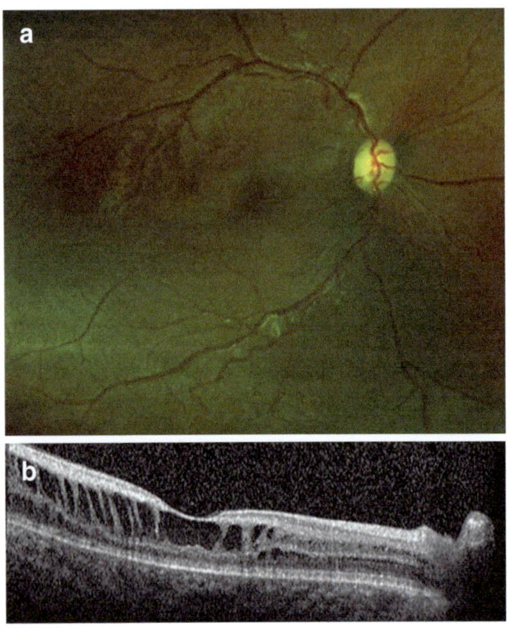

Fig. 25.1 Type 1 is the foveal type where the juvenile X-linked retinoschisis presents clinically apparent foveal schisis and no peripheral retinoschisis on clinical examination and on color photograph (**a**) while the SD-OCT (**b**) shows the schisis does not extend beyond what is noted on clinical examination

Retinoschisis can also be categorized as exudative and non-exudative. Eyes with exudative retinoschisis have hard exudates on examination [12] (Fig. 25.5). It is unclear if the lipid in these patients is secondary to resolving hemorrhage, vascular incompetence, both, or neither. The inner retina may develop retinal holes or tears, or it may fragment over time, leaving membranous remnants. Some use the term "vitreous veils" to describe these, although they are retinal or retinal and vitreal in nature and not only vitreous. In addition, the inner retina may or may not have retinal blood vessels. In some patients, the inner retinal vessels may cross into the vitreous, whereas in others the retinal vessels may course in the outer leaf of the retina. Vitreous hemorrhage is a common complication, occurring in 30–40% of eyes with JXLRS. Vitreous hemorrhage occurs when bridging vessels rupture or secondary to neovascularization.

Patients may also develop optic disc and retinal neovascularization and may thus present with a vitreous hemorrhage. The retina may also be dragged nasally, possibly secondary to the dehiscence of the NFL temporally [13]. Additionally, in some patients, the peripheral retina may also have a metallic sheen, retinal pigment epithelium (RPE) changes, intraretinal blood cysts, or sheathed and occluded vessels [6]. A tapetal reflex associated with the Mizuo-Nakamura phenomenon has also been described.

25.2.3 Disease Natural Course

The natural course of JXLRS varies considerably. Visual acuity deterioration usually appears gradually in the first and second decades of life and stays relatively stable until the fifth or sixth decade. However, some patients may experience a sudden vision loss secondary to the

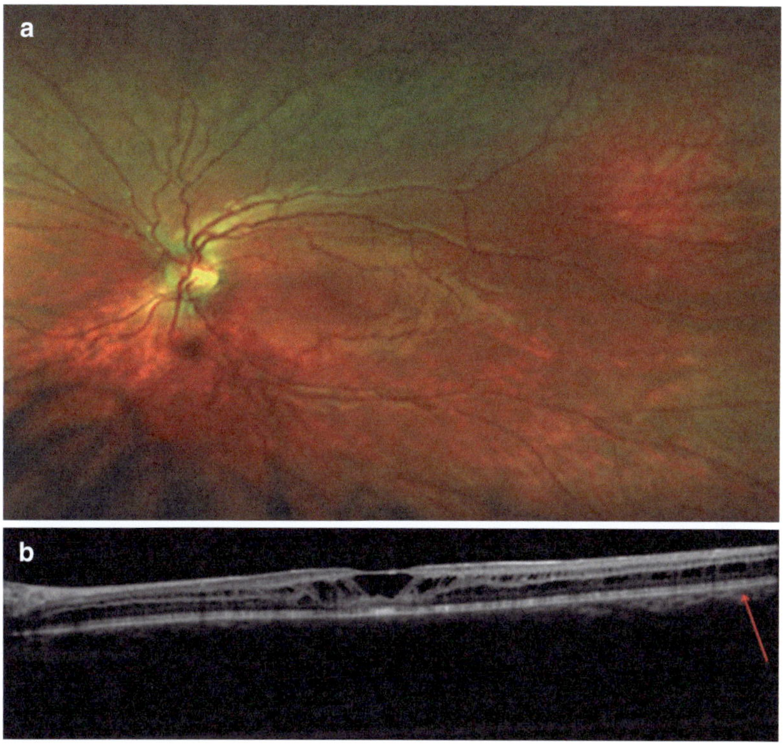

Fig. 25.2 Type 2 is the foveolamellar where the juvenile X-linked retinoschisis presents with foveal schisis on clinical examination and on color photograph (**a**) and lamellar schisis (**b**) (red arrow) on SD-OCT, which extends beyond the schisis noted on clinical examination

development of complications as retinal detachment (RD) and/or vitreous hemorrhage. On the other hand, spontaneous resolution of bullous peripheral retinoschisis has been reported with apposition of the inner and outer retinal layers, occasionally leaving a pigment line. Often, the classic radiating striae are seen at earlier age regress gradually and are replaced by a blunted foveal reflex later on with older patients [14]. Macular atrophy is one of the most common causes of vision loss in older patients due to RPE changes that also affect the peripheral retina. Sometimes, a large posterior schisis cavity can develop when the intraretinal septae in the fovea break down and the microcysts coalesce causing further vision loss.

Rhegmatogenous RD (RRD) may either develop secondary to outer retinal breaks in the presence of concurrent inner retinal breaks or from full-thickness retinal breaks occurring during vitreous detachment. On the other hand, tractional RD (TRD) may also develop from the retinoschisis cavity and/or posterior hyaloidal contraction. It is worth noting that chronic retinoschisis cavities without RD can exhibit a pigmented demarcation line, and not all patients with JXLRS and chronic RD exhibit a pigment line. Thus, a pigment line cannot solely be used to include or exclude a chronic RD in these patients.

25.2.4 Diagnostic Investigations

25.2.4.1 Optical Coherence Tomography

Although diagnosis is based on clinical examination, yet spectral domain OCT (SD-OCT) has revealed that the area of retinoschisis markedly extends beyond the ophthalmoscopically visible spoke-wheel pattern (Figs. 25.2 and 25.3). Cystoid changes may involve various retinal layers from the NFL to the nuclear layer (Fig. 25.1). In older patients, SD-OCT might show absence of retinoschisis, retinal thinning, and epiretinal membranes (ERM) that increase the difficulty to differentiate from other forms of macular dystrophy.

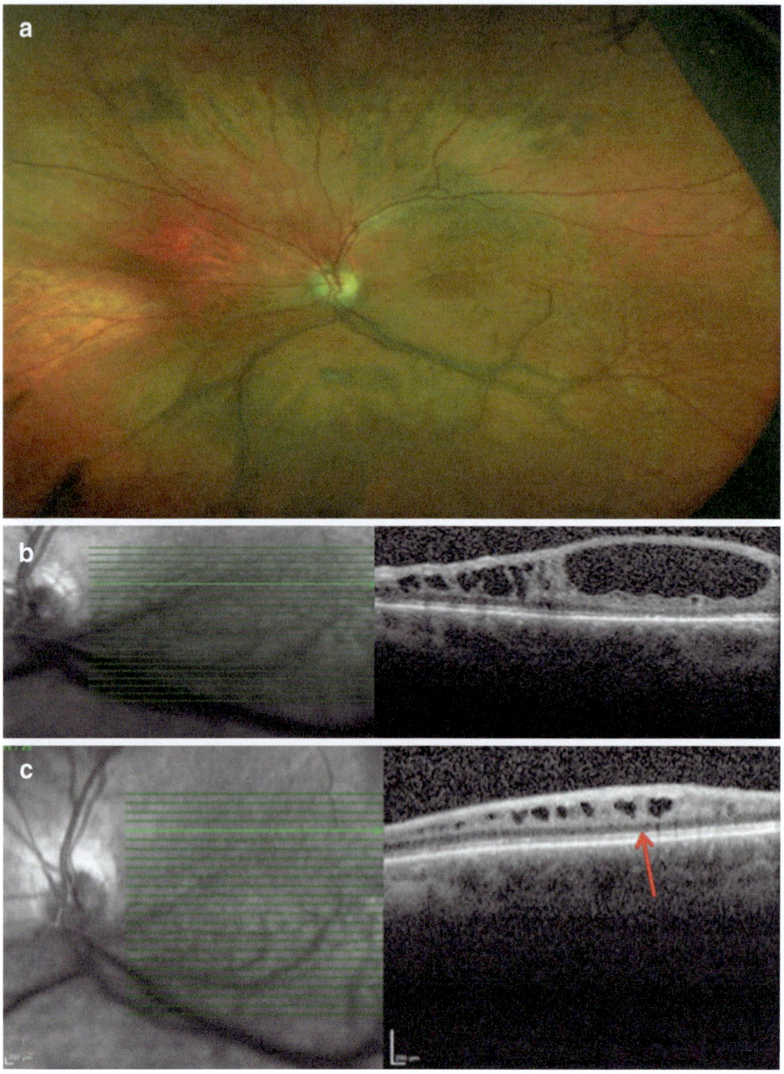

Fig. 25.3 Type 3 is the complex type where the juvenile X-linked retinoschisis presents with foveal (**a**), peripheral (**b**), and lamellar (red arrow) components (**c**)

25.2.4.2 Fluorescein Angiography

There is no leakage associated within the cystic-like spaces unlike macular edema-associated vascular diseases. However, hyperfluorescence may occur secondary to either diffuse pigmentary changes or vascular leakage within peripheral schisis. Some patients may even demonstrate non-perfusion in both schitic and non-schitic areas [15]. Fundus autofluorescence shows foveal alterations due to altered light transmission in the area of retinoschisis which is a characteristic sign.

25.2.4.3 Electrophysiology

The characteristic ERG sign is called "negative" ERG elicited by a bright flash of light in the dark-adapted retina in which the a-wave is larger than the b-wave in contrast to the normal findings. Electronegative ERG is found, even in eyes with schisis confined to the fovea. In the early stages of disease, at younger age, patients may have a normal a-wave, although with progressive involvement of the photoreceptors there is a reduction in the a-wave [16].

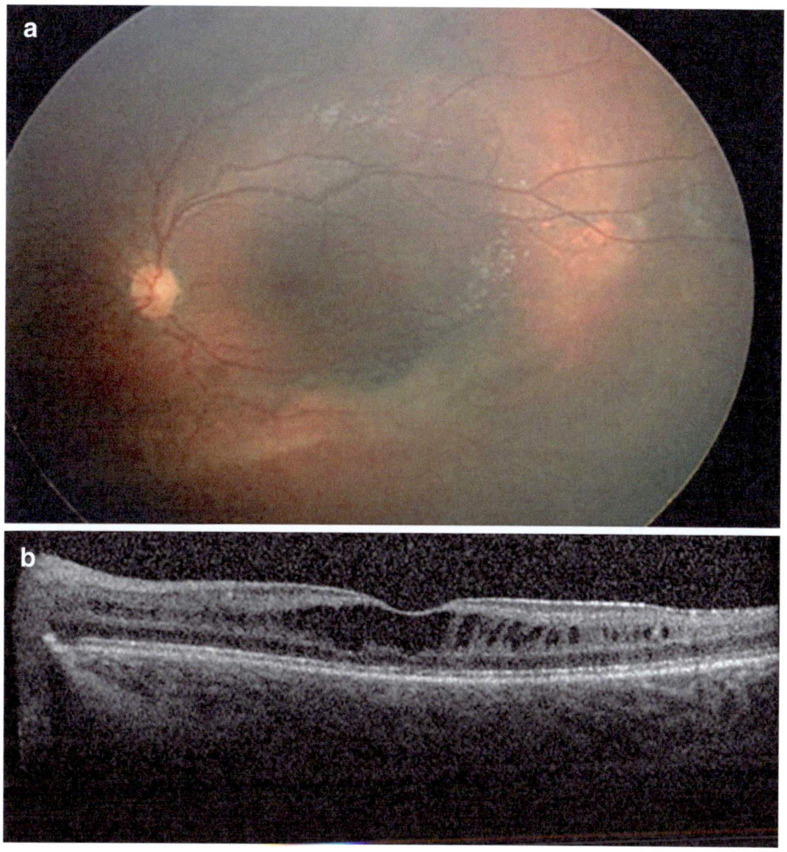

Fig. 25.4 Type 4 where the juvenile X-linked retinoschisis presents with foveal and peripheral retinoschisis only in the color photograph (**a**). The foveal schisis noted on SD-OCT (**b**) does not extend beyond what is apparent clinically

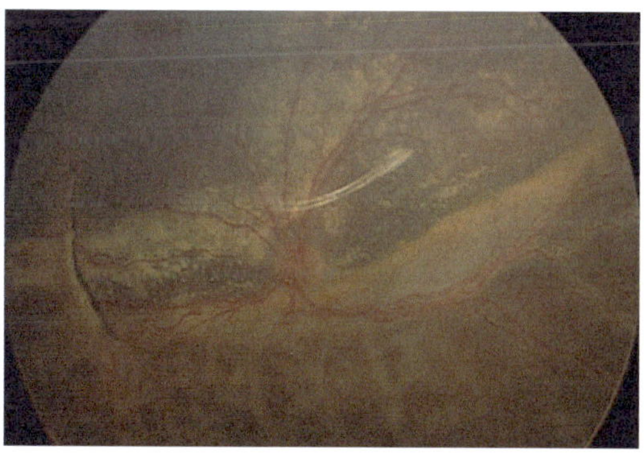

Fig. 25.5 Exudative juvenile X-linked retinoschisis with peripheral bullous schisis overhanging the macula and hard exudate

25.2.4.4 Genetic Testing

Genetic testing of the RS1 gene or use of a multigene panel that includes RS1, and to others within the family.

25.2.5 Treatment

JXLRS is a complex disease with multiple and variable pathological changes, complications, and presentations, thus the management plan will be decided on an individual basis and with a complete understanding of this disorder natural course. The decision is further complicated by the availability of several medical and surgical options. In most cases, treatment is limited to prescription of low-vision aids.

25.2.5.1 Medical Intervention for Retinoschisis (Foveal and Peripheral)

Currently, there are no clinical trials that support specific medical interventions for foveal JXLRS. Few reports have found success with topical or oral carbonic anhydrase inhibitors for both foveal and peripheral retinoschisis [17]

within no clear consensus. Ocriplasmin has also been found in a report to lead to resolution, but the schisis recurred [18].

25.2.5.2 Surgical Intervention

Prophylactic Intervention

Prophylactic treatment of peripheral retinoschisis is controversial. First, spontaneous regression of retinoschisis cavities has been reported [19]. Second, peripheral retinoschisis has low rates of progression to TRD of about 10%, and RRD of about 10–20%. Thus eyes, with or without inner wall retinal breaks, that do not progress or extend into the macula should be observed [20]. Therefore, prophylactic laser barricade for stable peripheral retinoschisis should be avoided due to the high rates of iatrogenic retinal breaks and progression to RRDs [21].

However, barricade laser photocoagulation—guided by OCT, if available—with low power (less than 200 mW), long duration burns (greater than 300–400 ms) for progressive peripheral retinoschisis may be an alternative option in young patients that are unable to tolerate prolonged anesthesia or refuse surgery. Although, prophylactic inner wall retinectomy or drainage has also been reported, yet again in the absence of progression it should be avoided due to the risk of RRD or proliferative vitreoretinopathy (PVR) [22].

Vitreoretinal Surgery

The surgical intervention decision will always depend on many factors namely; progression of vision loss, patient's age, retinoschisis location and configuration, status of the other eye, status of the macula, presence or absence of RD and its extent, and the severity of the pathology.

Indications and Decision-Making

Peripheral Retinoschisis in the Absence of RD

A young patient with either stable or slowly progressive vision changes in the weaker eye may warrant observation and more extensive discussion with the family. On the other hand, a monocular patient with progressive vision loss in the better eye due to advancing peripheral retinoschisis will likely undergo a surgical intervention rather than observation.

Peripheral retinoschisis cavities with thin inner leaflets and inner retinal holes are more stable than cavities with smooth uninterrupted inner leaflets. Although the exact reason is unknown, free communication of fluid between the intraschisis cavity and vitreous with inner wall breaks may create a more stable vitreoretinal interface by equilibrating the push-pull forces between the schisis and vitreous cavities, respectively. Thus, progressive bullous retinoschisis overhanging, but not involving, the macula may be amenable to vitrectomy. It is worth mentioning, that surgical intervention for progressive peripheral retinoschisis involving the macula may have anatomic success but visual success may be more unpredictable.

Peripheral Retinoschisis in the Presence of RD Without Macular Involvement

The posterior hyaloid in pediatric eyes is intimately adherent to the retina [23], its incomplete separation increases the risk of PVR with posterior hyaloidal contraction-related RD [13]. Therefore, better first to evaluate patients with rhegmatogenous schisis RDs for primary scleral buckling. Outer wall breaks are difficult to find but are often located at the posterior edge of the schisis RD cavity.

Peripheral Retinoschisis in the Presence of RD with Macular Involvement

If the rhegmatogenous or tractional schisis-related RD involves the macula, then vitrectomy is the choice due to difficulty in achieving proper support of posterior outer wall breaks with an encircling buckle. Additional indications include vitreous hemorrhage and exudative RD [24].

Foveoschisis in the Absence of RD

Classically should be observed or offered medical treatment. Given the difficulty in removing all of the posterior hyaloid in pediatric patients there exists the risk of creating full-thickness retinal breaks associated with the adherent posterior hyaloid intraoperatively or even hyaloidal contraction postoperatively as well. However, several reports suggest successful resolution of macular schisis with PPV, with internal limiting membrane (ILM) peeling with or without foveal sparing, and gas tamponade [25].

Vitrectomy Principles and Techniques

- As mentioned, the presence of a demarcation line does not solely indicate the existence of a RD, as it is present in patients with long-standing retinoschisis.
- Some authors advocate the use of preoperative ocriplasmin for posterior hyaloidal separation in progressive bullous peripheral retinoschisis, rhegmatogenous schisis, and tractional schisis RDs [26]. However, the use of triamcinolone, and/or perfluorocarbon (PFO) are also useful common adjuncts for both vitreous dissection and identification of outer wall breaks.
- Try to preserve the inner leaflet as much as possible in the hope of using future gene therapy in re-approximating the inner and outer leaflets. However, if the posterior hyaloid cannot be separated from the inner schisis leaflet due to either an intimate adherence or thin inner leaflet, a limited inner wall retinectomy may be performed with or without light laser over the retinectomy and outer wall breaks [24]. If vitreous traction remains in rhegmatogenous schisis RD, we proceed with an inner wall retinectomy and drain through the existing outer wall break with a large bore cannula followed by silicone oil (SO) tamponade.
- A similar approach is utilized in PVR schisis RDs with careful peeling of the overlying proliferation in a posterior to anterior fashion using a combination of the Trese spatula and max grip forceps with or without PFO to both provide and control the degree of counter traction on the retina.
- In tractional schisis RDs in which a shallow macular detachment is present but there is no outer wall break, vitrectomy is beneficial with careful hyaloidal dissection and internal drainage of the schisis cavity with a small gauge needle.
- In type 2 or 3 JXLRS (unlike type 4), try to avoid inner wall retinectomies and dissect the anterior proliferation overlying the schisis cavity, as the lamellar cavities are more difficult to separate from the deeper layers of the retina. However, it is not an absolute contraindication.
- Surgical technique for peripheral retinoschisis drainage, could be through a 23- or 25-gauge transconjunctival 3-port vitrectomy approach. In the 3-port technique, use an anterior segment infusion cannula if the bullous schisis is retrolenticular. After careful core and posterior vitreous hyaloidal separation, a small gauge cannula (42-gauge) is utilized to make a partial thickness, inner wall drainage retinotomy in the schisis cavity to promote drainage under fluid–air exchange.
- Use 80% SO exchange for primary tamponade for several reasons: to achieve long-term stabilization of the schisis RD, to avoid postoperative positioning that is difficult to perform in children, to aid in dampening the potential for recurrent PVR, and to reduce elevated intraocular pressure and long-term corneal decompensation that can occur with SO [27].

25.3 Myopic Foveoschisis

The term myopic foveal retinoschisis was first introduced in 1999 by Takano and Kishi [2] in patients with high myopia and posterior staphyloma. Today, MF is one of the major causes of visual loss in highly myopic eyes. MF is found to be asymptomatic in considerable percentage of patients who remain unaware of the development of MF due to its silent and slow nature [30]. Clinically, the macular changes could be visible on slit lamp biomicroscopy as microcystic appearances and almost always occurring in the presence of a posterior staphyloma, as mentioned above by Baba et al. [28]. However, OCT should be the main diagnostic tool for confirming the presence of MF [29] (Fig. 25.6). There is a consensus today that interventions are indicated for patients with documented declined visual acuity, progressive visual symptoms, metamorphop-

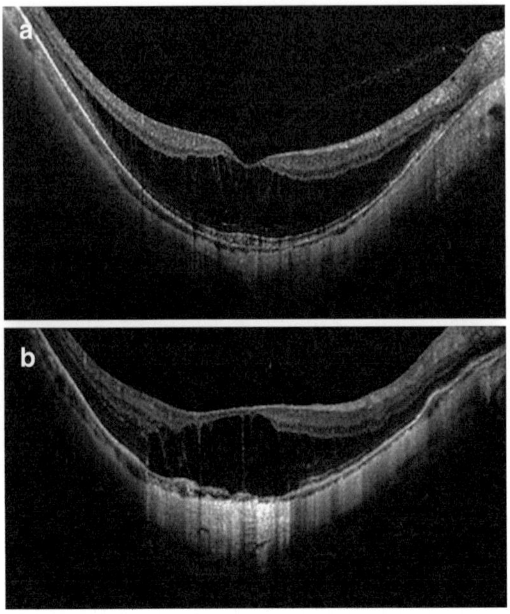

Fig. 25.6 Myopic foveoschisis (**a**, **b**); SD-OCT images showing splitting of the retinal layers with a relatively inner thicker layer and outer thinner layer

sia, and no major atrophic changes in the foveal area on OCT. The surgical technique involves either vitrectomy with ILM peel and gas tamponade or macular buckle or their combination. Figures 25.7 and 25.8 show SD-OCT scans of the macular area before and after vitrectomy and fovea sparing ILM peeling in highly myopic eye in a female patient. The pathogenesis and management of myopic foveoschisis is discussed in details in Chap. 26 page 273.

25.4 Vitreomacular Traction Syndrome

VMTS develops secondary to persistent anterior-to-posterior traction on the macula from persistent vitreomacular adhesions [30]. VMTS may result in a wide variety of retinal distortions as ERM, retinal blood vessel avulsion, retinal hole, cystoid macular edema, or TRD [31] (Fig. 25.9). It was first reported by Hotta et al. in 2004 [3], and later in 2013, the International Vitreomacular Traction Study Group [32] included foveoschisis as part of its pathological staging/classification of VMTS. All of the following criteria must be seen on at least 1 B-mode OCT scan for an eye to be classified as having VMT: (1) perifoveal vitreous cortex detachment from retinal surface; (2) macular attachment of vitreous cortex within 3-mm radius of fovea; and (3) association of attachment with foveal surface distortion, intraretinal structural changes, foveal elevation above RPE, or combination thereof, but no full-thickness interruption of all retinal layers. VMTS also know to develop cystic spaces that coalesce to form retinoschisis and foveoschisis. The main difference between VMTS associated foveoschisis and myopic foveoschisis is the absence of elongated axial length, in addition to other features of myopic maculopathy. The pathogenesis and management of VMTS associated foveoschisis is discussed in details in Chap. 23 page 243.

25.5 Pit Macular Syndrome

A significant proportion of patients with optic nerve pits may develop macular schisis, especially if the pit is on the temporal portion of the nerve head [33]. These patients appear to develop retinoschisis with an outer layer detachment confined to the central macular region. The fluid is thought to originate in the vicinity of the optic nerve and extends through the schisis, eventually arriving at the outer layer detachment [33]. The source of the fluid in optic disc pit maculopathy has been the focus of controversy, because of the paucity of available histopathologic material and because of the lack of any apparent route for the fluid to go from the nerve to the macula.

Imumura et al. in 2010 [34], demonstrated through OCT image analysis of 16 patients the possible pathogenesis of maculopathy in patients with optic nerve pits. In their study, fluid apparently emanating from the optic nerve pit extended directly into various layers of the retina, including the sub-ILM space, ganglion cell layer, inner nuclear layer, outer nuclear layer, or subretinal space; the outer nuclear layer appeared to be most commonly affected (Fig. 25.10). In 13 eyes (81%), fluid was present in more than 1 layer of the retina. RD was common (11 of 16 cases), and in 10 of the 11 cases, intraretinal fluid overlying the area of RD was observed. However, an outer

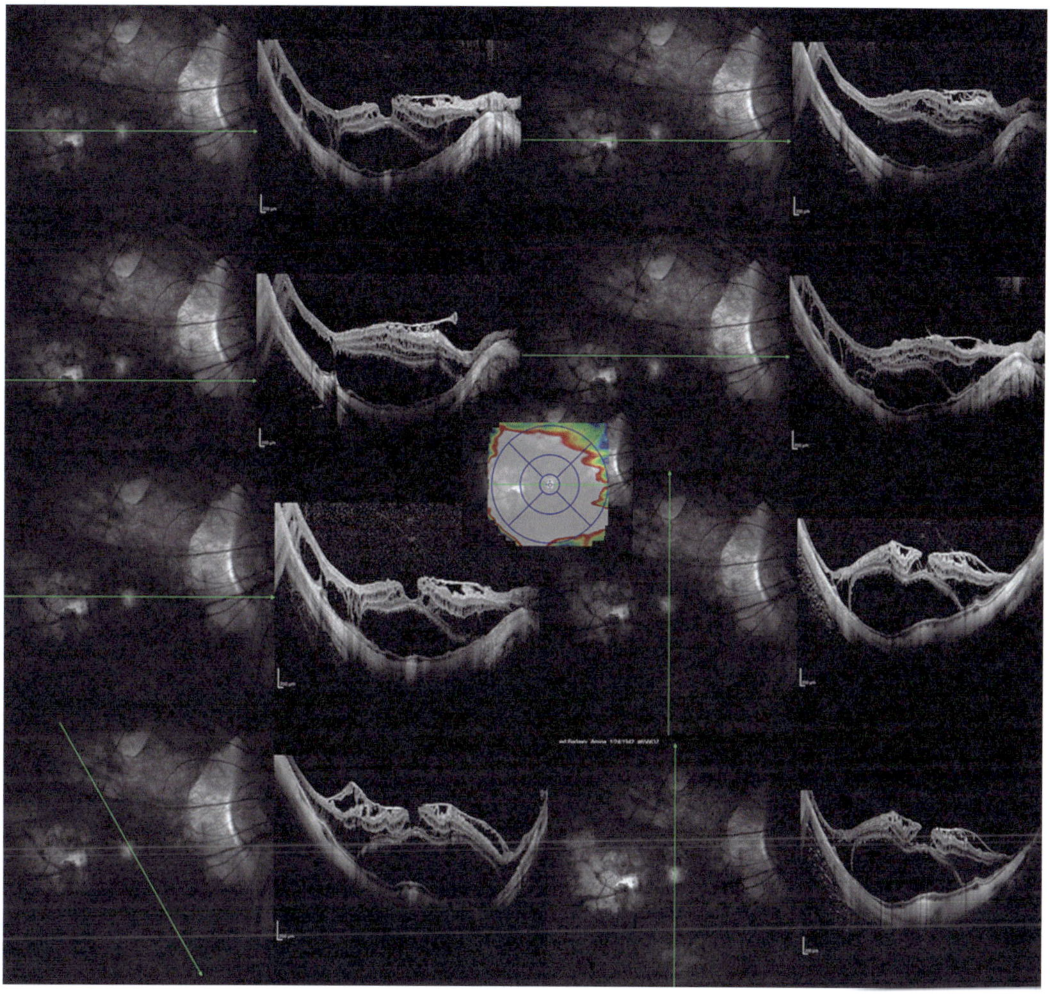

Fig. 25.7 SD-OCT scans of highly myopic eye with foveoschisis showing posterior staphyloma, and a large area of foveoschisis reaching the vascular temporal arcades

layer hole was observed in only three cases; thus, in most eyes, subretinal fluid (SRF) existed without the appearance of an outer retinal hole.

Accordingly, these OCT findings [34] show that fluid can go from optic nerve pit into different retinal layers where the fluid enters and accumulates dictating the appearance of the resultant maculopathy. This same hypothesis can be extended to explain the findings after failed surgery. Vitrectomy with intraocular gas and laser photocoagulation attempts to create a barrier to the passage of fluid from the region of the pit into the central macula. Laser photocoagulation causes full-thickness scarring of the retina in conjunction with scarring at the outer retina that serves to create adherence between the retina and RPE.

Surgical intervention classically includes complete posterior hyaloid removal, limited ILM flap removal (about one disc diameter temporal to the disc), inversion of the ILM flap to cover the disc and pit, stuffing the ILM inside the pit (may need perfluorocarbon liquid assistance), one raw of light laser at the temporal disc margin, slow fluid–air exchange mainly on the nasal retina, and finally SF6 20% gas flush in the vitreous cavity. The patient is initially placed in a prone position for few hours following the surgery, following by supine, or at least non-prone position for 5 days. The management of optic disc pit associated foveoschisis is discussed in details in Chap. 27 page 295.

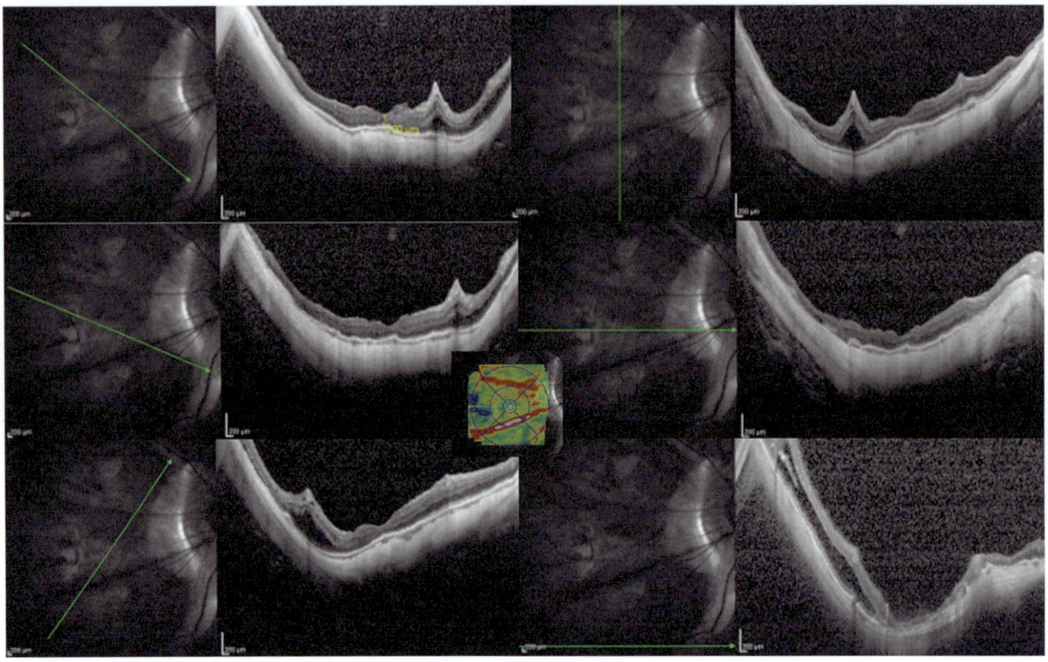

Fig. 25.8 SD-OCT scans of the eye in Fig. 25.7 following vitrectomy and foveal sparing ILM peeling showing resolution of most of the schitic cavities with small remnant fold below the foveal area

Fig. 25.9 Vitreomacular traction syndrome; SD-OCT images showing partial posterior hyaloids detachment, foveal adhesions, and anteroposterior foveal traction in non-myopic eyes causing cystic changes in (**a**) and early foveal schisis in (**b**)

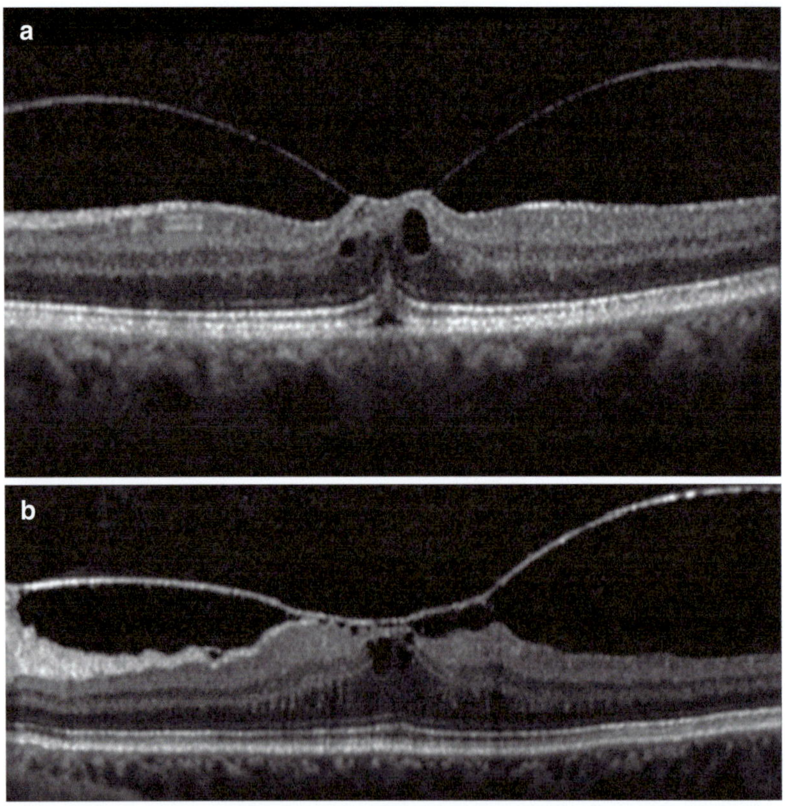

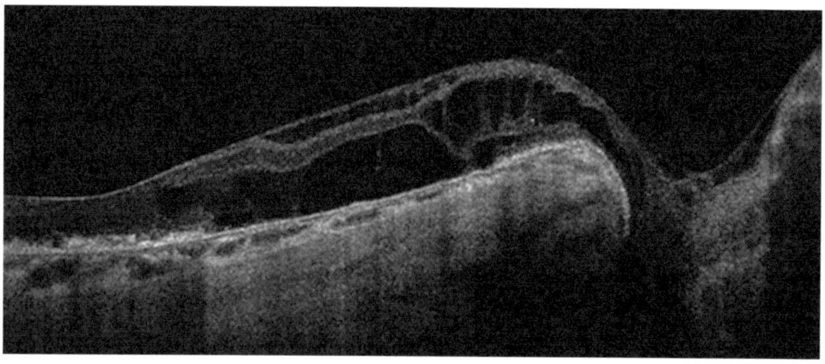

Fig. 25.10 Swept Source OCT scan for an eye with optic nerve head pit showing intraretinal fluid affecting multiple layers and extending toward the pit site to communicate with vitreous cavity

25.6 Idiopathic Foveomacular Retinoschisis

This type of foveoschisis is diagnosed by exclusion, being not inherited and not associated with myopia, VMTS, optic pit, or glaucoma. All cases are old, having unilateral foveoschisis, hyperopia with short axial length, complete posterior vitreous detachment, and weak leakage from the optic disc on fluorescein angiography [35]. Because of unilaterality, the cause likely is not a systemic factor such as an inherited condition but rather a topical abnormality. The involvement of morphologic abnormalities of the optic disc seems not to be the case because no pit macular syndrome or glaucoma is present. However, weak hyperfluorescence from the optic disc is observed on fluorescein angiography images, indicating the possibility of an optic disc abnormality that is not clearly seen on OCT.

In other words, the relatively short axial length may be associated with the presence of retinoschisis because the uveal effusion syndrome with an extremely short axial length is characterized by an exudative RD as a result of the thickened sclera with inhibited choroidal outflow. This theory is supported by some case reports that have described retinoschisis with microphthalmus. Vitrectomy with fovea-sparing ILM peeling achieved morphologic and visual improvements in the cases with visual loss [36, 37].

References

1. Haas J. Ueber das Zusammenvorkommen von Veraenderungen der Retina und Choroidea. Arch Augenheilkd. 1898;37:343–8.
2. Takano M, Kishi S. Foveal retinoschisis and retinal detachment in severely myopic eyes with posterior staphyloma. Am J Ophthalmol. 1999;128:472–6.
3. Hotta K, Hotta J. Retinoschisis with macular retinal detachment associated with vitreomacular traction syndrome. Retina. 2004;24:307–9.
4. Bonnet M. Serous macular detachment associated with optic nerve pits. Graefes Arch Clin Exp Ophthalmol. 1991;229:526–32.
5. Ober MD, Freund KB, Shah M, et al. Stellate nonhereditary idiopathic foveomacular retinoschisis. Ophthalmology. 2014;121:1406–13.
6. George ND, Yates JR, Moore AT. X-linked retinoschisis. Br J Ophthalmol. 1995;79:697–702.
7. Gieser EP, Falls HF. Hereditary retinoschisis. Am J Ophthalmol. 1961;51:1193–200.
8. Jager GM. A hereditary retinal disease. Trans Ophthalmol Soc. 1953;73:617–9.
9. Wu WW, Wong JP, Kast J, et al. RS1, a discoidin domain-containing retinal cell adhesion protein associated with X-linked retinoschisis, exists as a novel disulfide-linked octamer. J Biol Chem. 2005;280:10721–30.
10. Sieving PA, Bingham EL, Roth MS, et al. Linkage relationship of X-linked juvenile retinoschisis with Xp22.1-p22.3 probes. Am J Hum Genet. 1990;47:616–21.
11. Prenner JL, Capone A Jr, Ciaccia S, et al. Congenital X-linked retinoschisis classification system. Retina. 2006;26:S61–4.
12. Rao P, Robinson J, Yonekawa Y, et al. Wide-field imaging of nonexudative and exudative congenital X-linked retinoschisis. Retina. 2016;36:1093–100.

13. Joshi MM, Drenser K, Hartzer M, et al. Intraschisis cavity fluid composition in congenital X-linked retinoschisis. Retina. 2006;26:S57–60.
14. Deutman AF. Sex-linked juvenile retinoschisis. In: Deutman AF, editor. The hereditary dystrophies of the posterior pole of the eye. Assen: Van Gorcum; 1971. p. 48–98.
15. Sikkink SK, Biswas S, Parry NR, et al. X-linked retinoschisis: an update. J Med Genet. 2007;44:225–32.
16. Miyake Y, Shiroyama N, Ota I, et al. Focal macular electroretinogram in X-linked congenital retinoschisis. Invest Ophthalmol Vis Sci. 1993;34:512–5.
17. Verbakel SK, van de Ven JP, Le Blanc LM, et al. Carbonic anhydrase inhibitors for the treatment of cystic macular lesions in children with x-linked juvenile retinoschisis. Invest Ophthalmol Vis Sci. 2016;57:5143–7.
18. Patel A, Morse L. Ocriplasmin for foveal in X-linked retinoschisis. Retin Cases Brief Rep. 2015;9:248–51.
19. George NDL, Yates JRW, Bradshaw K, et al. Infantile presentation of Xlinked retinoschisis. Br J Ophthalmol. 1995;79:653–7.
20. Ferrone PJ, Trese MT, Lewis H. Vitreoretinal surgery for complications of congenital retinoschisis. Am J Ophthalmol. 1997;123:742–7.
21. Brockhurst R. Photocoagulation in congenital retinoschisis. Arch Ophthalmol. 1970;84:158–65.
22. Turut P, Francois P, Castier P, et al. Analysis of results in the treatment of peripheral retinoschisis in sex-linked congenital retinoschisis. Graefes Arch Clin Exp Ophthalmol. 1989;227:328–31.
23. Sebag J. Age-related differences in the human vitreoretinal interface. Arch Ophthalmol. 1991;109:966–71.
24. Regillo CD, Tasman WS, Brown GC. Surgical management of complications associated with X-linked retinoschisis. Arch Ophthalmol. 1993;111:1080–6.
25. Byeon SH, Lee SC, Koh HJ, et al. Surgical removal of the internal limiting membrane in progressive macular change in X-linked juvenile retinoschisis. Retin Cases Brief Rep. 2007;1:156–9.
26. Wong SC, Capone A Jr. Microplasmin (ocriplasmin) in pediatric vitreoretinal surgery: update and review. Retina. 2013;33:339–48.
27. Scott IU, Flynn HW, Azen SP, et al. Silicone oil in the repair of pediatric complex retinal detachments: a prospective, observational, multicenter study. Ophthalmology. 1999;106:1399–407; discussion 1407–1408
28. Baba T, Ohno-Matsui K, Futagami S, Yoshida T, Yasuzumi K, Kojima A, et al. Prevalence and characteristics of foveal retinal detachment without macular hole in high myopia. Am J Ophthalmol. 2003;135(3):338–42.
29. Panozzo G, Mercanti A. Optical coherence tomography findings in myopic traction maculopathy. Arch Ophthalmol. 2004;122(10):1455–60.
30. Jaffe NS. Vitreous traction at the posterior pole of the fundus due to alterations in the vitreous posterior. Trans Am Acad Ophthalmol Otolaryngol. 1967;71:642–52.
31. Smiddy WE, Michels RG, Glaser BM, et al. Vitrectomy for macular traction caused by incomplete vitreous separation. Arch Ophthalmol. 1988;106:624–8.
32. Duker JS, Kaiser PK, Binder S, de Smet MD, Gaudric A, Reichel E, Sadda SR, Sebag J, Spaide RF, Stalmans P. The International Vitreomacular Traction Study Group classification of vitreomacular adhesion, traction, and macular hole. Ophthalmology. 2013 Dec;120(12):2611–9.
33. Gass JD. Serous detachment of the macula. Secondary to congenital pit of the optic nerve head. Am J Ophthalmol. 1969;67:821–41.
34. Imamura Y, Zweifel SA, Fujiwara T, Freund KB, Spaide RF. High-resolution optical coherence tomography findings in optic pit maculopathy. Retina. 2010;30(7):1104–12.
35. Marukoi I, Morizane Y, Kimura S, Shiode Y, Hosokawa M, Sekiryu T, Iida T, Shiraga F. Clinical characteristics of idiopathic foveomacular retinoschisis. Retina. 2016;36(8):1486–92.
36. Sonmez K, Ozcan PY. Angle-closure glaucoma in a patient with the nanophthalmos-ocular cystinosis-foveoschisis-pigmentary retinal dystrophy complex. BMC Ophthalmol. 2012;12:23.
37. Yu S, Gao Y, Liang X, Huang Y. Acquired retinoschisis resolved after 23 gage pars plana vitrectomy in posterior microphthalmos. BMC Ophthalmol. 2014;14:65.

Myopic Traction Maculopathy: Guidelines to Treatment

26

Barbara Parolini, Michele Palmieri, Alessandro Finzi, Gianluca Besozzi, Angela Lucente, Ugo Nava, Sajish Pinackatt, and Rino Frisina

Glossary and Terminology

We followed the definitions of retinoschisis suggested by Benhamou et al. [1]. We hereby provide the choices of glossary and terminology that were made in this study, in order to avoid any possible misinterpretation.

Schisis Splitting of the neurosensory retina. Since, in most cases, the schisis interested the whole macula and not just the fovea, and since it could be found not only in the fovea but also (or only) in the extrafoveal area (Fig. 26.1), we avoided the term Foveomacular schisis or Foveoschisis and selected to use maculoschisis.

Inner Maculoschisis Inner Maculoschisis (I-MS) is as a splitting of the inner retinal layers, at different levels, from the internal limiting membrane (ILM) to the inner nuclear layer (Fig. 26.2). The ILM can be detached from the nerve fibers layer and connected to it with a column-like structure.

B. Parolini (✉) · M. Palmieri · A. Lucente · U. Nava
Eyecare Clinic, Brescia, Italy

A. Finzi · S. Pinackatt
Department of Ophthalmology, Istituto Clinico S. Anna, Brescia, Italy

G. Besozzi
Department of Ophthalmology, Vito Fazzi Hospital, Lecce, Italy

R. Frisina
Department of Ophthalmology, University of Padova, Padova, Italy

A. Jain et al. (eds.), *Cutting-edge Vitreoretinal Surgery*,
https://doi.org/10.1007/978-981-33-4168-5_26

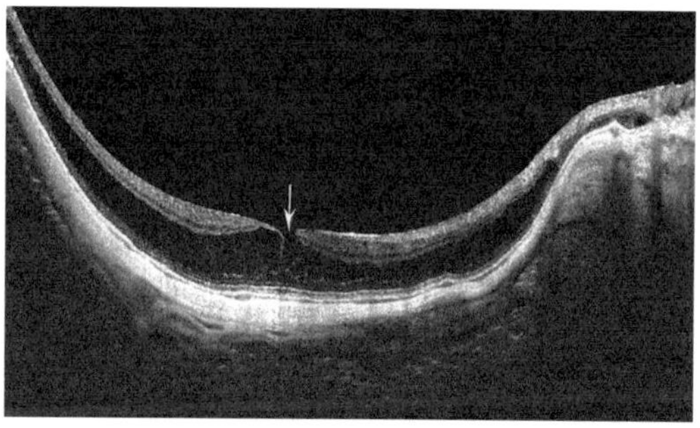

Fig. 26.1 Eye affected by outer maculoschisis involving the whole macula in a 49-year-old female. The arrow indicates an associated inner lamellar macular hole

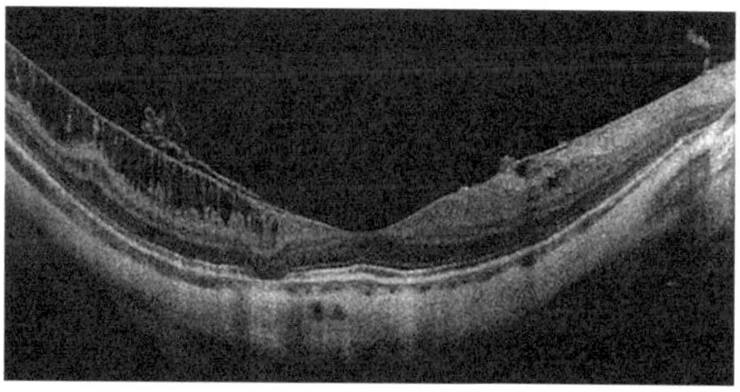

Fig. 26.2 Eye affected by inner maculoschisis in a 44-year-old female

Outer Maculoschisis Outer Maculoschisis (O-MS) is a splitting of the outer retinal layers (Fig. 26.1), from the outer plexiform layer, that changes in a column like structure, to the outer nuclear layer to the external limiting membrane and the photoreceptors layer.

Inner Lamellar macular hole Inner Lamellar Macular Hole (I-LMH) is a splitting of the foveal layers, developing from the internal limiting membrane (Fig. 26.1). The depth and width of the I-LMH may vary significantly.

Outer Lamellar Macular Hole Splitting in the layer of the photoreceptors (Figs. 26.3 and 26.4). The location and the width of the Outer Lamellar Macular Hole (O-LMH) may vary significantly.

Macular detachment We defined macular detachment (MD) as cases with neurosensory detachment (Fig. 26.4) with separation of the photoreceptors from the retinal pigment epithelium (RPE).

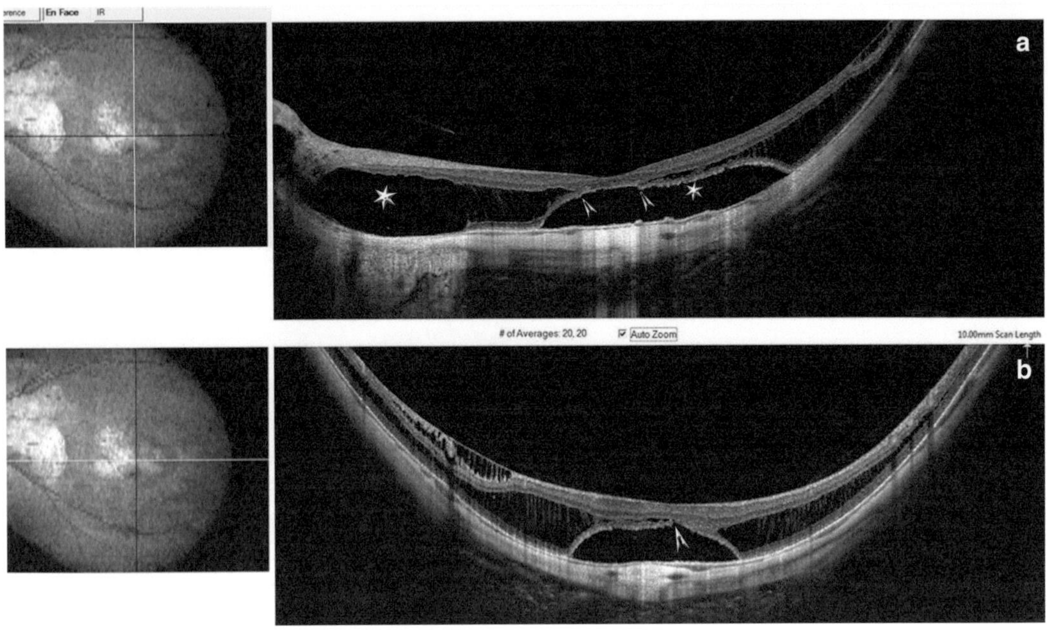

Fig. 26.3 Eye affected by inner and outer maculoschisis and by foveal detachment in a 59-year–old female. The arrow indicates an associated outer lamellar macular hole. The star indicates the areas of detachment. (**a**) horizontal scan, (**b**) vertical scan

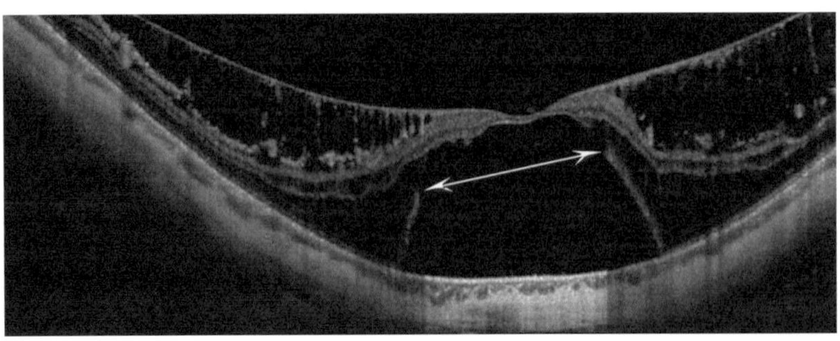

Fig. 26.4 Eye affected by inner and outer maculoschisis and by foveal detachment in a 62-year-old male. The arrow indicates the extension of an associated outer lamellar macular hole

26.1 Definition

Myopic Traction Maculopathy is a complex disease that affects high myopic eyes with and without posterior staphyloma. Despite different studies have been published, there is no agreement on the definition, neither a complete knowledge of the natural history and the pathogenesis, nor a unique classification of the disease. Moreover, the surgical treatment is still controversial.

In literature, different definitions of MTM may be found, from macular schisis-like thickening of the retina, to foveal detachment, to macular foveoschisis (MF), to foveoschisis, to shallow macular detachment.

The first description of MTM was given by Phillips in 1958 [2], who reported a posterior retinal detachment, without macular hole in patients with myopic staphyloma, assuming a tractional pathogenesis of what they called "retinomacular schisis."

In 1999, Takano and Kishi first published the optical coherence tomography (OCT) characteristics and findings of "foveal retinomacular schisis" [3].

Panozzo et al. [4] first described this condition as "myopic traction maculopathy" (MTM) and established that MTM may affect patients with high myopia and posterior staphyloma in 9–34% [4].

Shimada et al. [5] described different stages of the MF, leading to a foveal detachment, through the formation of an outer lamellar hole.

Recently the authors have proposed a new classification of MTM and defined MTM as a progressive disease that first involves the innermost layers of the retina with an Inner Macular Schisis (I-MS) and gradually progresses involving the outermost retinal layers until a macular detachment appears, while the schisis disappear. The MTM Staging System has been published [6].

26.2 Epidemiology

MTM is thought to affect 9% of high myopic eyes [7]. About 50% of patients affected progresses to major complications such as Full-thickness macular hole (FTMH) or macular detachment within 2 years [8].

Panozzo et al. reported that 9–34% of high myopic eyes with posterior staphyloma may be affected by MTM [4].

26.3 Pathogenesis: The Game of Forces

The pathogenesis of MTM is multifactorial and it is still not fully understood. The rigidity of ILM, the progression of the staphyloma and the antero-posterior traction caused by epiretinal affections seem to contribute to the evolution of MTM.

Anatomically, the retina is a multilayered multicellular structure which is held together, as a unique tissue, by *tangential centripetal* forces, mainly exerted by the Muller cells and by the external and internal limiting membranes.

In progressive myopia, different *centrifugal* forces tend to modify the shape and the location of the retina and the fovea from the ideal one, racing against the unique centripetal intraretinal force. These centrifugal forces may be exerted by the vitreous and the sclera, with two main different directions: tangential or perpendicular to the retinal tissue.

The progressive deformation of the sclera due to staphyloma induces an increasing stretching of the choroid–RPE–retina complex toward lateral and posterior orbit. The vitreous, as well as the sclera, may also generate both tangential and perpendicular centrifugal force; the latter toward the vitreous cavity.

This "Game Of Traction" leads to different clinical pictures and to a combination of inner maculoschisis, outer maculoschisis, inner LMH, outer LMH, foveal to macular detachment, macular detachment with a FTMH, FTMH on flat retina. Figure 26.5 describes the interaction of the different forces exerted on the retina in progressive myopia.

Early stages of MTM seem to involve first the innermost retinal layers and presenting as an I-MS. Then the progression of the disease depends on the prevalent centrifugal forces exerted on the retina.

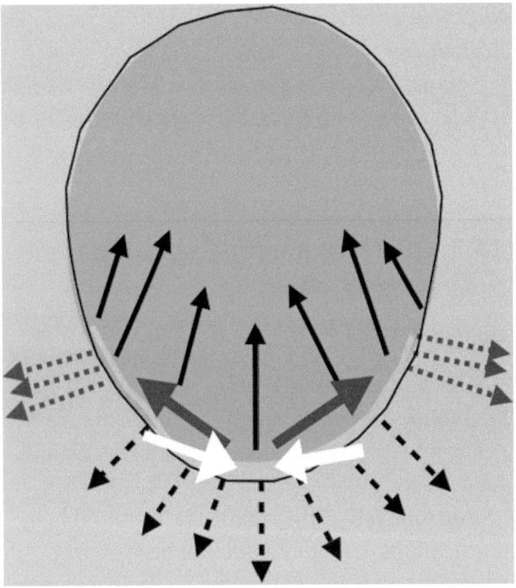

arrow color	type of force	direction of vector	exerted by	action
white	centri petal	to the fovea	intraretinal structure	holds the retina together
line black	centri fugal	to the anterior vitreous	vitreous	pull the retina anteriorly
dark grey	centri fugal	to the lateral orbit	vitreous	stretch and open the fovea
dotted grey	centri fugal	to the lateral orbit	lateral sclera	stretch and open the fovea
dashed black	centri fugal	to the posterior orbit	posterior sclera	pull the retina posteriorly

Fig. 26.5 Schematic representation of the different forces exerted on the retina in an eye with pathologic myopia. One centripetal force (white) maintains the shape and attachment of the retina. Different centrifugal forces tend to detach or stretch the retina

If the prevalent centrifugal forces are perpendicular (Fig. 26.6), I-MS progresses and involves the outer layers becoming an IO-MS, then an O-MS until an MD appears. While the outer component further progresses to MD, the inner component of schisis is progressively relieved, because the intraretinal force becomes progressively prevalent when the retina detaches from the RPE.

Once the macula is detached, a disruption and splitting of the ellipsoid zone band might occur generating an O-LMH.

On the other hand, if the prevalent centrifugal forces are tangential, the patient will develop an I-LMH and eventually a FTMH (Fig. 26.7). The delamination of the retinal layers can be asymmetric in the different macular quadrants and the I-LMH may show different shapes based on the direction of the main vector of traction. The observation that a myopic LMH evolves into an FTMH was already made [9, 10].

When both the perpendicular and the tangential forces act together, a macular detachment with either lamellar (Fig. 26.8a, b) or FTMH (Fig. 26.8b, c) will appear.

Epiretinal abnormalities such as epiretinal membranes or vitreoretinal tractions from anomalous adhesion between vitreous cortes and retina, may also be associated with to every manifestation of MTM and contribute to the disease progression.

The natural course is not completely well-known due to the limited number of studies about it. Some patients remain stable for a year while others progress. MTM spontaneous resolution has been reported. However, it seems clear that the progressive nature of the disease is a consequence of its pathogenesis [11]. The Authors have observed cases of spontaneous resolution that restarted to progress years after the resolution (REF).

26.4 Clinical Manifestations and Diagnosis

The onset of MTM may vary among patients and may be totally asymptomatic in early stages [12, 13].

As a consequence of the lack of symptoms, the knowledge of the natural history is not easily

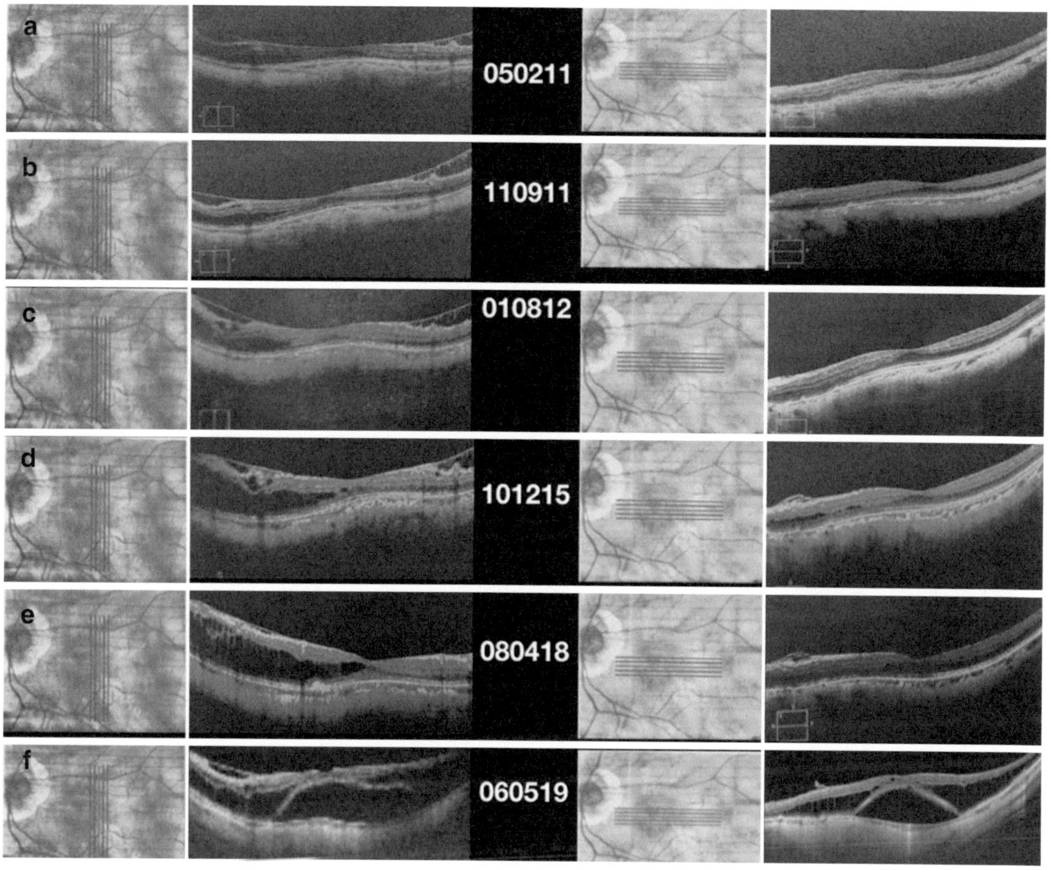

Fig. 26.6 Natural evolution of MTM with prevalent forces perpendicular to the retina in a female patient. (**a**) OCT taken at the age of 43 years on February 5, 2011, showing MTM in the form of inner-outer schisis and normal fovea. BCVA was 0.8 Decimal. (**b**) OCT taken at the age of 43 years on September 11, 2011, showing MTM in the form of inner-outer schisis and normal fovea. BCVA was 0.8 Decimal. (**c**) OCT taken at the age of 44, on August 1, 2012, showing MTM in the form of predominantly outer schisis and normal fovea. BCVA was 0.7 Decimal. (**d**) OCT taken at the age of 47 years, showing MTM in the form of inner-outer schisis. BCVA was 0.7 Decimal. (**e**) OCT taken at the age of 50 years, showing MTM in the form of predominantly outer schisis. The inner component of the schisis is less apparent. The schisis is visible only in the area where the concavity of the sclera is more evident and pronounced. BCVA was 0.7 Decimal. (**f**) OCT taken at the age of 51 years, showing MTM in the form of schisis detachment with normal fovea. BCVA was 0.2 Decimal

predictable [14] and the disease could be underestimated. The symptoms reported by patients are blurred vision, reduce visual acuity, central scotoma, and, more rarely, metamorphopsia [4].

Indirect ophthalmoscopy and biomicroscopy are limited in detecting signs of MTM, because of the retinal transparency and the chorioretinal changes [3]. However, typical changes of progressive myopia may be revealed: chorioretinal atrophy, peripapillary atrophy, staphyloma, lacquer cracks, and myopic CNV.

OCT is the key instrument to diagnose this disease [15]. However, the OCT 2D B-scan has limitations. This is demonstrated by the fact that the vertical and horizontal scans of these eyes can be completely different (Fig. 26.4). We should imagine the posterior pole of the eye with progressive myopia as a three-dimensional concave structure, with an inner side, consisting of the vitreous cavity, and an outer side consisting of the sclera. Thus, combining a 3D MRI with OCT reconstruction better images the posterior pole of

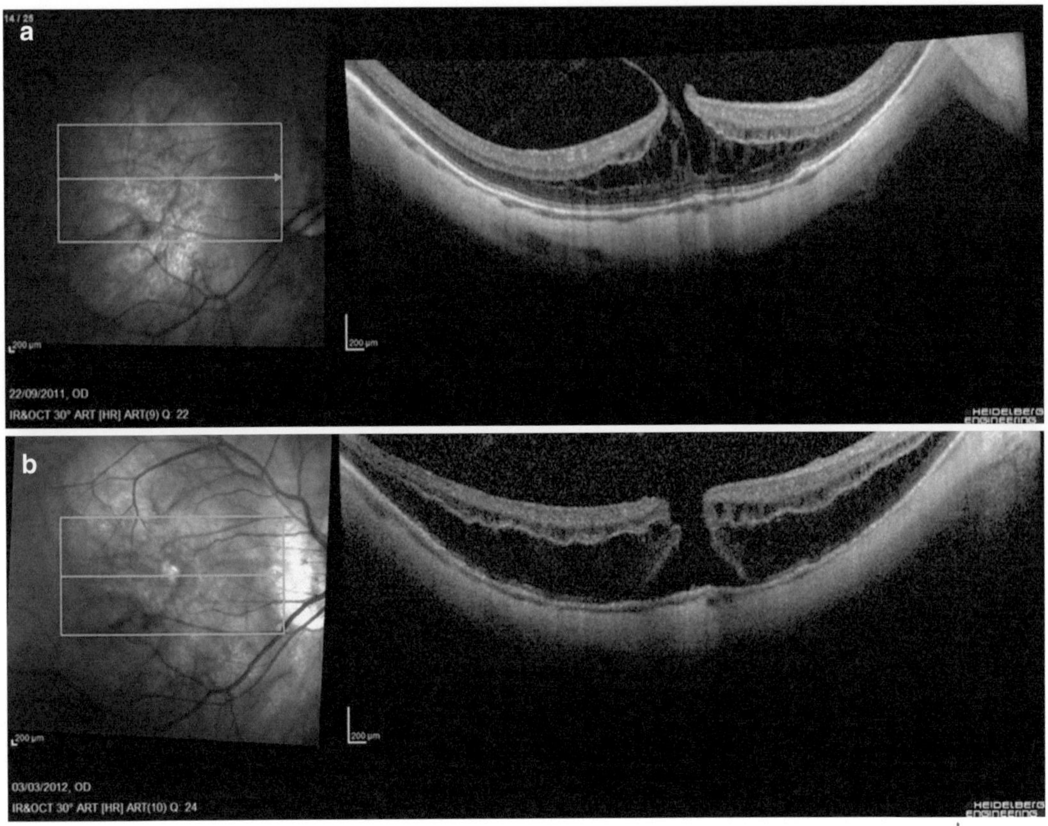

Fig. 26.7 Example of natural progression of MTM due to tangential forces. (**a**) OCT taken at the age of 42 years, showing an O-MS and an I-LMH with VMT. (**b**) 3 years later, the OCT shows a progression to an FTMH with predominantly O-MS and no evident epiretinal abnormalities

myopic eyes and it is more appropriate to study MTM (Fig. 26.9).

Maculoschisis is a separation of the inner plexiform layer or at the inner limiting membrane or of the outer retinal layers, between the outer plexiform and the outer nuclear layer [1, 16]. The splitting of retinal layers appears as highly reflective multiple columnar vertical or vertical oblique structures, with a hyporeflective space between these structures [1]. It is easily distinguishable from cystic spaces which are hyporeflective but rounded or oval.

Posterior retinal detachment or, according to other definitions foveal detachment, can be another common aspect of MTM [11]. Foveal detachment is a separation between the RPE and the photoreceptors layers [13, 17], usually limited to the posterior pole, and may be associated with an FTMH. Many authors confirm that foveal detachment occurs after the formation of the MF and may precede the formation of a macular hole [18].

OCT might also show the presence of an outer lamellar hole (O-LMH) as a disruption of the ellipsoid zone band on a detached fovea. The O-LMH represents a real splitting in the photoreceptors and is visible in the area of foveal detachment. Defects in the photoreceptors inner and outer segments may contribute to visual loss associated with MTM and may have predictive value for postoperative visual recovery [19].

The use of microperimetry should also be considered to analyze foveal functionality [20].

Epimacular abnormalities may usually be detected as the hyper-reflective lines overlying the inner macular schisis and seem to be important contributors to the separation of the inner layers of the neural retina which in turn leads to macular schisis [16].

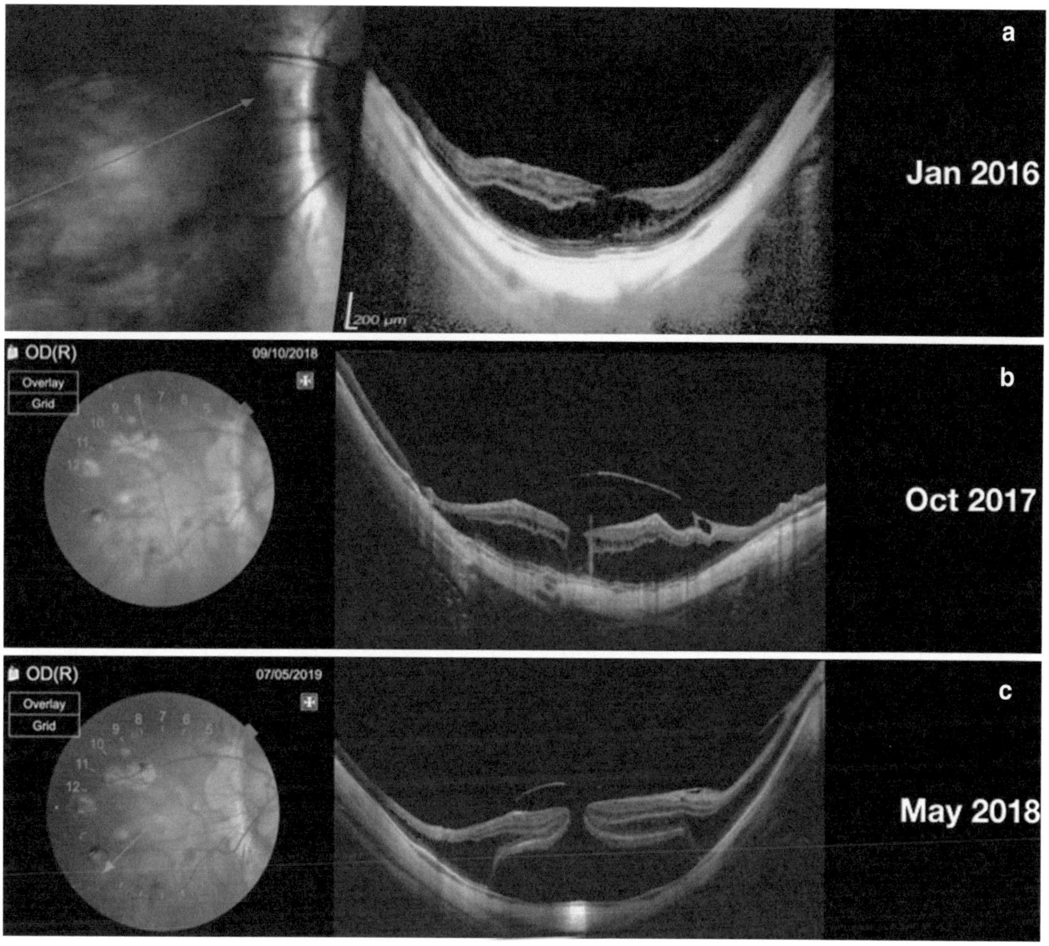

Fig. 26.8 Evolution of MTM in a highly myopic eye of a female. (**a**) OCT scan, taken at the age of 53 years, shows O-MS in the macula with normal fovea. (**b**) OCT scan, taken at the age of 55 years, shows O MS in the macula with the development of an I-LMH and visible epiretinal abnormalities. (**c**) OCT scan, taken 6 months after the previous one, shows O-MS with development of macular detachment and FTMH

26.5 Management

One of the most critical aspects of MTM is management.

The current approach to MTM is to follow-up patients and surgery is recommended in case of serious visual impairment and evolved macular detachment with macular holes. This management limits the functional outcomes of surgery.

Asymptomatic patients should be followed with observation every 12–18 months, since BCVA in this group is still good and the progression is slow. However, patients suffering a vision loss or a worsening of metamorphopsia, patients affected by a symptomatic I-LMH or a FTMH and patients affected by macular detachment should be directed to surgery.

26.5.1 Surgical Approach

The first surgical approaches to MTM were directed to solve the most severe and final stage of MTM, the retinal detachment associated with a macular hole. The aims of these interventions were to restore anatomy and did not guarantee an acceptable functional recovery.

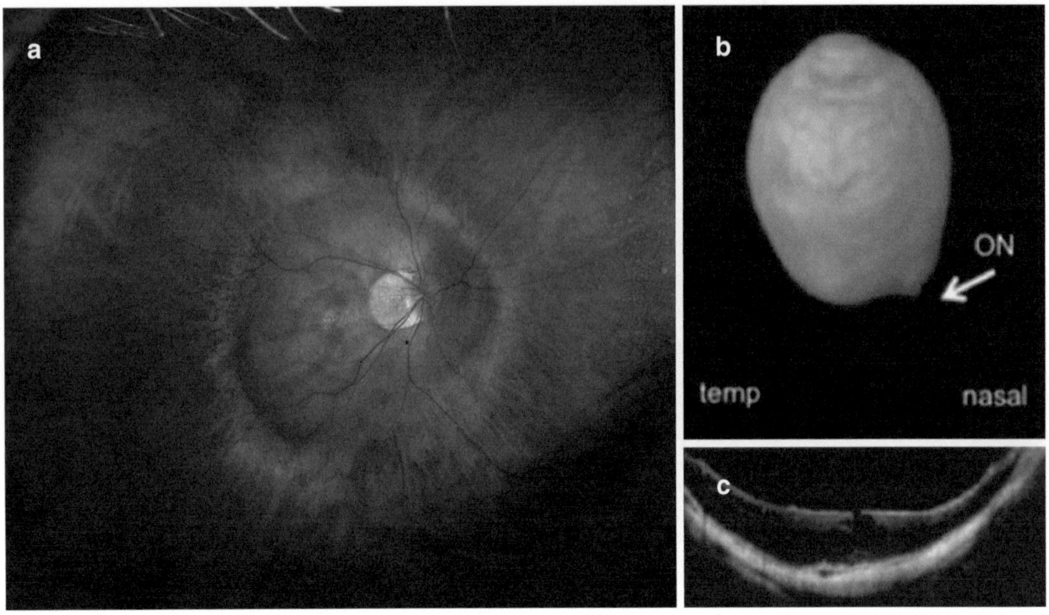

Fig. 26.9 Eye affected by outer maculoschisis. (**a**) Wide field IR image showing a Type 1 Staphyloma involving the posterior pole. (**b**) MRI imaging showing the whole shape of the eyeball. The white arrow indicates the Optic Nerve (ON). (**c**) OCT scan showing the predominantly outer schisis associated with an I-LMH

The idea of preventing axial elongation and scleral growth by the placement of material over the posterior part of the eye was proposed by surgeons many years before the description of MTM. Shevelev [21] first proposed, in 1930, the transplantation of fascia lata for scleral reinforcement.

In 1957, Schepens Okamura and Brockhurst described the macular buckling procedures [22].

From 1957 to the 1980s, the gold standard for the treatment of macular detachment with macular hole was definitely the macular buckle (MB) [22–31].

The first article that considered pars plana vitrectomy (PPV) for the Macular Hole Macular Detachment (MHMD) goes back to 1982 [32] by Gonvers. Many authors published afterward [33, 34]. Since then, PPV has been proposed as the intervention of choice, with the rationale of eliminating the tangential tractions, allowing the retina to relax. Therefore, MB was abandoned for a while, mainly due to the challenges and complications linked to the surgical technique.

However, PPV had limited efficacy. Indirectly this lack of success was revealed by the list of papers proposing different approaches with different tamponades. PPV with gas was linked to a high rate of failure or relapse. In 1999, Wolfensberger et al. [35] proposed the use of silicone oil associated with the laser treatment of the hole and obtained 92% of retinal reattachment, but, as expected, poor increase in vision.

The increasing use of peeling the ILM improved the range of success of PPV, as demonstrated in 2001 by Kadonoso et al. [36].

Thereafter, Lu et al. [37] in 2002, compared various methods of PPV, associating the injection of gas, with and without laser treatment of the macular hole, and injection of silicone oil without laser treatment, demonstrating the superiority of the first method, with the results of 93%, 58%, 57%, respectively, giving a key role to laser treatment for anatomic success. It must be highlighted, however, that functional results were very poor.

In 2006, Chen [38] reported a retinal reattachment success rate of 50–60% after PPV and gas injection.

Panozzo et al. [15], in 2007, carried out the first large-scale work on MTM. The study consisted of 24 eyes (including 5 with foveal detachment and 19 with MF), followed for 5 years, and treated with the sole purpose of removing the vitreous-retinal traction without using tamponade. The authors reported that 95.8% of the eyes had complete resolution of MTM stable in time. Four of the 5 eyes with macular detachment and 1 eye with maculoschisis developed, however, a macular hole that did not hesitated in a new macular detachment and an eye remained unchanged. As for the visual recovery, 70% improved, 30% remained unchanged.

Different authors [39, 40] presented promising results with the use of heavy silicone oil in the treatment of eyes with persistence of idiopathic macular hole after PPV and gas injection. However, after removal of heavy silicone oil, retinal detachment was reported.

In 2011, Mete et al. [41] compared the results of standard silicone oil 1000 cSt and heavy silicone oil in the ability of reattach the retina and closing the hole in 42 cases of MHMD. The anatomic results were similar, with a macular reattachment rate of 76.5% and 81.8% for silicone oil and for heavy silicone oil, respectively. The frequent relapses of macular detachment in both groups were always linked to reopening of the hole. Mete et al. concluded that there was a high recurrence rate of retinal detachment and an unsatisfactory final BCVA with both tamponades.

The success of PPV in high myopia remained limited with any tamponade, mainly because of high rate of retinal detachment recurrence, failure to close the hole in MHMD, and risk to induce an iatrogenic macular hole in MTM.

The unsatisfactory results of PPV left open the way to a new course of publications on buckling the macula, which started again, after 20 years, in 2000 with Sasoh [42].

In 2001 Ripandelli [43], and later in 2005 Theodassiadis [44], described MB success with a sponge and with a solid silicone exoplant, respectively. Although the reattachment rate with macular buckling was reported to be very high, the rate of hole closure was unknown because of lack of study with OCT.

The point was that surgeons dealing with MHMD realized the limitation of PPV. However, MB, although more efficient, remained difficult and linked to complications.

Some authors started to find a way to make the macular buckling technique easier, first of all with different buckle designs.

Tanaka, Ando, and Usui [45] published in 2005 the successful approach of a new semirigid rod-exoplant in MHMD recurrences after PPV. The exoplant consisted of a T-shaped semirigid silicone rubber rod internally reinforced with titanium wires and an indenting head at one end.

In 2009, Parolini presented the 2 years results of a new design of MB, at the Heatam meeting in Amsterdam. The idea was to propose an L-shaped buckle, made with a titanium stent inserted into a silicone sleeve, with the aim to obtain a macular indentation but allowing an anterior suture. The shape resembled the Ando plomb with the difference of using a titanium stent (MRI compatible), not stainless steel wire, and soft silicone sponge, not solid silicone, to indent the macula.

In 2009, B. Ward et al. [46] examined the buckling of the posterior pole, with sclera reinforcement, as a tool for myopia control and followed the course of untreated fellow eyes. Ward concluded that the experience with 59 cases showed effective axial myopia control and an acceptable safety profile for posterior pole buckling. No case of visual acuity loss occurred with the procedure.

In 2012, Tian J et al. [47] applied the technique of macular buckling in 5 cases of MHMD after initial failure of pars plana PPV with ILM peeling and silicone oil tamponade. In this study, the retina was reattached after buckling. However, visual acuity did not improve and anatomical macular holes only closed in two patients. This could be related to extensive and long term and marked atrophy of the RPE/choriocapillaris complex in the macular area.

More recent literature [48, 49] added to PPV the technique of inverted ILM flaps reporting a higher success rate to close the holes [50].

Alkabes [51] recently published a 16-year review on MB for MTM and compared the results with PPV. She clearly confirms that MB was the first technique considered to treat MHMD.

26.5.2 Guidelines to MTM Treatment

The surgical treatment of MTM is still controversial. The goals of surgery need to be anatomical and functional. The anatomical goals should be retinal attachment; hole closure; atrophy prevention. The functional goals should be to improve or maintain central vision and the central visual field. However, in eyes with progressive myopia we should ideally aim not only to treat but also to prevent the outset or the progression of MTM, since progressive myopia is a degenerative and progressive disease.

The authors have proposed new management guidelines of MTM, based on the new MTM Staging System (MSS).

The aim of their study was to clarify how to choose among four options of management: observation, PPV, MB, or combined surgery (MB + PPV).

The choice of treatment was made by looking at the forces exerted on the retina (Fig. 26.5), with the intention to counteract the centrifugal forces that tend to detach the retina from the eyewall, perpendicularly, and/or tend to split the retina, tangentially, in the macula. In their study, the authors used PPV, MB, or combined surgery to treat 157 eyes affected by different stages of MTM.

Observing the anatomical results of the different treatments, they concluded that PPV better addressed the tangential tractions on the inner retinal surface, i.e., the modulation of the macular pattern, while the MB addressed the perpendicular tractions on the retina induced by scleral elongation, i.e., the modulation of the retinal pattern.

Treating a prevalent tangential traction with a MB brings to potential complications as well as treating a prevalent perpendicular traction with PPV. If only one component of traction is treated, the opposite component will manifest itself in time. Thus, whenever a combination of perpendicular and tangential forces is treated only with a MB, the perpendicular component is solved and the retinal pattern will improve, but the tangential force inducing alteration of the macular pattern remains unchanged and might even worsen.

For example, if a patient affected by a mild maculoschisis, with mild ERM and without preoperative I-LMH undergoes MB, the tangential tractions induced by the buckle, pushing the retina vertically and anteriorly, lead to a iatrogenic splitting of the fovea (Fig. 26.10).

In the same way, when O-MS or a foveal detachment are treated only with PPV (Fig. 26.11) the schisis and detachment have a low chance to resolve or end up in iatrogenic macular hole.

Parolini assessed that inner and outer schisis should be followed with observation every 12–18 months, since BCVA in these groups is still good and the progression is slow, unless epiretinal abnormalities are associated. The symptomatic cases should be treated as cases of ERM without MTM. A high rate of anatomical success could be reached when PPV was used for schisis associated with lamellar of full-thickness macular hole.

MB should be considered and evaluated case by case when outer schisis is associated with a macular hole. MB and late PPV revealed particularly useful in cases of maculoschisis and lamellar macular hole, even in eyes with macular atrophy, obtaining a gain in visual function when the schisis and the I-LMH were resolved.

The recommendation by the author is to treat the schisis/detachment first, with MB, and then to treat the macular pattern with PPV, only if required by lack of recovery of visual acuity or by progression of the I-LMH.

The final anatomical resolution of the schisis is slower with MB alone, compared with combined MB + PPV.

The final restoration of the foveal profile in the presence of lamellar of FTMH was achievable only when PPV was added. However, even in these cases, PPV can be added at a later time only if needed, thus avoiding the possible side effects of PPV and restoring the foveal profile on an attached retina not affected by schisis nor detachment.

Macular detachments should be treated immediately with an MB alone. PPV might be added later on and only if needed.

Macular detachments associated with a macular hole (MHMD) should be immediately treated

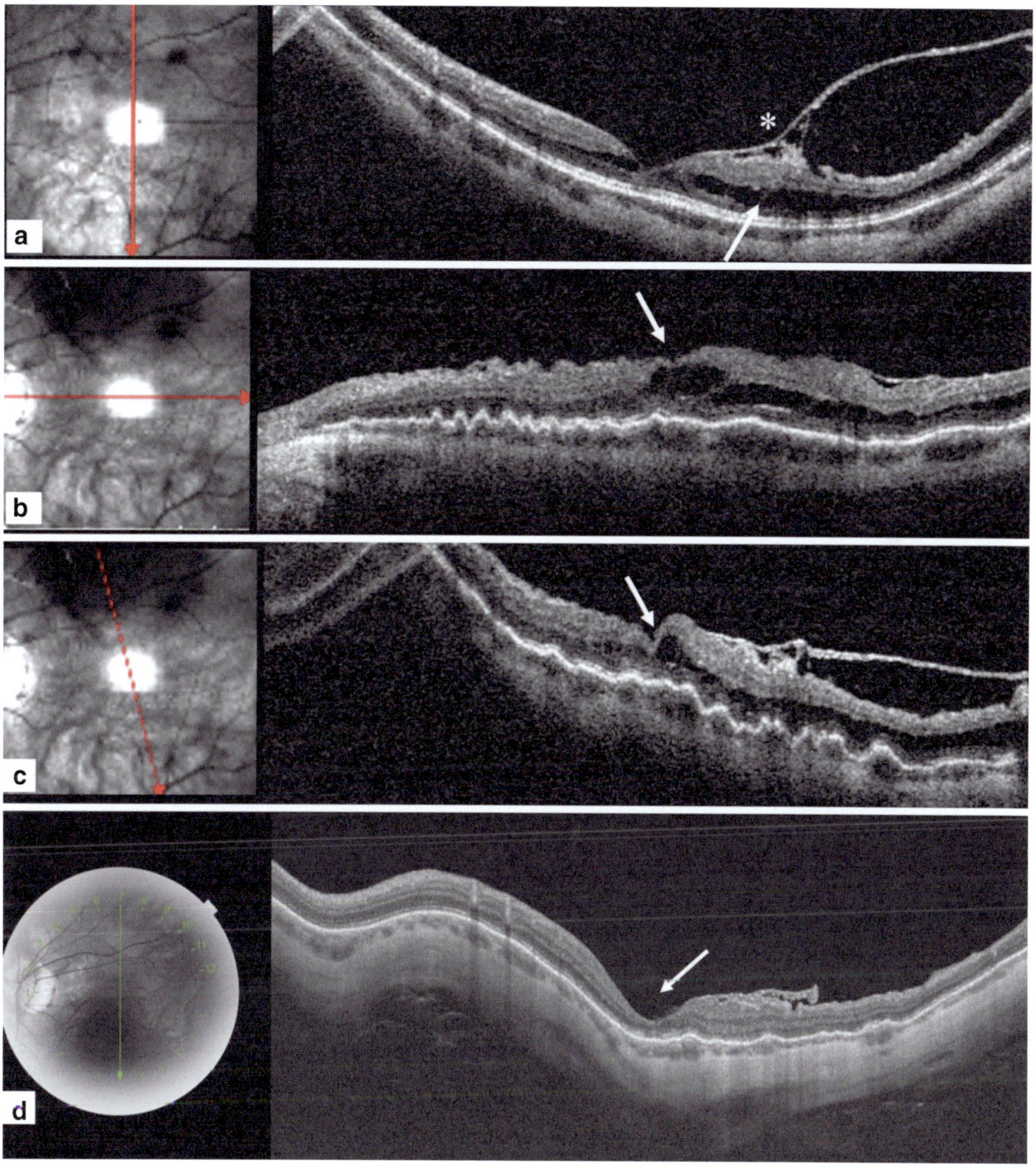

Fig. 26.10 Eye affected by outer maculoschisis with epiretinal abnormalities in a 45-year-old male. (**a**) Preoperative OCT showing the schisis (white arrow) and epiretinal abnormalities (star). (**b**) Horizontal OCT scan 2 months after MB, showing the worsening of the maculoschisis (white arrow). (**c**) Vertical OCT scan 2 months after MB, showing the worsening of the maculoschisis (white arrow) and a more evident traction with different vectors of the epiretinal abnormality. (**d**) Vertical OCT scan 12 months after MB showing resolution of the schisis (white arrow)

with combined MB + PPV in order to treat simultaneously the outer retina and the macular hole.

Both MB and combined surgery resolve the schisis. While the result of buckle is slow, progressive, and visible in months, the result of subsequent or combined PPV is visible within 1–2 weeks. The surgeon should choose, case by case, whether a quick result is better than a slow result, which allows to avoid the consequences of PPV.

Some cases of MHMD, were initially treated successfully only with MB and gas injection, obtaining both the retinal attachment and the

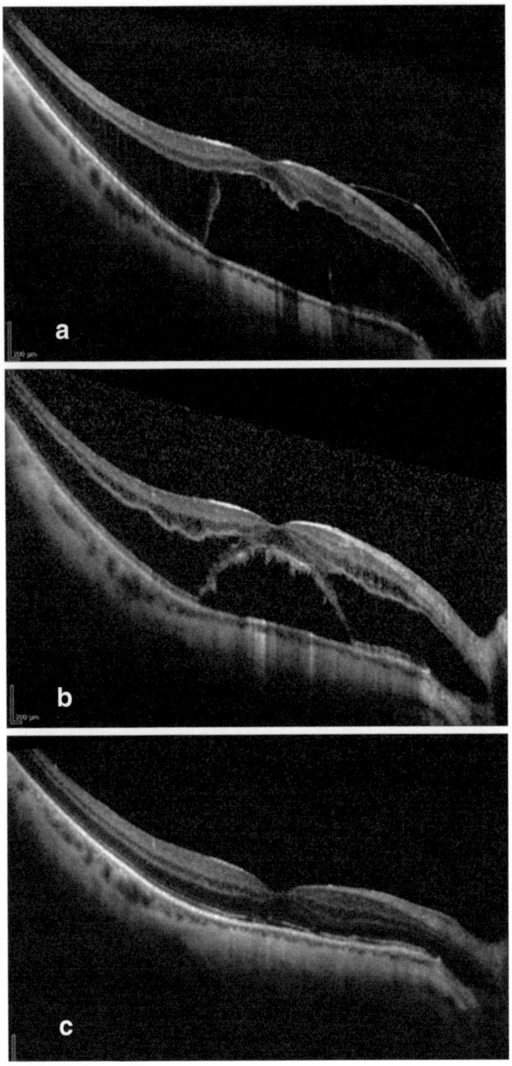

Fig. 26.11 Eye affected by maculoshisis and foveal detachment in a 55-year-old male. (**a**) Preoperative OCT showing the schisis and the foveal detachment with an O-LMH. (**b**) OCT scan 8 months after PPV surgery, showing the resolution of the O-LMH and the persistence of the foveal detachment and the schisis. (**c**) OCT scan, 2 weeks after MB. The O-MS and the foveal detachment are solved

complete hole closure. However, years after the first surgery, the authors observed an opening/reopening of FTMH (Figs. 26.12 and 26.13) due to the progression of the tangential traction.

In conclusion, the surgical treatment of MTM should be customized per patient depending on the stage of the disease.

26.5.3 Role of ILM Peeling

In literature, there is no agreement on the role of ILM peeling. On one hand, it was shown that ILM peeling with ILM flap increased the chance of anatomical success of MHMD [48, 50]. However, it was also well shown that ILM peeling increased the risk of iatrogenic FTMH [52] when cases of MD without FTMH were treated. Therefore, the removal of the inelastic ILM should be postponed to obtaining an attached macula by implanting an MB, in order to reduce this risk. Once the macula is flat, surgeons may perform PPV with or without ILM flap to release the tangential traction exerted by the ILM and to treat the FTMH, when present.

26.6 The Macular Buckle

26.6.1 Preoperative Assessment of the Eye and Patient

A complete slit lamp examination is mandatory. BCVA and microperimetry are useful methods to follow the postoperative functional change. Refraction should be checked in the treatment eye and in the fellow eye. An average 2.0 diopters hyperopic shift should be expected when implanting properly the MB. If the eye is still phakic, it is preferable to implant the buckle first and then proceed with the lens removal if needed. In cases of severe cataract compromising the intraoperative view, a choice can be made either to leave the eye aphakic and proceed with a second implant later, or preferably, to implant an IOL with a myopic residual target refraction. Any previous surgery linked to a change in refraction in the treated or fellow eye should be known, in order to plan the final refractive target. Axial length should be measured preoperatively and periodically after MB.

Any previous surgery should be known. A previous episcleral surgery or episcleral devices such as glaucoma valves could interfere with the implantation of the buckle.

Motility of the eye and diplopia should be assessed before surgery, in order to better judge if

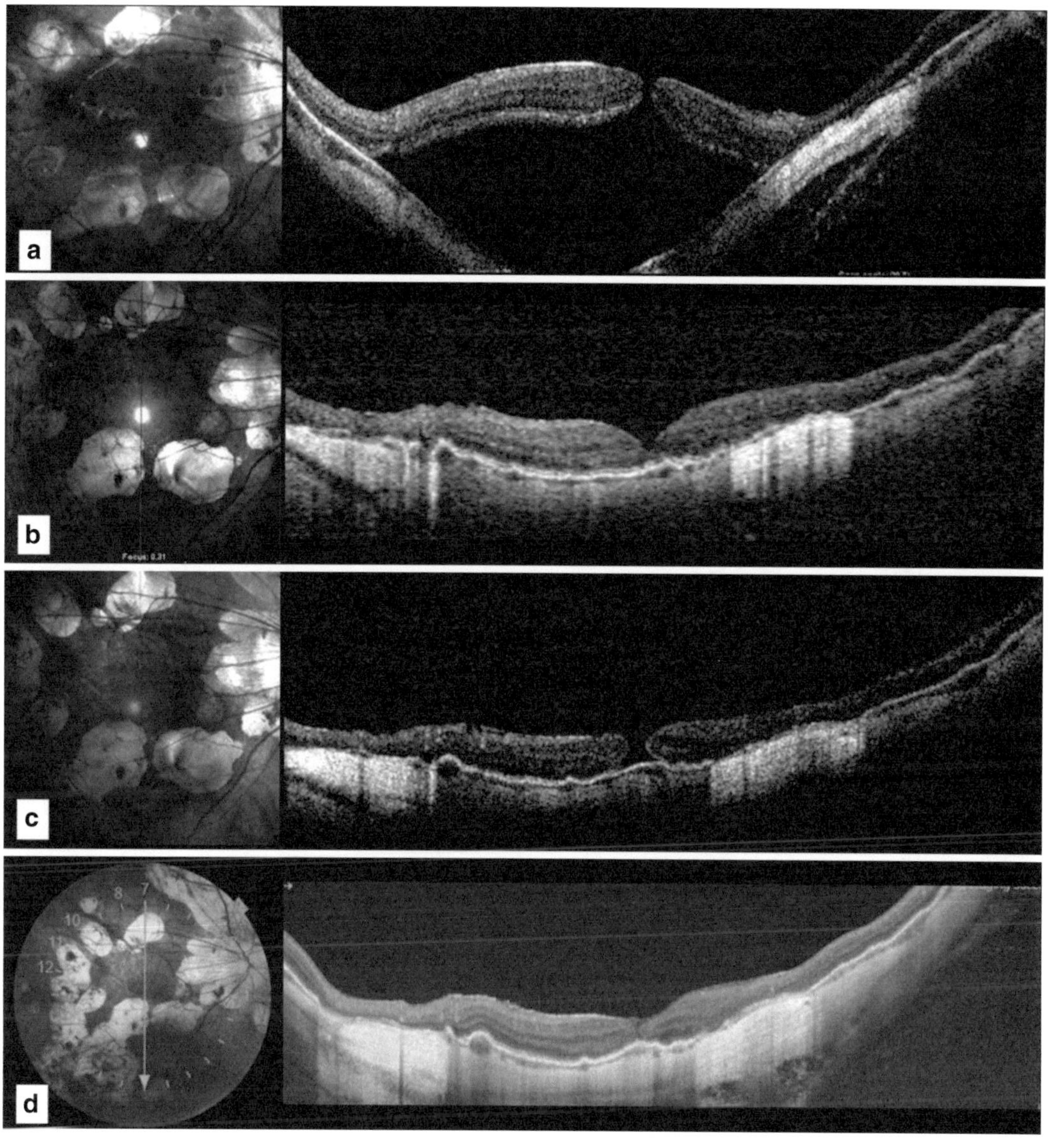

Fig. 26.12 Eye affected by macular detachment with full-thickness macular hole, in a 51–year-old female. (**a**) Preoperative OCT showing the macular detachment with an FTMH. (**b**) OCT scan 1 year after MB, showing the resolution of the detachment. The FTMH appears closed. The indentation is flat. (**c**) OCT scan, 3 years after MB. The eye developed a reopening of the FTMH due to residual tangential traction. (**d**) OCT 1 month after PPV and ILM peeling to solve the FTMH

possible postoperative limitation in the eye movement were induced by the buckle or were present preoperatively and in order to adequately manage them.

Preoperative MRI is not necessary. Collecting data on the original shape of the entire eye and the staphyloma could be helpful in a clinical study setting and postoperatively in order to verify the position of the buckle in relation to the optic nerve (Fig. 26.14).

The category of Myopic Maculopathy according to the International Photographic Classification and grading system [53] should be noted, to better understand the potential postoperative gain in visual function, based on the amount and location of atrophic areas. Suspect signs of

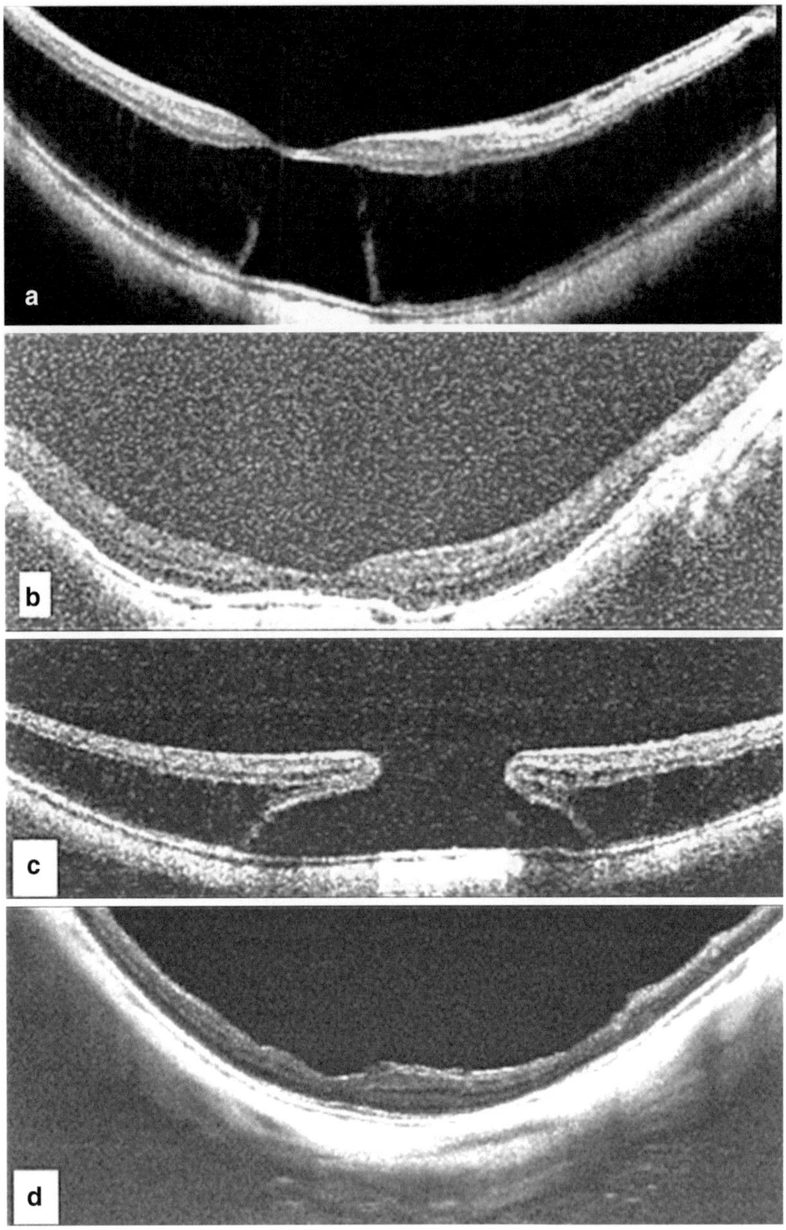

Fig. 26.13 Eye affected by maculoschisis with foveal detachment and outer lamellar macular hole, in a 39-year-old female. (**a**) Preoperative OCT showing the schisis and the foveal detachment with an O-LMH. (**b**) OCT scan 1 year after MB, showing the resolution of the O-LMH, of the foveal detachment and of the schisis. The indentation is flat. (**c**) OCT scan, 3 years after MB. The eye developed an FTMH due to residual tangential traction. (**d**) OCT 1 month after PPV and ILM peeling to solve the FTMH

CNV should be noted in order to promptly allow proper treatment. Wide field fundus photo offers an easier and more accurate classification of the staphyloma [54] (Fig. 26.9).

OCT is the gold standard examination and the main guide to MTM management. Vertical and horizontal OCT scans (at least 9 mm wide) and 3D reconstruction, when available, are useful in understanding the change in the shape of the posterior pole, not only from the preop to the postoperative time, but also during the follow-up.

26.6.2 Indication to the Treatment with Macular Buckle

Macular buckle is indicated to treat prevalent tractions that are perpendicular to the retinal

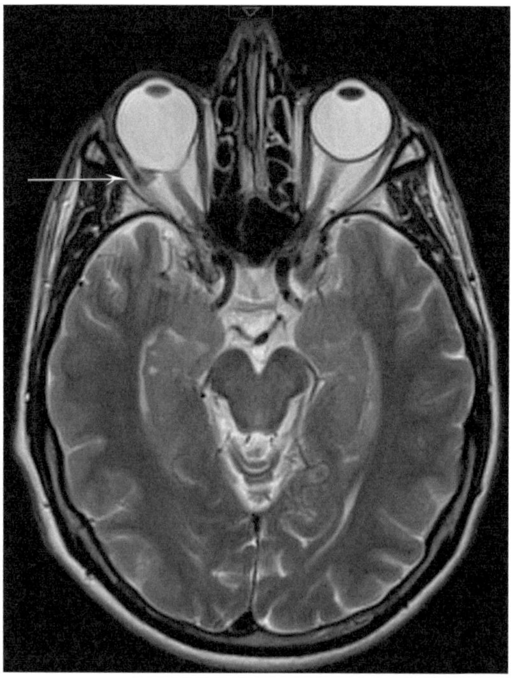

Fig. 26.14 MRI of a patient operated with macular buckle. The right eye is highly myopic and the section of the buckle is indicated by the white arrow

plane. Considering the pros and cons of the actual surgical technique, we advise applying *macular buckle alone* in cases of:

1. Outer maculoschisis with I-LMH
2. Maculoschisis associated with macular detachment
3. Complete macular detachment

Our advice is to apply *macular buckle in combination to PPV*, in the following cases:

1. FTMH associated with outer maculoschisis
2. FTMH associated with maculoschisis and macular detachment
3. Complete macular detachment with FTMH

Our advice is to apply *PPV a few months after macular buckle*, in case of I-LMH still symptomatic after treating the maculoschisis (or maculoschisis + macular detachment) with a buckle.

26.6.3 Anesthesia

MB surgery can be performed under general anesthesia but also under local anesthesia and sedation. In case of local anesthesia in high myopic eyes, sub-Tenon with blunt cannulas is preferable over peribulbar with needle, to lower the risk of scleral perforation.

Parolini proposed a technique which implies to stabilize the globe by holding the superior and the lateral rectus muscle. Therefore, as in any episcleral surgery when traction is applied to the muscle, attention needs to be paid intraoperatively to an acute drop in heart rate.

26.6.4 Postoperative Care

Postoperative care resembles the one of any episcleral surgery. The eye is red and swollen for at least 1 week. Steroid and antibiotic drops should be advised for the first 2 weeks. The follow-up should be scheduled at least at 1 day, 1 week, 1 month, 3–6–12–18–24 months, and then every year.

26.6.5 Complications of the Macular Buckle and Their Management

Some degree of diplopia (particularly in the temporal gaze on the side of the MB location) may occur in 6% of patients in the first postoperative weeks. It is advisable to counsel the patient to move the eye in different directions for 10 min, 3–4 times every day for the first month, in order to lower the chance of formation of fibrotic membranes around the buckle and around the muscles, Tenon's and conjunctival complex. This advice will lower the chance of postoperative diplopia.

Pain is limited and easily treatable in the first week with proper therapy.

Diplopia and pain were mostly linked to the excessive size of the first models of MB.

Exposure of the lateral arm of the buckle through the conjunctiva might occur months or years after surgery. Minimal exposure can be treated by covering the lateral arm with pericardium or donor sclera. In case of recurrent exposure, the buckle can be removed safely.

26.6.6 Effect of Macular Buckle over Time and Effect of Buckle Removal

If the buckle is removed within 3 months after surgery, the MTM could relapse with sudden vision loss (Fig. 26.15). When the buckle is removed

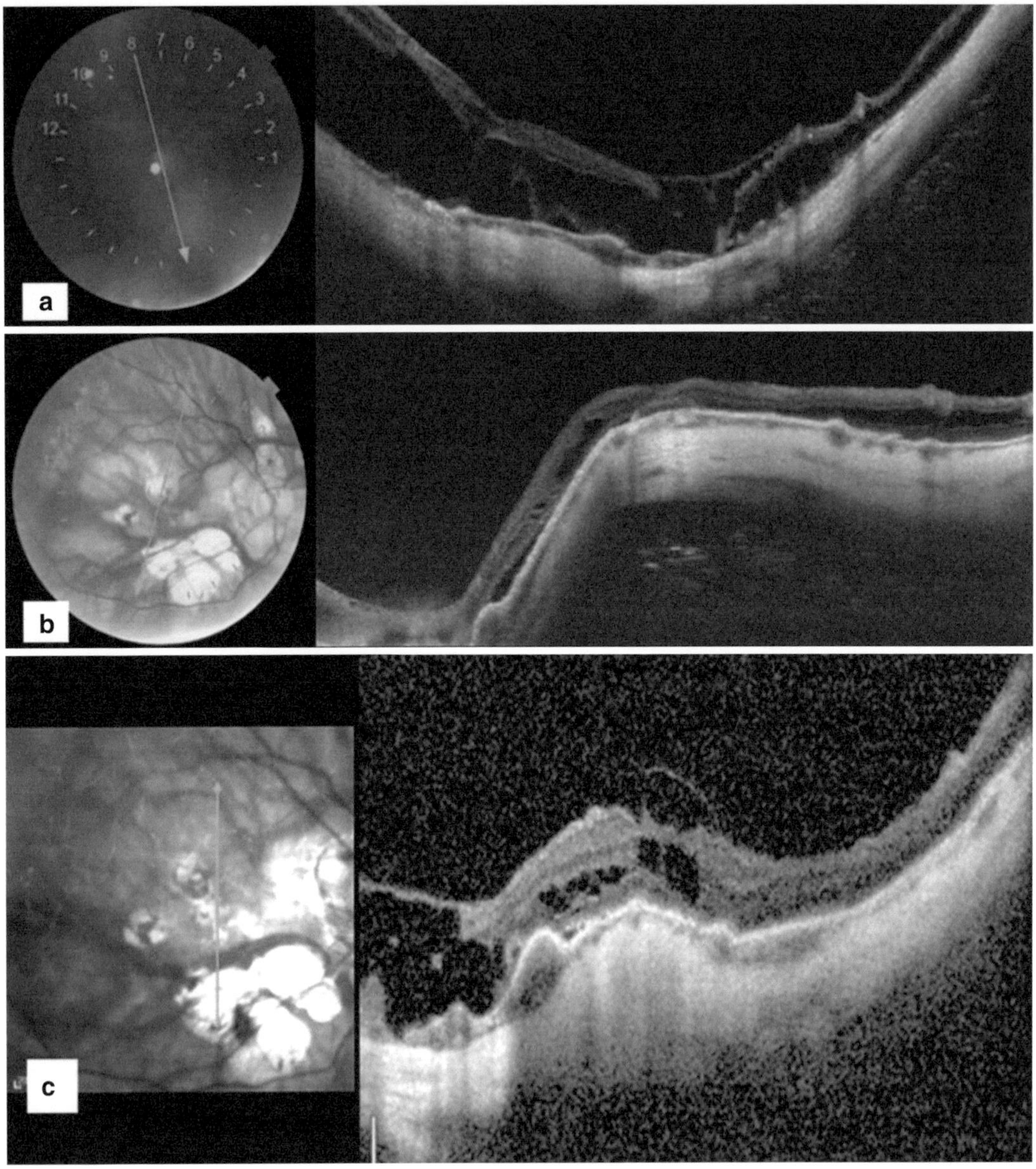

Fig. 26.15 Eye affected by maculoschisis and areas of detachment. (**a**) Preoperative OCT showing a schisis with areas of MD and an O-LMH. (**b**) Postoperative OCT after combined MB + PPV surgery without ILM peeling showing a successful resolution of the schisis and the O-LMH. The shape is now convex over the buckle. (**c**) Recurrence of MTM, immediately after MB removal, due to pain. The MB had been implanted only 2 months before removal

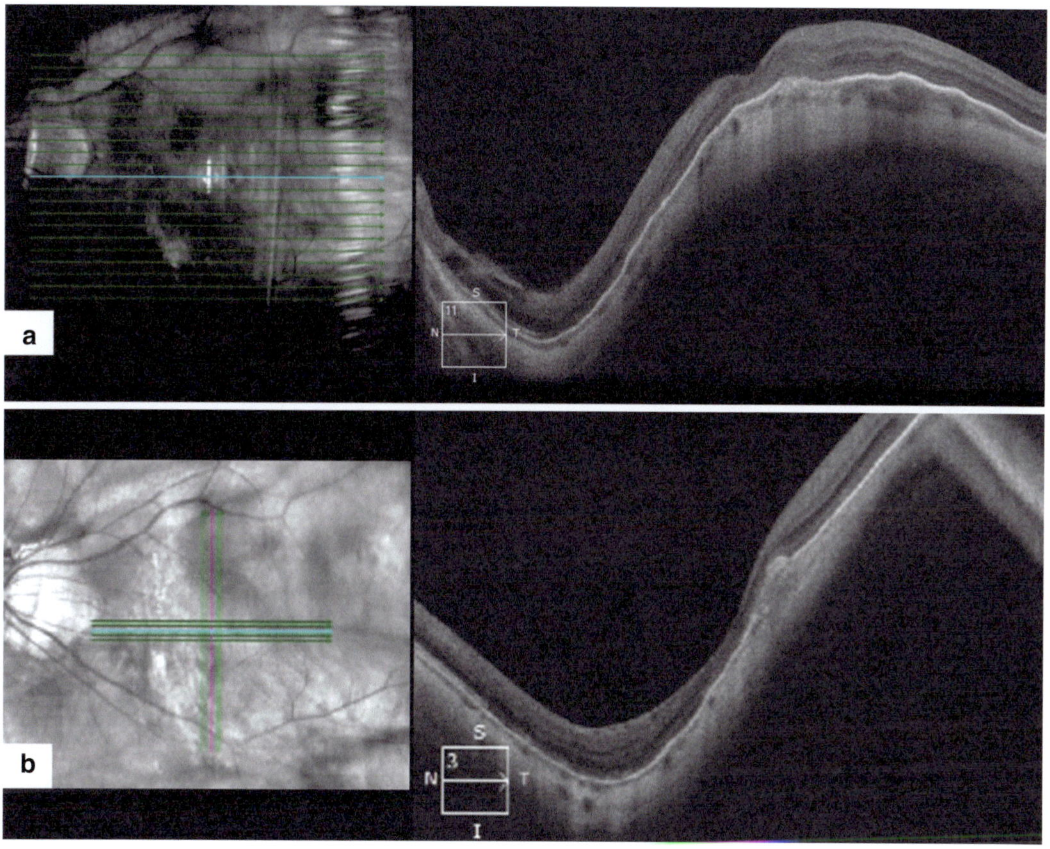

Fig. 26.16 (**a**) Postoperative OCT showing the convex shape of the posterior pole, 4 years after MB implantation. (**b**) OCT scan 2 months after MB removal. The shape of the posterior pole is convex and the fovea and choroid appear thinner. The juxtafoveal CNV occurred 1 year after MB implantation

years after surgery, the anatomical benefit remains although the indentation becomes less pronounced (Fig. 26.16). We advise not to remove the buckle whenever possible or to for at least 6 months.

The buckling effect is always more evident in the first month, then a mild release of indentation is visible (Fig. 26.19). However, the new scleral shape, obtained 2 months after surgery, seems to remain unchanged in most of the cases when the buckle is not removed.

The ideal final shape of the sclera and retina complex is horizontal (Fig. 26.17).

26.6.7 Evolution of the Surgical Technique

Different models of macular buckle have been proposed in the years. The first technique consisted of suturing a sponge to the sclera behind the macula. This technique has been abandoned because too difficult and links to a high rate of complications.

Different models have been proposed to overcome this difficulty such as the model of Devine, Ando, and Landolfo [55].

The idea was to be able to move the sutures anteriorly in a safer and more accessible location.

The first model of MB proposed by Parolini was created by inserting a stainless steel wire into a silicone sponge, 7 mm wide and 5 mm thick (507 Labtician). The sponge could be bent to an L-shape, with a short side, called head, to buckle the macula, and a long side, called arm, to allow an anterior suture. The MB was inserted by pushing the head behind the macular sclera, through the superotemporal quadrant, leaving

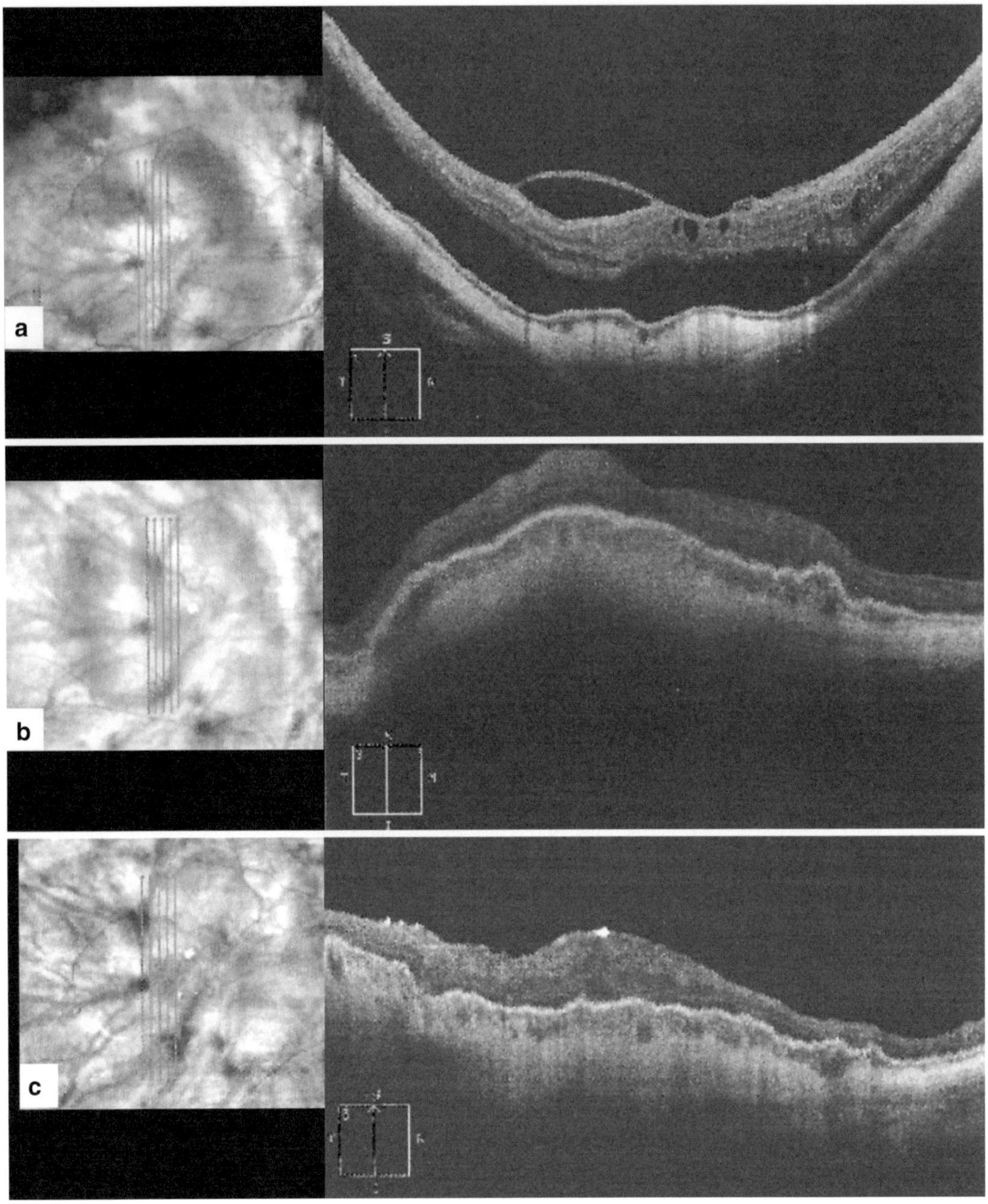

Fig. 26.17 (**a**) Preoperative OCT showing the concave shape of the posterior pole, in an eye with macular detachment in a posterior staphyloma. (**b**) OCT scan 1.5 months after MB implantation. The shape of the posterior pole is convex and the fovea and choroid appear thicker. (**c**) Vertical OCT scan 6 months after MB implantation. The shape of the posterior pole is horizontal

the arm parallel to lateral without the need of detaching any muscles. The sutures needed to stabilize the arm were placed anteriorly at the level of the insertion of the lateral rectus muscle. The first results were presented at the EVRS meeting in 2009 and at the Heatam meeting in 2009. Later, in 2011, the model was modified (Figs. 26.18 and 26.19) by substituting the stainless steel stent with a titanium stent covered by a silicone sleeve (70 Labtician), in order to avoid

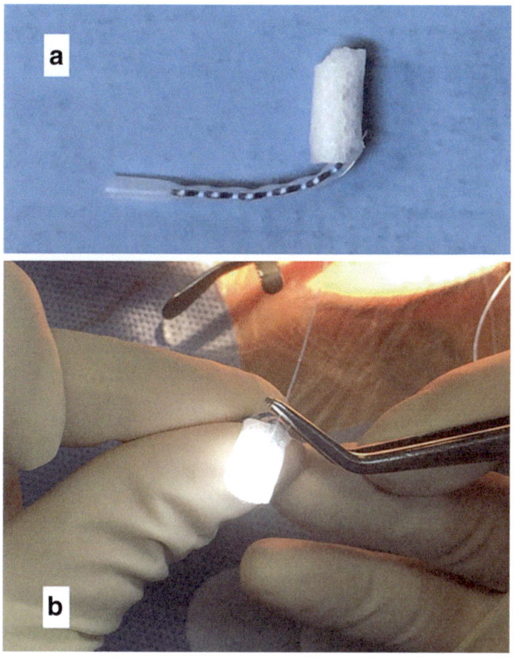

Fig. 26.18 Example of macular buckles used by the author. (**a**) A titanium stent was covered by a silicone sleeve in the arm of the MB, while the head was covered by a silicone sponge. (**b**) MB with a fiber optic light inside the head, to control the final position of the buckle using scleral transillumination

the extrusion induced by the sponge. The solid silicone covering the head of the buckle was replaced with a soft sponge, with the aim to avoid atrophy of the RPE induced by acute angles of solid silicone. Moreover, to assess the final position of the MB, the use of a panoramic microscope and two optic fibers positioned into the pars plana and into the head of the buckle was adopted (Figs. 26.18 and 26.19). The scleral transillumination helps the surgeon to manage the exact position of the buckle and center it underneath the fovea and in particular underneath the macular hole, if present. The size of the head of the buckle should be 7 mm by 8–10 mm to avoid the risk of inducing pain, diplopia, or limitations to eye movement.

The MB is positioned in the superotemporal quadrant with the lateral arm parallel either to the lateral or to the superior rectus muscle. The first option leads to buckle the macula from the temporal side to the nasal side. The second option leads to buckle the macula from 12 o'clock to 6 o'clock and parallel to the optic nerve. This position reduces the risk of optic nerve touch, extrusion, and diplopia.

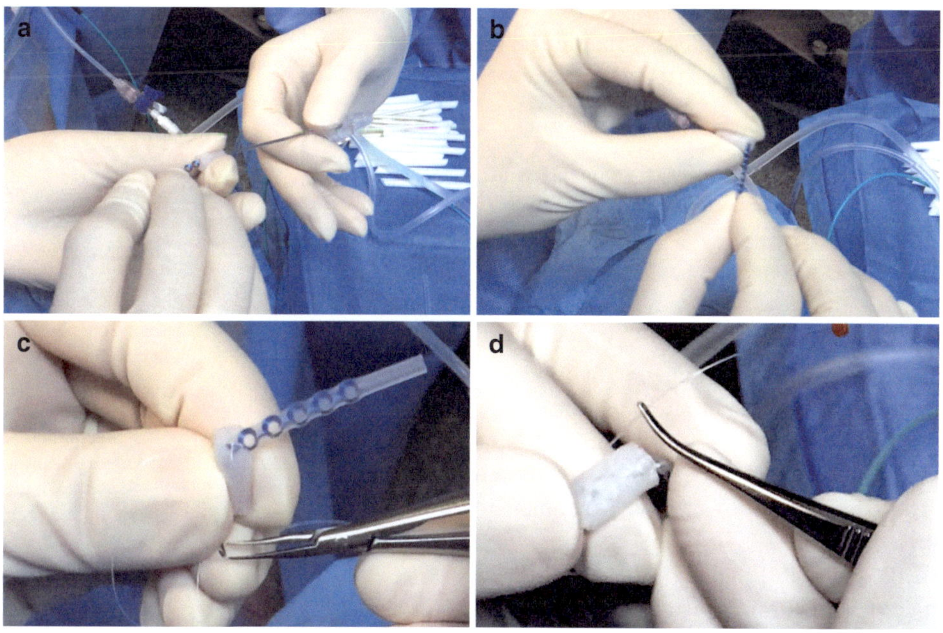

Fig. 26.19 Key steps to assemble a macular buckle. (**a**) Insertion of the titanium stent inside a soft silicone sponge. (**b**) Bending of the arm of the MB. (**c**) Fixing the silicone sponge to the arm. (**d**) Insertion of a fiber optic light inside the head of the MB

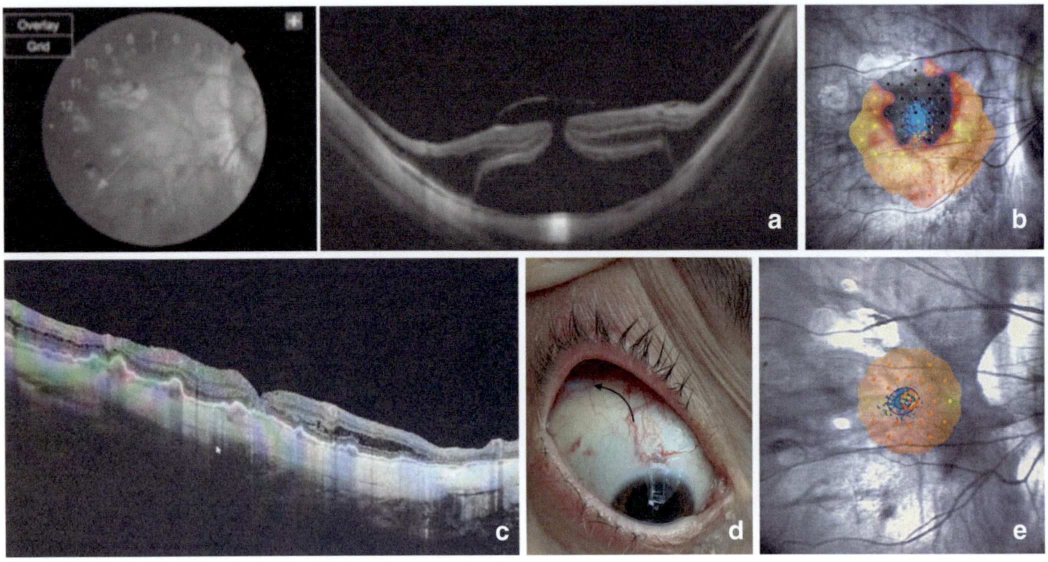

Fig. 26.20 Case report of 56-year-old female affected by MTM. (**a**) SD-OCT showing an MD with an FTMH. (**b**) Preoperative microperimetry. (**c**) Postoperative OCT 1 month after combined MB + PPV surgery with ILM inverted flap technique. (**d**) Postoperative picture of the anterior segment. The arrow shows the arm of the MB barely visible beneath the conjunctiva. (**e**) Postoperative microperimetry

The final shape of the posterior sclera should be as horizontal as possible, resembling the normal posterior pole. An excessive change in the shape of the macula, with a final convex profile, could induce metamorphopsia, unwanted tangential, or excessive refractive modifications. Therefore, the most suitable shape for the head of the buckle is a flat one, in order to reach a flat scleral surface.

26.7 Case Report

Here we report a case of a 56-year-old female affected by MTM in her right eye (Fig. 26.20a, b). This patient was followed up for 3 years before surgery, showing a progressive worsening of both BCVA and her clinical picture. At last follow-up, SD-OCT showed an FTMH with an MD. The patient was directed to a combined surgery.

An MB and a PPV with ILM inverted flap technique were performed. Figure 26.20-C shows the postoperative results 1 month after surgery. A complete macular flattening was obtained, with a complete closure of an FTMH. Figure 26.20-D shows the anterior segment of our patient, with the arm of the MB visible beneath the conjunctiva.

Disclosure No competing interests.
No financial disclosure.

References

1. Benhamou N, Massin P, Haouchine B, Erginay A, Gaudric A. Macular retinoschisis in highly myopic eyes. Am J Ophthalmol. 2002;133(6):794–800.
2. Phillips C. Retinal detachment at the posterior pole. Br J Ophthalmol. 1958;42:749–53.
3. Takano M, Kishi S. Foveal retinoschisis and retinal detachment in severely myopic eyes with posterior staphyloma. Am J Ophthalmol. 1999;128(4):472–6.
4. Panozzo G, Mercanti A. Optical coherence tomography findings in myopic traction maculopathy. Arch Ophthalmol. 2004;122(10):1455–60. https://doi.org/10.1001/archopht.122.10.1455.
5. Shimada N, Yoshida T, Sugamoto Y, et al. Progression from macular retinoschisis to retinal detachment in highly myopic eyes is associated with outer lamellar hole formation progression from macular retinoschisis to retinal detachment in highly myopic eyes is associated with outer lamellar hole formation. Br J Ophthalmol. 2008;92(6):762–4. https://doi.org/10.1136/bjo.2007.131359.

6. Frisina R, Gius I, Palmieri M, Finzi A, Tozzi L, Parolini B. Myopic Traction Maculopathy: Diagnostic and Management Strategies. Clin Ophthalmol. 2020;14:3699–708. https://doi.org/10.2147/OPTH.S237483. PMID: 33173268; PMCID: PMC7646438.
7. Wallman J. Myopia and the control of eye growth. Introduction. In: Ciba found symposium; 1990.
8. Tkatchenko TV, Shen Y, Tkatchenko AV. Mouse experimental myopia has features of primate myopia. Investig Ophthalmol Vis Sci. 2010;51(3):1297–303. https://doi.org/10.1167/iovs.09-4153.
9. Dell'Omo R, Virgili G, Bottoni F, et al. Lamellar macular holes in the eyes with pathological myopia. Graefes Arch Clin Exp Ophthalmol. 2018;256(7):1281–90. https://doi.org/10.1007/s00417-018-3995-8.
10. Zampedri E, Romanelli F, Semeraro F, Parolini B, Frisina R. Spectral-domain optical coherence tomography findings in idiopathic lamellar macular hole. Graefes Arch Clin Exp Ophthalmol. 2017;255(4):699–707. https://doi.org/10.1007/s00417-016-3545-1.
11. Shimada N, Tanaka Y, Tokoro T, Ohno-Matsui K. Natural course of myopic traction maculopathy and factors associated with progression or resolution. Am J Ophthalmol. 2013;156(5):948–957.e1. https://doi.org/10.1016/j.ajo.2013.06.031.
12. Ouyang PB, Duan XC, Zhu XH. Diagnosis and maculopathy treatment of myopic traction. Int J Ophthalmol. 2012;5(6):754–8. https://doi.org/10.3980/j.issn.2222-3959.2012.06.19.
13. Gaucher D, Haouchine B, Tadayoni R, et al. Long-term follow-up of high myopic foveoschisis: natural course and surgical outcome. Am J Ophthalmol. 2007;143(3):455–62. https://doi.org/10.1016/j.ajo.2006.10.053.
14. Ichibe M, Baba E, Funaki S, Yoshizawa T, Abe H. Retinoschisis in a highly myopic eye without vision impairment. Retina. 2004;24(2):331–3.
15. Panozzo G, Mercanti A. Vitrectomy for myopic traction maculopathy. Arch Ophthalmol. 2007;125(6):767–72. https://doi.org/10.1001/archopht.125.6.767.
16. Fujimoto M, Hangai M, Suda K, Yoshimura N. Features associated with foveal retinal detachment in myopic macular retinoschisis. Am J Ophthalmol. 2010;150(6):863–70. https://doi.org/10.1016/j.ajo.2010.06.023.
17. Fang X, Weng Y, Xu S, et al. Optical coherence tomographic characteristics and surgical outcome of eyes with myopic foveoschisis. Eye. 2009;23(6):1336–42. https://doi.org/10.1038/eye.2008.291.
18. Sun CB, Liu Z, Xue AQ, Yao K. Natural evolution from macular retinoschisis to full-thickness macular hole in highly myopic eyes. Eye. 2010;24(12):1787–91. https://doi.org/10.1038/eye.2010.123.
19. Sayanagi K, Ikuno Y, Soga K, Tano Y. Photoreceptor inner and outer segment defects in myopic foveoschisis. Am J Ophthalmol. 2008;145(5):902–8. https://doi.org/10.1016/j.ajo.2008.01.011.
20. Ripandelli G, Rossi T, Scarinci F, Scassa C, Parisi V, Stirpe M. Macular vitreoretinal interface abnormalities in highly myopic eyes with posterior staphyloma: 5-year follow-up. Retina. 2012;32(8):1531–8. https://doi.org/10.1097/IAE.0b013e318255062c.
21. Shevelev M. Operation against high myopia and scleralectasia with aid of the transplantation of fascia lata on thinned sclera. Russ Oftalmol J. 1930;11(1):107–10.
22. Schepens CL, Okamura ID, Brockhurst RJ. The scleral buckling procedures. I. Surgical techniques and management. AMA Arch Ophthalmol. 1957;58(6):797–811.
23. Calabria GA, Pruett RC, Refojo MF, Schepens CL. Sutureless scleral buckling. An experimental technique. Arch Ophthalmol. 1970;83(5):613–8.
24. Theodossiadis GP, Theodossiadis PG. Optical coherence tomography in optic disk pit maculopathy treated by the macular buckling procedure. Am J Ophthalmol. 2001;132(2):184–90.
25. Theodossiadis GP, Sasoh M. Macular buckling for retinal detachment due to macular hole in highly myopic eyes with posterior staphyloma. Retina. 2002;22(1):129.
26. Rosengren B. The silver plomb method in amotio retinae: clinical experience and results. Bibl Ophthalmol. 1966;70:253–6.
27. Klöti R. Silver clip for central retinal detachments with macular hole. Mod Probl Ophthalmol. 1974;12:330–6.
28. Maćkowiak A. Retinal detachment surgery for giant tear or macular hole. The oblique encircling silastic band without evacuation of subretinal flui. Jpn J Ophthalmol. 1970;18:245.
29. Mateo C, Burés-Jelstrup A, Navarro R, Corcóstegui B. Macular buckling for eyes with myopic foveoschisis secondary to posterior staphyloma. Retina. 2012;32(6):1121–8. https://doi.org/10.1097/IAE.0b013e31822e5c32.
30. Parolini B, Frisina R, Pinackatt S, Mete M. A new L-shaped design of macular buckle to support a posterior staphyloma in high myopia. Retina. 2013;33(7):1466–70. https://doi.org/10.1097/IAE.0b013e31828e69ea.
31. Siam AL. Management of central retinal detachment due to a macular hole. Br J Ophthalmol. 1973;57(5):351–4.
32. Gonvers M, Machemer R. A new approach to treating retinal detachment with macular hole. Am J Ophthalmol. 1982;94(4):468–72.
33. Vallat M. Surgical treatment of retinal detachment from macular hole. Graefes Arch Clin Exp Ophthalmol. 1986;224(3):238–9.
34. Oshima Y. Complete epiretinal membrane separation in highly myopic eyes with retinal detachment resulting from a macular hole. Am J Ophthalmol. 1998;126(5):669–76.
35. Wolfensberger TJ, Gonvers M. Long-term follow-up of retinal detachment due to macular hole in myopic eyes treated by temporary silicone oil tamponade and laser photocoagulation. Ophthalmology. 1999;106(9):1786–91. https://doi.org/10.1016/S0161-6420(99)90344-5.

36. Kadonosono K, Yazama F, Itoh N, et al. Treatment of retinal detachment resulting from myopic macular hole with internal limiting membrane removal. Am J Ophthalmol. 2001;131(2):203–7.
37. Lu L, Li Y, Cai S, Yang J. Vitreous surgery in highly myopic retinal detachment resulting from a macular hole. Clin Exp Ophthalmol. 2002;30(4):261–5.
38. Chen Y. Treatment of retinal detachment resulting from posterior staphyloma-associated macular hole in highly myopic eyes. Retina. 2006;26(1):25–31.
39. Rizzo S. Successful treatment of persistent macular holes using "heavy silicone oil" as intraocular tamponade. Retina. 2006;26(8):905–8.
40. Cheung B. Results of high-density silicone oil as a tamponade agent in macular hole retinal detachment in patients with high myopia. Br J Ophthalmol. 2007;91(6):719–21.
41. Mete M, Parolini B, Maggio E, Pertile G. 1000 cSt silicone oil vs heavy silicone oil as intraocular tamponade in retinal detachment associated with myopic macular hole. Graefes Arch Clin Exp Ophthalmol. 2011;249(6):821–6.
42. Sasoh M, Yoshida S, Ito Y, Matsui K, Osawa S, Uji Y. Macular buckling for retinal detachment due to macular hole in highly myopic eyes with posterior staphyloma. Retina. 2000;20(5):445–9.
43. Ripandelli G, Coppé AM, Fedeli R, Parisi V, D'Amico DJ, Stirpe M. Evaluation of primary surgical procedures for retinal detachment with macular hole in highly myopic eyes: a comparison [corrected] of vitrectomy versus posterior episcleral buckling surgery. Ophthalmology. 2001;108(12):2258–64. discussion 2265
44. Theodossiadis GP, Theodossiadis PG. The macular buckling procedure in the treatment of retinal detachment in highly myopic eyes with macular hole and posterior staphyloma: mean follow-up of 15 years. Retina. 2005;25(3):285–9.
45. Tanaka T, Ando F, Usui M. Episcleral macular buckling by semirigid shaped-rod exoplant for recurrent retinal detachment with macular hole in highly myopic eyes. Retina. 2005;25(2):147–51.
46. Ward B, Tarutta EP, Mayer MJ. The efficacy and safety of posterior pole buckles in the control of progressive high myopia. Eye. 2009;23(12):2169–74. https://doi.org/10.1038/eye.2008.433.
47. Tian J, Tang L-S, Guo X-J, Luo Y-H. Episcleral macular buckling for posterior retinal detachment in silicone oil filled eyes associated with myopic macular hole. Int J Ophthalmol. 2013;6(2):165–8. https://doi.org/10.3980/j.issn.2222-3959.2013.02.11.
48. Sasaki H, Shiono A, Kogo J, et al. Inverted internal limiting membrane flap technique as a useful procedure for macular hole-associated retinal detachment in highly myopic eyes. Eye. 2017;31(4):545–50. https://doi.org/10.1038/eye.2016.263.
49. Yuan J, Zhang L-L, Lu Y-J, Han M-Y, Yu A-H, Cai X-J. Vitrectomy with internal limiting membrane peeling versus inverted internal limiting membrane flap technique for macular hole-induced retinal detachment: a systematic review of literature and meta-analysis. BMC Ophthalmol. 2017;17(1):219. https://doi.org/10.1186/s12886-017-0619-8.
50. Kinoshita T, Onoda Y, Maeno T. Long-term surgical outcomes of the inverted internal limiting membrane flap technique in highly myopic macular hole retinal detachment. Graefes Arch Clin Exp Ophthalmol. 2017;255(6):1101–6. https://doi.org/10.1007/s00417-017-3614-0.
51. Alkabes M, Mateo C. Macular buckle technique in myopic traction maculopathy: a 16-year review of the literature and a comparison with vitreous surgery. Graefes Arch Clin Exp Ophthalmol. 2018;256(5):863–77. https://doi.org/10.1007/s00417-018-3947-3.
52. Figueroa MS, Ruiz-Moreno JM, Gonzalez del Valle F, et al. Long-term outcomes of 23-gauge pars plana vitrectomy with internal limiting membrane peeling and gas tamponade for myopic traction maculopathy. Retina. 2015;35(9):1836–43. https://doi.org/10.1097/IAE.0000000000000554.
53. Guo X, Xiao O, Chen Y, et al. Three-dimensional eye shape, myopic maculopathy, and visual acuity: the zhongshan ophthalmic center–brien holden vision institute high myopia cohort study. Ophthalmology. 2017;124(5):679–87. https://doi.org/10.1016/j.ophtha.2017.01.009.
54. Hsiang HW, Ohno-Matsui K, Shimada N, et al. Clinical characteristics of posterior staphyloma in eyes with pathologic myopia. Am J Ophthalmol. 2008;146(1):102–10. https://doi.org/10.1016/j.ajo.2008.03.010.
55. Lvaar A. Macular hole induced retinal detachment: treatment with an armed silicone implant. Ophthalmic Surg. 1986;17(12):810–2.

Management of Maculopathy Due to Optic Disc Pit

27

Dhananjay Shukla

27.1 Introduction

Optic disc pits are rare, congenital cavitary anomalies of the optic nerve head [1]. They are included among the *atypical* optic nerve colobomas (not occurring In line with embryonic fissure) because of their sporadic, unilateral nature, and frequently temporal location on the optic disc [2]. Optic pits remain asymptomatic, often till third or fourth decade of life, when vision declines due to thickening of the adjoining macula with schisis or serous detachment (25–75% of cases); macular involvement occurs almost exclusively with temporally located optic pits [1–4]. Optic pit maculopathy (OPM) was initially presumed to be a serous detachment of macula, a concept which persists in literature, notwithstanding the prescient description of macular schisis by Lincoff and colleagues without the aid of optical coherence tomography (OCT) [4, 5]. The macular schisis is now considered central to the development of maculopathy: the splitting starts at the macular edge of the optic pit as fluid enters the outer retinal layers, and dissects through the inner retinal layers, also gaining access to subretinal space [3, 4, 6, 7]. Though the origin of the fluid causing maculopathy is not established, an increasing majority of researchers believe that synchitic vitreous enters papillomacular retina through the dysplastic tissue of pit [5–7]. Vitreomacular traction, both anteroposterior and tangential, appears to play a major role in the passage of fluid into macula [5, 6, 8].

27.2 Natural History and Indications for Treatment

Sobol and colleagues followed up 15 patients (15 eyes) with optic pit maculopathy for an average duration of 9 years [8] They reported that 80% of the eyes end up with a vision of 20/200 or less—in spite of spontaneous resolution of fluid in 26% eyes—largely due to retinal pigment epithelial degeneration, inner retinal cysts, and formation of lamellar and full-thickness macular holes. The visual loss occurred within 6 months of the serous detachment [8]. Most authorities had been unanimous so far about the need for urgent intervention in view of the poor visual prognosis of untreated optic pit maculopathy [1, 4]. The most recent and the largest surgical study on the subject however specified that maculopathy without subretinal fluid (SRF), especially with good vision, can be safely observed. Once SRF develops, chances of spontaneous recovery are reduced 5 times and worsening occurs 3 times more commonly [3]. Besides SRF, other indications of early surgery include spread of schisis into multiple layers of

D. Shukla (✉)
Retina-Vitreous Service, Ratan Jyoti Netralaya, Gwalior, India

A. Jain et al. (eds.), *Cutting-edge Vitreoretinal Surgery*,
https://doi.org/10.1007/978-981-33-4168-5_27

macula, interruption of the outer retinal bands, and development of outer lamellar holes, which tend to worsen visual outcomes after surgery [3, 4, 9–11].

27.3 Evolution of Treatment Options

Once the treatment is indicated by progressive visual loss with corresponding increase in maculopathy, treatment options include barrage laser photocoagulation of the optic pit, pneumatic retinopexy, macular scleral buckling, and vitrectomy. Postel and colleagues were one of the first to compare the anatomical success of these procedures [12]. They reported that laser demarcation of the optic pit did not significantly improve the macular reattachment/flattening over the natural course of the disease; pneumoretinopexy improved outcomes in two-thirds of the cases; while macular buckling and vitrectomy were successful in most of the cases. Currently, small gauge vitrectomy is the default option for vitreoretinal surgeons due to its relative ease and less invasiveness as compared to posterior scleral buckling [4]. The other area of certainty is lack of benefit from laser photocoagulation alone [4, 12]. However, for young patients with moderate visual loss and favorable macular anatomy (no multilayered schisis, SRF, outer lamellar hole, or retinal pigment epithelial atrophy), the charm of a noninvasive procedure remains, in the form of pneumoretinopexy. Akiyama et al. attempted SF_6 gas injection in 8 patients, with 50% reattachments, the rest were successfully treated with vitrectomy [13]. Recently, Lei et al. improved the success rate of pneumoretinopexy to 100% in another small case series with a few tweaks: they used long-duration tamponade (C_3F_8), followed it up with laser barrage, kept the patients in the prone position for 2 weeks, and reinjected gas as required [14]. However, it is important to emphasize that performing a safe and adequate laser demarcation of the pit at the papillomacular bundle with suitably low power (especially in a child), as well as injecting and positioning a large, single gas bubble over the optic pit margin in the presence of non-syneretic gel vitreous in the young subjects may pose considerable real-world problems. These considerations, and the relative ease of small-gauge vitrectomy, have led to a lack of enthusiasm in surgeons at large in standalone pneumoretinopexy [3, 4].

27.4 Surgical Technique

27.4.1 Vitrectomy

Notwithstanding the dispute about the origin of macular fluid, the role of vitreopapillary traction in initiating and sustaining macular hydration is beyond controversy [15]. Pars plana vitrectomy is therefore the default treatment of optic pit maculopathy, with success rates ranging from 75–100% in the largest and most recent interventional studies [3, 10, 16–19]. The undisputed key step in vitrectomy is the detachment of posterior hyaloid (PVD) after core vitrectomy, and maybe the only procedure required in most cases [3, 4, 16, 18, 19]. The accessory procedures employed to reduce failures, recurrences, and complications of vitrectomy have been numerous and varied. The described bouquet of surgical adjuvants and variants include a choice of tamponade (none, air, short- or long-acting gases, or silicone oil), laser demarcation of the optic pit, partial/complete removal of the internal limiting membrane (ILM) from macula, draining the submacular fluid, filling the pit with various tissues (ILM, scleral plug, fibrin glue, etc.), removing the tissue/condensed vitreous from the optic pit, and most recently, inner retinal fenestration [4].

27.4.2 Gas Tamponade

The agents most frequently used are short-acting gases like air, sulfur hexafluoride (SF_6) and long-lasting gases like perfluoropropane (C_3F_8). The second largest surgical study on optic pits (MACPIT Study) reported excellent results (86% reattachment rates) with both the types of gases [20]. Nonetheless, unless prone positioning is strictly followed, use of gases other than air could predispose the young subjects to avoidable cataract formation. Further, complete resolution of macular fluid in most cases takes about a year, which counters the utility of even long-acting gases or silicone oil [3, 4, 19, 20]. Hirakata and colleagues reported about 90% anatomical success without any gas or laser [16]. Teke and Citirik concurred that use of gas did not affect the final outcomes, with the rider that resolution of maculopathy might be faster in patients with gas tamponade [10]. The largest and most recent study till date similarly reported no additional benefit from the use of tamponade [3].

27.4.3 Laser Demarcation of the Optic Pit

There has been a great variability in the literature on the timing and wavelength of the laser used to cordon off the optic pit; however, the dreaded nerve fiber layer damage and consequent visual field defects have not been reported irrespective of the wavelength and timing of the barrage photocoagulation [4]. Since the irrelevance of laser to surgical outcomes was first documented [16], it has been endorsed by the most recent, largest, and longest surgical studies [17–20]. Withholding laser makes intuitive sense since the demarcation does not affect fluid seepage through inner retinal layers of the papillomacular isthmus, unless it reaches upward from RPE and compacts (thus damaging) the inner retina, making laser probably a no-win situation.

27.4.4 ILM Peeling

Retinal surgeons are trigger-happy with ILM peeling during any macular surgery and optic pits are no exception; except that in some cases, the central macula is wafer-thin due to large outer lamellar holes. We reported excellent outcomes in such cases, and encountered no intra-operative macular holes (Fig. 27.1). In spite of full-thickness macule holes developing in 4 out of 7 cases, we obtained excellent anatomical AND visual outcomes, without further intervention in most cases. In such thinned out macula and in presence of adherent gel vitreous, PVD induction is probably more traumatic and liable to cause macular holes: indeed, two studies reported paramacular/macular holes in 25% and 33% of cases, respectively, without ILM peeling [19, 21]. However, any risk factor for macular hole formation is better avoided as it can lead to poor visual outcomes [10], and therefore ILM peeling may better be reserved for surgical failures rather than as a primary surgical procedure, as shown by the latest and largest studies [4, 17, 18, 20].

27.4.5 Plugging the Pit

Besides peeling ILM, retinal surgeons have another fetish, closing the holes. So the optic pit has been plugged with a variety of autologous tissue, ranging from platelet-rich plasma, scleral graft, ILM flap, or fibrin glue [22–25]. The plug is most commonly reserved for primary surgical failures, justifying the add-on procedure, especially in view of the gratifying outcomes. On the contrary, others have reported that the removal of tissue from the pit increased the success rate of conventional vitrectomy, without the need for any scleral plug [26].

27.4.6 Draining the Macular Fluid

Here is a key issue with persistently labelling the pit maculopathy as retinal detachment: endo-drainage of the *subretinal* fluid appears a justified, acceptable procedure [27–29]. Since we became aware of the essentially intraretinal location of macular fluid [5], and the redundancy of any tamponade to settle it [16], inflicting the trauma of a drainage retinotomy into an already compromised macula has become futile and unacceptable [2, 4]. On the other hand, the surgeon's itch to reattach the retina can be safely satisfied by drainage through the pit, for whatever it is worth [4, 11, 29, 30].

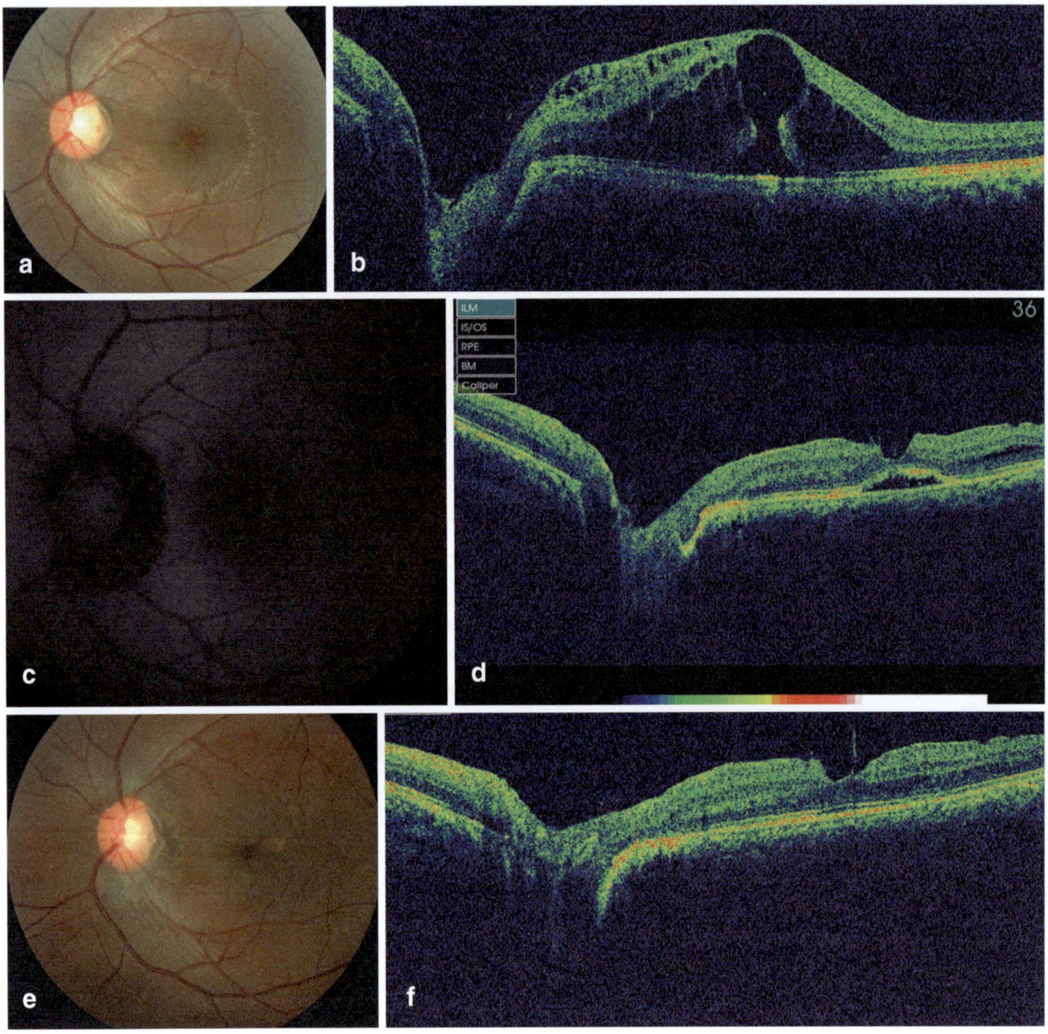

Fig. 27.1 Optic pit maculopathy: A forbidding case turns out well. (**a**) This 19-year-old man was aware of reduced vision (6/18) in the left eye for about a month. There was a tiny pit at 3:00 meridian at the temporal rim of the left optic disc, with adjoining macular elevation and a suspected macular hole. (**b**) Optical coherence tomography (OCT) revealed a severe presentation: a massive macular schisis (850 μ) with large outer retinal dehiscence and a wafer-thin roof (33 μ), betraying a chronic course in spite of the short history. (**c**) Autofluorescence imaging 3 months after vitrectomy (including peeling of internal limiting membrane, barrage laser, and gas) reveals normalizing signals except at center, where residual fluid retains hyperautofluorescence. The pigment epithelial atrophy secondary to barrage photocoagulation at the disc margin stands out as confluent rows of hyperautofluorescent signals. (**d**) In spite of the residual subretinal fluid centrally, continuity of the photoreceptor layer and external limiting membrane on OCT ensured visual recovery to 6/6 at 3 months. Also, note that the (heavy) laser scars (see **c**) adjoining the disc edge leave the papillomacular bundle unscathed; the patient complained of no scotomas. (**e**, **f**) One year postoperatively, the patient maintained excellent vision, with near-perfect recovery of foveal contours and integrity of outer retinal bands on OCT, despite the dissociated nerve fibers visible around the central macula

27.4.7 Inner Retinal Fenestration

Investigators, starting with the redoubtable late JDM Gass himself, have long argued that cerebrospinal fluid (not vitreous) is the source of macular fluid associated with optic pit [31]; but nobody took the argument far enough to attempt *draining the macular schitic fluid into vitreous cavity*, contrary to the conventional wisdom of blocking the entry of fluid from the vitreous cavity into macula. Spaide and colleagues first proposed this contrarian hypothesis through a case study where they only created a partial thickness fenestration radial to the pit through the inner retinal layers after core vitrectomy [32]. Eight years later, they supported the hypothesis by the largest-so-far single-surgeon case series with 3 years' follow-up and 94% success rate, without laser, ILM peeling or even PVD induction [21]. Others, however, could not replicate their remarkable success [3, 32, 33]. The authors themselves conceded that the fenestration was useful mainly for the eyes with fluid entry through inner retina [21]. Others have demonstrated that fluid enters into macula from the pit predominantly through outer retina layers, and then dissects into inner retina and subretinal space [3, 34].

27.4.8 Macular Scleral Buckling

Theodossiadis and colleagues reported another radical approach, which consisted of external fixation of a posterior scleral sponge across the macula without any laser or gas [35]. This technique claimed to address both the putative sources of fluid in pit maculopathy (vitreous and CSF) and improvement in both visual acuity and fields. They recently summed up their long-term results with an excellent anatomical success rate of about 85% over a follow-up of 13 years [36]. In spite of the appeal of an external approach in the young subjects with clear crystalline lenses (minimal risk of cataract) and adherent gel vitreous (difficult and potentially traumatic PVD induction), the inherent difficulty and long learning curve of the macular buckle have prevented most retinal surgeons from leaving their comfort zone of vitrectomy [3, 4, 12, 35].

27.5 Summary

Optic pit is a rare congenital defect, which intermittently conduits fluid vitreous or CSF into macular retina; but becomes visually symptomatic only decades later, when enough fluid accumulates in multiple layers of macula. Though young subjects with only intraretinal fluid and good vision can be observed initially, treatment is required in all cases where progressive visual decline is documented. Untreated patients should be periodically followed up with fundus photography, OCT, and autofluorescence imaging. Vitrectomy is the default and definitive treatment. Though barrage photocoagulation and pneumoretinopexy could be attempted in young patients hesitant for surgery, they should be viewed as stopgap arrangements to defer rather than avoid surgery. While simple core vitrectomy with PVD induction is the most evidence-based primary intervention, additional procedures like laser demarcation, ILM peeling, plugging the pit, and gas tamponade are justified in surgical failures. Before labelling a case as failed procedure, it is advisable to wait for 6–12 months to allow the chronic schitic cavities to settle down. Finally, the surgeons should also be aware of the situations where surgery is unlikely to help: chronic schisis leading to full-thickness retinal cysts (Fig. 27.2) or macular hole (as seen on OCT), and extensive geographic atrophy in the posterior pole (as confirmed on AF imaging). With a judicious use of the advanced modern imaging technology and surgical techniques, the management of this rare entity has become more consistent, reproducible, and rewarding for the vitreoretinal surgeon.

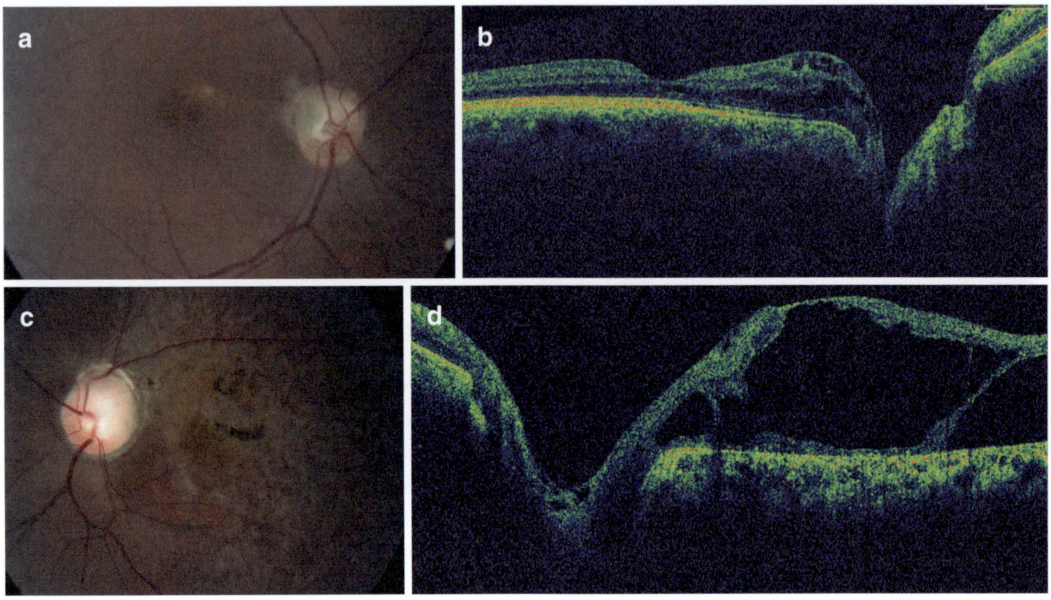

Fig. 27.2 Bilateral optic disc pits: Both of which are better left alone. (**a**) This 22-year-old man presented with poor vision in the left eye (LE) for a few years. The best-corrected visual acuity (BCVA) was 6/6p in the right eye. Note the temporal optic pit with subretinal precipitates supero-nasal to the fovea; the macula appears flat clinically. (**b**) OCT RE shows a localized multilayered schisis along the optic pit rim adjoining macula. The central fovea shows a few small cysts; there is no macular elevation, and the outer retinal bands are intact. (**c**) LE, for which the patient presented, was legally blind with BCVA of 3/60. The extensive retinal pigment epithelial mottling suggested a spontaneous collapse of macular schisis and detachment secondary to optic pit. The elevation of the superior and inferior temporal arcade vessels betrays the residual elevation of a thinned-out, glass-like retina. (**d**) OCT LE revealed massive, moth-eaten schitic cavities with widespread destruction of most of the sensory retinal layers and Muller's cells. This photograph appeared in the Official Newsletter of the Vitreoretinal Society—India (a nonprofit publication with member-only circulation), September 2018 issue, in Panel Discussion: Controversies in surgical management of optic pit maculopathy, anchored by the author (Dhananjay Shukla), pages 15–20. The permission to reproduce the photograph has been obtained by the author

References

1. Brodsky MC. Congenital optic disk anomalies. Surv Ophthalmol. 1994;39:89–112.
2. Jain N, Johnson MW. Pathogenesis and treatment of maculopathy associated with cavitary optic disc anomalies. Am J Ophthalmol. 2014;158:423–35.
3. Steel DHW, Suleman J, Murphy DC, Song A, Dodds S, Rees J. Optic disc pit maculopathy: a two-year nationwide prospective population-based study. Ophthalmology. 2018;125:1757–64.
4. Shukla D, Leila M. Surgical management of optic pit maculopathy: controversies and caveats. Exp Rev Ophthalmol. 2017;12:3–9.
5. Lincoff H, Lopez R, Kreissig I, et al. Retinoschisis associated with optic nerve pits. Arch Ophthalmol. 1988;106:61–7.
6. Rutledge BK, Puliafito CA, Duker JS, et al. Optical coherence tomography of macular lesions associated with optic nerve head pits. Ophthalmology. 1996;103:1047–53.
7. Imamura Y, Zweifel SA, Fujiwara T, et al. High-resolution optical coherence tomography findings in optic pit maculopathy. Retina. 2010;30:1104–12.
8. Sobol WM, Blodi CF, Folk JC, Weingeist TA. Long-term visual outcome in patients with optic nerve pit and serous retinal detachment of the macula. Ophthalmology. 1990;97:1539–42.
9. Steel DHW, Williamson TH, Laidlaw DAH, et al. Extent and location of intraretinal and subretinal fluid as prognostic factors for the outcome of patients with optic disk pit maculopathy. Retina. 2016;36:110–8.
10. Teke MY, Citirik M. 23 gauge vitrectomy, endolaser, and gas tamponade versus vitrectomy alone for serous macular detachment associated with optic disc pit. Am J Ophthalmol. 2015;160:779–85.
11. Shukla D, Kalliath J, Tandon M, et al. Vitrectomy for optic disk pit with macular schisis and outer retinal dehiscence. Retina. 2012;32:1337–42.

12. Postel EA, Pulido JS, McNamara JA, Johnson MW. The etiology and treatment of macular detachment associated with optic nerve pits and related anomalies. Trans Am Ophthalmol Soc. 1998;96:73–93.
13. Akiyama H, Shimoda Y, Fukuchi M, et al. Intravitreal gas injection without vitrectomy for macular detachment associated with an optic disk pit. Retina. 2014;34:222–7.
14. Lei L, Li T, Ding X, et al. Gas tamponade combined with laser photocoagulation therapy for congenital optic disc pit maculopathy. Eye. 2015;29:106–14.
15. Yokoi T, Nakayama Y, Nishina S, et al. Abnormal traction of the vitreous detected by swept-source optical coherence tomography is related to the maculopathy associated with optic disc pits. Graefes Arch Clin Exp Ophthalmol. 2016;254:675–82.
16. Hirakata A, Inoue M, Hiraoka T, et al. Vitrectomy without laser treatment or gas tamponade for macular detachment associated with an optic disc pit. Ophthalmology. 2012;119:810–8.
17. KKESH Study Group. Pars plana vitrectoy with juxtapapillary laser photocoagulation versus vitrectomy without juxtapapillary laser photocoagulation for the treatment of optic disc maculopathy: the results of the KKESH international collaborative retina study group. Br J Ophthalmol. 2016;100:478–83.
18. Ryat JS, Rudnisky CJ, Waite C, et al. Long-term outcomes for optic disk pit maculopathy after vitrectomy. Retina. 2015;35:2011–7.
19. Bottoni F, Cereda M, Secondi R, et al. Vitrectomy for optic disc pit maculopathy: a long-term follow-up study. Graefes Arch Clin Exp Ophthalmol. 2018;256:675–82.
20. Avci R, Kapran Z, Ozdek Ş, et al. Multicenter study of pars plana vitrectomy for optic disc pit maculopathy: MACPIT study. Eye. 2017;31:1266–73.
21. Ooto S, Mittra RA, Ridley ME, et al. Vitrectomy with inner retinal fenestration for optic disc pit maculopathy. Ophthalmology. 2014;121:1727–33.
22. Todorich B, Sharma S, Vajzovic L. Successful repair of recurrent optic disk pit maculopathy with autologous platelet rich plasma: report of a surgical technique. Retin Cases Brief Rep. 2017;11(1):15–7.
23. Travassos AS, Regadas I, Alfaiate M, et al. Optic pit: novel surgical management of complicated cases. Retina. 2013;33:1708–14.
24. Nawrocki J, Bonińska K, Michalewska Z. Managing optic pit. The right stuff! Retina. 2016;36:2430–2.
25. de Oliveira PRC, Berger AR, Chow DR. Use of evicel fibrin sealant in optic disc pit-associated macular detachment. Ophthalmic Surg Lasers Imaging Retina. 2017;48:358–63.
26. Gregory-Roberts EM, Mateo C, Corcóstegui B, et al. Optic disk pit morphology and retinal detachment: optical coherence tomography with intraoperative correlation. Retina. 2013;33:363–70.
27. Ziahosseini K, Sanghvi C, Muzaffar W, et al. Successful surgical treatment of optic disc pit maculopathy. Eye. 2009;23:1477–9.
28. Jalil A, Stavrakas P, Dhawahir-Scala FE, et al. Drainage of subretinal fluid in optic disc pit maculopathy using subretinal 42-gauge cannula: a new surgical approach. Graefes Arch Clin Exp Ophthalmol. 2010;248:751–3.
29. Shukla D. Endodrainage of macular schisis through optic disc pit. Arch Ophthalmol. 2012;130:808–9.
30. García-Arumí J, Guraya BC, Espax AB, et al. Optical coherence tomography in optic pit maculopathy managed with vitrectomy-laser-gas. Graefes Arch Clin Exp Ophthalmol. 2004;242:819–26.
31. Gass JDM. Serous detachment of the macula: secondary to congenital pit of the optic nerve head. Am J Ophthalmol. 1969;67:821–41.
32. Spaide RF, Fisher Y, Ober M, et al. Surgical hypothesis: inner retinal fenestration as a treatment for optic disc pit maculopathy. Retina. 2006;26:89–91.
33. Slocumb RW, Johnson MW. Premature closure of inner retinal fenestration in the treatment of optic disk pit maculopathy. Retin Cases Brief Rep. 2010;4:37–9.
34. Roy R, Waanbah AD, Mathur G, et al. Optical coherence tomography characteristics in eyes with optic pit maculopathy. Retina. 2013;33:771–5.
35. Chatziralli I, Theodossiadis P, Theodossiadis GP. Optic disk pit maculopathy: current management strategies. Clin Ophthalmol. 2018;12:1417–22.
36. Theodossiadis GP, Chatziralli IP, Theodossiadis PG. Macular buckling in optic disc pit maculopathy in association with the origin of macular elevation: 13-year mean postoperative results. Eur J Ophthalmol. 2015;25:241–8.

Part VII

Ocular Trauma

Posterior Segment Complications of Ocular Trauma

28

S. Natarajan, Ritu Shah, and Astha Jain

28.1 Open Globe Injuries

Open globe injuries (OGIs) are a major cause of vision-threatening ophthalmic emergency, especially in working age population. The mean estimated incidence of OGIs is ~3.5 cases in 100,000 annually, leading to 200,000 OGIs per year worldwide [1]. They are further classified as globe rupture, or laceration which involves penetrating and perforating injuries and intraocular foreign body.

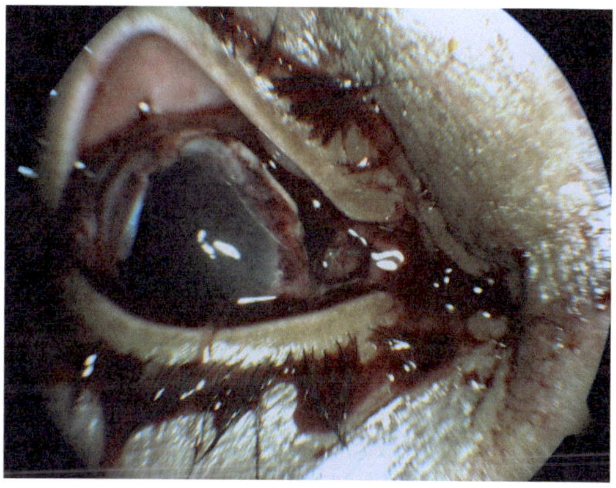

Fig. 28.1 Slit lamp photograph showing conjunctival chemosis and globe rupture post-blunt ocular trauma. Multiple scleral ruptures were discovered intraoperatively on globe exploration

28.1.1 Globe Rupture

A globe rupture occurs when there is full-thickness defect of cornea, sclera, or both the structures by blunt or penetrating trauma (Fig. 28.1). Globe rupture usually results from high-velocity blunt objects striking the eye which eventually may raise IOP leading to tissue tearing and decompression via a rupture of the eye wall [2]. The rupture site is most commonly near the globe's equator, posterior to the insertion of the rectus muscles as the sclera here is weakest and thinnest. In eyes with a previous surgical incision, the rupture usually occurs at the previous incision. It is necessary to keep a high index of suspicion for occult globe rupture in cases of OBT. Signs of high suspicion include low IOP of 5 or less at presentation, visual acuity of light perception or less, abnormally shallow or deep anterior chamber, dislocation of lens, presence of RAPD, dense VH preventing the view of the fundus or an RD [3]. The visual prognosis is usually

Electronic Supplementary Material The online version of this chapter (https://doi.org/10.1007/978-981-33-4168-5_28) contains supplementary material, which is available to authorized users.

S. Natarajan (✉) · R. Shah
Aditya Jyot Eye Hospital, Mumbai, India
e-mail: drritu@adityajyoteyehospital.org

A. Jain
Aditya Jyot Foundation for Twinkling Little Eyes, Mumbai, India

Aditya Jyot Eye Hospital, Mumbai, India

A. Jain et al. (eds.), *Cutting-edge Vitreoretinal Surgery*,
https://doi.org/10.1007/978-981-33-4168-5_28

poor. Poor visual acuity at presentation is a predictor of poor visual outcome. An urgent intervention in form of globe exploration and closure of the wound is required. The rupture can be associated with conditions like hyphema, dislocation of lens, traumatic cataract, vitreous hemorrhage, or retinal detachments. The primary closure of the wound can be combined with lensectomy and vitrectomy as required or a secondary surgery can be planned at a later date. Pre- and postoperative antibiotic covers are essential to prevent endophthalmitis.

28.1.2 Penetrating and Perforating Injuries

By definition, penetrating injuries are those with one entry wound, i.e., the causative object does not pass through and through, while perforating injuries have both entry and exit wounds. The incidence is higher in males [4]. The causative agent is usually a high velocity or sharp object. The most important primary prevention includes wearing adequate and appropriate protective eyewear while doing vision-threatening activities.

Prompt evaluation and management are warranted. A thorough history regarding the type of object and mode and timing of injury and whether any protective eyewear was being worn at the time of injury should be recorded. In case the view of posterior segment is jeopardized due to media opacity like hyphema, cataract, or VH, a gentle USG and CT scan should be done to rule out retained intraocular foreign bodies (IOFB). MRI is contraindicated where a metallic foreign body is suspected.

The factors accounting for poor visual outcomes are poor visual acuity at time of presentation, presence of RAPD, time involved between injury and repair, severity of injury, size and location of wound, presence of VH, RD, and IOFB [5].

A prompt globe exploration and closure with or without vitrectomy should be done [6]. A single-step approach of wound closure and comprehensive reconstruction can be undertaken. Such an approach is specifically indicated in cases with IOFB and endophthalmitis. A two-step approach consists of watertight primary closure followed by vitrectomy and globe reconstruction at a second stage usually after 10–14 days. Strict asepsis has to be followed. General anesthesia is preferred. The goals of vitrectomy are to remove the media opacities as far as possible, remove the focus of infection or IOFB if any, remove the damaged vitreous and hence reduce the scaffold for further fibrocellular proliferation leading to PVR. The timing of vitrectomy varies from surgeon to surgeon. Early intervention in cases of traumatic detachments reduces the incidence of endophthalmitis and proliferative vitreoretinopathy (PVR). However, a later intervention may reduce chances of intraoperative hemorrhage and postoperative inflammation. Pre- and postoperative antibiotic coverage is a must. The infusion port during the vitrectomy is placed in the healthy sclera and should be free from incarceration. The flow in vitreous cavity should be free flow to avoid secondary retinal or choroidal detachments. An adequate visualization of posterior segment is essential. In cases of severe corneal trauma, a temporary keratoprosthesis or endoscope can be used. Vitrectomy is done with high-speed cutters and with low-to-moderate suction. The lens should be removed in case it is cataractous or required for anterior vitreous dissection. It is necessary to do a complete vitrectomy to prevent further fibrovascular proliferations. Special attention should be paid for any retinal incarceration. Such cases require complete relief of traction at incarcerated site. A relaxing retinectomy (RR) can also be done which is extended up to normal retina to ensure complete relaxation of the retina. The anterior incarcerated retina is then completely excised.

Severely injured eye might require enucleation, especially to prevent sympathetic ophthalmia (SO). However, prompt and tight surgical wound closure and adequate management of postoperative inflammation have decreased the incidence of SO and hence this argument is no more justified [7]. Despite repeated surgeries, the risk of SO has not risen above 0.1–0.3% during the last four decades [8]. It was only 20 years ago that Morris et al. reported on their attempts to reconstruct 11 eyes with severe ocular trauma that could not perceive light. The authors succeeded in restoring some function in 7 of 11 cases [9].

Although there may be cases that are not salvageable, an attempt to salvage the eye by primary repair rather than primary enucleation must be done. Primary enucleation should never be the first approach.

28.2 Closed Globe Injuries

28.2.1 Commotio Retinae/Berlins Edema

It is a transient opacification of the retina post-blunt trauma. It can be located at the posterior pole or in retinal periphery. When it involves the macula it is known as Berlin's edema (Fig. 28.2). It was first described by Berlin in 1873 [10].

Various theories have been proposed for its pathogenesis. Though originally postulated to be due to extracellular edema [10], there are recent reports on the histopathological studies which show disruption or fragmentation of the photoreceptor outer segment of the retina as the most common finding in patients with commotio retinae [11].

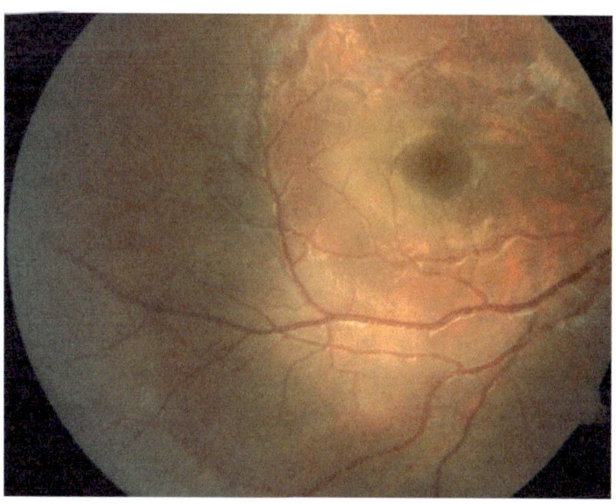

Fig. 28.2 Fundus image showing edema at the macular region (Berlin's edema) seen post blunt trauma to the eye

The OCT shows increased retinal thickness with disruption of the IS/OS junction and corresponding hyperreflectivity [11] and damage to the external limiting membrane. Those with IS/OS junction defects are more likely to have irreversible photoreceptor damage [12]. There is no specific treatment for this condition. Oral steroids may be given to reduce the edema. The visual prognosis is usually good except in cases of choroidal ruptures, retinal detachments or atrophy and hypertrophy of RPE.

28.2.2 Vitreous Hemorrhage

It usually occurs due to traumatic disruption of the blood vessels in anterior segment or posterior segment due to external mechanical forces [13]. Among all traumatic causes, OBT accounts for the majority of traumatic VH being responsible for 29.6–64% of such cases with a male predominance [13, 14].

The visual acuity can vary from 20/200 or better to hand movements or even light perception [14]. Those presenting with low visual acuity and cataract or aphakia are considered as risk factors for poor prognosis [14]. Ultrasound (USG) is essential to rule out associated retinal detachments (RD), intraocular foreign body (IOFB), and occult scleral ruptures along with the position of the dislocated lens in which cases, urgent surgical intervention is required. Posterior vitreous detachment (PVD) and associated choroidal detachment can also be noted in USG.

There is no consensus regarding the timing of intervention. One can wait for up to 2–3 months for spontaneous resolution of the hemorrhage (head elevation and avoidance of strenuous activities are advised in this period). Small gauge transconjunctival pars planavitrectomy (PPV) can be planned in cases of nonresolving vitreous hemorrhage. Initially the vitreous from central region is removed anteriorly and then extending the excision up to the posterior hyaloid. A complete vitrectomy with PVD induction should be done. Long-standing VH can be associated with spontaneous PVD. A fresh hemorrhage appears reddish or yellowish while old blood is brownish. Active bleeding points if visualized can be managed by raising the IOP and fluid air exchange or with the help of endocautery. A thorough peripheral examination of the retina with the help of wide-angle viewing systems should be done intraoperatively to rule out any retinal breaks or dialysis in which case endolaser/cryo can be done simultaneously. Cryotherapy is preferred in case of anterior breaks and when residual vitreous obscures its view. It is necessary to clear the vitreous around the retinal breaks thoroughly in order to avoid undue traction around them later, which can lead to retinal detachments. Removal of subretinal blood also warrants elimination of the vitreous surrounding it. The blood can then be aspirated from the existing tear or a retinotomy with an extrusion cannula. The retinotomy is later treated with laser. The prognosis is usually good in simple cases of VH. However, in those associated with RD, IOFB, and globe ruptures, the visual prognosis may be affected depending on the extent of the effect.

28.2.3 Posterior Dislocation of Lens

Anteroposterior force generated due to blunt trauma leading to equatorial expansion can cause disruption of zonular fibers and hence dislocation of lens/IOL [15]. It may be associated with VH or RD, secondary glaucoma and traumatic vitreoretinopathy Ultrasound can aid in diagnosis. Surgery involves complete vitrectomy to free the nucleus/IOL of surrounding vitreous followed by its removal. Details of the surgery have been covered in Chap. 37.

28.2.4 Choroidal Rupture

It was first described by Von Graefe in 1854 [16]. It is a break in the choroid, Bruch's membrane, and RPE due to an expansile force created by rapid compression of the globe following blunt trauma. Sclera being inelastic resists the expansion but retina stretches during the injury. Bruch's membrane breaks due to lack of elasticity [17]. It occurs in 5–8% of all closed globe injuries [18].

Choroidal ruptures are of two types—direct and indirect. Those following direct trauma, i.e., directly at the site of trauma tend to be anterior and parallel to the ora serrata. The indirect ruptures are caused due to countercoup mechanism and usually involve the posterior pole most commonly located temporal to the optic nerve and affect macula. These account for nearly 60% of the cases [19].

The symptoms depend on the area affected. Macula involving cases usually present with decreased vision, scotomas, enlargement of the blind spot, or metamorphopsia. It appears as a crescent-shaped curvilinear reddish-yellow line usually parallel to the optic nerve. At times, it may not be visible initially due to overlying hemorrhage. The rupture can be partial thickness or full thickness. The late complication frequently include CNV (5–10%) [17]. Those closer to fovea are more prone to CNV. The visual prognosis for central ruptures is usually poor, especially if associated with retinal or subretinal hemorrhages, vitreous hemorrhage, or CNV.

Diagnosis is usually based on the history of blunt ocular trauma along with clinical findings. FFA shows early hypofluorescence due to rupture of choroidal vessels at the site followed by late staining due to leakage from adjacent capillaries. Hyperflourescence increasing in size and intensity can be seen in cases with CNVM. OCT shows discontinuity of the RPE along with thinning of the underlying choroid.

Treatment usually involves observation along with Amsler's monitoring. Anti-VEGFs are used in cases complicated with CNVM [17].

28.2.5 Optic Nerve Avulsion

Avulsion of optic nerve is one of the severe complications of ocular trauma. It is characterized by disinsertion of optic nerve from retina, choroid, and vitreous at the level of lamina cribrosa without rupture of nerve sheath [20]. Common sites include intraorbital and intracanalicular areas [21]. The lamina cribrosa is more prone to injury due to absence of myelin and other supportive connective tissues [22]. Although rare, it should be kept in suspicion when the vision loss is severe and dense [22].

The vascular changes are commonly associated due to close relation of optic nerve with retinal vasculature [21]. The visual prognosis depends on the initial vision after trauma. The visual loss is due to damage and break of the nerve fibers [22]. Partial avulsions usually carry better prognosis.

The diagnosis can be made clinically by seeing a cavity at the site of optic disc but the view is frequently obliterated due to associated vitreous or retinal hemorrhages. USG and CT can help in diagnosing such cases. USG shows hypolucent area in the region of optic nerve head [23] and CT scan shows vitreous prolapse into optic nerve sheath in a mushroom pattern. VEP can also point toward optic nerve involvement.

Vitrectomy can be done in cases with dense vitreous hemorrhage but the outcome is limited due to optic nerve involvement.

28.2.6 Traumatic Macular Holes

The incidence of traumatic macular hole is close to 1.4% among closed globe injury [24]. It is more common in the younger population [24] and can lead to visual loss, especially if associated with other retinal pathologies like commotio retinae, retinal or vitreous hemorrhage, choroidal ruptures, retinal tears, or dialysis. Traumatic macular holes tend to have a larger base diameter and thinner average retinal thickness than idiopathic ones and are usually not associated with PVD [25].

The exact causative mechanism is not known. Yokotsuka et al. postulated sudden vitreous separation as the primary cause [26] while Johnson et al. proposed the countercoup mechanism in 2001 [27].

Several case reports show high rate of spontaneous closure of traumatic macular holes usually between 2 weeks and 12 months [28]. The visual prognosis is usually good after spontaneous closure. The mechanism of closure is proliferation of glial cells or RPE from the hole's edge and stimulation of astrocytes migration to heal the hole [29]. Observation is advised for 3–6 months due to high rate of spontaneous closure. However, early vitrectomy can be planned in children to avoid amblyopia.

Vitrectomy and ILM peeling with intraocular tamponade is the treatment of choice for non-closing and large macular holes. Details of the procedure have been covered in Chap. 22. The final visual outcome depends on the size and duration of the macular hole.

28.2.7 Retinal Detachment

Traumatic RD usually occurs due to abrupt globe deformity following the impact of OBT. The force of the injury is an important predictor of the extent of vitreoretinal damage. Those with high myopia, aphakia, and fellow eye history of RD are more prone to such consequences [7]. Retinal dialysis is the most common retinal finding in cases of blunt trauma and the most common being that by a fist. In a series of 5360 eyes with RD, dialysis was the most frequent type of tear in detachments related to trauma [30]. It is described as disinsertion of retina from the ora serrata. The most common site is inferotemporal followed by superonasal. Apart from retinal dialysis, retinal tears are also noted, which can eventually lead to rhegmatogenous RD. Giant retinal tears (GRT) can also be present which can be either circumferential or radial.

Many patients are asymptomatic initially and present only after vision loss due to retinal detachments. Others may present with flashes, floaters, loss of peripheral visual field, or dimness of vision [30]. The absence of symptoms is related to the fact that many retinal dialyses occur in the absence of a PVD with a slow progression of subretinal fluid, and there is characteristic involvement of the superior visual field [31]. Thus, a thorough retinal peripheral examination with scleral depression is essential to identify dialysis before it progresses to retinal detachment. The dialysis typically opens up on scleral depression. Repeated examinations may be required in cases of VH or preretinal blood, which can obscure the view. There may be other associated findings like avulsion of the vitreous base, VH, traumatic cataract, retinal demarcation lines, and pars plana detachments. According to a study, demarcation lines were more common in inferotemporal dialyses suggesting some chronicity, whereas vitreous base avulsion and pars plana detachments were more common with superonasal dialyses suggesting more acute and severe trauma [30].

The diagnosis is usually by thorough clinical examination and can be aided by USG and wide field imaging. The dialysis and tears with no or minimal subretinal fluid can be safely treated with photocoagulation or cryopexy [32] (Fig. 28.3). The treatment should be initiated as soon as possible.

In cases with detachments, an urgent surgical intervention is warranted. Scleral buckling is usually preferred in such cases because PVD induction, which is difficult in young subjects, can be avoided by this procedure. Also, chances of iatrogenic breaks, secondary cataract formation, and complications related to intraocular tamponade of gas/oil can be avoided [33]. Circumferential silicon buckles are usually used based on the location and size of the break. Subretinal fluid may or may not be drained. Absorption of SRF in cases of chronic detachments tends to be slower.

The indications for primary vitrectomy in traumatic RD include VH, dislocated lens, PVR, giant retinal tear with everted flap, posterior tear, and subretinal hemorrhage. It is necessary to rule out choroidal hemorrhage prior to the surgery with USG. PPV helps in removal of media opacities like VH and allows a better view of the retina. The timing of vitrectomy is still controversial. Early vitrectomy poses a higher risk of intraoperative complications, bleeding, wound leakage, and bad visualization. Conversely, a delayed vitrectomy have a higher incidence and severity of postoperative complications, mainly PVR [34].

The prognosis is usually not very good due to longer intervals in treatment, frequent occurrence of PVR, and frequent macular involvement. Visual outcomes are better if the macula is attached at the time of repair. Worse presenting visual acuity, RAPD, presence of submacular hemorrhages, foveal choroidal rupture, macular hole, globe rupture, PVR, endophthalmitis, or IOFBs are all associated with poor visual outcome.

28.2.8 Traumatic PVR

PVR may develop in up to 70% of cases in open globe injuries especially in case of subretinal or vitreous hemorrhage, GRT, or large wound. It develops due to chronicity of the detachments along with fibrous tissue changes in the vitreous and usually occurs inferiorly first as cells gather in between the retina and oil bubble due to gravity. It eventually causes a pull on the retina and leads to retinal detachments (Fig. 28.4).

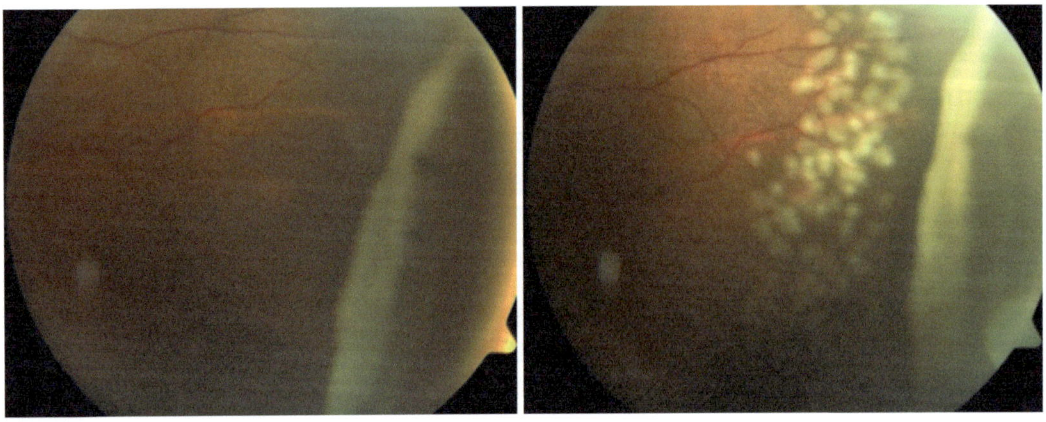

Fig. 28.3 Fundus image on the left shows retinal dialysis post blunt ocular trauma which was lasered as seen in the image on the right. The patient was sequentially observed and the retina remained stable post laser

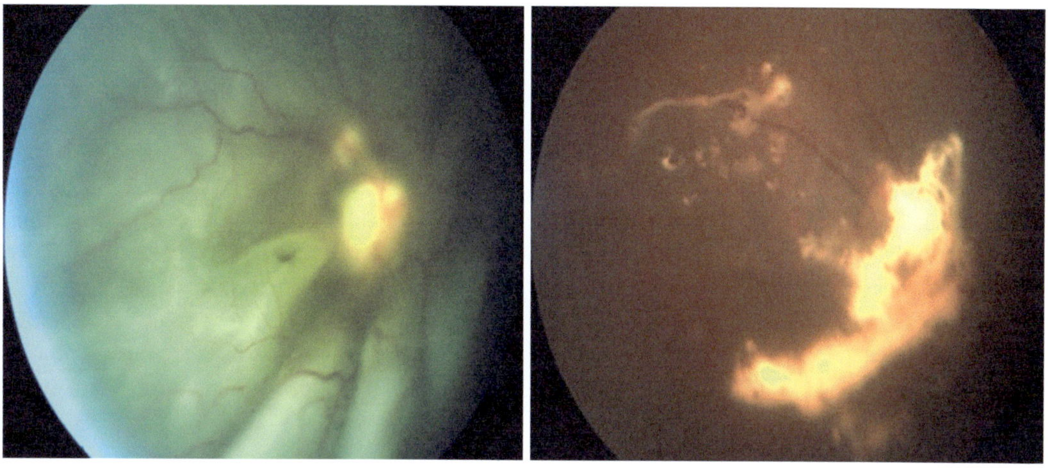

Fig. 28.4 Fundus image on the left shows traumatic retinal detachment with proliferative vitreoretinopathy in a patient with blunt ocular trauma. The right image is the postoperative fundus image with attached retina and silicone oil in situ

PFCL is an invaluable tool in these cases as it allows flattening of retina, facilitate intraocular manipulations, removal of epiretinal and fibroproliferative membranes, and provide adequate intraoperative retinal tamponade. It also helps in draining the SRF by anterior retinal breaks and stabilizes large breaks. Meticulous peeling of the epiretinal membranes and removal of any subretinal bands and gliosis with help of forceps and scissors is essential for successful reattachment of the retina. If needed, bimanual vitrectomy and membrane dissection should be done with the help of chandelier illumination.

In cases with persistent traction, relaxing retinotomy (RR) should be done. Almost 40% of the cases will need RR to reattach the retina [35]. Circumferential RR is preferred. Endodiathermy is applied to the edge of the retina to be incised prior to excision. Then, the retina is incised with help of microscissors or vitrectomy cutters up to the site of normal retina to relieve complete traction. The anterior retina is then excised. Injection of PFCL is then done to drain the remaining SRF and flatten the retina. Endophotocoagulation is done in 2–3 rows along the edge of RR. Slippage of retina in these cases can be avoided by direct PFCL–SOI exchange. Gases like SF6 or C3F8 and silicone oil are lighter tamponades with lower specific gravity and hence support the superior retina well but can pose a risk of inferior and posterior pole PVR due to accumulation of fibrous tissues [36]. Heavy tamponades in form of 5000 cst silicone oil or densiron are often required. They are especially preferred in inferior PVR. However, there are cases of recurrent superior detachments in a densiron filled eyes. Sandwich technique (use of densiron with silicone oil) is useful in such cases. Densiron is used in place of balanced salt solution in the infusion port using the dual-mode injection/extraction available in Alcon constellation vitrectomy system in complicated cases. This helps in draining of the persistent SRF while injecting densiron simultaneously. Densiron being heavier settles inferiorly under the silicone oil without mixing with it or losing its unique physical property. Hence, complete tamponade is obtained.

28.2.9 Chorioretinitis Sclopetaria

This relatively rare condition was first described in 1901 by Goldzieher [37]. Sclopetaria is a secondary outcome of a decelerating object passing at a high velocity adjacent to the sclera [38]. This results in concussion injury to the retina and choroid. The mechanism is thought to be the energy released by the projectile while passing close to the eyeball [37]. There is typically no penetration of the particle into the globe.

The area affected due to direct injury is usually the area adjacent to the path of the projectile. While indirect effect can be caused in other areas of choroid and retina due to propagation of the shock waves. Multiple areas of affection can be present.

The visual acuity at presentation depends on the area involved. The condition is frequently associated with ocular motility disorders, IOP changes due to intraocular inflammation, retinal, and macular edema. It is usually associated with poor visual prognosis.

The retina is rarely detached in such conditions due to inflammation in the necrotic edges of the rupture, which causes chorioretinal scar formation [37]. Hence, prophylactic cryopexy or photocoagulation is usually not required. The late complication of this condition involves formation of CNV.

28.2.10 Subretinal Hemorrhages

Visual loss is profound and immediate in cases with submacular hemorrhages (SMH) (Fig. 28.5). Permanent damages to neurosensory retina and retinal pigment epithelium are likely to occur due to iron toxicity to photoreceptors from hemoglobin breakdown. Early removal of SMH from the macular area is associated with better visual outcomes. Vitrectomy with modifications like a retinotomy, mechanical removal of subretinal clot, tissue-type plasminogen activator (tPA) use has been tried with variable final visual outcomes [39].

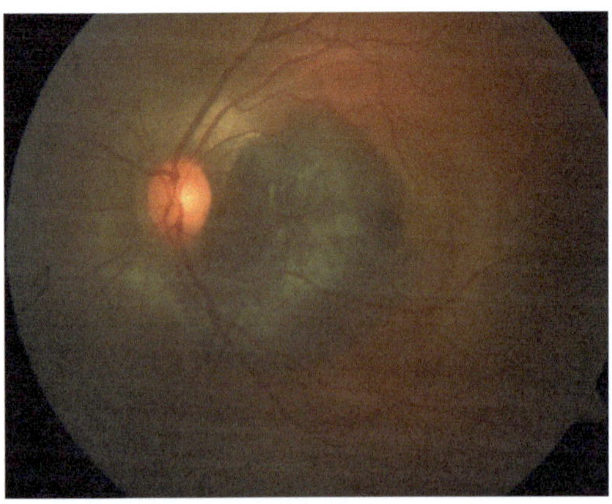

Fig. 28.5 Fundus image showing dense submacular bleed following trauma by a cricket ball

tPA along with pneumatic displacement (SF6 or C3F8) of the blood from fovea or pneumatic displacement alone is associated with better anatomical outcomes. Appropriate postoperative positioning also helps in faster displacement of blood. Better visual outcomes are expected in cases with good initial visual acuity, duration <2 weeks and hemorrhage not larger than three-disc diameters.

28.2.11 Posttraumatic Endophthalmitis

Posttraumatic infectious endophthalmitis occurs in 2–7% of all penetrating intraocular injuries and 7–31% of injuries with retained intraocular foreign bodies [40]. Due to initial injury, delay in primary repair and more virulent organisms (Bacillus or/staphylococcus species), they have worse outcomes than other types of endophthalmitis. Presentation >24 h after injury, IOFBs composed of steel, and organic or soil-contaminated IOFBs, large wounds, vitreous prolapse through the wound are all risk factors for endophthalmitis. The clinical signs include eyelid edema, congestion, purulent discharge, corneal edema, anterior chamber reaction, hypopyon, vitritis. The patient may present with out of proportion pain. The progression and severity depend on the virulence of the organism.

The indications for pars plana vitrectomy from the Endophthalmitis Vitrectomy Study were limited to postoperative infections and do not apply in cases of trauma and IOFBs associated with endophthalmitis [41]. Pars plana core vitrectomy along with preoperative and postoperative antibiotics on an urgent basis is needed. Empirical intravitreal vancomycin (1 mg/0.1 mL) and ceftazidime (2.25 g/0.1 mL) are used. Intravitreal amphotericin B (0.005 mg/0.1 mL) is reserved for infections with a strong suspicion of fungal infections. The use of adjunctive intravitreal steroids is controversial. In cases with corneal opacity/abscess, vitrectomy can be done open sky or needs to be combined with temporary keratoprosthesis which can then be replaced with donor cornea at the end of the surgery. The purpose of vitrectomy is to reduce the load of inflammation and infection, obtaining a sample for culture studies, irrigating toxins, and allowing better distribution of antibiotics. The peripheral vitreous removal and base excision is avoided in such cases due to friable nature of the retina. The topicals involve instillation of fortified antibiotics started on first postoperative day. Repeat intravitreal injections can be safely performed 48 h after the first injection. In cases of worsening inflammation or pain, repeat intravitreal injections or vitrectomy has to be considered.

Adequate intraocular samples (AC tap, vitreous tap, and vitrectomy cassette fluid) and IOFBs should be sent for microbiology investigations (Gram stain, aerobic, anaerobic, and fungal cultures). The most common species involved are *Bacillus, Staphylococcus epidermidis,* and *Streptococcus* species. *Bacillus*, in particular, tends to be aggressive and frequently cause rapid destruction of ocular tissues [42]. The prognosis is usually poor and depends on the virulence of the causative organism, timing and extent of the surgery, and presence of retinal detachment.

28.2.12 Suprachoroidal Hemorrhage

An expulsive choroidal hemorrhage is a dreadful complication rarely associated with traumatic globe rupture. Predisposing factors are age, systemic hypertension, diabetes, glaucoma, myopia, and recent intraocular surgery.

Symptoms are pain, headache, nausea, and vomiting. The clinical signs include low IOP, forward bulge of the iris and pupillary dilatation. The diagnosis can be made on USG that shows a round mound with low-to-medium point echoes. When choroidal mounds touch each other they are called kissing choroidals. USG also notes clot lysis and hence guides in timing and site of drainage during the surgery. The largest choroidal is the optimum site for drainage.

The ideal timing of vitrectomy is debatable. The surgery can be delayed for about 2 weeks. However, in cases of kissing choroidals and uncontrolled IOP one can intervene earlier. One should watch for liquefaction of clot lysis on USG, which is evident as reduced echogenicity. Surgical intervention is done in presence of anterior chamber infusion. The surgery includes choroidal drainage 4 mm posterior to the limbus in the quadrants having hemorrhage by either scleral cutdown or by an angled insertion of 23 or 25 gauge trochar cannula. Oozing out of dark chocolate brown fluid occurs suggestive of suprachoroidal hemorrhage. After choroidal drainage, a long infusion cannula is put and infusion is started only after seeing the tip. The goals of hemorrhagic choroidal drainage are to eliminate appositional or large, nonappositional choroidals, normalize IOP, and eliminate posterior pressure on the lens–iris diaphragm. Concurrent vitrectomy with PFCL and silicone oil tamponade is also required, especially in cases associated with vitreous hemorrhage or retinal detachments.

28.2.13 Sympathetic Ophthalmia

The incidence of SO ranges from 0.2 to 0.5% after penetrating ocular injuries. It is a bilateral diffuse granulomatous inflammation that usually occurs within days or months of penetrating ocular injuries (about 80% occurring in first 3 months and 90% within first year) [43]. The injured eye is called the exciting eye and the other eye developing inflammation later is called the sympathizing eye. There is no age or racial predisposition but it occurs more commonly in males following ocular trauma. The possible mechanism is thought to be of autoimmune origin.

The patient presents with pain, photophobia, and blurring of the vision in the sympathizing eye. The clinical signs include bilateral diffuse panuveitis showing mutton fat KPs on corneal endothelium and/or posterior synechae. The IOP may be raised secondary to inflammation. The patient may have associated vitritis, retinal vasculitis, papillitis, and choroiditis (seen as whitish lesions called "Dalen Fuch's nodules" in peripheral fundus). The predisposing factors include penetrating trauma, trauma near ciliary body, interval between repair more than 48 h, and larger wound.

The diagnosis is usually based on history taking and clinical examination. However, OCT, FFA, and ICGA can help in the diagnosis. FFA shows multiple hyperfluorescent spots seen in venous phase till late phases. In severe cases, there may be pooling of exudates suggestive of exudative retinal detachment. ICGA shows multiple hypofluorescent spots that become more distinct in late phases. B scan shows choroidal thickening and exudative detachment of the retina.

Systemic corticosteroids are the mainstay of treatment. Additionally, topical steroids and cycloplegics are used to control the anterior chamber reaction and prevent posterior synechae formation. The steroids are followed by systemic immunomodulatory agents like cyclosporine, azathioprine, or cyclophosphamide.

Secondary enucleation of the exciting eye to reduce inflammation in the sympathizing eye does not necessarily lead to a better visual outcome or to a reduced need for medical therapy [44].

References

1. Negrel AD, Thylefors B. The global impact of eye injuries. Ophthalmic Epidemiol. 1998;5:143–69.
2. Lee C-H, Lee L, Kao L-Y, Lin K-K, Yang M-L. Prognostic indicators of open globe injuries in children. Am J Emerg Med. 2009;27(5):530–5.
3. Russell SR, Olsen KR, Folk JC. Predictors of scleral rupture and the role of vitrectomy in severe blunt ocular trauma. Am J Ophthalmol. 1988;105(3):253–7.
4. May DR, Kuhn FP, et al. The epidemiology of serious eye injuries from the United States Eye Injury Registry. Graefes Arch Clin Exp Ophthalmol. 2000;238:153–7.
5. Agrawal R, Rao G, Naigaonkar R, Ou X, Desai S. Prognostic factors for vision outcome after surgical repair of open globe injuries. Indian J Ophthalmol. 2011;59:465–70.
6. Mittra RA, Mieler WF. Controversies in the management of open-globe injuries involving the posterior segment. Surv Ophthalmol. 1999;44:215–25.
7. Shukla M, Ahuja OP, Jamal N. Traumatic retinal detachment. Indian J Ophthalmol. 1986;34:29–32.
8. Eagling EM. Perforating injuries involving the posterior segment. Trans Ophthalmol Soc UK. 1975;95:335.
9. Morris R. Management of ocular trauma: treatment options for eyes with no light perception. Proceedings of the 12th Congress of the Societas Ophthalmologica Europae, Stockholm. 1999.
10. Berlin R. Zursogenannten. commotio retinae. Klin Monatsbl Augenheilk. 1873;1:42–78.
11. Blight R, Hart JC. Structural changes in the outer retinal layers following blunt mechanical non-perforating trauma to the globe: an experimental study. Br J Ophthalmol. 1977;61:573–87.
12. Saleh M, Letsch J, Bourcier T, Munsch C, Speeg-Schatz C, Gaucher D. Long-term outcomes of acute traumatic maculopathy. Retina. 2011;31:2037–43.
13. Yeung L, Chen TL, Kuo YH, et al. Severe vitreous hemorrhage associated with closed-globe injury. Graefes Arch Clin Exp Ophthalmol. 2006;244(1):52–7.
14. AlHarkan DH, Kahtani ES, Gikandi PW, Abu El-Asrar AM. Vitreous hemorrhage in pediatric age group. J Ophthalmol. 2014;2013:497083.
15. Marcus DM, Topping TM Jr, Frederick AR. Vitreoretinal management of traumatic dislocation crystalline lens. Int Ophthalmol Clin. 1995;35(1):139–50.
16. Patel MM, Chee YE, Elliot D. Choroidal rupture: a review. Int Ophthalmol Clin. 2013;53(4):69–78.
17. Ament CS, Zacks DN, Lane AM, et al. Predictors of visual outcome and choroidalneovascular membrane formation after traumatic choroidalrupture. Arch Ophthalmol. 2006;124(7):957–66.
18. Glazer LC, Han DP, Gottlieb MS. Choroidal rupture and optic atrophy. Br J Ophthalmol. 1993;77(1):33–5.
19. Wood CM, Richardson J. Indirect Choroidalruptures: aetiological factors, patterns of ocular damage and final visual outcome. Br J Ophthalmol. 1990;74(4):208–11.
20. Mumcuoglu T, Durukan HA, Erdurman C, Hurmeric V, Gundogan FC. Functional and structural analysis of partial optic nerve avulsion due to blunt ocular trauma. Case report. Indian J Ophthalmol. 2010;58:524–6.
21. Babitha V, Prasannakumary C, Ramesan E, Raju KV. Optic nerve avulsion: a rare presentation of blunt trauma. Muller J Med Sci Res. 2017;8:97–9.
22. Mackiewicz J, Tomaszewska J, Jasielska M. Optic nerve avulsion after blunt ocular trauma- case report. Ann Agric Environ Med. 2016;23:382–3.
23. Simsek T, Simsek E, Ilhan B, Ozalp s SB, Zilelioglu O. Traumatic optic nerve avulsion. J Pediatr Ophthalmol Strabismus. 2006;43:367–9.
24. Kuhn F, Morris R, Witherspoon CD, Mann L. Epidemiology of blinding trauma in United States eye injury registry. Ophthalmic Epidemiol. 2006;13(3):209–16.
25. Huang J, Liu X, Wu Z, Sadda S. Comparision of full thickness macular holes and idiopathic macular holes by optical coherence tomography. Graefes Arch Clin Exp Ophthalmol. 2010;248(8):1071–5.

26. Yokotsuka K, Kishi S, Tobe K, Kamei Y. Clinical characteristics of traumatic macular holes. Jpn J Ophthalmol. 1991;45:1121–4.
27. Johnson RN, McDonald HR, Lewis H, et al. Traumatic macular hole: observations, pathogenesis and results of vitrectomy surgery. Ophthalmology. 2001;108(5):853–7.
28. Kusaka S, Fujikado T, Ikeda T, Tano Y. Spontaneous disappearance of traumatic macular holes in young patients. Am J Ophthalmol. 1983;77:922–4.
29. Azevedo S, Ferreira N, Meireles A. Management of pediatric traumatic macular holes-case report. Case Rep Ophthalmol. 2013;4(2):20–7.
30. Ross WH. Traumatic retinal dialyses. Arch Ophthalmol. 1981;99(8):1371–4.
31. Hagler WS. Retinal dialysis: a statistical and genetic study to determine pathogenic factors. Trans Am Ophthalmol Soc. 1980;78:686–733.
32. Schachat AP, Wilkinson CP, Hinton DR, Sadda SR, Wiedemann P. Ryan's retina. 6th ed. Beijing: Elsevier; 2018.
33. Chang JS, Marra K, Flynn HW Jr, Berrocal AM, Arroyo JG. Scleral buckling in the treatment of retinal detachment due to retinal dialysis. Ophthalmic Surg Lasers Imaging Retina. 2016;47(4):336–40.
34. Kuhn F. Strategic thinking in eye trauma management. Ophthalmol Clin N Am. 2002;15(2):171–7.
35. Fivgas GD, Capone A. Pediatric rhegmatogenous retinal detachment. Retina. 2001;21(2):101–6.
36. Alkawas AA, Maaly EA, Ibrahim BM, Al-Humiari MA. Densiron-68 in the treatment of retinal detachment associated with inferior proliferative vitreoretinopathy or caused by lower or posterior breaks. Egypt Retina J. 2017;4:9–14.
37. Dubovy SR, Guyton DL, Green WR. Clinicopathologic correlation of chorioretinitissclopetaria. Retina. 1997;17(6):510–20.
38. Richards RD, West CE, Meisels AA. Chorioretinitissclopetaria. Am J Ophthalmol. 1968;66(5):852–60.
39. Rishi E, Gopal L, Rishi P, Sengupta S, Sharma T. Submacular haemorrhage: a study amongst Indian eyes. Indian J Ophthalmol. 2012;60:521–5.
40. Duch-Samper AM, Menezo JL, Hurtado-Sarrio M. Endophthalmitisfollowing penetrating eye injuries. Acta Ophthalmol Scand. 1997;75:104–6.
41. Forster RK. The endophthalmitis vitrectomy study. Arch Ophthalmol. 1995;113:1555–7.
42. Alfaro DV, Roth D, Liggett PE. Posttraumatic endophthalmitis. Causative organisms, treatment, and prevention. Retina. 1994;14:206–11.
43. Arevalo JF, Garcia RA, Al-Dhibi HA, Sanchez JG, Suarez-Tata L. Update on sympathetic ophthalmia. Middle East Afr J Ophthalmol. 2012;19(1):13–21.
44. Kilmartin DJ, Dick AD, Forrester JV. Prospective surveillance of sympathetic ophthalmia in the UK and Republic of Ireland. Br J Ophthalmol. 2000;84(3):259–63.

29 Surgical Techniques of Intraocular Foreign Body Removal

Diana M. Laura, Nika Bagheri, and Dante J. Pieramici

Penetrating ocular injuries with intraocular foreign bodies (IOFB) is a relatively common ocular trauma, seen in 17–41% of open globe injuries [1]. It is most frequently seen in patients aged 20s–40s, and most commonly in young men [2, 3]. Reported mechanisms include, most commonly, hammering, use of power tools, and weapon-related injuries [1, 4, 5], and less commonly assault, motor vehicle accidents, and firework injuries [6, 7]. Visual prognosis of IOFB injury, while variable, may be poor, and contributes significantly to the burden of eye disease with 25% of patients having a final visual acuity <20/200 [8]. Herein we describe trauma of the posterior segment with IOFB requiring vitreoretinal expertise.

Electronic Supplementary Material The online version of this chapter (https://doi.org/10.1007/978-981-33-4168-5_29) contains supplementary material, which is available to authorized users.

D. M. Laura
Bascom Palmer Eye Institute, University of Miami, Miami, Florida, USA

N. Bagheri (✉) · D. J. Pieramici
California Retina Consultants and Research Foundation, Santa Barbara, CA, USA
e-mail: nbagheri@californiaretina.com

A. Jain et al. (eds.), *Cutting-edge Vitreoretinal Surgery*,
https://doi.org/10.1007/978-981-33-4168-5_29

29.1 Preoperative Considerations

29.1.1 History

A good clinical history is critical for acute management and surgical planning. The history should emphasize the timing of injury, the mechanism of injury, which may help in identifying the nature and likelihood of the IOFB, whether eye protection was worn at the time, and if any interventions occurred since injury. High-velocity machinery such as metal grinding should increase the physician's suspicion for intraocular foreign body, even if the eye is relatively quiet immediately after injury. The physician should inquire about the patient's baseline visual acuity to assess the severity of damage. When considering timing of surgery and operative management, it is also essential to ask when the patient last had anything to eat or drink and if the patient has any allergies to medications [4, 7]. The history should also include confirmation of recent tetanus immunization. Careful documentation is especially important in cases of ocular trauma, as such records will often be requested for disability and legal matters.

29.1.2 Examination

Once the physician completes a thorough history, an ophthalmic examination should be performed.

This includes inspection of the external periocular area for cutaneous foreign bodies or lacerations. Subsequently, visual acuity and pupillary evaluation as well as external, slit lamp, and fundus examinations should be performed although they may be limited by degree of injury [7]. Care should be taken to avoid applying pressure on the globe with tonometry, scleral depression, or ultrasound if rupture is suspected to avoid expulsion of intraocular contents [9].

Ocular injuries secondary to IOFBs are commonly associated with anterior segment injuries, such as corneal and/or scleral perforation and hyphema, lens injury, including violation of lens capsule and subsequent traumatic cataract or zonular disruption with lens subluxation/dislocation, and posterior segment injuries, including vitreous hemorrhage and retinal breaks/detachment [4, 7]. Endophthalmitis may be present in open globe injuries, and diagnosis may be difficult due to trauma-induced inflammation [10]. Pain out of proportion to the degree of injury and purulent exudate from the injury site may aid in the identification of endophthalmitis in this scenario [10, 11].

Many studies have evaluated prognostic factors for visual outcome in ocular trauma. The ocular trauma score (OTS) assigns numerical raw points to six variables, and predicts the visual prognosis by arranging the sum of the raw points into five categories. The six variables include initial visual acuity, rupture, endophthalmitis, perforating injury, retinal detachment, and relative afferent pupillary defect [12]. The OTS does not explicitly address cases of trauma with IOFB, although it still provides prognostic value. The Ocular Trauma Classification Group reported a system for classifying ocular trauma at presentation according to four variables: type based on mechanism of injury, grade based on presenting visual acuity, pupil based on the presence or absence of a relative afferent pupillary defect, and zone based on the anteroposterior extent of injury [13]. IOFB is a category under type of injury, although presenting visual acuity and presence of a relative afferent pupillary defect were the most significant predictors of final visual acuity [14]. Greven et al. evaluated 59 consecutive patients with surgical removal of IOFB after ocular trauma and found poor prognostic factors include poor vision on presentation, the mechanism of injury, presence of an afferent pupillary defect, and vitreous hemorrhage [5].

29.1.3 Imaging

Ocular imaging is critical in the management of IOFBs, and the mode of imaging used to appropriately visualize the foreign body may vary by its composition. Imaging modalities used include B-scan ultrasonography, X-ray, computed tomography (CT), and magnetic resonance imaging (MRI).

Ultrasonography is useful for IOFBs, as it is relatively inexpensive and provides real-time, high-resolution images in multiple cross sections. Obtaining multiple views can help approximate the size of the IOFB [7]. It may also help to determine the exact IOFB location and extent of intraocular damage [15]. A study of porcine eyes showed an IOFB detection rate of 93% while, in contrast, plain X-rays detected an IOFB only 40% of the time [16]. It is crucial, however, to not apply too much force onto the eye with the ultrasound probe and risk causing further damage. Disadvantages to ultrasound include limitations in detecting vegetable matter, such as wood, as it can resemble blood or vitreous. Ultrasonography may require a skilled operator to differentiate true foreign bodies from artifacts [17].

Plain X-rays, while inexpensive and fast, are low yield in screening for IOFBs due to low sensitivity and inaccurate localization [4, 18]. As a result, a non-contrast CT scan of the orbits with thin cuts (1.0 mm) is the preferred modality of imaging in globe rupture. It provides not only a view of the bilateral globes, but also the surrounding orbital and facial bones and the retrobulbar space [4]. Both conventional and spiral CT can be used in the imaging of IOFBs, with conventional being more common due to increased availability. Studies indicate, however, that spiral CT may be advantageous due to shorter duration, less radiation, and multiplanar reconstruction ability [19]. CT is particularly advantageous because it does not require patient cooperation or any contact with the globe. Limitations of all CT scans include poor visualization of plastic or wood foreign bodies, especially if the cuts are not appropriately thin [7].

Though some metals are MRI compatible, the use of MRI imaging in this type of injury is typically only implemented once the presence of a metallic IOFB is ruled out with a thorough history and orbital X-ray or CT to prevent tissue damage from the movement of magnetic foreign bodies [7].

29.1.4 Preoperative Care

Correct preoperatively management is imperative to prevent further damage and infection. Up-to-date tetanus vaccination should be verified and enhanced in accordance with the Centers for Disease Control and Prevention. Patients should receive broad-spectrum antibiotics if open globe is suspected. Antibiotics should cover bacteria encountered most commonly in open globe injuries, particularly *Bacillus*, *Clostridium*, and coagulase-negative *Staphylococcus* species [10]. Studies indicate that oral levofloxacin has adequate ocular penetration and can be used in this scenario [20]. While being transported and awaiting surgery, patients should wear a rigid shield (i.e., Fox shield) over the injured eye and avoid strenuous activities or Valsava maneuvers. Generally, IOFBs should be removed as soon as possible (within 24 h) to reduce the risk of endophthalmitis. However, there is evidence from Iraq and Afghanistan that an alternative is closure of the wound, placement on systemic antibiotics, and then later removal of the IOFB. There were no cases of endophthalmitis in these cases [21].

29.2 Types of Intraocular Foreign Bodies

The most common IOFBs are metallic [22, 23]. CT is the preferred imaging modality for metallic IOFBs (Figs. 29.1, 29.2, and 29.3). On ultrasound, these are echo-dense with shadowing posterior to the foreign body. Though MRI is generally contraindicated, some metals, such as platinum, are MRI compatible [24]. Important manifestations to remember with iron or copper-containing IOFBs include siderosis bulbi and chalcosis, respectively. Siderosis bulbi clinically manifests as iris heterochromia, cataract, secondary glaucoma and retinal pigmentary degeneration [25]. ERG changes of siderosis bulbi are an increased "a" wave followed by a reduced "b" wave [7]. Clinical signs of chalcosis include Kayser-Fleischer ring, copper particles on the iris or in the anterior chamber, and sunflower cataract [7].

Multiple series indicate that the frequency of glass IOFB ranges approximately 3–18% [7, 22, 23]. The most common cause of injury in these cases is motor vehicle accidents [26]. Glass typically appears hyperdense on CT, hypointense on T2-weighted MRI, and hyperechoic on ultrasound (Fig. 29.4, Videos 29.1 and 29.2) [7]. Of note, glass is inert and does not necessarily need to be removed depending on its location and likelihood of complication.

IOFBs comprised of vegetable matter are typically encountered working outside, such as landscaping or gardening (Fig. 29.5). Typically, these are hypodense on CT and hypointense on MRI [27]. In cases of organic IOFBs, one should always be cautious of posttraumatic fungal endophthalmitis.

Explosives, particularly fireworks, are another cause of open globe and IOFB injuries and mainly occur in the setting of no eye protection (Fig. 29.6). In a study of 99 patients with firework-related eye injuries, approximately 10% had IOFB [6].

29.3 Surgical Instruments

The objectives of IOFB removal are to retrieve the IOFB from the globe in a minimally invasive manner and to repair the lesions created in the IOFB trajectory [28]. Instruments typically used include external magnets, forceps, and rare earth intraocular magnets.

Intraocular forceps are most useful when the IOFB is nonmagnetic, large, or in the anterior

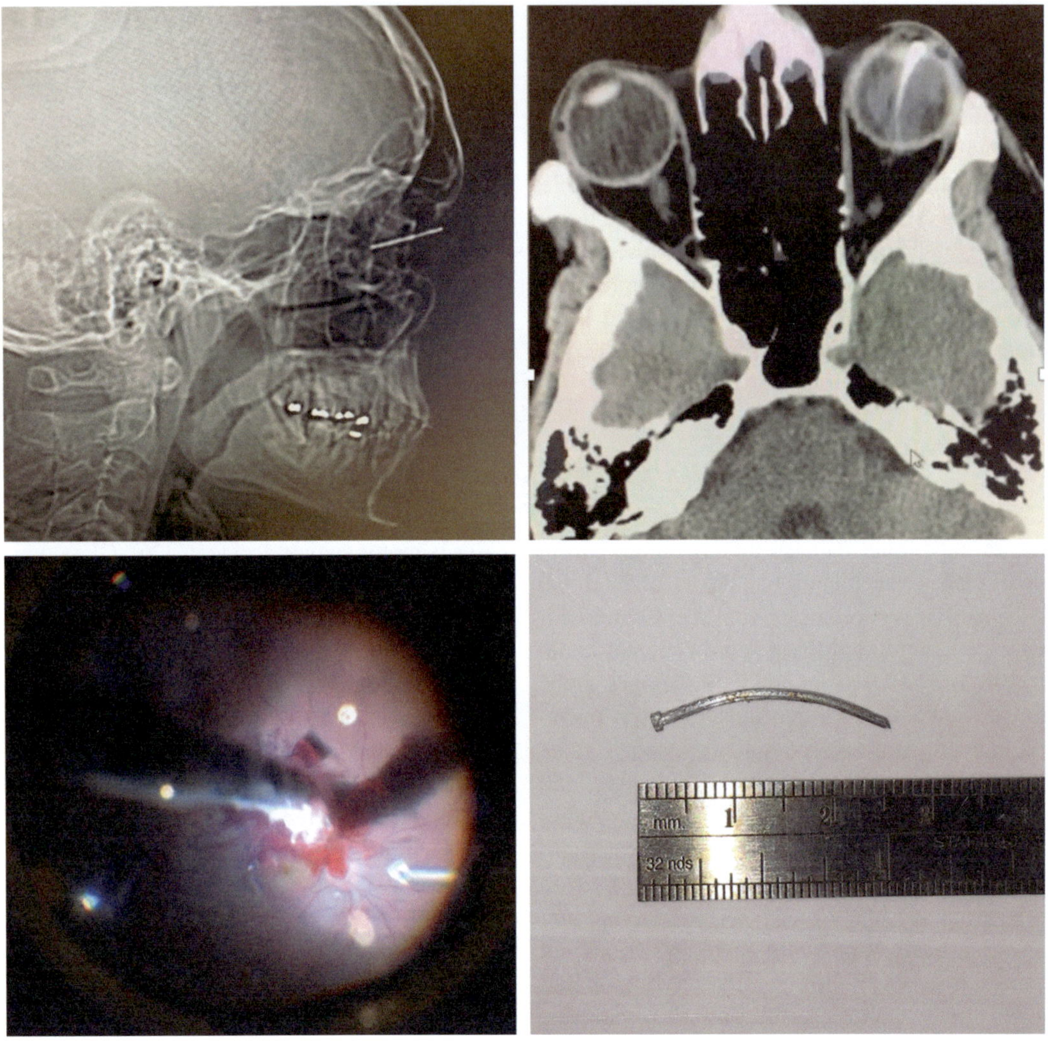

Fig. 29.1 Non-contrast computerized tomography of orbits, sagittal scout image, demonstrating nail within the left globe (top left). Axial non-contrast computerized tomography of orbits with evidence of large perforating metallic foreign body (top right). Intraoperative fundus photo of the left eye during pars plana vitrectomy showing perforating metallic foreign body along the inferior arcade (bottom left). After removal, the foreign body measures approximately 25 mm in length (bottom right). Image courtesy of Kim D. Tran, MD

chamber. Rare earth intraocular magnets allow for easier engagement and alignment of the IOFB compared to forceps, but removing the IOFB with magnet alone can cause it to become engaged in the sclera during extraction [7].

Historically, external magnets were used to extract almost all metallic IOFBs. This method led to uncontrolled IOFB removal and high risks of retinal detachment and development of proliferative vitreoretinopathy [28]. When using this instrument, the sclera overlying the IOFB or the pars plana 180 degrees away from the IOFB is incised. The underlying choroid is cauterized and incised to expose the vitreous base, if at the pars plana, or the retina, if at the site of IOFB. The magnet is then activated over the incision, attracting the IOFB and its removal through the sclerotomy [7].

The most common and current technique of foreign body removal is a pars plana vitrectomy (PPV), which provides good visualization of an IOFB in the posterior segment as well as any

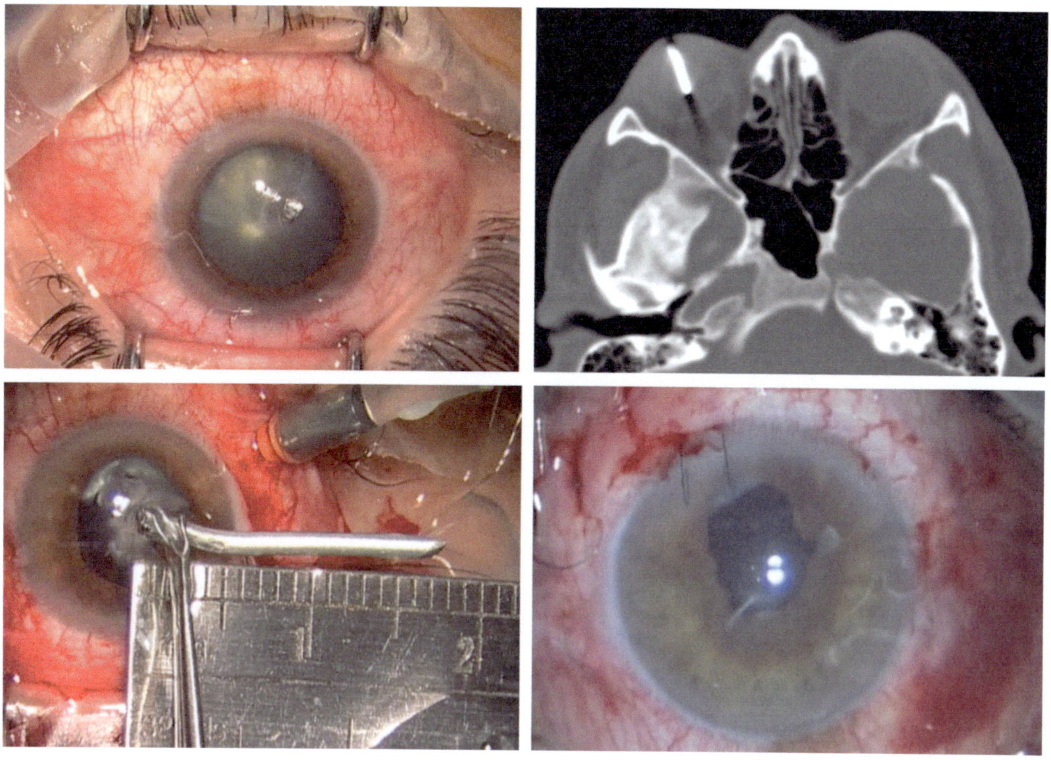

Fig. 29.2 Surgeon's view of the right eye demonstrating a metallic foreign body penetrating the central cornea and crystalline lens (top left). Axial non-contrast computerized tomography of orbits demonstrating large metallic foreign body within the globe and vitreous cavity (top right). After 23 gauge pars plana vitrectomy and lensectomy, the foreign body is removed and measures 17 mm in length (bottom left). Postoperative appearance of right eye following implantation of secondary intraocular lens in the ciliary sulcus (bottom right). Image courtesy of Jonathan S. Chang, MD, and Jayanth Sridhar, MD

retinal lesions/breaks [5, 28, 29]. It also allows for the collection of a vitreous sample that can be sent for gram stain and culture [7]. Additionally, studies report that eyes that underwent IOFB removal with PPV and forceps had better anatomic outcomes and fewer complications (including PVR and retinal detachment) than those that underwent extraction with an external magnet [30]. This approach, however, is more frequently associated with unintentional dropping of IOFB on the macula compared to removal through a sclerotomy with an external electromagnet [28].

In PPV, the IOFB is freed from the surrounding vitreous by dissecting around it to lyse any adhesions prior to extraction. In cases when the IOFB is embedded in the retina or choroid, the posterior hyaloid and vitreous in this area should be excised to potentially prevent peripheral retinal breaks during IOFB removal [5, 7, 9].

Small IOFBs, measuring less than 0.1 mm, suspended in the vitreous can often be extracted with the vitreous cutter. Ferromagnetic IOFBs of this size can also be removed using intraocular rare earth magnets. IOFBs that are 1–3 mm in size can be removed with either active compression or retractable basket forceps. Larger IOFBs measuring 3–5 mm can be removed with large foreign body forceps. For these and for IOFBs composed of glass, one may consider using diamond-coated forceps [31]. Many types of forceps may be employed in IOFB removal, and having the proper instrument design for the type and shape of IOFB makes the case much more straightforward. Bapaye et al. recently introduced a novel

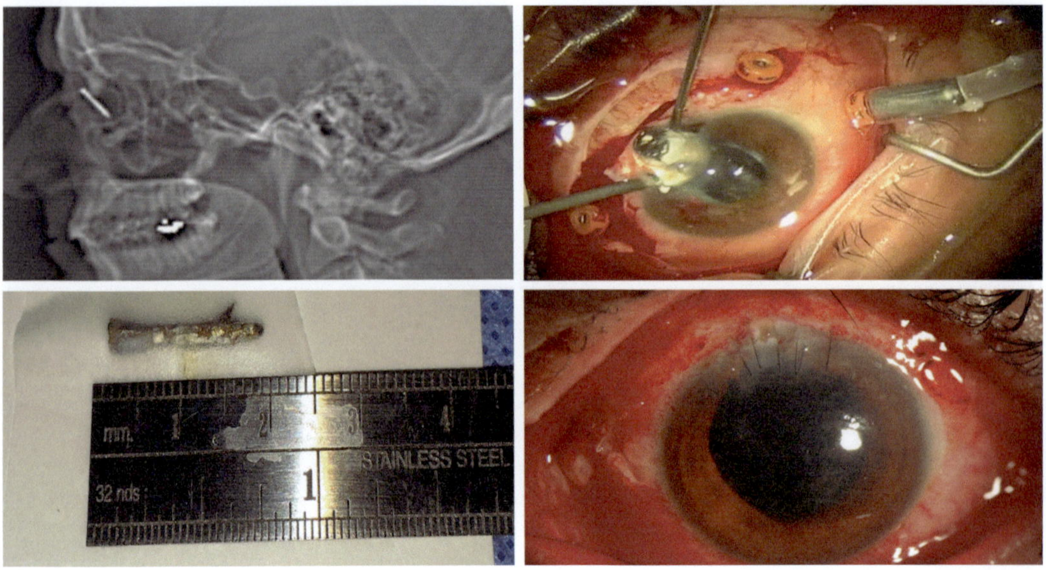

Fig. 29.3 Non-contrast computerized tomography of orbits, sagittal scout image, demonstrating nail within left globe (top left). Surgeon's view of left eye showing removal of large nail from original limbal wound during 23 gauge pars plana vitrectomy and lensectomy (top right). Nail measures about 17 mm in length (bottom left). Postoperative appearance of left eye with intact limbal sutures superiorly and aphakia (bottom right). Image courtesy of Jonathan S. Chang, MD, and Jayanth Sridhar, MD

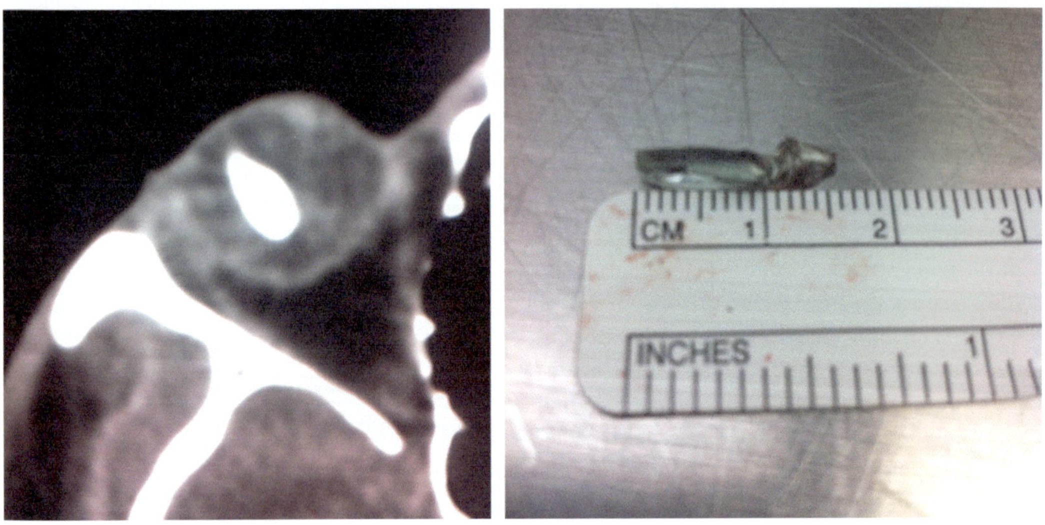

Fig. 29.4 Computerized tomography axial scan of the orbit with hyperdense glass intraocular foreign body (left). Large glass intraocular foreign body after removal (right). Image courtesy of Victor M. Villegas, MD

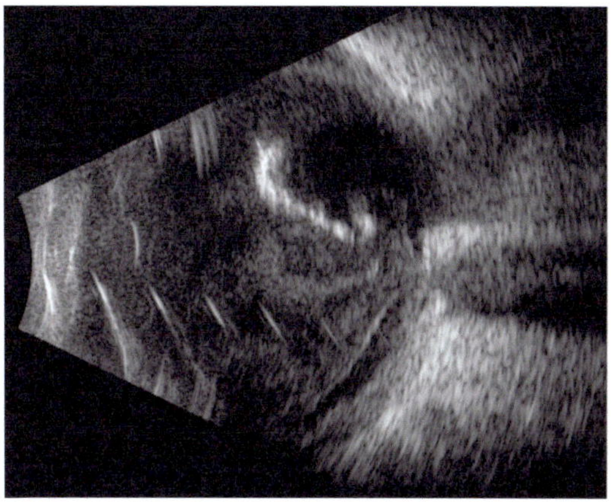

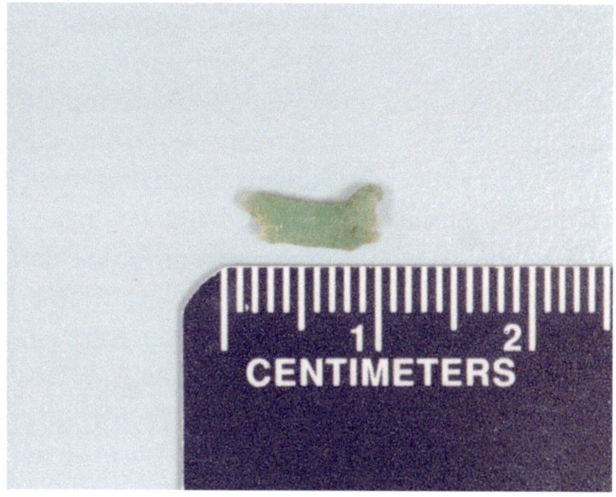

Fig. 29.5 B-scan ultrasonography (left) of 43-year-old gentleman who presented with fusarium endophthalmitis and intraocular foreign body after ruptured globe repair. He was found to have weed wacker nylon upon removal (right). Image courtesy of Jonathan H. Tzu, MD, and Basil K. Williams, MD

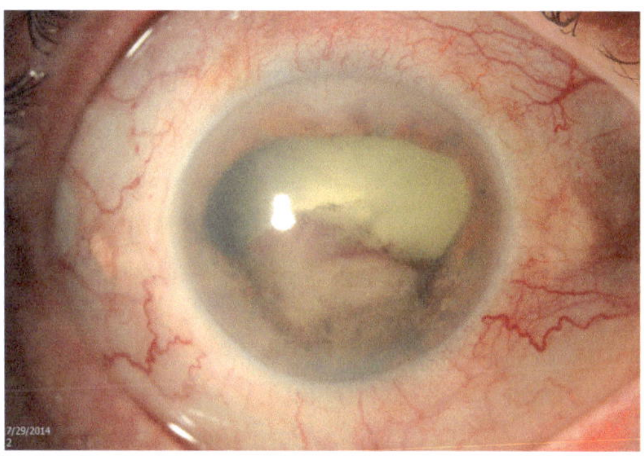

Fig. 29.6 Slit lamp photograph of 62-year-old gentleman status post fireworks injury causing hyphema, traumatic cataract, and retinal detachment. Image courtesy of Jonathan H. Tzu, MD, and Basil K. Williams, MD

grasping forceps "the claw" with four retractable prongs that more easily grasp irregular IOFBs of various shapes and sizes without crushing or splintering [32].

In general, smaller foreign bodies can be removed at the sclerotomy site. When foreign bodies measure greater than 4x4x4 mm, formation of a T-shaped sclerotomy may be required [4]. Alternatively, large IOFBs may be removed through the anterior chamber via a limbal incision. This is an option when the lens has been severely damaged and needs removal in-conjunction with the IOFB removal and vitrectomy.

29.4 Intraoperative Complications

29.4.1 Identification

Foreign body extraction from the posterior segment may lead to iatrogenic retinal tears and vitreous hemorrhage intraoperatively. For example, removal of the posterior hyaloid in areas of infectious retinitis may create retinal breaks [7]. Intraoperative removal of a perforating IOFB may result in rapid retinal detachment. Additionally, the potential of a dropped IOFB during its extraction is common and well described. A fallen IOFB can cause damage to the macula or optic disc and create retinal breaks and hemorrhages [28]. For this reason, it may be best to remove the core vitreous and specifically vitreous attached to the IOFB, but leave the posterior hyaloid to serve as a cushion in the case of an IOFB drop. After IOFB removal from the eye, the posterior hyaloid is then separated and removed. Alternatively, viscoelastic or PFO may be used to protect the posterior segment but this is not often necessary. Before the conclusion of the case, all patients undergoing PPV should undergo a complete scleral depressed retinal examination to evaluate for any pathology, including retinal breaks, retinal detachments, and choroidal detachments.

29.4.2 Prevention and Management

A complete vitrectomy should be performed to minimize any traction while removing the IOFB. To avoid postoperative retinal detachment, all retinal breaks identified should be treated with endolaser with consideration of intraocular tamponade. A lensectomy may be considered at the time of primary repair for optimal access in cases of pars plana or anterior retinal involvement, especially if high risk for proliferative vitreoretinopathy. Meticulous hemostasis may be achieved with endodiathermy. To minimize the risk of intraoperative optic nerve or macular damage from dropped IOFBs during extraction, perfluorocarbon liquid (PFCL) may be instilled. A retrospective study of 42 patients who underwent 23 gauge PPV with instillation of perfluorocarbon liquid (PFCL) found this technique is a safe method of protecting the macula from unexpected falling of a metallic IOFB during its removal [28].

Proper placement of the sclerotomy site for IOFB removal helps maintain a stable globe with appropriate intraoperative fluidics. If a bimanual approach or hand-off technique is needed, an illuminating chandelier may be used. Ravani et al. describe success with a midline sclerotomy approach for IOFB removal in phakic eyes using a chandelier illuminator to minimize lens trauma [33]. Prior to removal, the sclerotomy site should be enlarged to the appropriate width. If possible, care should be taken to grasp the IOFB along its length in a direction that minimizes the sclerotomy size. An intraocular magnet is a good way to align a magnetic IOFB along its long axis so that intraocular forceps in the fellow hand can be used to grasp it for removal in the proper alignment. Once the IOFB is removed, the sclerotomy site should be sutured to minimize hypotony. If lensectomy is performed, the IOFB may be removed via clear corneal incision. In the event of choroidal hemorrhage, rapid closure is advised. Increasing the infusion pressure and careful endodiathermy may help maintain good hemostasis. In cases of concurrent endophthalmitis, silicone oil tamponade may be considered as it does not support microbial growth [34].

29.5 Postoperative Considerations

29.5.1 Endophthalmitis

As previously mentioned, detection of endophthalmitis in cases of IOFB may be difficult, as posttraumatic and/or postoperative inflammation and pain may obscure infectious endophthalmitis. Clinical signs may include aqueous cell and flare, hypopyon, and vitreous cell. Prompt treatment is imperative for improved outcomes. Increased pain after stabilization from injury or surgery may be an important indicator of developing postoperative endophthalmitis.

According to the United States Eye Injury Registry, 3.4% of open globe injuries are associated with endophthalmitis [10, 35]. The presence of an IOFB raises the risk of developing endophthalmitis after trauma, particularly if the IOFB is made of organic material [7]. A review of the National Eye Trauma Registry showed that of 492 eyes with IOFB, 6.9% had infectious endophthalmitis with the majority (91%) apparent at the time of IOFB removal. The risk of developing endophthalmitis was markedly higher in patients with delayed repair over 24 hours of injury, as well as in older patients over 50 years of age [36]. Other risk factors for postoperative endophthalmitis include intraocular lens implantation [37], contaminated wound [38], and lens capsule rupture [38].

Whether it is detected preoperatively or postoperatively, management of endophthalmitis involves culture of the wound as well as intravitreal antibiotics, namely intravitreal vancomycin hydrochloride (1 mg/0.1 mL normal saline) and ceftazidime (2.25 mg/0.1 mL normal saline) [10]. In cases of fungal endophthalmitis, intravitreal voriconazole (50 mcg/0.1 mL normal saline) is used [10]. For high-risk cases with organic IOFB, administration of intravitreal or intracameral antibiotics and voriconazole at the time of primary surgical repair may help with prophylaxis. Patients will typically receive systemic antibiotics as part of the ruptured globe injury, and topical antibiotic therapy maybe used as adjuvant treatments.

29.5.2 Retinal Detachment

Retinal detachment is a serious complication of IOFB and extraction surgery. Several studies indicate that postoperative retinal detachment is associated with poor visual prognosis, though not as poor as preoperative retinal detachment [7]. In older studies, PPV decreased the risk of postoperative RD following IOFB removal from 79% to 11–23%, and more recent studies with PPV confirm a frequency of secondary RD in this range [28].

Few risk factors for postoperative retinal detachment have been identified. One study demonstrated that the presence of endophthalmitis and IOFBs over 4 mm in size were associated with an increased risk of post-vitrectomy retinal detachment [39]. In patients who have a retinal detachment at the time of surgery, removal of IOFB is associated with an increased risk of iatrogenic retinal breaks, potentially leading to a postoperative retinal detachment [7]. Given that these retinal detachments are associated with high risk for proliferative vitreoretinopathy (see below), consideration should be given for long-acting gas or silicone oil tamponade [40].

29.5.3 Proliferative Vitreoretinopathy

Proliferative vitreoretinopathy (PVR) is the most common cause of secondary retinal detachment and is associated with the formation and contraction of membranous scar tissue on the retinal surface. It has a complex pathophysiology and is associated with poor visual outcomes. Currently, there are no proven pharmacologic therapies to prevent or reduce PVR. Risk factors associated with PVR include size of IOFBs, vitreous hemorrhage, choroidal detachment, as well as the size and number of retinal tears [7].

29.5.4 Sympathetic Ophthalmia

Sympathetic ophthalmia (SO) is a granulomatous panuveitis that develops following penetrating ocular trauma or surgery in one eye. The incidence is between 0.28 and 1.9% after penetrating ocular trauma [41]. SO is thought to be an autoimmune reaction to exposed ocular antigens, and presents clinically as a decrease in vision, pain, and photophobia. Delaying or deferring enucleation may increase the risk of SO, and these risks should be discussed in cases of open globe ocular trauma. For most patients, however, current treatment strategies with steroids and immunosuppressive medications are effective in maintaining good vision [7]. Given the very small risk of and effective treatments for SO, most eyes should undergo initial repair (if anatomically feasible) even when the vision measures no light perception.

29.5.5 Pain Management

While patients are awaiting surgery for IOFB open globe injuries, pain may be managed with oral acetaminophen tablets, as this is generally well tolerated without any side effects. Patients may be given up to 1 g depending on the degree of pain. Nausea should also be addressed preoperatively as coughing or vomiting may increase intraocular pressure and risk further expulsion of intraocular contents.

Intraoperative surgical anesthesia may vary depending on the availability of anesthesia services. Depending on the extent of ocular injury, anesthesiologist monitored sedation and a peribulbar or retrobulbar block may be given prior to repair. Retrobulbar blocks are usually comprised of both lidocaine, which has a rapid onset of action but shorter duration, and bupivacaine, which has a slower onset of action but is longer duration. The effects of the block typically last 4–8 h. General anesthesia may be preferred as risks of a retrobulbar block are avoided, including, expulsion of intraocular contents when there is a large unstable posterior wound, increased intraocular pressure, and potentially exposing the retina to toxic levels of lidocaine. If good closure is achieved a subtenon block may be given at the end of the case for postoperative comfort.

While lidocaine and bupivacaine are typically used, an alternative pharmacologic option may be levobupivicaine. A study of 135 patients undergoing vitreoretinal surgery of similar duration under local anesthesia compared 0.5% levobupivacaine, 0.5% bupivacaine, and 2% lidocaine [42]. The authors found that the duration of motor and sensory block was longer in the levobupivacaine and bupivacaine groups than the lidocaine group. Furthermore, intraoperative pain was less in the levobupivacaine group than the lidocaine and bupivacaine groups. Thus, levobupivacaine may be an excellent option for retrobulbar anesthesia in vitreoretinal surgery.

Postoperatively, analgesia may be titrated depending on the complexity of the surgical case. Patients may start with oral acetaminophen and increase to acetaminophen with codeine as needed. Intraoperative steroids (125 mg IV methylprednisolone) or a methylprednisolone dose pack may help with inflammation and pain in the postoperative period.

One study of a pain management protocol following vitreoretinal surgery focused on the use of pre-emptive pain management [43]. In their protocol, patients were grouped based on complexity of surgery. Group A was minor procedures including pneumatic retinopexy and removal of scleral buckle. Group B was moderate procedures, including an uncomplicated 25G or 23G vitrectomy, and group C was higher level retinal procedures including complex vitrectomies lasting more than 2 hours, scleral bucking and cryotherapy, or unexpected complications during surgery. Eighty eight percent of their 100 patients experienced no or mild pain on the following regimen: acetaminophen 1 g 6 h after retrobulbar block and then every 6 hours as needed for group A; IV Parecoxib (a COX-2 inhibitor) 40 mg prior to discharge, acetaminophen 1 g 6 h after retrobulbar block, and acetaminophen 500 mg + codeine 30 mg every 6 h after as needed for group B; IV Parecoxib 40 mg prior to discharge, acetaminophen 1 g 6 h after retrobulbar block, and of oxycodone 5–10 mg every 4 h as well as acetaminophen 1 g every 6 h as needed for group C.

29.5.6 Aesthetics

Primary repair of ocular trauma is the preferred approach for the majority of cases. While prognostic factors are important in assessing the severity of eye injury, primary closure should always be the goal as visual recovery may occur even in patients presenting with no light perception vision. After primary closure, depending on the patient's final vision and level of comfort, a scleral shell or evisceration or enucleation may be considered. Patients who develop a blind painful eye are often the most grateful after removal. Working with an ocularist may help obtain an agreeable aesthetic outcome that enhances the patient's quality of life.

29.5.7 Prevention

Visual outcome following penetrating IOFB injury and subsequent extraction is often poor. Monocular precautions to help prevent injury to the remaining eye is important to discuss and emphasize with patients. Patients with a known trauma to one eye are at higher risk for recurrent eye trauma [44]. Polycarbonate lenses for daily protection of the uninjured eye as well as protective eyewear during certain contact sports or while at work (i.e., welding and construction) should be encouraged. All monocular patients should, at a minimum, have an annual dilated fundus exam to maintain good health in the uninjured eye. Of note, pediatric patients require special care for amblyopia prevention.

References

1. Guevara-Villarreal DA, Rodriguez-Valdes PJ. Posterior segment intraocular foreign body: extraction surgical techniques, timing, and indications for vitrectomy. J Ophthalmol. 2016;2016:2034509.
2. Choragiewicz T, Nowomiejska K, Wertejuk K, et al. Surgical treatment of open globe trauma complicated with the presence of an intraocular foreign body. Klin Ocz. 2015;117(1):5–8.

3. Jonas JB, Knorr HL, Budde WM. Prognostic factors in ocular injuries caused by intraocular or retrobulbar foreign bodies. Ophthalmology. 2000;107(5):823–8.
4. Yeh S, Colyer MH, Weichel ED. Current trends in the management of intraocular foreign bodies. Curr Opin Ophthalmol. 2008;19(3):225–33.
5. Greven CM, Engelbrecht NE, Slusher MM, Nagy SS. Intraocular foreign bodies: management, prognostic factors, and visual outcomes. Ophthalmology. 2000;107(3):608–12.
6. Kong Y, Tang X, Kong B, et al. Six-year clinical study of firework-related eye injuries in North China. Postgrad Med J. 2015;91(1071):26–9.
7. Loporchio D, Mukkamala L, Gorukanti K, et al. Intraocular foreign bodies: a review. Surv Ophthalmol. 2016;61(5):582–96.
8. Kuhn F, Morris R, Witherspoon CD, Mann L. Epidemiology of blinding trauma in the United States Eye Injury Registry. Ophthalmic Epidemiol. 2006;13(3):209–16.
9. Katz G, Moisseiev J. Posterior-segment intraocular foreign bodies: an update on management. Retin Physician. 2009;6(3):32–4.
10. Bhagat N, Nagori S, Zarbin M. Post-traumatic infectious endophthalmitis. Surv Ophthalmol. 2011;56(3):214–51.
11. Alfaro DV, Roth D, Liggett PE. Posttraumatic endophthalmitis. Causative organisms, treatment, and prevention. Retina. 1994;14(3):206–11.
12. Kuhn F, Maisiak R, Mann L, et al. The ocular trauma score (OTS). Ophthalmol Clin N Am. 2002;15(2):163–5, vi.
13. Pieramici DJ, Sternberg P Jr, Aaberg TM Sr, et al. A system for classifying mechanical injuries of the eye (globe). The Ocular Trauma Classification Group. Am J Ophthalmol. 1997;123(6):820–31.
14. Pieramici DJ, Au Eong KG, Sternberg P Jr, Marsh MJ. The prognostic significance of a system for classifying mechanical injuries of the eye (globe) in open-globe injuries. J Trauma. 2003;54(4):750–4.
15. McNicholas MM, Brophy DP, Power WJ, Griffin JF. Ocular trauma: evaluation with US. Radiology. 1995;195(2):423–7.
16. Bryden FM, Pyott AA, Bailey M, McGhee CN. Real time ultrasound in the assessment of intraocular foreign bodies. Eye (Lond). 1990;4(Pt 5):727–31.
17. Zacks DN, Hart L, Young LH. Ultrasonography in the traumatized eye: intraocular foreign body versus artifact. Int Ophthalmol Clin. 2002;42(3):121–8.
18. McElvanney AM, Fielder AR. Intraocular foreign body missed by radiography. BMJ. 1993;306(6884):1060–1.
19. Lakits A, Prokesch R, Scholda C, Bankier A. Orbital helical computed tomography in the diagnosis and management of eye trauma. Ophthalmology. 1999;106(12):2330–5.
20. Sakamoto H, Sakamoto M, Hata Y, et al. Aqueous and vitreous penetration of levofloxacin after topical and/or oral administration. Eur J Ophthalmol. 2007;17(3):372–6.
21. Colyer MH, Weber ED, Weichel ED, et al. Delayed intraocular foreign body removal without endophthalmitis during Operations Iraqi Freedom and Enduring Freedom. Ophthalmology. 2007;114(8):1439–47.
22. Fulcher TP, McNab AA, Sullivan TJ. Clinical features and management of intraorbital foreign bodies. Ophthalmology. 2002;109(3):494–500.
23. Zhang Y, Zhang M, Jiang C, Qiu HY. Intraocular foreign bodies in China: clinical characteristics, prognostic factors, and visual outcomes in 1,421 eyes. Am J Ophthalmol. 2011;152(1):66–73.
24. Marshall MW, Teitelbaum GP, Kim HS, Deveikis J. Ferromagnetism and magnetic resonance artifacts of platinum embolization microcoils. Cardiovasc Intervent Radiol. 1991;14(3):163–6.
25. Zhu L, Shen P, Lu H, et al. Ocular trauma score in Siderosis Bulbi with retained intraocular foreign body. Medicine (Baltimore). 2015;94(39):e1533.
26. Ghoraba H. Posterior segment glass intraocular foreign bodies following car accident or explosion. Graefes Arch Clin Exp Ophthalmol. 2002;240(7):524–8.
27. Ho VT, McGuckin JF Jr, Smergel EM. Intraorbital wooden foreign body: CT and MR appearance. AJNR Am J Neuroradiol. 1996;17(1):134–6.
28. Rejdak R, Choragiewicz T, Moneta-Wielgos J, et al. Intraoperative macula protection by perfluorocarbon liquid for the metallic intraocular foreign body removal during 23-gauge vitrectomy. J Ophthalmol. 2017;2017:6232151.
29. Wani VB, Al-Ajmi M, Thalib L, et al. Vitrectomy for posterior segment intraocular foreign bodies: visual results and prognostic factors. Retina. 2003;23(5):654–60.
30. Mester V, Kuhn F. Ferrous intraocular foreign bodies retained in the posterior segment: management options and results. Int Ophthalmol. 1998;22(6):355–62.
31. Karjosukarso DW, van Gestel SHC, Qu J, et al. An FEVR-associated mutation in ZNF408 alters the expression of genes involved in the development of vasculature. Hum Mol Genet. 2018;27(20):3519–27.
32. Bapaye M, Shanmugam MP, Sundaram N. The claw: a novel intraocular foreign body removal forceps. Indian J Ophthalmol. 2018;66(12):1845–8.
33. Ravani R, Chawla R, Azad SV, et al. Midline sclerotomy approach for intraocular foreign body removal in phakic eyes using endoilluminator: a novel technique. Indian J Ophthalmol. 2018;66(5):687–90.
34. Ahmed Y, Schimel AM, Pathengay A, et al. Endophthalmitis following open-globe injuries. Eye (Lond). 2012;26(2):212–7.
35. Danis RP. Endophthalmitis. Ophthalmol Clin N Am. 2002;15(2):243–8.

36. Thompson JT, Parver LM, Enger CL, et al. Infectious endophthalmitis after penetrating injuries with retained intraocular foreign bodies. Natl Eye Trauma Syst Ophthalmol. 1993;100(10):1468–74.
37. Andreoli CM, Andreoli MT, Kloek CE, et al. Low rate of endophthalmitis in a large series of open globe injuries. Am J Ophthalmol. 2009;147(4):601–8.e2.
38. Essex RW, Yi Q, Charles PG, Allen PJ. Post-traumatic endophthalmitis. Ophthalmology. 2004;111(11):2015–22.
39. El-Asrar AM, Al-Amro SA, Khan NM, Kangave D. Retinal detachment after posterior segment intraocular foreign body injuries. Int Ophthalmol. 1998;22(6):369–75.
40. Silicone Study Group. Vitrectomy with silicone oil or perfluoropropane gas in eyes with severe proliferative vitreoretinopathy: results of a randomized clinical trial. Silicone Study Report 2. Arch Ophthalmol. 1992;110(6):780–92.
41. Ozbek Z, Arikan G, Yaman A, et al. Sympathetic ophthalmia following vitreoretinal surgery. Int Ophthalmol. 2010;30(2):221–7.
42. Akay F, Toyran S, Oztas Z, Koksal S. Long-term choroidal thickness changes after acute solar retinopathy. Ophthalmic Surg Lasers Imaging Retina. 2015;46(7):738–42.
43. McCloud C, Harrington A, King L. A pre-emptive pain management protocol to support self-care following vitreo-retinal day surgery. J Clin Nurs. 2014;23(21–22):3230–9.
44. Wong TY, Klein BE, Klein R. The prevalence and 5-year incidence of ocular trauma. The Beaver Dam Eye Study. Ophthalmology. 2000;107(12):2196–202.

Part VIII

Endophthalmitis

30 Management of Endophthalmitis

Thirumalesh MB, Jivitesh Singh, and Astha Jain

30.1 Introduction

Endophthalmitis is an inflammatory condition of the eye which occurs due to an infectious process from bacteria, fungi, or, on rare occasions, parasites involving intraocular cavities (the aqueous and/or vitreous humor), sparing the sclera. It is the most feared complication because of its potential for vision loss. In comparison, when inflammation spreads throughout the globe involving all the layers including the Tenon's capsule with or without involvement of the peri-ocular tissues, the condition is known as pan-ophthalmitis.

Cataract surgery is the most common procedure associated with exogenous endophthalmitis because of large number of surgeries carried out everywhere in the world. Other procedures associated with risks of endophthalmitis include corneal surgeries (penetrating keratoplasty, keratoprosthesis insertion, refractive corneal surgeries), retina procedures (intravitreal injections, vitrectomies), glaucoma surgical procedure (blebs, glaucoma valve placements). Endophthalmitis is a potentially devastating complication that leads to permanent severe vision loss in about one-third of cases [1].

30.2 Clinical Presentation

The predominant symptoms seen in a study of around 100 patients exhibited decreased vision (94%) and pain (75%). On ocular examination, there is difficulty to visualize the fundus due to pupillary fibrin membrane and hypopyon in anterior chamber and exudates in vitreous cavity [2]. The mean time between cataract surgery and diagnosis of endophthalmitis was 13 days (median, 9 days; range, 1–39 days). Visual acuity at the time of diagnosis was <5/200 in 61 of 73 (83.6%) patients, including light perception in 11 of 73 (15.1%) [3].

30.3 Classification and Types of Endophthalmitis

It may be categorized by clinical course (acute versus chronic), by etiology (infectious versus non-infectious), by the route the causative agent enters the globe (exogenous and endogenous) and by the organisms involved (bacteria, fungi, parasites and rarely, viruses).

T. MB (✉) · J. Singh
Narayana Nethralaya, Bengaluru, India

A. Jain
Aditya Jyot Foundation for Twinkling Little Eyes, Mumbai, India

A. Jain et al. (eds.), *Cutting-edge Vitreoretinal Surgery*, https://doi.org/10.1007/978-981-33-4168-5_30

30.3.1 Based on Time of Presentation

Endophthalmitis can be classified into three types based on time of presentation. The endophthalmitis that occurs early is more fulminant and the organisms are more virulent. The Hyperacute/Fulminant endophthalmitis presents 2–4 days postoperatively, and is most frequently due to streptococci, *Staphylococcus aureus,* or Gram-negative organisms. The Acute enophthalmitis which is moderately severe, occurs 5–7 days postoperatively, and is frequently due to *Staphylococcus epidermidis*, coagulase-negative cocci, or more rarely, fungal species. Infection which persists beyond 6 weeks despite treatment is termed as Chronic infection. *Propionibacterium acnes*, *Staphylococcus epidermidis*, or fungal infections are the most common cause for chronicity.

30.3.2 Based on the Route the Causative Agent Enters the Globe

Endophthalmitis is classified as exogenous where the causative organism enters the eye by direct inoculation after either any intraocular surgery or trauma. Endogenous endophthalmitis is mainly due to hematogenous spread of infection.

30.3.2.1 Post-cataract Surgery Endophthalmitis

Post-cataract endophthalmitis is the major type of endophthalmitis seen worldwide. Most cases are attributable to Gram-positive bacteria, Coagulase-negative *Staphylococcus*, *Staphylococcus aureus*, and *Streptococcus* sp. Eyelids and ocular flora remain the most common source for these bacterial pathogens [4].

Worldwide incidence of endophthalmitis post-cataract surgery is 0.02– 0.11%. Studies from the Bascom Palmer Institute in Florida covering 3 separate time periods (1984–1994, 1995–2001, 2002–2009) show a decrease in post-cataract surgery endophthalmitis from 0.08% to 0.05% to 0.025%, respectively [5]. The decreasing trend of incidence is attributable to progressive improvements in microsurgical and aseptic techniques.

The infectious process undergoes an initial incubation phase which may be clinically imperceptible, lasts at least 16–18 h, during which a critical amount of pathogen proliferates and break down the aqueous barrier; this is followed by fibrin exudation and cellular infiltration by neutrophilic granulocytes. The acceleration phase follows primary infection of the posterior segment and leads to inflammation of the anterior chamber and an immune response with macrophages and lymphocytes infiltrating into the vitreous cavity within about 7 days.

30.3.2.2 Endophthalmitis Seen with Glaucoma Procedure

Glaucoma filtering bleb surgeries present with late-onset endophthalmitis in about 1.8% occurring from 3 months to 27 years postoperatively [6]. Acute onset endophthalmitis immediately following trabeculectomy is rarely seen (0.6%). High incidence of late-onset endophthalmitis has been reported after the use of the antimetabolites 5-fluorouracil (5–8%) and mitomycin C (MMC) (2.7–3%) [7].

Filtering blebs of eyes treated with mitomycin C have attenuated epithelium, loosely arranged hypocellular, subepithelial connective tissue, and are devoid of blood vessels. The resulting cystic, ischemic, and particularly thin-walled bleb has a greater potential risk of infection compared to a filtering bleb where no antiproliferative agents have been used [8]. The presence of a thin walled, cystic bleb is the determining factor in creating a direct access to the eye for an organism either by the high permeability of the cystic wall or by the relatively frequent coexistence of a conjunctival leak. Endophthalmitis risks also vary significantly with the location of the bleb. Endophthalmitis was seen to develop in 8% of patients where an inferior approach was used for the filtering bleb and in only 1.1% in whom a superior approach was used [7].

30.3.2.3 Endophthalmitis Post Keratoplasty

Endophthalmitis occurs in approximately 0.2% of keratoplasty cases in the acute postoperative period but in up to 0.7% if later cases are included [9]. Risk of endophthalmitis in cornea procedures like penetrating therapeutic keratoplasty (TPK) after a perforated corneal ulcer remains high due to contributing factors that include pathogen exposure, corneal perforation, systemic immune dysfunction, and both topical and oral steroid use. The majority of endophthalmitis following TPK is bacterial and mainly due to *Streptococcus* sp. and *Staphylococcus* sp. [10]. Gram-negative organisms, *Proteus mirabilis* and *Serratia marcescens* can cause approximately a quarter of infections [10].

30.3.2.4 Exogenous Endophthalmitis Secondary to Trauma

Longer time between injury and examination, poorer visual acuity at presentation, virulence of organisms, lens capsule breach, rural area address, and the presence of an intraocular foreign body (IOFB) are related to endophthalmitis [11].

Bacillus sp., mainly *Bacillus cereus* has been reported as responsible for up to 65% of post-traumatic endophthalmitis [12]. Virulence is attributable to bacterial toxins—hemolysins, lipases, enterotoxins, and proteases [13]. Infections are responsible for the rapid destruction of ocular tissue and visual loss. It may often cause loss of the eye in hours to a few days after injury due to severe inflammation and tissue destruction.

30.3.2.5 Postinjection Endophthalmitis

The risk of endophthalmitis is approximately 0.05% per injection [14], and because anti-VEGF injections need to be repeated at regular intervals for age-related macular degeneration, the risk of endophthalmitis is accumulative. Retrospective study based in the United States discovered a higher rate of endophthalmitis after intravitreal corticosteroid injections than after anti-VEGF injections (0.13% versus 0.02%) [15]. Patients with post-injection endophthalmitis typically present within 5 days after the injection.

The microbiology profile of post-injection endophthalmitis composed of coagulase-negative staphylococci (65%), streptococci viridans (30%), *S. aureus* (0–5%), and others (0–4%) [15, 16]. This is almost similar to the microbiology profile of post-cataract endophthalmitis except that the incidence of viridans streptococci is three times greater. This finding was contributed due to practice of giving intravitreal injections in outpatient settings. *Streptococcus viridans* is a commensal of the oral cavity. This also highlights the importance of not talking and wearing a face mask while giving intravitreal injections in either outpatient or inpatient setting.

30.3.2.6 Postvitrectomy Endophthalmitis

Post-vitrectomy endophthalmitis is less frequently see when compared to post-cataract endophthalmitis, but the microbiology profile is akin, with the majority of cases affected by coagulase-negative staphylococci. Vitrectomies are performed for various retinal conditions (e.g., retinal detachment and vitreous hemorrhage), and recent studies report an incidence of endophthalmitis of 0.02–0.06% following vitrectomy.

30.3.2.7 Recurrent Endophthalmitis

Propionibacterium acne is an anaerobic, pleomorphic, Gram-positive bacillus, a normal commensal of the conjunctival sac. It is resistant to the killing mechanisms of polymorphonucleocytes and monocytes, hence it persists intracellularly after phagocytosis [17]. Endophthalmitis with P acnes manifests as a chronic, low grade, delayed, and often recurrent postoperative granulomatous uveitis.

30.3.2.8 Endogenous Endophthalmitis

An endogenous cause is responsible for roughly 2–8% of all endophthalmitis [18]. Ocular complaints composed of (90%) decreased vision, 50% eye pain (50%). On examination, 35% have a hypopyon, and 33% have vitritis. Fever (37%) and flu-like symptoms (20%) are the common systemic associations [19]. Prompt diagnosis and treatment are essential to obtain the best visual outcomes. The underlying infection should also be investigated and managed, although it remains unidentified in many cases. Endogenous endophthalmitis is the result of hematogenous spread of infective organisms from a distant focus in body. Although a systemic source of infection may not always be present. Major risk factors for EE are immunocompromised states (chronic corticosteroid use, malignancy, organ transplant, diabetes mellitus), intravenous drug use, indwelling catheter, or dental procedures.

Gram-negative bacteria, *Klebsiella pneumoniae* is responsible for most cases of endogenous endophthalmitis in liver abscess and pneumonia affected patients of Asian origin [20]. *Staphylococcus aureus* and streptococci sp. and fungi are the frequent causative agents in North America and Europe [18]. *Candida* species, mostly *Candida albicans* is responsible for endogenous fungal endophthalmitis in hospitalized patients [18]. Risk factors for the development of *Candida* endogenous fungal endophthalmitis include diabetes, antibiotic use, gastrointestinal surgery, indwelling catheters, intravenous drug abuse, and immunosuppression [21].

When suspecting endogenous endophthalmitis, it requires a systemic workup for the source of infection, although in 44% of cases no source is found [2]. EE has been most commonly associated with liver abscesses, sinus infections, endocarditis, meningitis, or the presence of indwelling catheters (Figs. 30.1 and 30.2). A key diagnostic finding associated with an endogenous cause is the presence of a white infiltrate originating in the choroid and sometimes erupting into the vitreous cavity.

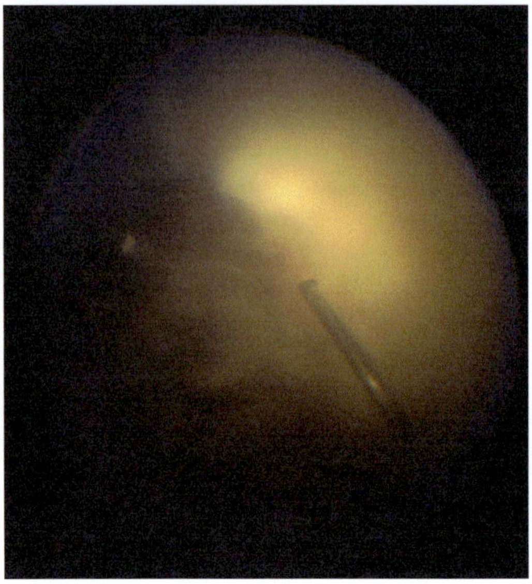

Fig. 30.1 Case of endogenous endophthalmitis in a 75-year-old female with a liver abscess on presentation. A large white-yellow colored bacterial colony is seen at the temporal quadrant, which is obscuring the view of retina beneath. After clearing the central vitreous with core vitrectomy, the partly necrotic and damaged retina can be visualized

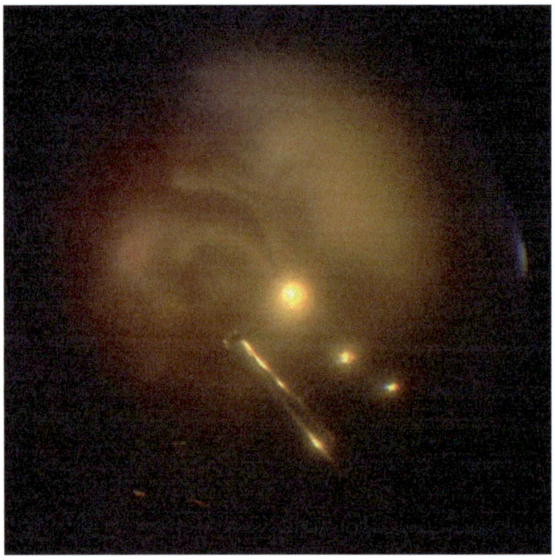

Fig. 30.2 Same case of endogenous endophthalmitis after vitrectomy. A clearer view of retina with optic disc can be visualized with reflection from the air while doing fluid air exchange

30.3.3 Based on Etiology

Endophthalmitis could be sterile or infectious.

Sterile endophthalmitis also known as toxic anterior segment syndrome (TASS) is characterized by a noninfectious anterior chamber inflammatory reaction that can have multiple etiologies. Sterile endophthalmitis is seen to occur within 24 h post-operative period. Absence of vitritis is the most important feature of TASS because it involves primarily anterior segment, while endophthalmitis involves both anterior as well as posterior segments.

There are multiple reasons for TASS, including residual chemicals from sterilization processes, toxicity of the polymethylmethacrylate (PMMA) monomers or intraocular lens rubbing onto the iris and ciliary body especially when IOL is placed in the sulcus [22, 23]. Autoimmunity to the lens cortical remnants can cause a mild-to-severe inflammation with hypopyon, in the absence of infection. Causes of infectious endophthalmitis is as described above.

30.4 Etiological Variation in Developed Versus Developing Nations

A retrospective analysis carried out between January 1997 and December 2006 from India of 955 patients presenting during a 10-year period found 92.6% to be exogenous endophthalmitis and only 7.4% endogenous endophthalmitis [24]. In a retrospective evaluation of 120 eyes of 114 patients, analyzing acute endophthalmitis trends between 1991 and 2004, found that of 120 cases, 59% were exogenous and 41% endogenous in origin [25].

Generally, studies have found coagulase-negative *Staphylococcus* is the top pathogen [3]. In two reports from India, the incidence of Gram-positive and Gram-negative bacteria were almost equal and more cases of *Pseudomonas aeruginosa* endophthalmitis were identified [26].

Bacillus organisms are spore-forming Gram-positive rods, ubiquitous in soil, water, and dust. Endophthalmitis caused by *Bacillus* species often results in poor visual outcomes. *Bacillus* sp. infections are responsible for the rapid destruction they can cause, with visual loss and often loss of the eye in hours to a few days after injury [12]. In a retrospective series carried in the United States only and 8 of 22 patients with *Bacillus* sp. endophthalmitis ultimately had visual acuity better than 6/60 [12]. *Bacillus* sp. have been reported as responsible for 15–46% of post-traumatic endophthalmitis but are only rarely isolated from post-surgical endophthalmitis cases [12]. In an Indian study, a variety of species were isolated and some infections were caused by a mixture of *Bacillus* sp. [27].

30.5 Diagnosis

The anterior chamber aspirate is obtained through a paracentesis using a 25–27 gauge needle attached to a tuberculin syringe to aspirate about 0.1 mL of aqueous humor. The anterior chamber reforms in 3–5 min.

The vitreous specimen can be obtained as an aspirate through a needle or using a vitreous biopsy as a part of a full therapeutic vitrectomy. It is imperative to note that simple needle aspiration may not provide sufficient volume for analysis and may cause unwarranted pull on the vitreous due to presence of dense vitreous associated with endophthalmitis.

Samples should be sent immediately for Gram's and KOH staining; however, the injection of broad-spectrum antibiotics should not be withheld, as the Gram stain is positive in around 60% of the cases. In case fungal etoilogy is proved on KOH/ Gram stain, comes out as positive, an antifungal agent should be added.

The samples should be inoculated in aerobic, anaerobic, and fungal culture media to look for any growth. Anaerobic media should be watched for at least 14 days if *Propionibacterium* sp. is suspected. Careful procedures can reveal a positive culture and prove the presence of endophthalmitis in 56–82% of samples.

30.6 Management

30.6.1 Role of Intravitreal Antibiotics

Systemic antibiotics are not an ideal treatment for endophthalmitis like other bodily infections because of the blood–retinal barrier. The majority of antibiotics have a poor penetration into the vitreous cavity when administered intravenously or orally; retrobulbar injections reach higher intraocular concentrations than subconjunctival injections [28].

We are facing a global healthcare crisis due to emerging resistance to commonly used antimicrobial agents. Increasing antimicrobial resistance may arise from widespread agricultural use of antibiotics as a part of poultry feed to animals, the overuse of antibiotics in hospitals and easy availability at outpatient clinics, and intrinsic genetic factors. Gram-positive organisms were reported to be 100% susceptible to vancomycin as reported by the Endophthalmitis Vitrectomy Study (EVS). But more recently, a review (1990–2015) reported 27 cases of endophthalmitis caused by Gram-positive organisms with reduced vancomycin susceptibility and vancomycin resistance [29].

Intravitreal antibiotic injections can rapidly achieve therapeutic drug levels directly at the sites of infection. The ideal drug should exhibit a good antibacterial activity against both Gram-positive and Gram-negative organisms, while causing no toxicity for ocular structures. Vancomycin has bactericidal activity against nearly all Gram-positive bacteria including methicillin-resistant *Staphylococcus aureus* or methicillin-resistant *Staphylococcus epidermidis* and cephalosporin-resistant streptococci, *Bacillus cereus*, and coagulase-negative staphylococci. It is also active in cases of recurrent endophthalmitis due to P acnes. It does not have any retinal toxicity with intravitreal injections of up to 2 mg [30]. Aminoglycosides including amikacin and gentamycin have been used for Gram-negative bacteria-associated endophthalmitis. Amikacin has four times less retinal toxicity than gentamicin at 0.4 mg/0.1 mL [31]. Ceftazidime is a third-generation cephalosporin which is an alternative to amikacin for Gram-negative endophthalmitis. It is bactericidal against the majority of Gram-negative bacteria, as well as *Pseudomonas aeruginosa*. Retinal toxicity of ceftazidime has been studied in primates at the concentration of 2.25 mg/0.1 mL, is considered safe and recommended for intravitreal injection [32]. Intravitreal antifungal agents of choice include amphotericin-B (0.005 mg/0.1 cc) or voriconazole (0.1 mg/0.2 cc).

Intravitreal imipenem (50 μg/0.1 mL) can be used as an alternative where organisms show resistance to ceftazidime. It has been reported to successfully treat 11 cases out of 56 ceftazidime resistant cases where patients achieved better anatomic useful vision outcomes. All cases were sensitive to imipenem [33]. In another study, vitrectomy was done using 0.025% povidone-iodine in the infusion fluid in four eyes with endophthalmitis. Resolution of endophthalmitis ensued in all cases with improvement in visual acuity and no reported complications. The 0.025% PI-BSS PLUS is bactericidal and nontoxic when used as an irrigation solution in vitrectomy. Use of povidone-iodine in irrigating fluid or as an intravitreal injection is a possible prophylactic and therapeutic future option [34].

30.6.2 Role of Vitrectomy

Vitrectomy has a vital role in the treatment of fulminant endophthalmitis. Vitrectomy facilitates the removal of infecting pathogens and their toxins, clears the dense vitreous membranes that could form and subsequently lead to tractional detachment of the retina, provides a vitreous sample for culture. However, the absence of vitreous can increase drug toxicity. Two factors mainly responsible are firstly, the drug comes in direct contact with retina and achieves higher concentration which can be retino-toxic. Secondly, the clearance of the antibiotic from the vitreous cavity is faster. These two factors mandate multiple injections that are necessary to obtain the same drug half-life and efficacy, thereby increasing the risk of retinal toxicity [35].

The Endophthalmitis Vitrectomy Study (EVS) was the first large multicentric randomized study, which provided us with the guidelines about the use of intravitreal antibiotics with pars plana vitrectomy (PPV) or vitreous tap. The EVS reported that in a subgroup of patients with presenting visual acuity of hand motions or better, there was no difference in the visual outcome with immediate PPV or vitreous tap. Nevertheless, in the subgroup of patients with presenting visual acuity of light perception only, visual outcomes were better with immediate PPV compared to vitreous tap [36]. It also concluded that omission of systemic antibiotic treatment can reduce toxic effects, costs, and length of hospital stay [36].

With the introduction of 23G and 25G vitrectomy, there is a prospect to perform a complete and safe PPV (Fig. 30.3). This involves commencing in the anterior segment while gradually working the way toward posterior segment. This includes if required, clearing the anterior chamber of fibrin and cellular material. Vitrectomy is started behind the lens and then gradually proceeds deeper. A thorough core vitrectomy along with posterior vitreous separation and removal of the macular hypopyon is recommended (Fig. 30.4). Vitreous base shaving ought to be done conservatively with low vacuum settings and care, not to induce any iatrogenic tears in the already necrotic retina. Silicone oil injection has an important role in necrotic retina with multiple holes and retinal detachment, where it can provide a tamponading effect to keep the retina in place [37].

Kuhn and Gini in their series of 47 patients which they treated for postoperative endophthalmitis, 91% achieved a visual acuity of 20/40 or better compared to 53% in the EVS [36]. None of the treated patients had a retinal detachment compared to 8.3% in the EVS. No patient suffered from phthisis compared to 6% EVS [36, 38]. Early intervention with a complete PPV is expected to offer prevention of further retinal damage and better visual outcomes especially in cases with poor media clarity and no red reflex irrespective of visual acuity [37].

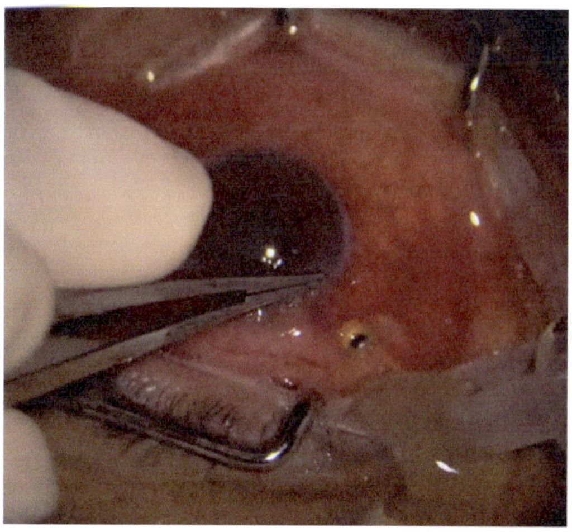

Fig. 30.3 Acute endophthalmitis presenting 48 h after vitrectomy for macular hole surgery. A straw-colored fluid is seen egressing out of the port opposite to the infusion port once infusion is turned on. Free flow of fluid is attributable due to vitreous being replaced with gas in first sitting of vitrectomy

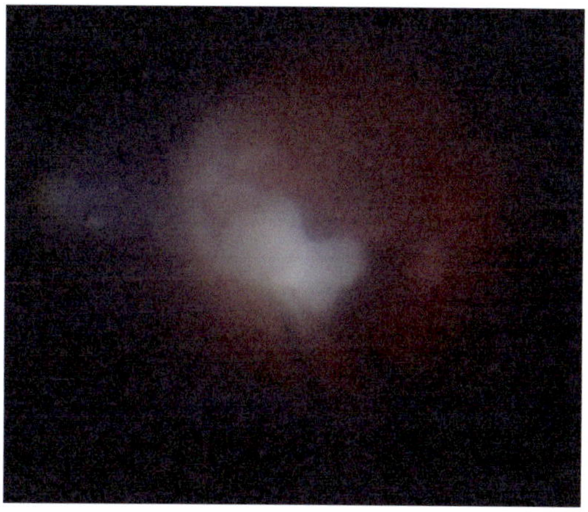

Fig. 30.4 Acute endophthalmitis in a gas-filled eye 48 h post vitrectomy. A white color microbial colony is seen over the posterior pole near to the disc in a hazy media, it was cleared using pars plana vitrectomy

In cases of endophthalmitis due to *Propionibacterium* sp. and *Candida* sp., PPV with explantation of the IOL and capsular bag itself is often necessary for an effective resolu tion. This is because capsular bag and IOL serve as a nidus for growth and sequestration of these organisms responsible for recurrent attacks of endophthalmitis [39].

30.7 Prophylaxis and Prevention

It has been proven beyond doubt that the use of intra-cameral antibiotics reduces the risk for postoperative endophthalmitis. Patients who receive intracameral injections of cefuroxime at the conclusion of cataract surgery have sixfold lower risk than those not receiving intracameral cefuroxime. The rate of postoperative endophthalmitis with intracameral injection at the end of surgery (0.055%) than in those without cefazolin injection (0.63%). Intracameral injection of cefazolin (1 mg in 0.1 mL solution) in cataract surgery has validated prophylactic efficacy in diminishing the rate of postoperative endophthalmitis without toxic effects on the cornea or retina [40]. 0.5% moxifloxacin can also be used as an alternative to cephalosporins at the last step of cataract surgery. It was found to be effective in reducing the risk for endophthalmitis [41].

References

1. Gower EW, Lindsley K, Tulenko SE, Nanji AA, Leyngold I, McDonnell PJ. Perioperative antibiotics for prevention of acute endophthalmitis after cataract surgery. Cochrane Database Syst Rev. 2017;2:CD006364. http://www.ncbi.nlm.nih.gov/pubmed/28192644
2. Cornut P-L, Thuret G, Creuzot-Garcher C, Maurin M, Pechinot A, Bron A, et al. Relationship between baseline clinical data and microbiologic spectrum in 100 patients with acute postcataract endophthalmitis. Retina. 2012;32(3):549–57. http://www.ncbi.nlm.nih.gov/pubmed/21968507
3. Lalwani GA, Flynn HW, Scott IU, Quinn CM, Berrocal AM, Davis JL, et al. Acute-onset endophthalmitis after clear corneal cataract surgery (1996–2005). Ophthalmology. 2008;115(3):473–6. http://www.ncbi.nlm.nih.gov/pubmed/18067969
4. Bannerman TL, Rhoden DL, McAllister SK, Miller JM, Wilson LA. The source of coagulase-negative staphylococci in the Endophthalmitis Vitrectomy study. Arch Ophthalmol. 1997;115(3):357. http://www.ncbi.nlm.nih.gov/pubmed/9076208
5. Eifrig CWG, Flynn HW, Scott IU, Newton J. Acute-onset postoperative endophthalmitis: review of incidence and visual outcomes (1995-2001). Ophthalmic Surg Lasers. 2002;33(5):373–8. http://www.ncbi.nlm.nih.gov/pubmed/12358290
6. Mandelbaum S, Forster RK, Gelender H, Culbertson W. Late onset endophthalmitis associated with filtering blebs. Ophthalmology. 1985;92(7):964–72. http://www.ncbi.nlm.nih.gov/pubmed/3895104
7. Higginbotham EJ, Stevens RK, Musch DC, Karp KO, Lichter PR, Bergstrom TJ, et al. Bleb-related endophthalmitis after trabeculectomy with mitomycin C. Ophthalmology. 1996;103(4):650–6. http://www.ncbi.nlm.nih.gov/pubmed/8618766
8. Brown RH, Yang LH, Walker SD, Lynch MG, Martinez LA, Wilson LA. Treatment of bleb infection after glaucoma surgery. Arch Ophthalmol. 1994;112(1):57. http://www.ncbi.nlm.nih.gov/pubmed/8285894
9. Chen JY, Jones MN, Srinivasan S, Neal TJ, Armitage WJ, Kaye SB, et al. Endophthalmitis after penetrating keratoplasty. Ophthalmology. 2015;122(1):25–30. http://www.ncbi.nlm.nih.gov/pubmed/25264028
10. Kunimoto DY, Tasman W, Rapuano C, Recchia F, Busbee B, Pearlman R, et al. Endophthalmitis after penetrating keratoplasty: microbiologic spectrum and susceptibility of isolates. Am J Ophthalmol. 2004;137(2):343–5. http://www.ncbi.nlm.nih.gov/pubmed/14962427
11. Essex R, Yi Q, Charles P, Allen P. Post-traumatic endophthalmitis. Ophthalmology. 2004;111(11):2015–22. http://www.ncbi.nlm.nih.gov/pubmed/15522366
12. Miller JJ, Scott IU, Flynn HW, Smiddy WE, Murray TG, Berrocal A, et al. Endophthalmitis caused by bacillus species. Am J Ophthalmol. 2008;145(5):883–8. http://www.ncbi.nlm.nih.gov/pubmed/18295182
13. Callegan MC, Kane ST, Cochran DC, Novosad B, Gilmore MS, Gominet M, et al. *Bacillus* endophthalmitis: roles of bacterial toxins and motility during infection. Investig Opthalmol Vis Sci. 2005;46(9):3233. http://www.ncbi.nlm.nih.gov/pubmed/16123424
14. Fileta JB, Scott IU, Flynn HW. Meta-analysis of infectious endophthalmitis after intravitreal injection of anti-vascular endothelial growth factor agents. Ophthalmic Surg Lasers Imaging Retin. 2014;45(2):143–9. http://www.ncbi.nlm.nih.gov/pubmed/24635156
15. VanderBeek BL, Bonaffini SG, Ma L. The association between intravitreal steroids and post-injection endophthalmitis rates. Ophthalmology. 2015;122(11):2311–2315.e1. http://www.ncbi.nlm.nih.gov/pubmed/26281823
16. Mccannel CA. Meta-analysis of endophthalmitis after intravitreal injection of anti–vascular endothelial growth factor agents. Retina. 2011;31(4):654–61. http://www.ncbi.nlm.nih.gov/pubmed/21330939
17. Cummins CS, Johnson JL. Corynebacterium parvum: a synonym for Propionibacterium acnes? J Gen Microbiol. 1974;80(2):433–42. http://www.ncbi.nlm.nih.gov/pubmed/4826546
18. Durand ML. Endophthalmitis. Clin Microbiol Infect. 2013;19(3):227–34. http://www.ncbi.nlm.nih.gov/pubmed/23438028
19. Jackson TL, Paraskevopoulos T, Georgalas I. Systematic review of 342 cases of endogenous bacterial endophthalmitis. Surv Ophthalmol. 2014;59(6):627–35. http://www.ncbi.nlm.nih.gov/pubmed/25113611
20. Sik Chung K, Keun Kim Y, Goo Song Y, Oh Kim C, Hoon Han S, Sik Chin B, et al. Clinical review of endogenous endophthalmitis in Korea: a 14-year review of culture positive cases of two large hospitals. Orig Artic. 2011;52:630–4. http://www.eymj.org
21. Binder MI, Chua J, Kaiser PK, Procop GW, Isada CM. Endogenous endophthalmitis. Medicine (Baltimore). 2003;82(2):97–105. http://www.ncbi.nlm.nih.gov/pubmed/12640186

22. Hunter JW. Early postoperative sterile hypopyons. Br J Ophthalmol. 1978;62:470–3. http://bjo.bmj.com/
23. Holyk PR, Eifrig DE. Effects of monomeric methylmethacrylate on ocular tissues. Am J Ophthalmol. 1979;88(3 Pt 1):385–95. http://www.ncbi.nlm.nih.gov/pubmed/484667
24. Ramakrishnan R, Bharathi MJ, Shivkumar C, Mittal S, Meenakshi R, Khadeer MA, et al. Microbiological profile of culture-proven cases of exogenous and endogenous endophthalmitis: a 10-year retrospective study. Eye. 2009;23(4):945–56. http://www.nature.com/articles/eye2008197
25. Krause L, Bechrakis NE, Heimann H, Kildal D, Foerster MH. Incidence and outcome of endophthalmitis over a 13-year period. Can J Ophthalmol. 2009;44(1):88–94. http://www.ncbi.nlm.nih.gov/pubmed/19169320
26. Madhavan H, Jambulingam M, Parameswaran S, Lysa S, Selvaraj M. A study on the incidence, microbiological analysis and investigations on the source of infection of postoperative infectious endophthalmitis in a tertiary care ophthalmic hospital: an 8-year study. Indian J Ophthalmol. 2010;58(4):297. http://www.ncbi.nlm.nih.gov/pubmed/20534919
27. Das T, Kunimoto D, Sharma S, Jalali S, Majji A, Nagaraja Rao T, et al. Relationship between clinical presentation and visual outcome in postoperative and posttraumatic endophthalmitis in South Central India. Indian J Ophthalmol. 2005;53(1):5. http://www.ncbi.nlm.nih.gov/pubmed/15829741
28. Barza M. Factors affecting the intraocular penetration of antibiotics. The influence of route, inflammation, animal species and tissue pigmentation. Scand J Infect Dis Suppl. 1978;14:151–9. http://www.ncbi.nlm.nih.gov/pubmed/100873
29. Relhan N, Albini TA, Pathengay A, Kuriyan AE, Miller D, Flynn HW. Endophthalmitis caused by gram-positive organisms with reduced vancomycin susceptibility: literature review and options for treatment. Br J Ophthalmol. 2016;100(4):446–52. http://www.ncbi.nlm.nih.gov/pubmed/26701686
30. Pflugfelder SC, Hernández E, Fliesler SJ, Alvarez J, Pflugfelder ME, Forster RK. Intravitreal vancomycin. Arch Ophthalmol. 1987;105(6):831. http://www.ncbi.nlm.nih.gov/pubmed/3495255
31. D'Amico DJ, Caspers-Velu L, Libert J, Shanks E, Schrooyen M, Hanninen LA, et al. Comparative toxicity of intravitreal aminoglycoside antibiotics. Am J Ophthalmol. 1985;100(2):264–75. http://www.ncbi.nlm.nih.gov/pubmed/4025468
32. Campochiaro PA, Green WR. Toxicity of intravitreous ceftazidime in primate retina. Arch Ophthalmol. 1992;110(11):1625. http://www.ncbi.nlm.nih.gov/pubmed/1444923
33. Dave VP, Pathengay A, Nishant K, Pappuru RR, Sharma S, Sharma P, et al. Clinical presentations, risk factors and outcomes of ceftazidime-resistant gram-negative endophthalmitis. Clin Exp Ophthalmol. 2017;45(3):254–60. http://www.ncbi.nlm.nih.gov/pubmed/27616274
34. Nakashizuka H, Shimada H, Hattori T, Noguchi T, Kokubo N, Yuzawa M. Vitrectomy using 0.025% povidone–iodine in balanced salt solution plus for the treatment of postoperative endophthalmitis. Retina. 2015;35(6):1087–94. http://www.ncbi.nlm.nih.gov/pubmed/25946690
35. Shen Y-C, Wang M-Y, Wang C-Y, Tsai T-C, Tsai H-Y, Lee Y-F, et al. Clearance of intravitreal voriconazole. Investig Ophthalmol Vis Sci. 2007;48:2238–41. http://iovs.arvojournals.org/pdfaccess.ashx?url=/data/journals/iovs/933237/
36. Forster RK. The endophthalmitis vitrectomy study. Arch Ophthalmol. 1995;113(12):1555. http://archopht.jamanetwork.com/article.aspx?doi. https://doi.org/10.1001/archopht.1995.01100120085015.
37. Kuhn F, Gini G. Vitrectomy for endophthalmitis. Ophthalmology. 2006;113(4):714. http://www.ncbi.nlm.nih.gov/pubmed/16581433
38. Kuhn F, Gini G. Ten years after... are findings of the endophthalmitis vitrectomy study still relevant today? Graefes Arch Clin Exp Ophthalmol. 2005;243(12):1197–9. http://www.ncbi.nlm.nih.gov/pubmed/16136321
39. Aldave AJ, Stein JD, Deramo VA, Shah GK, Fischer DH, Maguire JI. Treatment strategies for postoperative Propionibacterium acnes endophthalmitis. Ophthalmology. 1999;106(12):2395–401. http://www.ncbi.nlm.nih.gov/pubmed/10599678
40. Romero P, Méndez I, Salvat M, Fernández J, Almena M. Intracameral cefazolin as prophylaxis against endophthalmitis in cataract surgery. J Cataract Refract Surg. 2006;32(3):438–41. http://www.ncbi.nlm.nih.gov/pubmed/16631053
41. Melega MV, Alves M, Cavalcanti Lira RP, Cardoso da Silva I, Ferreira BG, Assis Filho HL, et al. Safety and efficacy of intracameral moxifloxacin for prevention of post-cataract endophthalmitis: randomized controlled clinical trial. J Cataract Refract Surg. 2019;45(3):343–50. https://linkinghub.elsevier.com/retrieve/pii/S0886335018309672

Part IX

Uveitis

Vitrectomy in Uveitis

31

Amit Palkar, Niharika Singh, Ekta Rishi,
and Pukhraj Rishi

31.1 Introduction

Vitrectomy in uveitis is unlike routine vitreoretinal surgery. Almost a decade after the development of pars plana vitrectomy (PPV) technique, the first report of PPV for the treatment of uveitis was published in 1981 [1]. Ever since, numerous case reports and case series have identified a wide spectrum of indications for PPV in uveitic eyes. In systematic reviews, the visual outcome following PPV has consistently demonstrated an improvement in 70% of eyes, no change in 20% of eyes, and worsening in 10% of eyes over the past four decades [2, 3]. PPV is beneficial both in diagnosis and in treatment of uveitis. It requires important preoperative considerations and perioperative control of inflammation, though there are times the surgeon must operate in inflamed eyes. Vitrectomy in uveitic eyes may not necessarily be a generic procedure, and often requires a tailored and rationalized approach weighing the risks and benefits involved. This chapter discusses the use of vitrectomy in the management of uveitic eyes.

A. Palkar · N. Singh · E. Rishi · P. Rishi (✉)
Shri Bhagwan Mahavir Vitreoretinal Services,
Sankara Nethralaya, Chennai, Tamil Nadu, India

A. Jain et al. (eds.), *Cutting-edge Vitreoretinal Surgery*,
https://doi.org/10.1007/978-981-33-4168-5_31

31.2 Indications

Vitrectomy in uveitis can be of diagnostic or therapeutic purpose (Fig. 31.1).

31.2.1 Diagnostic Vitrectomy

Approach to a patient presenting with uveitis, involves a good clinical history, comprehensive ocular examination, identification of pattern of clinical signs, formulating differential diagnosis, and tailoring investigations to rule in or rule out conclusive etiology of uveitis. Often specific diagnosis for nearly half of all uveitis patients cannot be determined. Administration of immunosuppressive therapy or anti-infective therapy may not alleviate the inflammation, rather may do more harm. In such cases, a diagnostic pars plana vitrectomy may help to determine the definite cause and guide further treatment.

Generally accepted indications for diagnostic PPV include atypical uveitis that responds poorly to conventional therapy, suspected infectious endophthalmitis (viral, bacterial, fungal, or parasitic), or suspected intraocular malignancy [4] (Table 31.1).

Diagnostic vitrectomy also has a positive therapeutic effect by removal of vitreous opacities mixed with inflammatory mediators and toxic elements. Moreover, it helps alleviate vitreoretinal traction, facilitate diffusion of intra-

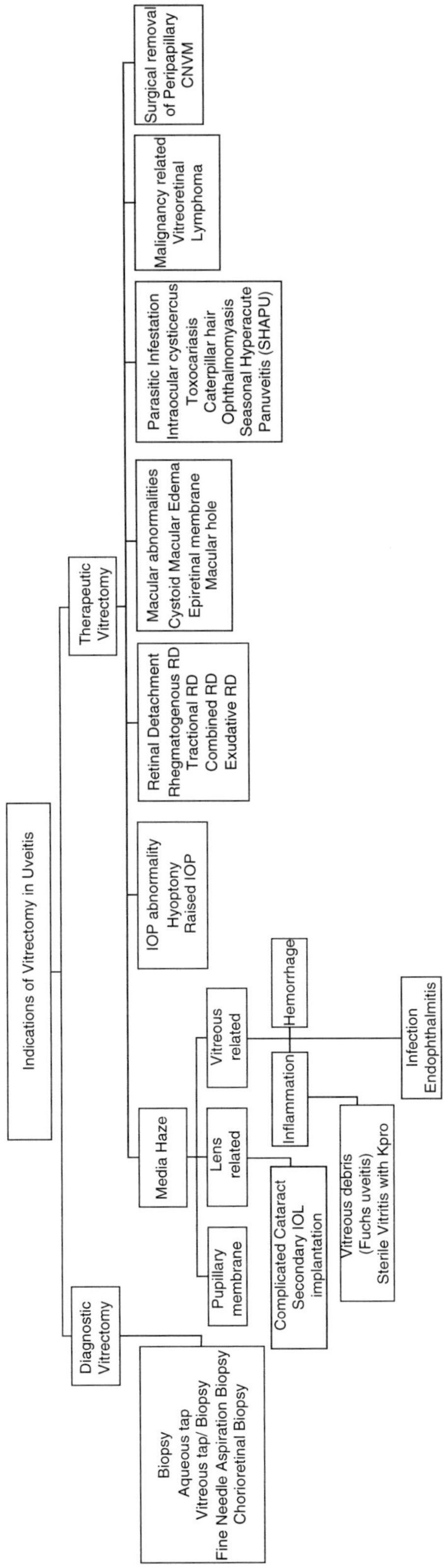

Fig. 31.1 Diagnostic and therapeutic indications of vitrectomy in uveitis

Table 31.1 Indications of diagnostic vitrectomy

Infectious	Noninfectious
1. Endophthalmitis (a) Postsurgical endophthalmitis (acute and chronic) (b) Traumatic endophthalmitis including intraocular foreign body (c) Endogenous endophthalmitis (d) Sterile endophthalmitis 2. Vitritis 3. Retinitis 4. Chorodits 5. Retinal vasculitis	Primary intraocular lymphoma Carcinoma metastasis including leukemia infiltration Choroidal melanoma

ocular drugs and allow better clarity for fundus examinations [5–9]. A meta-analysis estimated the success rate of diagnostic vitrectomy at 44% (95% CI [39–50%]) in determining the etiology of uveitis that was initially unknown [10]. This depends on several factors: patient selection, the severity of intraocular inflammation, timing of surgery, preoperative treatment, and its timing in relation to the surgery, the nature of the ocular disease, and analysis performed. Regardless, approximately 10% (95% CI [2–22%]) postoperative diagnostic vitrectomy patients may need secondary vitrectomy surgery for postoperative retinal detachment (RD), epiretinal membrane formation, or proliferative vitreoretinopathy.

31.2.1.1 Preoperative Evaluation

Diagnostic PPV is reserved for cases with severe sight-threatening disease because of the risk of complications and, where ocular and systemic evaluations are inconclusive of an etiology for the ocular inflammation. It should not be used to confirm an established systemic diagnosis of CSF positive or MRI proven CNS lymphoma with intraocular inflammation. An informed consent should be obtained, discussing the goal of the procedure and the potential vision-threatening complications of cataract formation, retinal detachment, proliferative vitreoretinopathy, or postoperative endophthalmitis. It is imperative to ensure transportation of the vitreous sample, requisition of appropriate laboratory test, credibility of the laboratory, communication with the pathologist, and/or microbiologist ahead of time and interpretation by experienced personnel, in order to yield valuable diagnostic value. Preoperative steps such as discontinuing steroids or avoiding the use of antibiotics until surgery can be useful in improving the "yield" of biopsies. The site of biopsy should be predecided in accordance to the area of most infiltration or exudation, based on clinical examination or imaging. Biopsies must be planned just as any other intraocular surgery.

31.2.1.2 Technique

A specimen of vitreous can be obtained by a vitreous tap or a diagnostic vitrectomy. Vitreous tap is an outpatient procedure while a diagnostic vitrectomy is performed in an operation theater. Diagnostic vitrectomy provides a larger sample of vitreous.

Vitreous Tap

Subconjunctival injection of 0.1 mL of 2% lignocaine is given at the site of entry into the vitreous cavity. Topical proparacaine 1% or lidocaine 4% with local massage with cotton tip applicator at the site of entry can provide adequate topical anesthesia. The periorbita is cleaned with povidone iodine and povidone iodine 5% drops are applied in the conjunctival cul de sac. After applying the lid speculum, the globe is stabilized with a cotton tip applicator or conjunctival forceps. A 2-cc disposable syringe with a 23–25G needle is used to obtain the specimen. Pars plana entry is made in the superior or inferior temporal quadrants at 3 mm from limbus in aphakes/pseudophakes and 3.5 mm in phakic eyes. The direction of the needle is toward the center of the globe. Under direct visualization, 0.1–0.2 cc of syneretic vitreous fluid is aspirated from the mid-vitreous cavity. In case of a dry tap, the direction of the needle is changed in the vitreous cavity under direct visualization until a pocket of liquid vitreous can be tapped. Automated self-sealing transconjunctival 23- or 25-gauge disposable vitreous cutters are available which have inbuilt infusion and aspiration. Sterile air or fluid may be injected through the infusion syringe to maintain intraocular volume. Straight needle aspiration of an undiluted vitreous specimen runs a risk of vitreoretinal traction and retinal detachment. This can be circumvented by guillotine mechanism of a vitreous cutter which obviates the risk.

Diagnostic Vitrectomy

Diagnostic Vitrectomy is performed under peribulbar or general anesthesia. A standard three-port transconjunctival 23- or 25-gauge vitrectomy with a three-way stopcock attached to the aspiration line is preferred. Alternately, a two-port vitrectomy can be performed with an illuminated infusion placed in one port and the vitreous cutter through the other. A syringe is connected to the stopcock to allow manual aspiration of uncontaminated vitreous in the aspiration line for analysis. At first, an undiluted vitreous sample is collected through the aspiration line with a 3- or 5-cc syringe directly connected to the vitreous cutter, with the infusion off. This syringe is manually aspirated by an assistant. Alternately, undiluted vitreous sample can still be collected with air infusion on, thereby simultaneously maintaining the intraocular pressure.

The infusion is kept off until the sample is withdrawn. The infusion cannula may help to maintain the intraocular pressure following biopsy, preventing sudden hypotony by intermittently turning on the infusion to prevent the eye from collapsing. If a sterile cassette and tubing were used for the surgery, the complete set, including the vitreous cutter, tubing, and the cassette can be sent for analysis. Usually, approximately 1 to 2 mL of core vitreous can be collected safely. Once an adequate vitreous sample is obtained, the infusion saline is turned on. The remaining vitreous can be removed as necessary, limiting oneself to a core vitrectomy or proceeding to complete vitrectomy. In areas with significant debris, more specimens can be collected in other syringes. The remaining vitreous wash fluid collected in the vitrector cassette can also be sent to the laboratory. A complete vitrectomy may provide a better diagnostic sample because vitreous cellularity is greater in the cortex rather than in the core, particularly in cases of vitreous inflammation and lymphoma [11]. In selected situations with retinal and/or choroidal involvement, a diagnostic vitrectomy can be combined with a biopsy of the involved tissue.

The clinical yield of vitreous specimens depends on the gauge and cutting speed of the vitrector. 20G, 23G, 25G, and 27G can all yield sufficient amounts of vitreous samples but may influence cellular integrity factored by the cutting speed of vitrector and the vacuum employed. Larger gauge can yield adequate sample with high-speed cutting as high as 1500 cuts per minute (cpm) but may mildly reduce fungal yield and markedly diminish the leukocyte viability [12]. Cell viability was found to begin to decrease at 600 cpm and viability was the lowest at a high cutting rate [13]. In order to diminish cellular damage, a cutting rate between 300 cpm and 500 cpm is desirable. Low vacuum settings contribute to higher cellular yields.

31.2.1.3 Processing Vitreous Samples

Processing of vitreous samples (Table 31.2) is guided by the clinical suspicion of either:

(a) Lymphoma or malignancy
(b) Infection

In case of limited cellularity in the sample, a paraffin cell block is prepared and stored.

31.2.2 Therapeutic Vitrectomy

In indicated cases, PPV has demonstrated significant visual gain compared to medical management and reduction in need of corticosteroids and immunosuppressive therapy, postoperatively. The common indications for therapeutic PPV in uveitic eyes are:

1. To clear the media haze
2. To treat macular abnormalities
3. To manage retinal detachment
4. To manage IOP abnormalities—raised IOP and hypotony
5. To manage parasitic infestations of the eye

PPV in uveitis is usually considered when inflammation becomes intractable and

Table 31.2 (A) Clinical suspicion of lymphoma or malignancy. (B) Clinical suspicion of Infection

Undiluted sample	Diluted sample
A.	
Smear using modified Wright Giemsa stain Polymerase chain reaction (PCR) analysis for gene rearrangements in the variable region of the heavy chain of immunoglobulin or the gamma chain of the T-cell receptor MYD88 L265P gene mutation testing Cytokine assay for interleukin (IL) 6 and IL-10, if indicated	Cytology analysis of Papanicolaou-stained slides In case of sufficient sample, centrifuged sediment embedded in a cell block for special stains (periodic acid Schiff), immunohistochemistry analysis, and flow cytometry
B.	
Smear—Gram stain, KOH mount Polymerase chain reaction (PCR) analysis of tuberculosis complex, herpes simplex virus, herpes zoster virus, cytomegalovirus, Toxoplasmosis species, or *Toxocara canis* antibody titers, based on clinical suspicion	Culture analysis—bacterial and fungal culture and antibiotic sensitivity

non-responsive to maximal medical therapy. However, any intraocular procedure induces intraocular inflammation. In the milieu of pre-existing inflammation, any surgery adds to the inflammation and to the risk of intraocular complications. In order to circumvent this problem, control of inflammation using a cover of systemic corticosteroids with or without immunosuppressive therapy (IMT), becomes mandatory in the perioperative period. Patients on IMT must have complete blood examination for cell counts, liver and renal functions. It is advisable to obtain a general physician evaluation and obtain a clearance for the administration of systemic corticosteroids and IMT. Prednisolone (1 mg/kg) in a weekly tapering regime is usually initiated preoperatively, or hiked up along with IMT, if already on therapy or without them. Continuation of systemic therapy postoperatively ensures adequate control of inflammation. A slow taper of systemic corticosteroids may be warranted in few cases, based on the postoperative inflammatory response.

Three months has been generally considered as the optimal duration of inflammation control prior to cataract surgery in patients with uveitis. However, there is less supporting evidence with regards to an optimal duration prior to PPV in uveitis patients. Delaying surgery to have adequate prior control of inflammation may not be a practical approach in certain situations like acute retinal necrosis with rhegmatogenous retinal detachment or infective endophthalmitis or for a diagnostic purpose that may guide sight-saving or lifesaving therapy in cases of vitreoretinal lymphoma. In such cases, prompt intervention is warranted. Perioperative intravenous or oral corticosteroids followed by a short postoperative oral steroid taper may prevent worsening inflammation. Utilization of microincision vitrectomy systems has demonstrated the advantage of reduced risk of inflammation, early recovery, and improved anatomical and visual outcomes.

31.2.2.1 Vitrectomy in Uveitis with Media Haze

Chronic intraocular inflammation usually leads to small non-dilating pupil with posterior synechiae, development of pupillary membranes, complicated cataract, dense posterior capsular opacities (PCO), thick membranes, and vitritis. In pseudophakic eyes, PCO may not be amenable to treatment with Nd:YAG laser alone. Small non-dilating pupil no more limits visualization during vitrectomy with wide-angle viewing systems. However, mechanical dilatation of pupil with hooks or rings may be helpful. Synechiae release under viscoelastic cover prior to the use of pupil dilators can enhance the surgical view. Small incisions are preferred to avoid intraoperative hypotony or intraocular pressure fluctuations. Often, viscoelastic elastic may visco-dissect the iris and anterior capsule of the lens and the injecting cannula may be used to lyse the adhesions. In severe plastered iris and a rigid pupil, pupilloplasty with multiple small nicks at the pupillary margin using intraocular scissors or vitrectomy probe may sometimes be necessary. Fine inflammatory membrane running over the iris surface and overlying the pupil in eyes with uveitis are common. Thick pupillary membranes need to be removed with a vitrectomy cutter or peeled with a microforceps initially to allow clear fundus visualization. In phakic eyes, surgical trauma to the anterior capsule must be carefully avoided. Many times, beneath the pupillary membrane, the crystalline lens is often devoid of significant opacities. This observation avoids needless removal of the crystalline lens while maintaining the compartmentalized nature of the globe.

Complicated cataract is a frequent sequela of uveitis and this is likely to hamper any vitreous surgery. Options exist for staged versus combined surgery. Phacoemulsification is the preferred approach to remove the lens opacity. A large anterior capsulotomy is preferred, along with good capsular polishing, as early and significant opacification of the lens capsule develops in uveitic eyes. "In the bag" placement of a foldable intraocular lens (IOL) is recommended [14]. IOL insertion is to be considered in all cases as it helps maintain compartmentalization and also reduces the risk of formation of iridocapsular adhesions. Silicone IOLs should be avoided and the benefits of heparin-coated IOLs are not well established.

Inflammatory membranes in the anterior vitreous and behind the posterior capsule of the lens are frequently encountered in patients with intermediate uveitis (IU) and sometimes in posterior uveitis. In pseudophakic eyes, these membranes are easily removed with the vitreous cutter. In phakic eyes, however, there is a potential risk of lens touch and needs more caution. Gentle suction in the aspiration mode to create a "safety zone" away from the crystalline lens, followed by removal with actuation of the cutter is sometimes helpful. Where such membranes are identified preoperatively, it is preferable to counsel the patient for the possible need for lens removal during surgery as there is a high-risk of lenticular injury. This avoids postoperative surprises to the patient both in terms of visual perception and in terms of costs.

The view of the fundus is obscured in uveitis either by the inflammatory debris in Fuchs' uveitis, membranes, and exudates of infective posterior uveitis or by endophthalmitis and vitreous hemorrhage, secondary to retinal neovascularization in IU or retinal vasculitis. Membranes are often mistaken during preoperative fundus examination and ultrasonography (USG) as posterior vitreous detachment (PVD). There is a higher prevalence of vitreoschisis in these situations. These vitreous changes must not be presumed as indicators of complete PVD. PVD induction is not mandatory in cases of endophthalmitis and is avoided to prevent iatrogenic breaks in the underlying inflamed and necrotic retina. Induction of PVD, however, is always desirable in cases of vitreous hemorrhage. Adequate and careful separation or dissection of the firm adhesions between the posterior hyaloid and the fibrovascular bridging tissue is needed. In the process, further hemorrhage may obscure view for subsequent steps in the surgery. Hemostasis in such an event is achieved by mechanical tamponade with the vitrectomy cutter or raising the bottle height/increasing infusion pressure. Vitreous hemorrhage in the postoperative period often resolves spontaneously in vitrectomized eyes. These eyes rarely need a vitreous lavage, where adequate addressal of new vessel disease is performed intraoperatively.

Dense vitritis obscures the view of the fundus and precludes monitoring retinal pathology and response to treatment. The three most important etiologies amongst south Asian patients related to vitritis in naïve eyes include Vitreoretinal Lymphoma (VRL), *Mycobacterium tuberculosis* and viral retinitis [15]. Sterile vitritis in eyes with permanent keratoprosthesis is an immune-mediated process either triggered by a reaction to the KPro device itself or to corneal antigens released during tissue necrosis that traverse holes in the KPro backplate into the posterior chamber, leading to inflammation. It is associated with sudden, painless decrease in vision accompanied with vitreous cells and membranes, with an attached retina (fundus exam or B-scan), and infectious endophthalmitis is often initially in the differential in these precious eyes. Sterile vitritis has been managed with peribulbar injection of triamcinolone or dexamethasone, followed by intensive topical steroid therapy. However, many patients are eventually treated preemptively with antibiotics and a vitreous tap for gram stain and culture. Some eyes may even undergo vitrectomy in conjunction with antibiotic treatment. After treatment of sterile vitritis, the course is usually benign. There is often near complete restoration of visual acuity with appropriate treatment [16].

31.2.2.2 Vitrectomy in Uveitis with Macular Abnormalities

Macular abnormalities in uveitis include cystoid macular edema (CME), epiretinal membrane (ERM), and macular hole (MH). Limited evidence is available supporting vitrectomy in managing structural changes of uveitic macular pathology, with inconsistent visual outcomes.

Inflammatory Cystoid Macular Edema

Cystoid Macular Edema (CME) is a major cause of visual loss in uveitis. Intermediate uveitis is the most frequent anatomic type of uveitis associated with the onset of macular edema [17]. CME develops following disruption to the BRB, release of inflammatory mediators, hyperpermeability of retinal vessels, Müller cell swelling due to increased potassium conductance, and mechanical tractional forces. OCT is now the preferred noninvasive imaging, making it patient friendly during frequent follow-up visits to monitor changes. Fluorescein Angiography (FA) sometimes helps differentiate inflammatory CME with the presence of disc leakage, from other causes of CME. Untreated inflammatory CME leads to chronic cysts, macular (pseudo) hole, macular ischemia, permanent photoreceptor damage, retinal atrophy, and fibrosis. Medical management with systemic or local (periocular or intraocular) corticosteroids or anti-VEGF therapy usually results in resolution of the CME.

Vitrectomy is reserved for recalcitrant CME. Theoretically, vitrectomy removes the inflammatory mediators contained within the vitreous sink while prospectively reducing the time inflammatory factors retained within the vitreous cavity. Concomitant release of mechanical traction due to epiretinal membranes with macular edema, is possible with vitrectomy. In 1992, Kaplan suggested that vitrectomy may provide an alternative to systemic immunosuppression in intermediate uveitis. Two randomized trials comparing PPV to medical therapy with systemic corticosteroids and/or immunomodulatory therapy demonstrated improvement in visual acuity at 6 months ($P = 0.01$) in chronic uveitic CME and 18 months ($P = 0.77$) in IU. However, this benefit is yet to be validated with large numbers in a multicentric trial [18, 19].

Epiretinal Membrane

Epiretinal Membrane (ERM) formation with or without CME is a well-known complication of chronic uveitis that is known to cause visual impairment. In the natural course of the disease, the ERM may just cause an increase in the mean retinal thickness with no significant visual change. But foveal ERM, focal ERM attachments with traction, and inner segment/outer segment disruption are associated with poorer vision. Progression of ERM with retinal distortion can be studied with OCT. ERM and ILM are attributed to macular pseudohole formation from concentric and tangential traction, which could eventually turn into a full-thickness macular hole (FTMH), when the ERM exert anterior–posterior vitreomacular traction (VMT).

Vitrectomy with ERM removal with or without internal limiting membrane (ILM) peeling improves the vitritis, restores the anatomy of the macula, and decreases retinal thickness, but may not significantly impact the visual acuity (VA). Unlike idiopathic ERMs, uveitic ERM may have pre-existing irreversible macular damage. Also, uveitic ERMs show the presence of inflammatory cells and the absence of RPE cells, unlike idiopathic ERMs and associated with elevated levels of IL-6 in vitreous [20]. Preservation of outer retinal layers may have a better visual prognosis with vitrecomy. There is no consensus regarding the timing of the surgery. The presence of inflammation is responsible for recurrence of ERM and controlled uveitis for at least 3 months have a low surgical recurrence rate [21].

Macular Hole

Uveitic macular holes are full-thickness Macular Hole (MH) that form in the setting of inflammatory eye conditions. MH is relatively a rare complication of posterior segment inflammation [22]. The estimated prevalence of MH to be 2.5% in a large review with uveitic macular hole [23, 24]. There is reported a predominance of MHs associated with Behcet's disease [25]. MH may have been under reported as media haze in uveitis limits biomicroscopic examination. With the advent of spectral-domain OCT, detection sensitivity has improved. Uveitic MH differs from idiopathic macular hole. Two mechanisms for the development of uveitic MH have been proposed: (1) An inflammatory focus on the macula may cause localized tissue necrosis and results in MH formation, or (2) Persistent hyaloidal traction, chronic CME, and epiretinal membrane traction may combine to exert sufficient force to cause hole formation.

Conventional surgery (Vitrectomy, ILM peel, and gas tamponade) is effective when combined with corticosteroids or immunosuppressive therapy despite elimination of tractional forces. They help in resolution of CME and subsequent closure of MH.

Outcomes of PPV for macular hole in uveitis may be often unpredictable. The anatomical closure of MH may not correlate with improved visual function. Also, there is no consensus or specified protocol for treating inflammation perioperatively and postoperative CME, it may confound visual improvement. In addition, spontaneous closure of UMH with visual recovery has been reported with medical management alone [25].

31.2.2.3 Vitrectomy in Uveitis with Retinal Detachment

The repair of retinal detachment in eyes with infective retinitis is a complex ordeal and must be performed using a combination of pars plana vitrectomy, internal tamponade (usually with silicone oil or a long-acting gas such as perfluoropropane), and photocoagulation with endolaser combined with or without scleral buckling. The most common causes of rhegmatogenous retinal detachment (RRD) in patients with infective retinitis are Acute Retinal Necrosis (ARN) and treated cytomegalovirus (CMV) retinitis. In the former, retinal detachment is part of the natural course of the disease; in the latter, it appears to be associated with healing usually after treatment with appropriate antiviral therapy. Another common cause associated with RRD is infective endophthalmitis.

31.2.2.4 Vitrectomy for Intraocular Pressure Management in Uveitis

Glaucoma in Uveitis

Elevated IOP is an important secondary complication that may result from ocular inflammatory sequelae or as a side effect of corticosteroids used to treat the inflammation. Uveitis can complicate with secondary angle closure, open-angle glaucoma, or combined mechanism glaucoma. IOP control is adequately achieved with medical management. Trabeculectomy is indicated when IOP is uncontrolled despite maximum-tolerated medical and laser therapy. However, it has been demonstrated that trabeculectomy with Mitomycin-C is less effective in reducing IOP in eyes with uveitic glaucoma than in eyes with primary open-angle glaucoma [26].

Glaucoma Drainage Device (GDD) Implantation is an option in eyes with active inflammation and conjunctival scarring and those with sustained-release steroid-induced increased IOP. Vitrectomy may be needed in case pars plana tube implantation of the GDD is planned. In refractory glaucoma of vitrectomized eyes, with poor visual potential, endocyclophotocoagulation may reduce the IOP.

Hypotony

Hypotony is typically described as IOP of <6 mmHg. Hypotony in acute uveitis is believed to be secondary to decreased ciliary body secretion (ciliary body shutdown) or increased uveoscleral outflow (prostaglandin-mediated or suprachoroidal effusions). Another mechanism for hypotony is related to traction on ciliary body caused by pars-plana membranes following chronic inflammation. These processes often are reversible with inflammation control. Hypotony in chronic uveitis is caused by inflammation and by structural complications like blunting or atrophy of ciliary processes resulting in decreased aqueous production, or cyclitic membranes, leading to ciliary body detachment or tractional cyclodialysis and thereby increasing outflow. Persistent hypotony, consequently causes hypotony maculopathy, optic nerve edema, and choroidal folds and often is associated with poor prognosis, ultimately leading to phthisis bulbi. Besides chronic uveitis, ocular trauma (such as cyclodialysis cleft), glaucoma surgery, retinal detachment, and proliferative vitreoretinopathy can give rise to chronic hypotony. It is prudent to identify the cause and mechanism of chronic hypotony. A high-frequency UBM imaging produces high-resolution imaging of the ciliary region with a depth of 3–6 mm and delineates the structural alteration at the ciliary body, the ciliary processes, presence of supraciliary effusions or pars plana membranes with traction and its extent [27, 28].

Planning a treatment involves adequate inflammation control and address the structural alteration. Treatment approaches include periocular or intraocular corticosteroid therapy, topical ibopamine (a nonselective dopaminergic agent), injection of viscoelastic material, or pars plana vitrectomy surgery with or without intraocular gas or silicone oil. Corticosteroid-induced intraocular pressure elevation, an adverse effect on the trabecular meshwork causes decreased aqueous outflow and ameliorates the ciliary body inflammation and aqueous secretion. However, aqueous secretion is mandatory when periocular or systemic corticosteroids are used.

Pars plana vitrectomy aims to stabilize and preserve the eyes, with perhaps some improvement in IOP and VA. Majority of eyes with chronic uveitis have cataract, posterior synechiae, and traction on ciliary region. Challenges begin from placement of infusion cannula in the presence of pars plana and ciliary membranes and visualization of the cannula to avoid inadvertent placement in the suprachoroidal space. It is essential to clear the axial opacities via the limbal route, first by placing the anterior chamber maintainer. Visualize the infusion cannula and then proceed. Local dissection of the fibrous tissue around the infusion cannula may be required with an MVR knife or vitrectomy cutter or a 6-mm infusion cannula can be used. After a complete vitrectomy, direct inspection of the ciliary region with depression using a cotton tip applicator. The ciliary membranes can be segmented using an intraocular scissors or cutter and removed. Care should be taken to avoid inadvertent damage to the ciliary body. Ciliary membranes should never be stripped or pulled as these have firm adhesions and may result in ciliary detachment. Endocautery use should be minimized during surgery as hemorrhage from ciliary processes is self-limiting, and excessive use of endocautery will destroy the remaining ciliary processes. Normal processes have well-defined crypts, a slightly corrugated appearance, and a deep brown color. A dysfunctional ciliary body may have complete absence of ciliary processes. Often a white fibrotic plaque with a variable degree of pigmentation is observed.

Once the vitrectomy is completed, the use of silicone oil depends on the status of the ciliary body examined intraoperatively. If ciliary processes are normal or have fewer clock hours with atrophy, removal of ciliary membrane alone may be enough to restore IOP. However, in case of complete ciliary atrophy with no ciliary processes, silicone oil injection may be considered. Silicone oil has been used in uveitic hypotony mainly for its tamponade effect on the ciliary body and macula and its space-occupying effect to prevent choroidal effusion [28]. There is no consensus as to whether the ciliary body will regain its function postoperatively and how many clock hours of healthy ciliary body or processes ensure adequate aqueous secretion to stabilize IOP.

Silicone oil undergoes early emulsification secondary to intraocular inflammation and therefore pre- and postoperative inflammation control is important and should be monitored. Eventually, if aqueous secretion is not restored, silicone oil gradually fills the anterior chamber

Table 31.3 Common parasitic infestations of eye requiring vitrectomy

Parasite group	Parasite	Clinical condition
Protozoans (unicellular)	*Toxoplasma gondii*	Toxoplasma retinochoroiditis
Metazoans helminths (multicellular)		
Nematodes (roundworms)	*Toxocara canis*/*Toxocara cati*	Toxocariasis
	Onchocerca volvulus	Onchocerciasis
	Dirofilaria repens *Gnathostoma spinigerum* Slender thread-like nematodes	Larva migrans ophthalmia syndrome Dirofilariasis Gnathostomiasis Diffuse unilateral subacute neuroretinitis (DUSN)
Cestodes (tapeworms)	*Taenia saginata* and *T. solium*	Cysticercosis

and decompensates the cornea with band-shaped keratopathy. If the IOP stabilizes, often patients maintain a good VA.

31.2.2.5 Vitrectomy in Parasitic Infestations

Intraocular parasitosis is highly prevalent in developing countries and provides several indications for surgical intervention [29].

A clinical suspicion is warranted in cases of panuveitis and posterior uveitis with iris holes or atrophy, intraocular caterpillar setae, hypopyon, hyphema, anterior chamber granuloma, live worm in AC or vitreous or subretinal space, intact mobile cyst in the vitreous or sequestered in the subretinal space and retinal signs of multifocal chorioretinitis with recurrent crops of retinitis, retinal vasculitis, retinal hemorrhages, and Diffuse Unilateral Subacute Neuroretinitis (DUSN). The common intraocular parasites which may require diagnostic or therapeutic vitrectomy are grouped into: (a) simple unicellular protozoans or (b) complex multicellular metazoans helminths (Table 31.3).

31.3 Conclusion

Vitreous surgery not only helps in establishing a diagnosis in eyes with uveitis, it also helps in their surgical management and visual improvement. However, the rare paradoxical relationship of surgery causing sympathetic ophthalmitis must also be borne in mind by the astute clinician [30]. Regardless, the benefits of surgery far outweigh the risks.

References

1. Algvere P, Alanko H, Dickhoff K, Lande Y, Saari KM. Pars plana vitrectomy in the management of intraocular inflammation. Acta Ophthalmol. 1981;59(5):727–36.
2. Becker M, Davis J. Vitrectomy in the treatment of uveitis. Am J Ophthalmol. 2005;140(6):1096–105.
3. Henry CR, Becker MD, Yang Y, Davis JL. Pars plana vitrectomy for the treatment of uveitis. Am J Ophthalmol. 2018;190:142–9.
4. Rishi P, Dhami A, Biswas J. Biopsy techniques for intraocular tumors. Indian J Ophthalmol. 2016;64(6):415–21.
5. Scott A, Mruthyunjaya P, McCallum R, Jaffe G. Diagnosticyield of vitreous biopsy in presumed sarcoidosis-related posterior segment inflammation. Graefes Arch Clin Exp Ophthalmol. 2012;250:1379–85.
6. Mruthyunjaya P, Jumper JM, McCallum R, et al. Diagnostic yield of vitrectomy in eyes with suspected posterior segment infection or malignancy. Ophthalmology. 2002;109:1123–9.
7. Bansal R, Gupta A, Gupta V, et al. Safety and outcome of microincision vitreous surgery in uveitis. Ocul Immunol Inflamm. 2016;25:775–84.
8. Svozilkova P, Heissigerova J, Brichova M, et al. The role of pars plana vitrectomy in the diagnosis and treatment of uveitis. Eur J Ophthalmol. 2011;21:89–97.

9. Ieki Y, Kiryu J, Kita M, et al. Pars plana vitrectomy for vitreous opacity associated with ocular sarcoidosis resistant to medical treatment. Ocul Immunol Inflamm. 2004;12:35–43.
10. Zhao XY, Xia S, Chen YX. Role of diagnostic pars plana vitrectomy in determining the etiology of uveitis initially unknown. Retina. 2020;40(2):359–69.
11. Mudhar HS, Sheard R. Diagnostic cellular yield is superior with full pars plana vitrectomy compared with core vitreous biopsy. Eye (Lond). 2013;27:50–5.
12. Ratanapojnard T, Roy CR, Gariano RF. Effect of vitrector cutting rate on vitreous biopsy yield. Retina. 2005;25:795–7.
13. Jiang T, Zhao Z, Chang Q. Evaluation of cytologic specimens obtained during experimental vitreous biopsy using B-cell lymphoma line. Eur J Ophthalmol. 2014;24:911–7.
14. Ganesh SK, Sudharshan S. Phacoemulsification with intraocular lens implantation in juvenile idiopathic arthritis. Ophthalmic Surg Lasers Imaging. 2010;44(1):104–8.
15. Rishi E, Rishi P, Therese KL, Ramasubban G, Biswas J, Sharma T, Bhende P, Susvar P, Agarwal M, George AE, Delhiwala K, Sharma VR. Culture and reverse transcriptase polymerase chain reaction (RT-PCR) proven Mycobacterium tuberculosis endophthalmitis: a case series. Ocul Immunol Inflamm. 2018;26(2):220–7.
16. Klufas MA, Yannuzzi NA, D'Amico DJ, Kiss S. Vitreoretinal aspects of permanent keratoprosthesis. Surv Ophthalmol. 2015;60(3):216–28.
17. Accorinti M, Okada AA, Smith JR, Gilardi M. Epidemiology of macular edema in uveitis. Ocul Immunol Inflamm. 2019;27(2):169–80.
18. Tranos P, Scott R, Zambarakji H, Ayliffe W, Pavesio C, Charteris DG. The effect of pars plana vitrectomy on cystoid macular oedema associated with chronic uveitis: a randomized, controlled pilot study. Br J Ophthalmol. 2006;90(9):1107–10.
19. Quinones K, Choi JY, Yilmaz T, Kafkala C, Letko E, Foster CS. Pars plana vitrectomy versus immunomodulatory therapy for intermediate uveitis: a prospective, randomized pilot study. Ocul Immunol Inflamm. 2010;18(5):411–7.
20. Sheybani A, Harocopos GJ, Rao PK. Immunohistochemical study of epiretinal membranes in patients with uveitis. J Ophthalmic Inflamm Infect. 2012;2(4):243–8.
21. Rao P, Todorich B, Yonekawa Y, Wang J, Sobrin L, Faia LJ. Surgical outcomes of epiretinal membranes in patients with a history of well-controlled preoperative uveitis. Ophthalmol Retina. 2018;2(3):192–6.
22. Nussenblatt RB. Macular alterations secondary to intraocular inflammatory disease. Ophthalmology. 1986;93(7):984–8. https://doi.org/10.1016/S0161-6420(86)33654-6.
23. Nicholson BP, Zhou M, Rostamizadeh M, et al. Epidemiology of epiretinal membrane in a large cohort of patients with uveitis. Ophthalmology. 2014;121(12):2393–8.
24. Branson SV, McClafferty BR, Kurup SK. Vitrectomy for epiretinal membranes and macular holes in uveitis patients. J Ocul Pharmacol Ther. 2017;33(4):298–303.
25. Bonnin N, Cornut PL, Chaise F, et al. Spontaneous closure of macular holes secondary to posterior uveitis: case series and a literature review. J Ophthalmic Inflamm Infect. 2013;3(1):34. https://doi.org/10.1186/1869-5760-3-349.
26. Iwao K, Inatani M, Seto T, et al. Long-term outcomes and prognostic factors for trabeculectomy with mitomycin C in eyes with uveitic glaucoma: a retrospective cohort study. J Glaucoma. 2014;23:88–94.
27. Kapur R, Birnbaum AD, Goldstein DA, et al. Treating uveitis-associated hypotony with pars plana vitrectomy and silicone oil injection. Retina. 2010;30(1):140–5.
28. Gupta P, Gupta A, Gupta V, Singh R. Successful outcome of pars plana vitreous surgery in chronic hypotony due to uveitis. Retina. 2009;29(5):638–43.
29. Rishi P, Agarwal M, Mahajan S, Rishi E. Management of intralenticular caterpillar setae. Indian J Ophthalmol. 2008;56(5):437–8.
30. Rishi E, Rishi P, Appukuttan B, Walinjkar J, Biswas J, Sharma T. Sympathetic ophthalmitis following vitreoretinal surgery: does antecedent trauma make a difference? Indian J Ophthalmol. 2015;63(9):692–8.

Viral Retinitis-Related Retinal Detachment

32

Aniruddha Agarwal and Vishali Gupta

32.1 Introduction

Among infectious causes of retinal involvement, viral retinitis is one of the most feared ophthalmic conditions, which is characterized by significant visual morbidity and a high risk of blindness [1–3]. Viral retinitis is an ophthalmic emergency, since early and appropriate therapy can avoid blinding complications and initiation of systemic therapy may also improve the mortality rates among these patients [4]. While viruses can lead to variable ophthalmic manifestations, *necrotizing retinitis* is the most common presentation of posterior uveitis, and is often caused by viruses from the herpes family (DNA viruses) [5–8].

Studies on viral retinitis have identified retinal detachment as one of the most common causes of permanent visual loss in these eyes [4, 9]. The risk is higher with systemic viremia in patients with human immunodeficiency virus (HIV) infection [1, 10]. Various other complications reported with viral retinitis include cataract, band-shaped keratopathy, uveitic glaucoma, and cystoid macula edema (CME), among others. Retinal detachment, by far, remains the most challenging complication of viral retinitis due to poor surgical results, guarded visual outcomes, and high risk of phthisis [11, 12].

Despite several advances in surgical techniques of rhegmatogenous retinal detachment repair, viral retinitis-associated retinal detachment continues to remain a management challenge due to high rates of failures, mainly attributed to the location and multiplicity of breaks, changes in the vitreous, significant retinal necrosis and difficulty in removing the hyaloid, presence of active retinitis and inflammation, challenges in identifying all the breaks, and achieving retinochoroidal adhesion at the regions of the breaks [11, 13–15]. In this chapter, various etiologies of viral retinitis-associated retinal detachment have been highlighted. In addition, the risk factors and incidence of retinal detachment have been described. Current management strategies for tackling retinal detachments in viral retinitis using modern techniques of pars plana vitrectomy and internal tamponade have been elaborated.

32.2 Viral Retinitis: Etiologies, Epidemiology, and Clinical Features

Viral retinitis is a serious vision-threatening entity, which is characterized by rapid progression and development of retinal necrosis. Viral retinitis occurs commonly among individuals who are immunocompromised, particularly in

A. Agarwal · V. Gupta (✉)
Advanced Eye Center, Department of Ophthalmology, Post Graduate Institute of Medical Education and Research (PGIMER), Chandigarh, India

A. Jain et al. (eds.), *Cutting-edge Vitreoretinal Surgery*, https://doi.org/10.1007/978-981-33-4168-5_32

patients with HIV infection and Acquired Immune Deficiency Syndrome (AIDS). Opportunistic infections occur among patients with patients, with CMV retinitis and herpetic progressive outer retinal necrosis (PORN) being the two most common types of viral uveitis in these patients [16]. Patients with solid organ transplantation and children with leukemias are also predisposed to develop viral retinitis [17]. Patients with diminished lymphocytic proliferative response, diminished cutaneous anergy, and relative or absolute increase in B-lymphocytes are also at risk of developing viral retinitis [18, 19]. However, necrotizing viral retinitis can occur in immunocompetent individuals as well, and the most common entity in this subset of patients is acute retinal necrosis (ARN). There are also a number of reports in the literature of viral retinitis developing after administration of intravitreal injections (most commonly corticosteroids), including CMV, HSV, and VZV retinitis. Sub-tenon injections have also been reported to cause CMV retinitis [20–23].

Necrotizing viral retinitis that predisposes to retinal detachment is most commonly caused by viruses that belong to the human herpes virus (HHV) family such as CMV, HSV, and VZV. HHV family of viruses are an important infectious cause of serious ocular inflammation. These viruses are known to persist in the latent form, and the reactivation can lead to keratitis, anterior uveitis, or retinitis (necrotizing and non-necrotizing). The most common viral entities that are associated with retinal detachment are ARN (that is caused by VZV, HSV-1, HSV-2, and rarely EBV and EMV), and CMV retinitis [24–27].

32.2.1 Acute Retinal Necrosis

ARN is a severe, vision-threatening ocular emergency, which is characterized by rapid evolution, progressive necrosis and destruction of the neurosensory retina, and occlusive retinal arteritis. This entity was initially described in 1971 by Urayama et al. in healthy young Japanese adults as an acute unilateral panuveitis with retinal periarteritis and diffuse necrotizing retinitis with retinal detachment [28]. ARN commonly occurs in young adults as well as elderly individuals and equally affects males and females. As mentioned previously, ARN is usually found in immunocompetent individuals. The risk factors for ARN include a young age, previous herpetic infections including varicella, shingles and HSV encephalitis, pre-existing chorioretinal scars, and, systemic and/or intravitreal corticosteroids [5, 6, 29–32].

The clinical features of ARN include redness, blurring of vision, photophobia, floaters, and ocular pain. Bilateral ARN is uncommon but can occur in up to one-third of patients with ARN. Patients usually present with anterior chamber inflammation and vitritis, typical lesions of peripheral necrotizing retinitis with focal areas of full-thickness necrotic lesions, circumferential extensions, and occlusive vasculitis with arteriolar narrowing and hemorrhages. Active lesions are yellow and necrotic, associated with retinal hemorrhages, occlusive vasculopathy (arterial), and rapidly progress circumferentially toward the posterior pole. In the healed stage, there is secondary retinal atrophy, proliferative vitreoretinopathy, and rhegmatogenous retinal detachment [5, 29, 31, 32]. The risk of retinal detachment increases with the size of the necrotizing lesion, which is typically quantified in terms of disc diameters [33]. More than 30% of patients with ARN can develop retinal detachment. Imaging evaluation of ARN lesions using optical coherence tomography (OCT) shows disorganization of the retinal structure that corresponds to the areas of retinal necrosis. In addition, there is marked inner and outer retina thinning within areas of retinal necrosis, consistent with retinal tissue loss. These lead to development of retinal breaks, and therefore, OCT is very useful in detecting retinal detachment early during the disease [34].

One of the goals of early treatment of ARN is to prevent progression of the lesions and avoid complications such as retinal detachment. As soon as ARN is diagnosed, therapy is begun immediately so that the lesions do not increase in size. Retinal detachment in ARN often leads to poor visual outcomes [6, 35].

32.2.2 Cytomegalovirus Retinitis

CMV retinitis is a form of necrotizing viral retinitis which typically occurs as an opportunistic infection in patients with HIV/AIDS, or in patients who are recipients of solid organ transplantation, long-term immunosuppressive therapy, or systemic corticosteroids [10, 17, 36–38]. More than 75% AIDS patients with CD4+ counts less than 50 cells/μL develop CMV retinitis [1]. Among patients with AIDS, CMV retinitis is the most frequent manifestation of CMV disease. Other states associated with CMV retinitis include patients on renal dialysis, advanced age, and uncontrolled diabetes mellitus.

Among individuals with HIV, CMV retinitis presents with absence of acute inflammatory signs such as redness, pain, and photophobia. Clinical features include mild anterior segment inflammation with few keratic precipitates and anterior chamber cells, and minimal vitritis. The retinal lesion typically presents as a single focus of full-thickness yellow-white necrotizing granular retinitis in the peripheral retina with a perivascular distribution that expands centrifugally. It is usually accompanied by retinal hemorrhage and vasculitis, usually in the form of retinal arteritis (*pizza pie retinopathy*). It can also present with a *brushfire* pattern of retinitis with more cheesy, granular appearance of the lesion, and minimal retinal hemorrhages. CMV retinitis can also present with an exuberant retinal vasculitis (*frosted branch angiitis*). Active lesions of CMV retinitis result in widespread necrosis and retinal tears, and development of retinal detachment [2, 10, 25, 36, 39, 40].

Studies of Ocular Complications of AIDS (SOCA) have demonstrated that mortality is significantly increased in HIV/AIDS patients with CMV retinitis, and have determined risks of ocular complications such as retinal detachment. Approximately 25–30% patients of CMV retinitis may develop retinal detachment, an incidence lesser than ARN. CD4+ T-cell counts less than 50 cells/μL is an important predictor of retinal detachment among patients with CMV retinitis [1, 2, 4, 10].

32.2.3 Other Viral Retinitis Predisposing to Retinal Detachment

Apart from HSV, VZV, and CMV retinitis, other miscellaneous viral infections may also result in rhegmatogenous retinal detachment in the post-inflammatory phase. West Nile Virus (WNV) fever is caused by a single-stranded RNA *Flavivirus* from the Flaviviridae family that is transmitted by infected mosquitoes. This condition is common in North America, Europe, Africa, as well as Asia. Majority of WNV infections are asymptomatic. Mild disease resulting in flu-like symptoms, headache, and myalgia may occur. WNV infection may result in posterior uveitis (chorioretinitis) that occurs in older patients, those with coexisting diabetes mellitus, with higher likelihood of presenting with encephalitis. The disease manifests as bilateral multifocal chorioretinitis. The lesions of WNV are very characteristic; classic curvilinear clustering of whitish scars with a "target-like" appearance that is located along the retinal nerve fibers. Rarely, WNV infection may be associated with retinal detachment requiring surgery [41, 42].

Retinitis associated with mumps and other agents such as rift valley fever virus may also be very rarely associated with retinal detachment [43, 44].

32.3 Incidence and Risk Factors of Retinal Detachment in Viral Retinitis

32.3.1 Risk of Retinal Detachment with Acute Retinal Necrosis

Patients with ARN caused due to viruses from the herpes family have a very high incidence of retinal detachment. Sternberg et al. in 1988 reported that more than 50% of patients with ARN develop retinal detachment [9]. In 2007, Lau et al. evaluated a cohort of patients without human immunodeficiency virus with ARN. The authors detected VZV as the leading cause of ARN, and showed that 80% (8/10) of eyes that could not be lasered prophylactically developed retinal detachment [5]. Similarly, Hillenkamp et al. evaluated a cohort of 27 patients without human immunodeficiency virus with ARN in a non-randomized, retrospective, interventional series (including three bilateral cases). Among patients treated with conventional therapy (intravenous acyclovir in combination with oral prednisolone), retinal detachment occurred in 18 of 20 eyes [29]. Muthiah et al. assessed patients with ARN that presented to ophthalmologists via the British Ophthalmological Surveillance Unit (BOSU) reporting system. The authors observed complications in 38.7% (12/31) of cases, with retinal detachment in 9/12 cases (75.0% of recorded complications) [6].

32.3.1.1 Retinal Detachment Risk with the Extent of Retinal Involvement

Recently, Butler et al. studied 41 eyes of 36 patients with clinically diagnosed ARN who were tested positive for HSV or VZV using polymerase chain reaction. In this series 59% of eyes developed retinal detachment. Interestingly, the authors observed that eyes with extensive involvement of the retina, i.e., retinitis involving ≥25% of the retina at presentation detached at nearly 12 times the rate compared to those with <25% retinal involvement [7]. Kim et al. also studied the incidence of retinal detachment based on the area of retinal involvement (zone as well as the extent) in 43 eyes of 35 patients. The authors observed that eyes with zone 1 (posterior) or extensive involvement had a higher rate of retinal detachment compared to other patients (30%; however, the patients received prophylactic laser therapy) [33].

32.3.1.2 Retinal Detachment Risk with Therapeutic Interventions

Tibbetts et al. studied the effect of therapy on the rates of retinal detachment; i.e., intravenous, oral, or intravitreal antiviral medications (including acyclovir, valacyclovir, famciclovir, valganciclovir, ganciclovir, and foscarnet), prophylactic laser retinopexy, aspirin, and oral steroids. However, the authors observed a prevalence of 50% retinal detachment and no variables including prophylactic laser therapy were associated with a decreased risk [35].

32.3.2 Risk of Retinal Detachment with Cytomegalovirus Retinitis

Early investigations by Jabs et al. revealed that 26% of patients (in a series of 145 patients with CMV retinitis) developed retinal detachment. The cumulative probability of a retinal detachment 1 year after the diagnosis of CMV retinitis was 50% [45]. Sandy et al. studied the incidence of outcome of retinal detachment in patients with CMV retinitis at two London (UK) AIDS centers. Of 147 patients with CMV retinitis, 47 eyes (28%) developed retinal detachments [46]. The Studies of Ocular Complications of AIDS (SOCA) Research Group have contributed significantly to our understanding of the incidence of retinal detachment among patients with CMV retinitis. The SOCA group observed that among 316 eyes with CMV retinitis at baseline, the risk of rhegmatogenous retinal detachment in the involved eye was 18.9% at 6 months and 37.9% at 1 year [4]. In 2010, the SOCA group studied the 5-year outcomes of patients with CMV retinitis and AIDS in the era of highly active anti-retroviral therapy (HAART). The authors observed that the rate of retinal detachment was 2.3/100 eye-years (EY) and varied from 1.2/100 EY for those with previously diagnosed retinitis and immune recovery to 4.9/100 EY for those with newly diagnosed retinitis [10]. Huang et al. described that among patients with AIDS and CMV retinitis, retinal detachments occurred in 12% of patients, and Goldberg et al. reported a similar incidence of 14% [36, 47].

Among individuals with CMV retinitis without HIV infection, Kuo et al. reported an incidence of retinal detachment of 3.7% per eye-year [38].

32.3.2.1 Retinal Detachment Risk with Therapeutic Interventions

Kempen et al. performed an investigation to determine if intravitreal therapy with antiviral therapy can reduce the risk of retinal detachment among individuals with CMV retinitis. The authors studied patients treated with the ganciclovir implant compared with those treated using systemic therapy alone (n = 511 patients with AIDS and CMV retinitis). No significant difference in the rate of retinal detachment was found between eyes treated with systemic therapy alone and those treated with ganciclovir implants. However, the use of HAART resulted in 60% reduction in the rate of retinal detachment [39]. Similarly, Young et al. performed a retrospective study to compare the rate of retinal detachment in a group of patients treated with intravitreal ganciclovir to the rate of retinal detachment in a group of patients treated with systemic ganciclovir (n = 186). The authors observed that intravitreal therapy performed better, and the risk of retinal detachment with systemic therapy was 14-fold higher than with intravitreal therapy [48].

32.4 Pathology of Retinal Detachment in Necrotizing Retinitis

Retinal detachment in patients with necrotizing retinitis most commonly occurs when the active inflammation has subsided, i.e., in the stage of convalescence and healing [11, 49]. The pathology of retinal detachment involves similar mechanisms in both CMV retinitis as well as ARN. During this stage, the areas of retinitis develop thinning and atrophy, with loss and disorganization of neurosensory retinal layers. In the regions of retinal atrophy, multiple retinal breaks develop, which are characteristically seen in patients with ARN and the retina appears *sieve-like* due to the multiple breaks [11, 12, 45, 49]. Due to retinal atrophy, it may be difficult to identify all the breaks. Often, the breaks may be posterior in location, and if there is accompanying inflammation, it may make the surrounding retina very friable and vulnerable to damage during surgery.

The pathology of retinal detachment due to atrophic breaks can be understood from optical coherence tomography of the lesions which can predict the development of retinal detachment [34].

32.5 Management of Retinal Detachment

32.5.1 Medical (Antiviral) Therapy for Viral Retinitis

The treatment of viral retinitis includes systemic antivirals administered either orally or intravenously, intravitreal antiviral agents, intraocular antiviral implants, and topical and systemic corticosteroids to control the inflammation. Prompt antiviral therapy helps in arresting the progression of retinal necrosis and decreasing the rates of complications such as retinal detachment, optic atrophy, fellow eye involvement, as well as decrease overall morbidity. Once the clinical diagnosis is established, therapy must be initiated promptly.

32.5.1.1 Therapy for Acute Retinal Necrosis

ARN is typically treated with intravenous (IV) acyclovir 10 mg/kg every 8 h or 1500 mg/m^2 per day for 5–10 days, followed by maintenance with oral acyclovir 800 mg 5 times daily for an additional 6 weeks [50, 51]. Due to the availability of newer antiviral agents, there is a recent trend toward shifting the patient to catheter-free therapy using oral antiviral agents such as valacyclovir or less commonly, famciclovir [52–55]. Treatment with either oral valacyclovir 1 g 3 times a day or oral famciclovir 500 mg 3 times daily can result in complete resolution of retinitis without the need for IV acyclovir therapy [52–54]. Intravitreal therapy can be tried for patients with macula-threatening ARN, or in refractory cases. Intravitreal foscarnet (2.4 mg/0.1 mL) has been used successfully to treat ARN [56]. Similarly, intravitreal ganciclovir (4 mg/0.1 mL) has also been effective in treating ARN [17, 57, 58].

32.5.1.2 Therapy for Cytomegalovirus Retinitis

Since CMV retinitis is most commonly seen in individuals with AIDS and very low CD4 counts, the primary aim of therapy in these patients is to reverse the immunodeficiency and augment the disease response by providing a cover of antiviral therapy. HAART has revolutionized the therapeutic management of patients with HIV and opportunistic infections such as CMV retinitis. Once HAART is initiated, specific anti-CMV therapy may be discontinued once the CD4 count is ≥100 cells/μL [59–63]. The antiviral agents used to target CMV include ganciclovir, valganciclovir, cidofovir, and foscarnet. Intravitreal injections of ganciclovir (4 mg/0.1 mL) can be also used as an adjunctive therapy, or a primary therapy in patients with CMV retinitis without HIV. Ganciclovir implants for treatment of CMV retinitis are no longer available [64–66].

32.5.2 Pars Plana Vitrectomy

Pars plana vitrectomy (PPV) has become the most commonly performed procedure for managing rhegmatogenous retinal detachments. With the availability of smaller gauge instruments and minimally invasive vitrectomy systems, the ease of performing vitrectomy has improved. Dugel et al. provided early evidence of the success rates of pars plana vitrectomy for viral retinitis-related retinal detachment in their series of 22 eyes of 19 patients. All these patients were diagnosed with AIDS and CMV retinitis, and were followed-up until the time of death. The authors performed PPV, fluid–air exchange, and internal tamponade, and observed an anatomical success of 89% with no intraoperative complications. However, optic nerve atrophy developed in 95% of patients postoperatively [67]. Weinberg et al. performed PPV, silicone oil tamponade, and endolaser for retinal detachment related to ARN caused by VZV in 5 eyes of 4 patients, and observed that these patients have severe retinal shortening and contracture, requiring relaxing retinotomies intraoperatively (often large ones). In their series, no re-detachment was observed and 4 eyes maintained ambulatory vision [68]. Overall, the anatomical success rate from retinal detachment surgery in ARN has been reported at 22–94% in the literature.

The basic steps of PPV remain the same in patients with viral retinitis. It is important to treat any active infection with IV or oral therapy, and control the inflammation prior to surgery. Standard 3-port approach is used for PPV (Fig. 32.1). With the introduction of modern 25-gauge vitrectomy systems, surgical techniques have become much safer. Pars plana lensectomy may be performed if there is significant cataract. Once the hyaloid is removed, adequate vitrectomy must be performed with vitreous base dissection to ensure the release of all tractional forces. In patients with viral retinitis-related retinal detachments, there may be a need for membrane peeling when severe inflammatory vitreal and retinal membranes are present. Procedures such as retinotomies and retinectomies are required in a significant proportion of patients [68, 69]. These procedures help to counter the traction caused by retinal shortening and prevent re-detachment. Usually, once fluid–air exchange is performed, it is best to do a meticulous endolaser photocoagulation around all the breaks, and often posterior to the edge of the lesions (Figs. 32.2 and 32.3) [12, 69–71]. It is important to check for any missed breaks, especially at the edges of the lesions.

For the purpose of internal tamponade, various reports describe the use of either long-acting gas (C_3F_8) or silicone oil (1000 cSt). In their series, Almeida et al. used silicone oil in 11 eyes out of 12, and used gas tamponade in 1 eye. None of the eyes developed re-detachment [69]. Canzano published a series of 6 eyes (five patients) where PPV was performed for CMV-related retinal detachment where the authors used gas tamponade alone. They observed that re-detachment was observed in one eye at 7 months after initial repair and was successfully reattached without using silicone oil [70]. While gas tamponade may be used in selective cases of

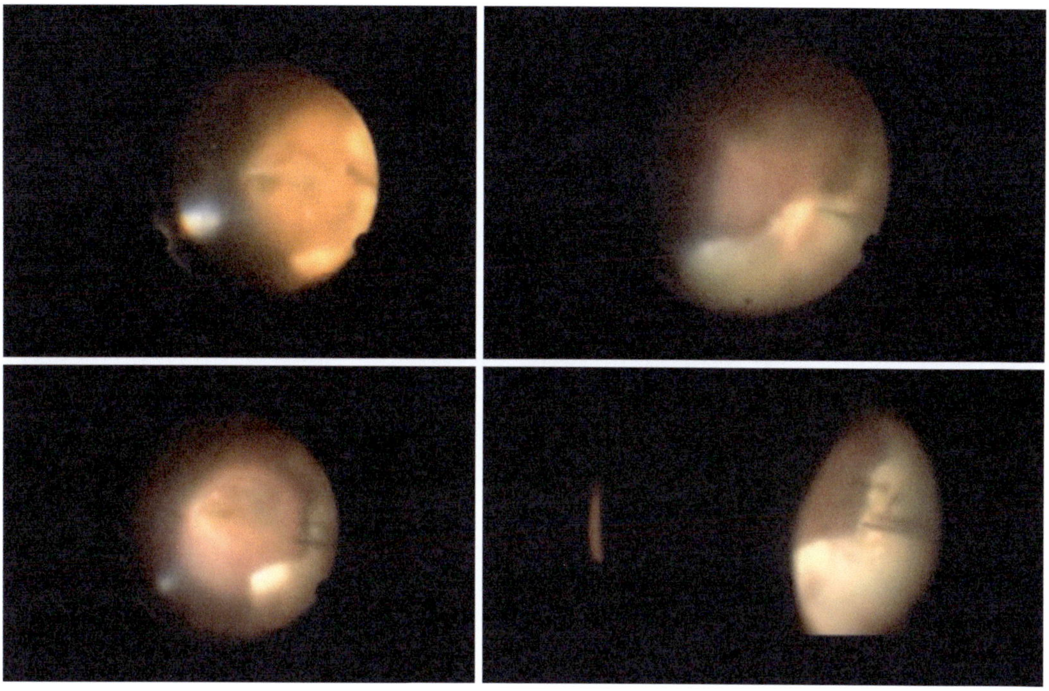

Fig. 32.1 The steps of pars plana vitrectomy (PPV) are shown in this figure. Standard 3-port vitrectomy is performed and the core vitreous is cleared and posterior hyaloid is removed (if not already detached). The vitreous over the retinitis lesions is carefully removed. It is important to protect the underlying necrotic retina

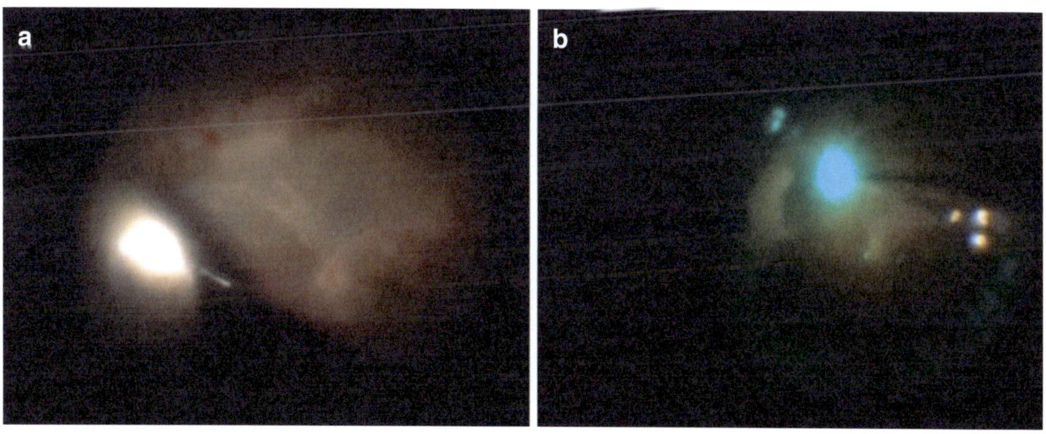

Fig. 32.2 Adequate peripheral dissection is performed by scleral depression (**a**). Laser photocoagulation is applied in a confluent manner, especially posterior to the retinitis lesions, making sure all the breaks are covered (**b**)

retinal detachment due to necrotizing viral retinitis, most surgeons would prefer the use of silicone oil for achieving tamponade [12, 71–73]. The choice of the tamponade depends on the degree and severity of the contracture and proliferative retinopathy, and surgeon's experience and choice. When silicone oil is being used in the management of retinal detachment, one can use 5000 cSt oil for longer tamponade in eyes with severe proliferation and contraction, high risk of hypotony, and need for a long-acting tamponade [13].

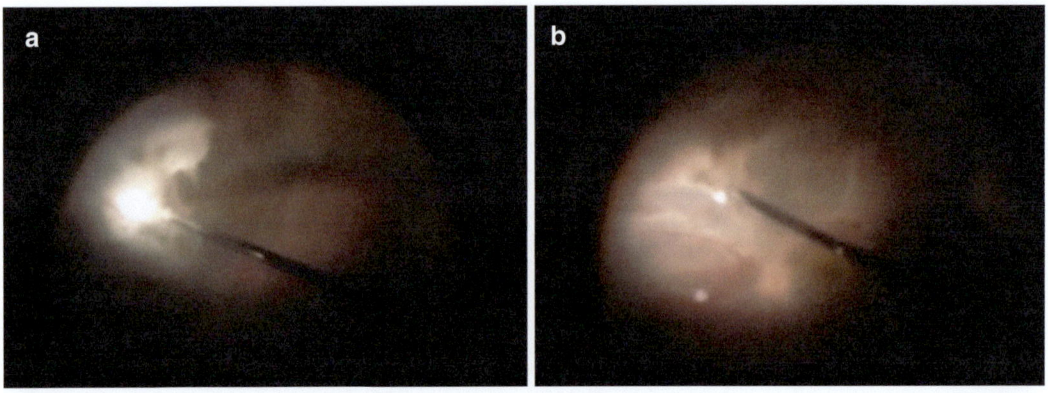

Fig. 32.3 The characteristic pattern of retinal breaks in viral retinitis-related retinal detachment consists of multiple atrophic holes in the healed area of retinitis (sieve-like retina) (**a**). These breaks must be marked using endocautery so that they are not missed after fluid–air exchange (**b**)

32.5.3 Scleral Buckling Procedures

Before the advent of PPV, scleral buckling procedures were performed for the management of retinal detachment associated with viral retinitis [74]. However, scleral buckle alone is insufficient in achieving anatomical attachment in these patients due to various factors including existence of multiple breaks (which may be posterior, or difficult to identify due to vitreous inflammation), abnormal vitreous forces, retinal contracture, epiretinal membranes, and other issues. Therefore, various surgeons compared the techniques of primary scleral buckling versus PPV with cryotherapy/laser therapy and internal tamponade. The final reattachment rate was 87.5% in the primary scleral buckle group and 100% in the non-buckle group in a series by Blumenkranz et al. The authors reported higher retinal reoperation and complication rates in the primary buckle group [75]. Subsequently, there has been an increasing trend toward combining scleral buckling along with PPV in order to achieve higher retinal reattachment rates. In the literature, several authors have described a combination of buckling-vitrectomy to achieve higher anatomical success in their cases. Scleral buckling is performed to augment the support to the anterior proliferation [15, 70, 76–79]. At times, surgeons may apply a 240-belt to support the anterior vitreous.

Various authors prefer to perform PPV without the use of a scleral buckling procedure in patients with retinal detachment resulting from viral retinitis. The advantages of avoiding scleral buckling include reduction of the intraoperative time, patient morbidity, and the risk of an accidental needle stick. In addition, many authors believe that an additional encirclage by scleral buckle may not necessarily improve the final retinal reattachment rate [80–82].

32.5.4 Prophylactic Laser Therapy

Because of the high frequency of retinal detachment associated with necrotizing retinitis, especially ARN, there has been an interest in determining whether laser procedures can be used prophylactically in these patients to prevent visual loss and ensuing complications resulting from retinal detachment in these cases. Prophylactic laser photocoagulation is applied in a confluent manner around the edge of attached uninfected retina posterior to the peripheral retinitis. This confluent laser results in inflammatory chorioretinal adhesion preventing detachment of the retina; however, it must be noted that laser therapy cannot prevent progression of the retinitis lesions. Various authors have reported a substantial decrease in the incidence of retinal detachment in their patients after prophylactic laser therapy [9, 32, 76, 83, 84].

The major challenges in laser therapy include difficulty in the application of laser if the media is hazy due to cataracts or vitritis. Laser therapy may fail, leading to retinal detachment, or worse, it may result in development of atrophic retinal holes. It may contribute to worsening of inflammatory response. Thus far, there are no randomized controlled trials studying the efficacy of prophylactic laser photocoagulation to prevent retinal detachment, and the published series include a limited number of patients with a retrospective study design. It may be possible that eyes with mild disease, limited areas of retinitis, clear media, and absence of vitreous opacities may do better with prophylactic laser therapy [85]. In the series published by Tibbetts et al. and Freeman et al., no differences in the rates of retinal detachment were observed, irrespective of prophylactic laser photocoagulation [12, 35]. Thus, stronger evidence is needed to understand the exact role of prophylactic laser therapy in viral retinitis.

32.6 Prognosis

Despite improved surgical techniques and success rates of anatomical reattachment of the retinal following detachment in viral retinitis, the overall visual prognosis remains guarded. In the postoperative period, several patients may develop optic atrophy or macular retinal atrophy leading to suboptimal visual gain. Failure of retinal attachment may occur, resulting in severe proliferative vitreoretinopathy and development of inoperable retinal detachments. Even in eyes with successful retinal attachment, macular pucker, epiretinal membranes, cataracts, band-shaped keratopathy, among others [5, 12, 29, 32, 46, 70, 80, 81, 86]. Macular holes and hypotony may also result, requiring additional surgical procedures [76]. Most series that include a long-term follow-up of patients developing retinal detachment, either due to ARN or due to CMV retinitis suggest an unfavorable prognosis unless the disease involvement is mild, extramacular, and amenable to early therapy [47, 82].

32.7 Conclusions

Viral retinitis can frequently lead to development of retinal detachment in both immunocompetent and immunocompromised individuals, leading to significant visual morbidity and high risk of blindness. ARN and CMV retinitis, therefore, remain a major challenge to the uveitis specialists as well as vitreoretina surgeons due to exuberant ocular inflammation, propensity to cause rapid retinal necrosis, high rates of surgical failure, and postoperative complications leading to suboptimal visual gain. Refinements in surgical techniques, and availability of better antiviral therapies have not only improved the anatomical and functional outcome in these eyes, but also improved the overall survival and mortality in these patients.

References

1. Holbrook JT, Jabs DA, Weinberg DV, et al. Visual loss in patients with cytomegalovirus retinitis and acquired immunodeficiency syndrome before widespread availability of highly active antiretroviral therapy. Arch Ophthalmol. 2003;121(1):99–107.
2. Thorne JE, Jabs DA, Kempen JH, et al. Causes of visual acuity loss among patients with AIDS and cytomegalovirus retinitis in the era of highly active antiretroviral therapy. Ophthalmology. 2006;113(8):1441–5. https://doi.org/10.1016/j.ophtha.2006.03.022.
3. Agarwal A, Singh R, Sharma A, Gupta V, Dogra MR. Ocular manifestations in patients with human immunodeficiency virus infection in the pre-HAART versus the HAART era in the North Indian population. Ocul Immunol Inflamm. 2017;25(3):396–404. https://doi.org/10.3109/09273948.2015.1133837.
4. Rhegmatogenous retinal detachment in patients with cytomegalovirus retinitis: the Foscarnet-Ganciclovir cytomegalovirus retinitis trial. The Studies of Ocular Complications of AIDS (SOCA) Research Group in collaboration with the AIDS clinical trials group (ACTG). Am J Ophthalmol. 1997;124(1):61–70.
5. Lau CH, Missotten T, Salzmann J, Lightman SL. Acute retinal necrosis features, management, and outcomes. Ophthalmology. 2007;114(4):756–62. https://doi.org/10.1016/j.ophtha.2006.08.037.
6. Muthiah MN, Michaelides M, Child CS, Mitchell SM. Acute retinal necrosis: a national population-based study to assess the incidence, methods of diagnosis, treatment strategies and outcomes in the UK. Br J Ophthalmol. 2007;91(11):1452–5. https://doi.org/10.1136/bjo.2007.114884.

7. Butler NJ, Moradi A, Salek SS, et al. Acute retinal necrosis: presenting characteristics and clinical outcomes in a cohort of polymerase chain reaction-positive patients. Am J Ophthalmol. 2017;179:179–89. https://doi.org/10.1016/j.ajo.2017.05.006.
8. Crapotta JA, Freeman WR, Feldman RM, et al. Visual outcome in acute retinal necrosis. Retina. 1993;13(3):208–13.
9. Sternberg P, Han DP, Yeo JH, et al. Photocoagulation to prevent retinal detachment in acute retinal necrosis. Ophthalmology. 1988;95(10):1389–93.
10. Jabs DA, Ahuja A, Van Natta M, et al. Course of cytomegalovirus retinitis in the era of highly active antiretroviral therapy: five-year outcomes. Ophthalmology. 2010;117(11):2152–61. https://doi.org/10.1016/j.ophtha.2010.03.031.
11. Irvine AR. Treatment of retinal detachment due to cytomegalovirus retinitis in patients with AIDS. Trans Am Ophthalmol Soc. 1991;89:349–63.
12. Freeman WR, Quiceno JI, Crapotta JA, Listhaus A, Munguia D, Aguilar MF. Surgical repair of rhegmatogenous retinal detachment in immunosuppressed patients with cytomegalovirus retinitis. Ophthalmology. 1992;99(3):466–74.
13. Davis JL, Serfass MS, Lai MY, Trask DK, Azen SP. Silicone oil in repair of retinal detachments caused by necrotizing retinitis in HIV infection. Arch Ophthalmol. 1995;113(11):1401–9.
14. Kawaguchi T, Spencer DB, Mochizuki M. Therapy for acute retinal necrosis. Semin Ophthalmol. 2008;23(4):285–90. https://doi.org/10.1080/08820530802111192.
15. Shah GK, Vander J. Rhegmatogenous retinal detachments with cytomegalovirus retinitis. Curr Opin Ophthalmol. 1998;9(3):6–10.
16. Kuppermann BD, Petty JG, Richman DD, et al. Correlation between CD4+ counts and prevalence of cytomegalovirus retinitis and human immunodeficiency virus-related noninfectious retinal vasculopathy in patients with acquired immunodeficiency syndrome. Am J Ophthalmol. 1993;115(5):575–82.
17. Agarwal A, Kumari N, Trehan A, et al. Outcome of cytomegalovirus retinitis in immunocompromised patients without Human Immunodeficiency Virus treated with intravitreal ganciclovir injection. Graefes Arch Clin Exp Ophthalmol. 2014;252(9):1393–401. https://doi.org/10.1007/s00417-014-2587-5.
18. Rochat C, Polla BS, Herbort CP. Immunological profiles in patients with acute retinal necrosis. Graefes Arch Clin Exp Ophthalmol. 1996;234(9):547–52.
19. Guex-Crosier Y, Rochat C, Herbort CP. Necrotizing herpetic retinopathies. A spectrum of herpes virus-induced diseases determined by the immune state of the host. Ocul Immunol Inflamm. 1997;5(4):259–65.
20. Dalessandro L, Bottaro E. Reactivation of CMV retinitis after treatment with subtenon corticosteroids for immune recovery uveitis in a patient with AIDS. Scand J Infect Dis. 2002;34(10):780–2.
21. Saidel MA, Berreen J, Margolis TP. Cytomegalovirus retinitis after intravitreous triamcinolone in an immunocompetent patient. Am J Ophthalmol. 2005;140(6):1141–3. https://doi.org/10.1016/j.ajo.2005.06.058.
22. Toh T, Borthwick JH. Acute retinal necrosis post intravitreal injection of triamcinolone acetonide. Clin Exp Ophthalmol. 2006;34(4):380–2. https://doi.org/10.1111/j.1442-9071.2006.01229.x.
23. Takakura A, Tessler HH, Goldstein DA, et al. Viral retinitis following intraocular or periocular corticosteroid administration: a case series and comprehensive review of the literature. Ocul Immunol Inflamm. 2014;22(3):175–82. https://doi.org/10.3109/09273948.2013.866256.
24. Kianersi F, Mohammadi Z, Ghanbari H, Ghoreyshi SM, Karimzadeh H, Soheilian M. Clinical patterns of uveitis in an Iranian tertiary eye-care center. Ocul Immunol Inflamm. 2015;23(4):278–82. https://doi.org/10.3109/09273948.2014.902474.
25. Pathanapitoon K, Kunavisarut P, Ausayakhun S, Sirirungsi W, Rothova A. Uveitis in a tertiary ophthalmology centre in Thailand. Br J Ophthalmol. 2008;92(4):474–8. https://doi.org/10.1136/bjo.2007.132175.
26. Llorenç V, Mesquida M, Sainz de la Maza M, et al. Epidemiology of uveitis in a Western urban multiethnic population. The challenge of globalization. Acta Ophthalmol. 2015;93(6):561–7. https://doi.org/10.1111/aos.12675.
27. Venkatesh P, Gogia V, Shah B, Gupta S, Sagar P, Garg S. Patterns of uveitis at the Apex Institute for Eye Care in India: results from a prospectively enrolled patient data base (2011–2013). Int Ophthalmol. 2016;36(3):365–72. https://doi.org/10.1007/s10792-015-0128-9.
28. Lee JH, Agarwal A, Mahendradas P, et al. Viral posterior uveitis. Surv Ophthalmol. 2017;62(4):404–45. https://doi.org/10.1016/j.survophthal.2016.12.008.
29. Hillenkamp J, Nölle B, Bruns C, Rautenberg P, Fickenscher H, Roider J. Acute retinal necrosis: clinical features, early vitrectomy, and outcomes. Ophthalmology. 2009;116(10):1971–5. https://doi.org/10.1016/j.ophtha.2009.03.029.
30. Cochrane TF, Silvestri G, McDowell C, Foot B, McAvoy CE. Acute retinal necrosis in the United Kingdom: results of a prospective surveillance study. Eye (Lond). 2012;26(3):370–7.; quiz 378. https://doi.org/10.1038/eye.2011.338.
31. Meghpara B, Sulkowski G, Kesen MR, Tessler HH, Goldstein DA. Long-term follow-up of acute retinal necrosis. Retina. 2010;30(5):795–800. https://doi.org/10.1097/IAE.0b013e3181c7013c.
32. Roy R, Pal BP, Mathur G, Rao C, Das D, Biswas J. Acute retinal necrosis: clinical features, management and outcomes--a 10 year consecutive case series. Ocul Immunol Inflamm. 2014;22(3):170–4. https://doi.org/10.3109/09273948.2013.819928.
33. Kim DY, Jo J, Joe SG, Lee JY, Yoon YH, Kim J-G. Clinical feature and visual prognosis of acute retinal necrosis according to the initially involved zone and extent: 10-year experience. Eur

J Ophthalmol. 2019;29(2):244–50. https://doi.org/10.1177/1120672118787438.
34. Invernizzi A, Agarwal AK, Ravera V, et al. Comparing optical coherence tomography findings in different aetiologies of infectious necrotising retinitis. Br J Ophthalmol. 2018;102(4):433–7. https://doi.org/10.1136/bjophthalmol-2017-310210.
35. Tibbetts MD, Shah CP, Young LH, Duker JS, Maguire JI, Morley MG. Treatment of acute retinal necrosis. Ophthalmology. 2010;117(4):818–24. https://doi.org/10.1016/j.ophtha.2009.09.001.
36. Huang G, Jiang Q, Li M, Lu Y, Wang Z. Retrospective study of cytomegalovirus retinitis complicated with acquired immunodeficiency syndrome. Int J Clin Exp Med. 2015;8(6):9537–42.
37. Kulshrestha MK, Goble RR, Murray PI. Cytomegalovirus retinitis associated with long term oral corticosteroid use. Br J Ophthalmol. 1996;80(9):849–50.
38. Kuo IC, Kempen JH, Dunn JP, Vogelsang G, Jabs DA. Clinical characteristics and outcomes of cytomegalovirus retinitis in persons without human immunodeficiency virus infection. Am J Ophthalmol. 2004;138(3):338–46. https://doi.org/10.1016/j.ajo.2004.04.015.
39. Kempen JH, Jabs DA, Dunn JP, West SK, Tonascia J. Retinal detachment risk in cytomegalovirus retinitis related to the acquired immunodeficiency syndrome. Arch Ophthalmol. 2001;119(1):33–40.
40. Vrabec TR. Posterior segment manifestations of HIV/AIDS. Surv Ophthalmol. 2004;49(2):131–57. https://doi.org/10.1016/j.survophthal.2003.12.008.
41. Khairallah M, Kahloun R. Ocular manifestations of emerging infectious diseases. Curr Opin Ophthalmol. 2013;24(6):574–80. https://doi.org/10.1097/ICU.0b013e3283654e09.
42. Yahia SB, Khairallah M. Ocular manifestations of West Nile virus infection. Int J Med SciInt. 2009;6(3):114–5.
43. Klomp HJ, Deutman AF, van Tongeren HA. Retinal abnormalities caused by Rift Valley fever virus. Ned Tijdschr Geneeskd. 1980,124(50):2122–5.
44. Laviano F, Zollo M. Diastasis in the course of epidemic parotitis. G Med Mil. 1956;106(4):490–3.
45. Jabs DA, Enger C, Haller J, de Bustros S. Retinal detachments in patients with cytomegalovirus retinitis. Arch Ophthalmol. 1991;109(6):794–9.
46. Sandy CJ, Bloom PA, Graham EM, et al. Retinal detachment in AIDS-related cytomegalovirus retinitis. Eye (Lond). 1995;9(Pt 3):277–81. https://doi.org/10.1038/eye.1995.54.
47. Goldberg DE, Wang H, Azen SP, Freeman WR. Long term visual outcome of patients with cytomegalovirus retinitis treated with highly active antiretroviral therapy. Br J Ophthalmol. 2003;87(7):853–5.
48. Young S, McCluskey P, Minassian DC, et al. Retinal detachment in cytomegalovirus retinitis: intravenous versus intravitreal therapy. Clin Exp Ophthalmol. 2003;31(2):96–102.
49. Freeman WR, Henderly DE, Wan WL, et al. Prevalence, pathophysiology, and treatment of rhegmatogenous retinal detachment in treated cytomegalovirus retinitis. Am J Ophthalmol. 1987;103(4):527–36.
50. Blumenkranz MS, Culbertson WW, Clarkson JG, Dix R. Treatment of the acute retinal necrosis syndrome with intravenous acyclovir. Ophthalmology. 1986;93(3):296–300.
51. Duker JS, Blumenkranz MS. Diagnosis and management of the acute retinal necrosis (ARN) syndrome. Surv Ophthalmol. 1991;35(5):327–43.
52. Aizman A, Johnson MW, Elner SG. Treatment of acute retinal necrosis syndrome with oral antiviral medications. Ophthalmology. 2007;114(2):307–12. https://doi.org/10.1016/j.ophtha.2006.06.058.
53. Aslanides IM, De Souza S, Wong DTW, et al. Oral valacyclovir in the treatment of acute retinal necrosis syndrome. Retina. 2002;22(3):352–4.
54. Figueroa MS, Garabito I, Gutierrez C, Fortun J. Famciclovir for the treatment of acute retinal necrosis (ARN) syndrome. Am J Ophthalmol. 1997;123(2):255–7.
55. Huynh TH, Johnson MW, Comer GM, Fish DN. Vitreous penetration of orally administered valacyclovir. Am J Ophthalmol. 2008;145(4):682–6. https://doi.org/10.1016/j.ajo.2007.11.016.
56. Wong R, Pavesio CE, Laidlaw DAH, Williamson TH, Graham EM, Stanford MR. Acute retinal necrosis: the effects of intravitreal foscarnet and virus type on outcome. Ophthalmology. 2010;117(3):556–60. https://doi.org/10.1016/j.ophtha.2009.08.003.
57. Kishore K, Jain S, Zarbin MA. Intravitreal ganciclovir and dexamethasone as adjunctive therapy in the management of acute retinal necrosis caused by Varicella zoster virus. Ophthalmic Surg Lasers Imaging. 2011;42:e87–90. https://doi.org/10.3928/15428877-20110901-06.
58. Luu KK, Scott IU, Chaudhry NA, Verm A, Davis JL. Intravitreal antiviral injections as adjunctive therapy in the management of immunocompetent patients with necrotizing herpetic retinopathy. Am J Ophthalmol. 2000;129(6):811–3.
59. Timperley A, Taha H, Das S. Management of cytomegalovirus retinitis in HIV infection in the era of highly active antiretroviral therapy. Int J STD AIDS. 2015;26(10):757–8. https://doi.org/10.1177/0956462415571374.
60. Stewart MW. Optimal management of cytomegalovirus retinitis in patients with AIDS. Clin Ophthalmol. 2010;4:285–99.
61. Whitcup SM. Cytomegalovirus retinitis in the era of highly active antiretroviral therapy. JAMA. 2000;283(5):653–7.
62. Bodaghi B, Michelson S. Cytomegalovirus: virological facts for clinicians. Ocul Immunol Inflamm. 1999;7(3–4):133–7.
63. Jabs DA, Ahuja A, Van Natta M, Dunn JP, Yeh S. Studies of the ocular complications of AIDS Research Group. Comparison of treatment regimens

for cytomegalovirus retinitis in patients with AIDS in the era of highly active antiretroviral therapy. Ophthalmology. 2013;120(6):1262–70. https://doi.org/10.1016/j.ophtha.2012.11.023.
64. Ghosh F, Hansson L-J, Bynke G, Békássy AN. Intravitreal sustained-release ganciclovir implants for severe bilateral cytomegalovirus retinitis after stem cell transplantation. Acta Ophthalmol Scand. 2002;80(1):101–4.
65. Campbell RJ, Chow B, Victor G, Kravcik S, Hodge WG. Treatment of CMV retinitis with intravitral ganciclovir in the HAART era. Can J Infect Dis. 2001;12(5):300–4.
66. Studies of Ocular Complications of AIDS Research Group. The AIDS Clinical Trials Group. The ganciclovir implant plus oral ganciclovir versus parenteral cidofovir for the treatment of cytomegalovirus retinitis in patients with acquired immunodeficiency syndrome: The Ganciclovir Cidofovir Cytomegalovirus Retinitis Trial. Am J Ophthalmol. 2001;131(4):457–67.
67. Dugel PU, Liggett PE, Lee MB, et al. Repair of retinal detachment caused by cytomegalovirus retinitis in patients with the acquired immunodeficiency syndrome. Am J Ophthalmol. 1991;112(3):235–42.
68. Weinberg DV, Lyon AT. Repair of retinal detachments due to herpes varicella-zoster virus retinitis in patients with acquired immune deficiency syndrome. Ophthalmology. 1997;104(2):279–82.
69. Almeida DR, Chin EK, Tarantola RM, et al. Long-term outcomes in patients undergoing vitrectomy for retinal detachment due to viral retinitis. Clin Ophthalmol. 2015;9:1307–14. https://doi.org/10.2147/OPTH.S87644.
70. Canzano JC, Morse LS, Wendel RT. Surgical repair of cytomegalovirus-related retinal detachment without silicone oil in patients with AIDS. Retina. 1999;19(4):274–80.
71. Ratanasukon M, Kittantong A, Visaetsilpanonta S, Somboonthanakij S. Pars plana vitrectomy with silicone oil or gas endotamponade in HIV-related rhegmatogenous retinal detachments in Thai patients. J Med Assoc Thail. 2007;90(6):1161–6.
72. Stier PA, Glazer LC, Garretson BR, Deutsch TA. Surgical repair of retinal detachment secondary to cytomegalovirus retinitis. Ophthalmic Surg Lasers. 1999;30(4):289–94.
73. Schoenberger SD, Kim SJ, Thorne JE, et al. Diagnosis and treatment of acute retinal necrosis: a report by the American Academy of Ophthalmology. Ophthalmology. 2017;124(3):382–92. https://doi.org/10.1016/j.ophtha.2016.11.007.
74. Clarkson JG, Blumenkranz MS, Culbertson WW, Flynn HW, Lewis ML. Retinal detachment following the acute retinal necrosis syndrome. Ophthalmology. 1984;91(12):1665–8.
75. Blumenkranz M, Clarkson J, Culbertson WW, Flynn HW, Lewis ML, Young GM. Visual results and complications after retinal reattachment in the acute retinal necrosis syndrome. The influence of operative technique. Retina. 1989;9(3):170–4.
76. McDonald HR, Lewis H, Kreiger AE, Sidikaro Y, Heckenlively J. Surgical management of retinal detachment associated with the acute retinal necrosis syndrome. Br J Ophthalmol. 1991;75(8):455–8.
77. Lim JI, Enger C, Haller JA, et al. Improved visual results after surgical repair of cytomegalovirus-related retinal detachments. Ophthalmology. 1994;101(2):264–9.
78. Davis JL. Management of CMV retinal detachments in the new era of antiretroviral therapy. Ocul Immunol Inflamm. 1999;7(3–4):205–13.
79. Baumal CR, Reichel E. Management of cytomegalovirus-related rhegmatogenous retinal detachments. Ophthalmic Surg Lasers. 1998;29(11):916–25.
80. García RF, Flores-Aguilar M, Quiceno JI, et al. Results of rhegmatogenous retinal detachment repair in cytomegalovirus retinitis with and without scleral buckling. Ophthalmology. 1995;102(2):236–45.
81. Nasemann JE, Mutsch A, Wiltfang R, Klauss V. Early pars plana vitrectomy without buckling procedure in cytomegalovirus retinitis-induced retinal detachment. Retina. 1995;15(2):111–6.
82. Ahmadieh H, Soheilian M, Azarmina M, Dehghan MH, Mashayekhi A. Surgical management of retinal detachment secondary to acute retinal necrosis: clinical features, surgical techniques, and long-term results. Jpn J Ophthalmol. 2003;47(5):484–91.
83. Althaus C, Loeffler KU, Schimkat M, Hudde T, Sundmacher R. Prophylactic argon laser coagulation for rhegmatogenous retinal detachment in AIDS patients with cytomegalovirus retinitis. Graefes Arch Clin Exp Ophthalmol. 1998;236(5):359–64.
84. Hudde T, Althaus C, Sundmacher R. Acute retinal necrosis syndrome. Argon laser coagulation for prevention of rhegmatogenic retinal detachment. Ophthalmologe. 1998;95(7):473–7.
85. Park JJ, Pavesio C. Prophylactic laser photocoagulation for acute retinal necrosis. Does it raise more questions than answers? Br J Ophthalmol. 2008;92(9):1161–2. https://doi.org/10.1136/bjo.2008.147181.
86. Mathur G, Ratra D, Bhuibhar SS, Roy R. Clinical outcomes of retinal detachment surgery following Cytomegalovirus Retinitis in patients on highly active anti-retroviral therapy for acquired immune deficiency syndrome. Ocul Immunol Inflamm. 2015;23(5):400–4. https://doi.org/10.3109/09273948.2014.999376.

Vitreoretinal Surgery for Parasitic Diseases

33

Harsha Bhattacharjee, Ajit Babu Majji,
Dipankar Das, and Jitendra Kumar

33.1 Introduction

Human ocular parasitic disease is of medical importance worldwide, because it may cause significant ocular morbidity and even blindness if diagnosis and treatments are not done in time. Poor environmental and sanitary conditions favor the parasitism between human and animals. The condition is more prevalent in tropical countries but international tourism has increased the risk of worldwide dissemination. No effective antiparasitic drug is available for cure of intravitreal parasitic infestation. Success of treatment depends upon early detection and complete removal of parasite from vitreous cavity.

Parasitic diseases as an indication for vitreoretinal surgery is rare and usually constitute less than 1% of vitreoretinal surgeries. The parasitic infections of the eye occur as zoonotic diseases with human as an intermediate host or accidental host [1–3]. Most parasites get access to gastrointestinal tract by accidental ingestion through vegetables or uncooked meat. Parasites get access to bloodstream from gastrointestinal tract and reach liver and other organs which in most cases serve as end organs. Most parasites access the eye through bloodstream either through choroidal blood flow into subretinal space and then into the vitreous cavity or through ophthalmic artery to retinal arteries and vitreous cavity or episcleral vessels into anterior chamber. Presence of the parasite can cause visual symptoms by secondary effects and may require vitreoretinal interventions [3]. The vitreoretinal surgery may be needed to deal with the parasitic infections or inflammation secondary to presence of parasite or long-term effects of the secondary complications like development of vitreous membranes, traction retinal detachment, or secondary rhegmatogenous retinal detachment. In this chapter, the author will provide the clinical aspects of intraocular parasite infections relevant to vitreoretinal surgery. Life cycle and pathology of individual parasitic infestations will not be described in detail; however, pathogenesis will be discussed as and when relevant.

33.2 Pathogenesis

Most frequent human vitreoretinal parasite disease encountered in Asia are Cysticercosis and Gnathostomiasis as regards to vitreoretinal surgery [4–13].

Toxoplasma infections both congenital and acquired forms are more common but from vitreoretinal surgical point of view is less relevant [1, 3]. Toxocara infections and hydatid cyst are less common in Asia [14–19]. Thelazia,

H. Bhattacharjee · D. Das · J. Kumar
Sri Sankaradeva Nethralaya, Guwahati, India

A. B. Majji (✉)
Centre for Sight, Hyderabad, India

A. Jain et al. (eds.), *Cutting-edge Vitreoretinal Surgery*,
https://doi.org/10.1007/978-981-33-4168-5_33

Baylisascaris, and malaria are very rare in occurrence [17, 18, 20, 21].

Cysticercosis is the most common platyhelminth infestation by cysticercus cellulosae larval form of pork tapeworm *Taenia solium*, contracted by ingestion of uncooked pork, vegetables, or water contaminated with eggs of *T. solium* [2]. Sites of predilection for the cysticerci to develop are central nervous system, subcutaneous tissue, skeletal muscles, heart muscle, and eye [2]. Ocular manifestations can be devastating as the cysticercosis increases in size, leading to blindness in 3–5 years, if no intervention is contemplated. Location of intraocular cysticercosis may be in vitreous cavity (up to 60%) and subretinal space (in 40%). Complications could be retinal detachment, proliferative vitreoretinopathy, vitreous inflammation (Fig. 33.1a–c), macular scar (Fig. 33.2a, b), and endophthalmitis-like picture [11, 13].

Gnathostoma is a nematode causing ocular infection in addition to skin (migratory cutaneous nodules), brain (meningitis, meningoencephalitis, and myeloencephalitis), gastrointestinal tract (abdominal mass), and respiratory system (bronchitis and pleurisy) [6, 22]. Ocular gnathostomiasis is rare but involves the eyelids, conjunctiva, cornea, anterior chamber, and vitreous cavity [6]. Most cases present as presence of parasite in the anterior chamber and few in vitreous cavity [22]. This parasitic infestation is mostly observed in Southeast Asian countries. Common definitive hosts are domestic cats, dogs, and wild mammals. Human is an incidental host [7]. The infection in the eye is due to third-stage larvae, which cannot mature in humans, but can remain viable for years [6]. The parasite is capable of migrating to various parts of the eye causing structural damage leading to severe intraocular inflammations, secondary glaucoma, formation of vitreous

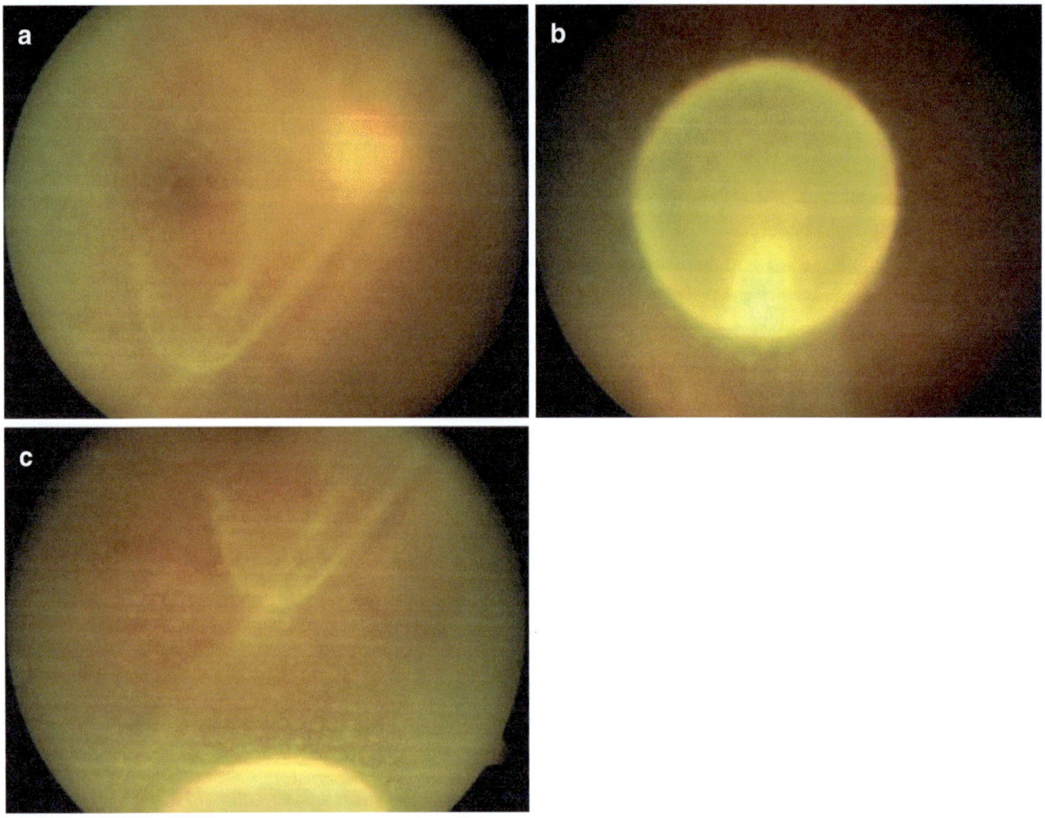

Fig. 33.1 (**a**) Color fundus photograph showing vitreous inflammation with hazy view of the disc and partial posterior vitreous detachment; (**b** and **c**) showing intravitreal cysticercosis inferiorly

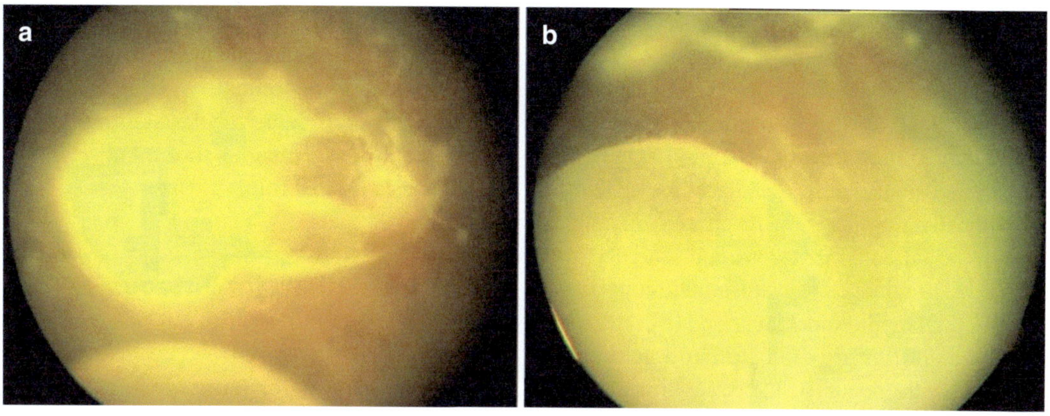

Fig. 33.2 Color fundus photographs showing submacular scarring with vitreous inflammation (**a**) and intravitreal cysticercosis (**b**)

band leading to vitreoretinal traction, and retinal detachment [6, 23].

Ocular toxocariasis is caused by *Toxocara canis* which is a nematode and a helminthic parasitic of dogs (and other canides). Human is paratenic hosts. This rare infection occurs following ingestion of embryonated egg particularly by kids and young adults (accidental) by eating contaminated soil, dogs' fur, or undercooked or raw meat of intermediate host (lamb or rabbit). The infection is also possible following handling of contaminated soil by bare unprotected fingers and hands where the skin is having some erosion. Ingested eggs develop to L3 Larva and migrate in human body and cause syndromic manifestation, which are clinically known as visual and ocular larva migrants. The larva induces reactive inflammatory process that encapsulates the organism and forms eosinophilic granuloma either in the posterior pole or in the periphery of the retina. Typically affecting children present with monocular vision loss, clinical manifestations of posterior uveitis (photophobia, floaters), and leucocoria. Often the cases are presented with chronic endophthalmitis. Toxocara granuloma is detectable by indirect ophthalmoscopy. Other reported clinical manifestations are papillitis, diffuse unilateral subacute neuroretinitis, and visible motile subretinal Nematode. The inflammatory mass resolves and may lead to fibrocellular membrane formation or tractional retinal detachment or combined tractional and rhegmatogenous retinal detachment [15, 24–27]. Diagnosis is mostly clinical. However, ELISA for detection of toxocara canis excretory/secretory (TES) antigens has diagnostic value.

Management consists of control of inflammation, elimination of offending organisms, and management of secondary retinal and vitreous complications. For controlling inflammation topical, periocular, and oral steroids are used. Cycloplegic has a role in anterior uveal involvement. Anthelmintics therapy (albendazole, thiabendazole) has a limited role. Twenty-five percent of cases require vitrectomy for cleaning persistent vitreous opacities and hemorrhage. Vitrectomy is also performed for treating rhegmatogenous retinal detachment or traction retinal detachment (caused by peripheral granuloma). Cryotherapy is used in treating peripheral granuloma and laser photocoagulation for the migrating visible larva [15, 28–31].

Toxoplasma gondii is the most common cause of parasitic infective retinochoroiditis, which usually is controlled by oral medication including pyrimethamine/sulfadiazine/ clindamycin in combination with corticosteroids or monotherapy [1, 3]. Vitreous surgery in *T. gondii* infection is used for severe or persistent vitreous inflammation in patients with active lesions. More common indication for pars plana vitrectomy is, however, for removal of persistent vitreous opacities in otherwise quiet eye [1].

Hydatid cyst is caused by echinococcus granulosus. Liver lesions are most common (60–70%), followed by lungs, kidney, spleen, brain, and other tissues [16]. Hydatid cysts occur rarely within the eye, although they are more common in the orbit. The cysts usually lie in the subretinal space but occasionally may develop in choroid or appear free in the vitreous cavity. Vitreous surgery may be needed to remove the cyst from vitreous cavity or subretinal or choroidal location [16].

Alaria species are diplostomatid nematodes that as adults occur in the small intestine of carnivorous mammals. Alaria species have life cycles that involve succession of three hosts: snail first intermediate host, tadpole or frog second intermediate host, and a carnivore is the definitive host. Humans become infective by eating intermediate or paratenic host containing metacercariae. The most common means of infection of humans is by eating inadequately cooked frog's legs. Treatment may include oral anthelmintics like praziquantel and albendazole or laser photocoagulation to destroy the subretinal or intraretinal worms away from macula. Vitrectomy to remove intravitreal or subretinal worms has also been reported to be effective [20].

Diffuse unilateral subacute neuroretinitis (DUSN) is characterized by progressive visual loss due to inflammatory changes in the retina, retinal vessels, retinal pigment epithelium, and optic nerve [18]. DUSN is attributable to infestation by a solitary intraretinal or subretinal nematode. Several species of nematodes have been suggested as the etiological agent for DUSN including *Toxocara canis*, *Baylisascaris procyonis*, and *Ancylostoma caninum*. Medical therapy, laser photocoagulation, and cryotherapy may be indicated. Vitreous surgery is rarely indicated to remove the nematode [17, 18].

Diagnosis is made on the basis of high index of suspicious, direct demonstration of parasite in the eye (live or dead) and specific clinical findings in the retina. Serology for antibody detection and molecular technique for parasitic DNA have a contributory role, species of the parasite can be diagnosed by instant direct compound microscopy (Fig. 33.3). Management principle is control of ocular inflammation, elimination of offending parasite, and management of secondary retinal and vitreoretinal complications [32–34]. Topical, oral, or periocular steroids have a role in controlling inflammation. Anti-parasitic therapy has a limited role.

33.3 Indications for Vitreous Surgery

- **Vitreous surgery for parasitic infestation of the eye may be indicated for the following reasons:**
- Persistent ocular inflammation.
- Residual vitreous exudates or membranes after subsidence of inflammation.
- Removal of intra- or subretinal or intravitreal parasites.
- For management of secondary complications like traction or rhegmatogenous retinal detachment.

33.3.1 Persistent Ocular Inflammation

Initial phases of parasitic inflammation may be associated with severe intraocular inflammation mimicking endophthalmitis, which may be needing vitreous surgery apart from medical management. Such an indication may arise in cases of *Toxocara* or *Toxoplasma* infections [3, 19]. Cysticercosis cyst can present with severe intraocular inflammation if there is an accidental rupture of the cyst [2, 12, 13].

33.3.2 Residual Vitreous Exudates or Vitreous Membranes

Residual vitreous exudates may persist in spite of the resolution of active infection in cases of toxocara or toxoplasma retinochoroiditis [3, 19]. Vitreous surgery is indicated to clear the vitreous exudates to improve the visual acuity. Vitreous membranes may form between the optic disc and the peripheral granuloma in toxocariasis as well

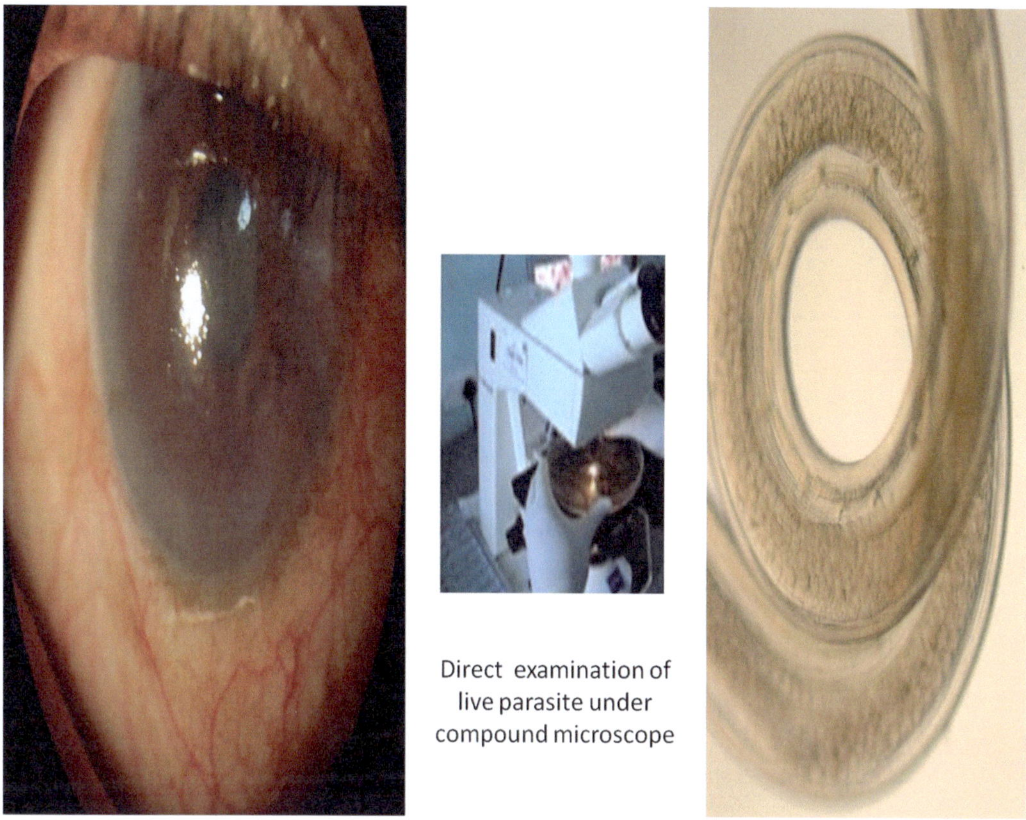

Fig. 33.3 Examination of live parasites under the objective of a compound microscope where all the internal structures are visible for instant reporting of the parasite. Courtesy Dr. D. Das [32]

as epiretinal membrane formation in macular area [15, 19]. Vitreous surgery is helpful in preventing secondary traction or rhegmatogenous retinal detachment in these cases.

33.3.3 Removal of Intravitreal, Intraretinal, or Subretinal Parasites

Common clinical condition requiring vitreous surgery is intravitreal (Fig. 33.4a, b) or subretinal cysticercosis (Fig. 33.5a, b) [8, 10, 11, 13]. DUSN due to varied etiological organisms forms other major groups requiring vitreous surgery [18]. Subretinal or intravitreal hydatid cyst is a rare clinical situation for vitreous surgery [16]. Intravitreal gnathostomiasis also forms an indication for vitreous surgery, especially in the Asian population [5–7].

33.3.4 Secondary Complications

Secondary complications include tractional retinal detachment or rhegmatogenous retinal detachment. Retinal detachment was found in 48.8% (22/45) eyes with intraocular cysticercosis in one of the studies [13].

In cases of toxocara infestation, retinal detachment is more often due to traction band development secondary to toxocara granuloma, with resultant retinal break formation leading to rhegmatogenous retinal detachment [19, 30].

33.4 Treatment of Posterior Segment Cysticercosis

Untreated intraocular cysticercosis when dies incite severe ocular inflammation. Hence, surgery is the treatment of choice.

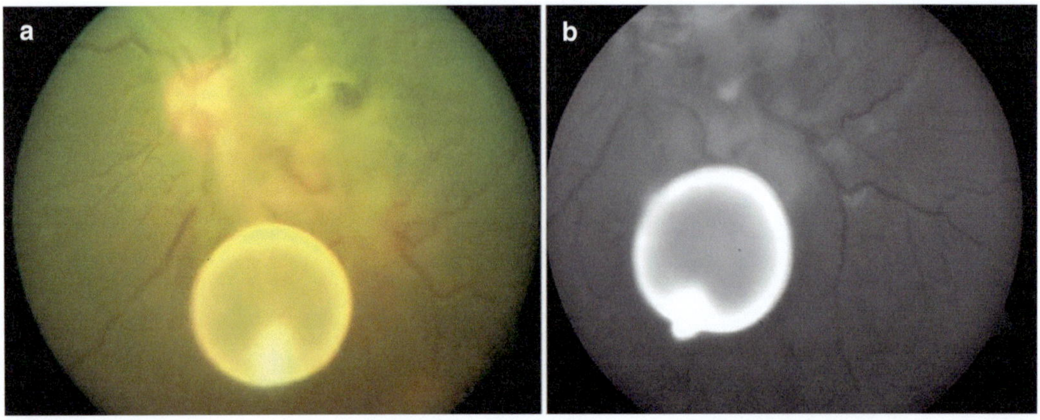

Fig. 33.4 Fundus photographs showing premacular scarring with partial posterior vitreous detachment and intravitreal cysticercosis (**a** and **b**)

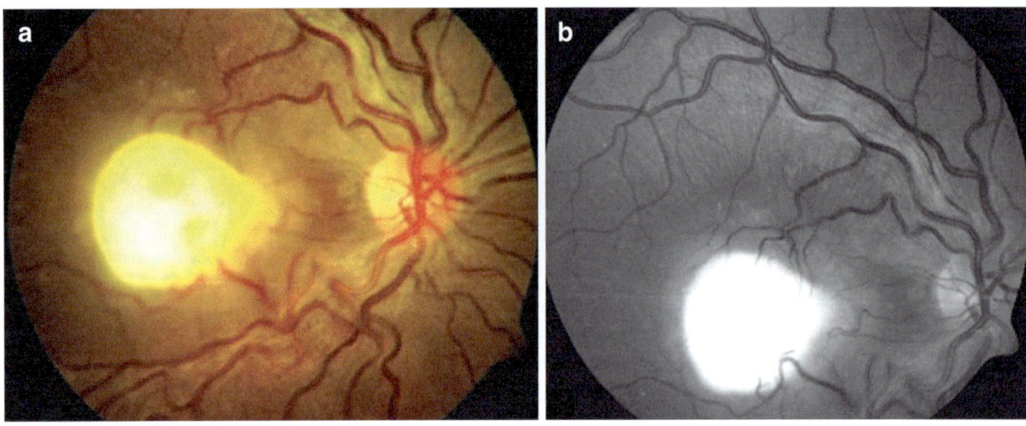

Fig. 33.5 Fundus photographs showing subretinal cysticercosis with retinal vessels coursing over the lesion (**a** and **b**). Note the vitreous cavity is free of inflammation

33.4.1 Intravitreal Cysts

Various modalities have been described in the surgical management of intravitreal cysticercosis such as diathermy, photocoagulation, and cryotherapy. But these methods have now become obsolete as it results in the release of toxins from the cyst causing severe intraocular inflammation in the vitreous cavity. Surgical removal of the cyst can be through either the transretinal or the transscleral route. Earlier, it was recommended that the cyst could be removed in toto through one of the ports because it will help in prevention of any rupture and release of any toxin from the cyst which is mainly responsible for severe vitritis [1].

In the modern day of advancement of vitreoretinal surgery (23G, 25G, and 27G vitrectomy) removal of the cysts using the vitreous cutter is advocated. Vitreous needs to be cleared in the anterior vitreous cavity and around the cysticercosis cyst. Delivery of intravitreal cysticercosis can follow two courses, The sclerotomy can be extended and the cyst can be delivered with the help of flute needle or active suction of vitreous cutter or with the help of intravitreal cryoprobe. Alternatively, one can do a 23-gauge sutureless vitrectomy with cysticercosis contents sucked and cyst can be cut and removed with the help of 23-gauge cutter. The maximum suction and high cut rate ensure that the cyst contents hardly come in contact with the ocular structures with minimum release of toxins. In case one cuts and aspirates the cystcercosis cyst in vitreous cavity, a wash with steroids is recommended to reduce the postoperative inflammation. Systemic corticosteroids are used before and after surgical removal of the cysticercosis cyst to prevent any possible chance of vitritis.

33.4.2 Subretinal Cyst

Earlier, small subretinal cysticercus was treated with photocoagulation. There are two different approaches to remove subretinal cyst anterior to equator and posterior to equator. Subretinal cysts that are anterior to the equator may be removed transsclerally [2]. The cyst has to be localized with indirect ophthalmoscopy, the exact site marked with diathermy. A radial sclerotomy of adequate size is made at this site, and preplaced sutures are placed. The choroid is exposed and obvious blood vessels cauterized. Then the cyst can be easily removed through the choroidal incision with gentle pressure on the globe.

For subretinal cysts posterior to the equator, a transvitreal approach is preferred. A retinotomy is made close to the cyst, avoiding the large retinal blood vessels. For submacular cysts, retinotomy is made preferentially along the horizontal raphe. A silicone tipped extrusion cannula is used to deliver the cyst into the vitreous cavity and removed as mentioned previously. Fluid–gas exchange is performed, and the retinotomy sealed with an endolaser. An encircling 2.5-mm band can be used to support the posterior vitreous base in eyes with peripheral vitreous traction.

33.4.3 Communicating Cysticercosis

Kumar et al. [35] first described these as viable intravitreal cysticercus cellulosae in communication with subretinal space. Multiple cysts in the same eye at different locations may be present. There may be a rhegmatogenous retinal detachment associated with it. Nowadays, treatment modality of communicating cysticercosis is pars plana vitrectomy. With timely pars plana vitrectomy, good visual acuity can be achieved in patients with intravitreal and subretinal cysticercosis without macular involvement.

33.5 Vitreous Surgery for Live Nematodes

The most common live nematode infestation of the eye is by Gnathostoma and Angiostrongylus. The clinical condition is characterized by clinical features of multiple iris holes, uveitis, subretinal track lesions, and rarely retinal detachment with multiple retinal holes. Vitreous surgery for removal of live worms involves standard 3-port pars plana vitrectomy and induction of posterior hyaloid detachment. The parasite can be aspirated into 19- or 20-gauge aspiration cannula or active suction by vitreous cutter. After removal of the worms, one should carefully do a retina examination and identify all the retinal lesions and endophotocoagulation around the lesions and intraocular tamponade with long-acting gases or silicone oil, depending on the intraocular condition. The worm obtained by surgery should be subjected to parasitology evaluation for species identification and patient should be subjected to systemic evaluation and appropriate systemic therapy.

33.6 Vitreous Traction Membranes and Epiretinal Membranes

Vitreous traction membranes may be extending from the disc to retinal periphery in patients with resolved toxocariasis warranting vitreous surgery. The vitreous surgery follows the general principles of vitrectomy for epiretinal and traction membranes except for in the area of healed granuloma. There will be a full-thickness retinochoroidal scar, where one needs to truncate and free the healed granulomatous area from rest of the retina and secure the area by 3–4 rows of contiguous laser photocoagulation burns. Depending on the amount of residual traction left around the healed granuloma, one should decide about whether to use or not to use any intraocular tamponading agents and whether to use long-acting gases or silicone oil. The vitreous sample and the membranes removed during surgery should be subjected to histopathological and serological evaluation.

33.7 Vitreous Exudates and Endophthalmitis Like Presentation

Parasitic infestations may present as endogenous endophthalmitis like picture, which may respond to initial therapy with antibiotics and steroids. As the clinical picture quietens, the diagnosis becomes clear. At times the persistent vitreous exudates may warrant PPV and the diagnosis may be made during surgery. The PPV in persistent vitreous exudates follows the same principles as that of post-uveitis vitrectomy. However, one needs to be careful while inducing posterior vitreous detachment. During vitrectomy or at the end of the surgical procedure one needs to be observant about possible live parasites either in the vitreous cavity or intraretinal space, which need to be dealt with as required.

33.8 Traction or Rhegmatogenous Retinal Detachment

Traction and combined traction and rhegmatogenous retinal detachments are not an uncommon finding in parasitic infections of the eye. The scars resulting from toxocara granuloma or cysticercosis entry point into vitreous cavity from subretinal space are likely to be dense and involving all layers of retina and choroid. The residual scars cannot be removed in toto. So every attempt should be made to isolate the area and relieve all the traction bands extending into the healed granulomatous scar. Photocoagulation around the scar should be done so that the rest of the retina will remain stable. Use of tamponading agents like long-acting gas or silicone oil will depend on the status of the retina, location of the scar, and relation of the scar to the surrounding retina. If there is any doubt about the complete clearance of traction, it is better to inject silicone oil.

33.9 Results

The success rate for removal of intraocular cysticercosis, either intravitreal or subretinal, is nearly 100% and success of attachment of retina with modern-day vitrectomy is about 85–90% [13]. Visual recovery depends on the location of the scar. If the scar is involving the macula, the visual acuity can be poor. Otherwise good visual recovery (better than 20/40) can be expected in 70% of the patients (Figs. 33.6a, b, 33.7a, b) [13]. Though literature is not concrete about the timing of the surgery, there is an indication toward early surgical intervention once diagnosed.

Reports on vitreous surgery for toxocariasis with vitreous traction membranes and traction detachment are rewarding with good anatomical outcome, with macular attachment in all eyes and relatively good visual acuities (better than 20/70) in 50% of the eyes (5 out of 10 eyes) [17].

Literature available on vitrectomy for live nematodes or trematodes in the vitreous cavity constitutes either single case reports or small case series, showing successful removal of parasites with good anatomical and visual outcomes [5–7, 16, 18, 20, 31, 36].

33.10 Complications

In addition to complications related to vitreous surgery, vitrectomy in cysticercosis carries an additional risk of cyst rupture and toxic reaction to cyst contents [13]. One should be thorough in irrigation and aspiration of vitreous cavity with triamcinolone to reduce possible postoperative inflammation. Recurrent epiretinal membrane formation is another risk factor frequently seen after removal of cysticercosis or after vitreous surgery for traction detachment in toxocariasis and following vitrectomy for live intraocular parasitic infestations [13, 17]. Recurrent retinal

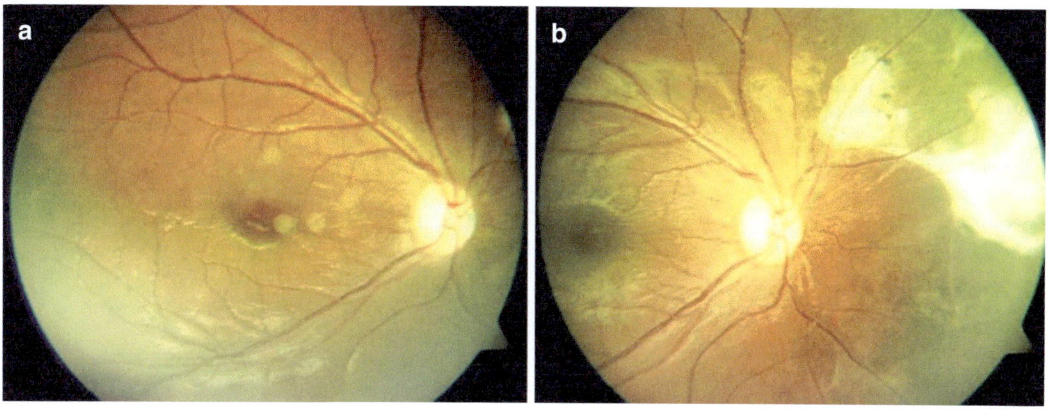

Fig. 33.6 Color fundus photographs showing residual subretinal scarring following vitreous surgery for subretinal cysticercosis. Note healthy condition of the macula. Postoperative visual acuity at 3 months follow-up was 20/20 (**a** and **b**)

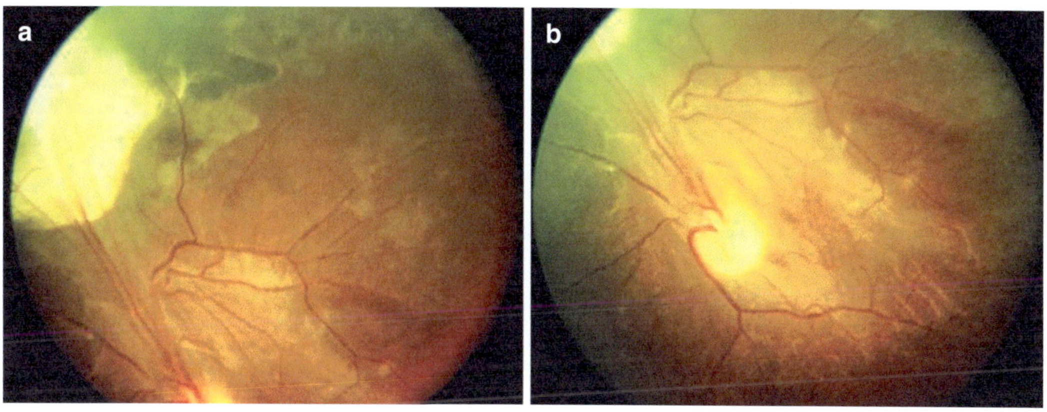

Fig. 33.7 Color fundus photographs showing peripheral residual scarring following vitreous surgery for subretinal cysticercosis (**a**). Note macular heterotopia (**b**). Postoperative visual acuity at 3 months follow-up was 20/200

detachment is another possible complication following vitrectomy for toxocara related traction retinal detachment and chorioretinal scars with traction retinal detachment associated with cysticercosis [13, 17]. Subretinal cysticercosis with scarring is prone to more frequent occurrence of recurrent retinal detachment [10].

33.11 Conclusion

Parasitic diseases as an indication for surgery constitute less than 1% of the surgeries in a vitreoretinal surgical unit. Intravitreal or subretinal cysticercosis and gnathostomiasis are frequent causes of indication for vitreous surgery in Asia. Indications for vitrectomy in parasitic diseases include persistent ocular inflammation, residual vitreous exudates or membranes, intravitreal or subretinal parasites, and for management of associated secondary complications like traction or rhegmatogenous retinal detachment. Anatomical outcomes are generally good after surgical intervention for parasitic diseases, but visual results are variable depending on the location of the residual scar. Management protocol of intravitreal infestation is yet to be standardized and management algorithm is awaiting finalization.

References

1. Engstrom RE, Holland GN, Nussenblatt RB, et al. Current practices in the management of ocular toxoplasmosis. Am J Ophthalmol. 1991;111:601–10.
2. Cano MR. Ocular cysticercosis. In: Ryan SJ, editor. Retina. 3rd ed. New York: Mosby; 2001. p. 1553–7.
3. Jabs DA, Nguyen QD. Ocular toxoplasmosis. In: Ryan SJ, editor. Retina. 3rd ed. New York: Mosby; 2001. p. 1531–44.
4. Ratra D, Phogat C, Singh M, et al. Intravitreal cysticercosis presenting as neovascular glaucoma. Indian J Ophthalmol. 2010;58:70–3.
5. Basak SK, Sinha TK, Bhattacharya D, et al. Intravitreal live Gnathostoma Spinigerum. Indian J Ophthalmol. 2004;52:57–8.
6. Biswas J, Gopal L, Sharma T, et al. Intraocular Gnathostoma Spinigerum. Retina. 1994;14:438–44.
7. Bhattacharjee H, Das D, Medhi J. Intravitreal gnathostomiasis and review of literature. Retina. 2007;27:67–73.
8. Nainiwal S, Chand M, Verma L, et al. Intraocular live cysticer-cus larva. Ophthalmic Surg Lasers Imaging. 2003;34:464–6.
9. George T, Mathai A, Challa JK, et al. Intravitreal cysticercosis: how did it get there? Aus New Zealand J Ophthalmol. 1998;26:159–60.
10. Luger MHA, Stilma JS, Ringens PJ, et al. In-toto removal of a subretinal cysticercus cellulosae by pars plana vitrectomy. Br J Ophthalmol. 1991;75:561–3.
11. Natarajan S, Malpani A, Nirmalan PK, et al. Management of intraocular cysticercosis. Graefes Arch Clin Exp Ophthalmol. 1999;237:812–4.
12. Messener KH, Kammerer WS. Intraocular cysticercosis. Arch Ophthalmol. 1979;97:1103–5.
13. Sharma T, Sinha S, Shah N, et al. Intraocular cysticercosis: clinical charecteristics and visual outcome after vitreoretinal surgery. Ophthalmology. 2003;110:996–1004.
14. Maguire AM, Green WR, Michels RG, et al. Recovery of intraocular Toxocara canis by pars plana vitrectomy. Ophthalmology. 1990;97:675–80.
15. Werner JC, Ross RD, Green WR, et al. Pars plana vitrectomy and subretinal surgery for ocular toxocariasis. Arch Ophthalmol. 1999;117:532–4.
16. Muftuoglu G, Cicik E, Ozdamar A, et al. Vitreoretinal surgery for a subretinal hydatid cyst. Am J Ophthalmol. 2001;132:435–7.
17. Amin HI, McDonald HR, Han DP, et al. Vitrectomy update for macular traction in ocular toxocariasis. Retina. 2000;20:80–5.
18. de Souza EC, Nakashima Y. Diffuse unilateral subacute neuroretinitis. Ophthalmology. 1995;102:1183–6.
19. Wilkinson CP. Ocular toxocariasis. In: Ryan SJ, editor. Retina. 3rd ed. New York: Mosby; 2001. p. 1545–52.
20. McDonald HR, Kazacos KR, Schatz H, et al. Two cases of intraocular infection with alaria mesocercaria. Am J Ophthalmol. 1994;117:447–55.
21. Lee J, Chung SH, Lee SC, et al. A technique for removal of a live nematode from the vitreous. Eye. 2006;20:1444–6.
22. Kean BH, Sun T, Ellsworth RM. Color altas and text book of ophthalmic parasitology. New York: Igaku-Shoin; 1991. p. 151–6.
23. Bathrick ME, Mango CA, Mueller JF. Intraocular gnathostomiasis. Ophthalmology. 1981;8:1293–5.
24. Biglan AW, Glickman LT, Lobes LA. Serum and vitreous toxocara antibody in nematode endophthalmitis. Am J Ophthalmol. 1986;224:218–20.
25. Belmont JB, Irvine A, Benson W, et al. Vitrectomy in ocular toxocariasis. Arch Ophthalmol. 1982;100:1912–5.
26. Hagler WS, Pollard ZF, Jarrett WH, et al. Results of surgery for ocular toxocara canis. Ophthalmology. 1981;88:1081–6.
27. Grand GM, Roper-Hall G. Pras plana vitrectomy for ocular toxocariasis. Retina. 1981;1:258–61.
28. Shields JA. Ocular toxocariasis: a review. Surv Ophthalmol. 1984;28:361–81.
29. Triester G, Machemer R. Results of vitrectomy for rare proliferative and hemorrhagic diseases. Am J Ophthalmol. 1977;84:394–412.
30. Small KW, McCuen BW, DE Juan E, et al. Surgical management of retinal traction caused by toxocariasis. Am J Ophthalmol. 1989;108:10–4.
31. Portal M. 2019. https://eyewikiaau.org/toxocariasis. Accessed 26 July 2019.
32. Das D, Ramchandra V, Istam S, et al. Update on ocular parasitic disease. Ind J Ophthalmol. 2016;64:794–802.
33. Jane C, Werner MU, Robin D, et al. Pars plana vitrectomy and subretinal surgery for ocular toxocariasis. Arch Ophthalmol. 1999;117:532–4.
34. Lombardo J. Subretinal cysticercosis. Optom Vis Sci. 2001;78(4):188–94.
35. Kumar A, Verma L, Khosla PK, Tewari HK, Jha SN. Communicating intravitreal cysticercosis. Ophthalmic Surg. 1989;20(6):424–6.
36. Sharma T, Sinha S, Shah N, Gopal L, Shanmugam MP, Bhende P, Bhende M, Shetty NS, Agrawal R, Deshpande D, Biswas J, Sukumar B. Intraocular cysticercosis: clinical characteristics and visual outcome after vitreoretinal surgery. Ophthalmology. 2003;110(5):996–1004.

Part X

Gene Therapy

Gene Therapy for Inherited Retinal Disease

34

Sharola Dharmaraj

34.1 Introduction

Inherited retinal diseases (IRDs) are a clinically and genetically heterogeneous group of disorders with 307 mapped chromosomal loci and 271 identified genes [1]. IRD affects 2 million people worldwide and is one of the commonest causes of childhood blindness [2]. Both syndromic and non-syndromic forms of IRDs are caused by mutations in genes involved in the structure and function of the visual pathway. Genetic testing involves gene identification and mutation detection. Despite the rapid discovery of pathogenic retinal genes a reliable molecu lar diagnosis is only available in half of these patients [3]. Significant advances in molecular genetics have enabled accurate diagnosis for IRDs furthering more appropriate therapeutic options.

Gene therapy uses viral vectors devoid of pathogenic components to deliver functional genes into the retinal cell to restore visual function. Single gene defects cause a vast majority of IRD. Gene augmentation in addition to cell replacement provides greater benefit in sustained cell loss. Gene therapy also includes optogenetics (gene delivery of light-activated tools to surviving cells in the retinal circuit), suppression gene therapy, and gene editing. More recently short interfering ribonucleic acid (siRNAs) have been used for downregulation of gene expression leading to functional inactivation of targeted genes. CRISPR (clustered regularly interspaced short palindromic repeats) technology allows for editing one or multiple sites within the genome. The advent of induced pluripotent stem cells and the CRISPR-Cas9 system offer a powerful additional strategy to treat IRD.

34.2 Genetics and Pathogenesis of Inherited Retinal Disease

Heritable retinal diseases represent a group of rare disorders with several heterogeneous mutations leading to photoreceptor loss and decreased visual acuity. These conditions are inherited in a recessive, dominant, and X-linked manner. In autosomal dominant disease there is a 50% chance of the offspring being affected when one parent is affected; while in recessive disease the risk is 25% of each offspring being affected. In X-linked disease females are unaffected carriers whereas males are affected. In genetically outbred populations, autosomal recessive retinitis pigmentosa accounts for 50–60%, dominant 30–40%, and X-linked 5–15% [4].

IRDs include photoreceptor degenerations (rod or cone dominated) and vitreoretinopathies. Abnormal embryonic development and defects

S. Dharmaraj (✉)
Moorfields Eye Hospital, London, UK

A. Jain et al. (eds.), *Cutting-edge Vitreoretinal Surgery*,
https://doi.org/10.1007/978-981-33-4168-5_34

in biochemical pathways lead to degeneration of photoreceptor and retinal pigment epithelial cells.

Non-syndromic and monogenic retinal disease account for a far greater percentage of IRDs than syndromic retinal disease.

Syndromic retinal disease include Alagille, Alstrom, Bardet-Biedl, Jeune, Joubert, Meckel-Gruber, neuronal ceroid lipofuscinosis, Primary ciliary dyskinesia, Refsum, Senior Loken, Stickler and Usher syndromes, familial exudative vitreoretinopathy, and peroxisomal disease. It is important to have complete clinical and genetic examinations in patients with IRD to diagnose all syndromic variants.

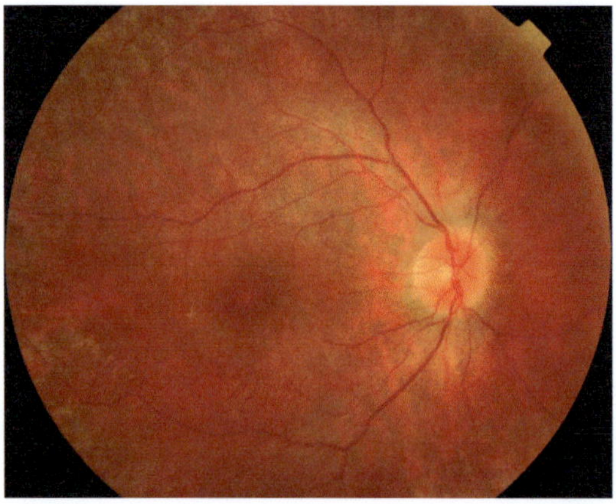

Fig. 34.1 *RPE65*-related Leber's congenital amaurosis

34.3 Inherited Retinal Disorders Where Gene Therapy Has Been Trialled

Retinitis pigmentosa (RP) the commonest retinal dystrophy (1 in 3500 live births) is characterised by progressive photoreceptor loss [5]. RP has a variable inheritance pattern associated with mutations in over 100 genes. Degeneration of rod photoreceptors causes nyctalopia, progressive loss of peripheral vision and motion detection. Retinal examination shows pigmentary retinopathy of varying degrees, attenuated vasculature and optic atrophy. Mutations in the gene coding MERTK (a receptor tyrosine kinase essential for removal of debris from photoreceptors) causes progressive rod–cone degeneration and safety of a viral vector has been demonstrated.

Leber congenital amaurosis (LCA) is a heterogeneous infantile retinal dystrophy presenting with profound visual loss nystagmus, sluggish pupillary responses and an extinguished electroretinogram (ERG). Mutations in several genes causing LCA have been identified, *CEP290* being the commonest. Mutations in *RPE65* cause early-onset severe retinal degeneration and LCA (Fig. 34.1). Successful genetherapy has been demonstrated by various groups of investigators.

Choroideremia is a chronic X-linked retinal degeneration (1 in 50,000 males) due to the deficiency of Rab-escort (REP1) protein causing degeneration of the retinal pigment epithelium and photoreceptors. Choroideremia presents in males with night blindness, progressive visual field restriction in late childhood leading to profound visual loss beyond the fourth decade. As the central photoreceptors are lost late it presents a potential window for treatment before these cells are irreversibly lost [6].

Stargardt disease is the most common form of juvenile-onset macular autosomal recessive disorder caused by mutations in ATP binding cassette subfamily A, member 4 (*ABCA4* gene). Patients present with central visual loss due to progressive accumulation of lipofuscin in the RPE cells.

X-linked juvenile retinoschisis (XLRS) presents with decreased vision in early childhood (1 in 10,000 men). Retinoschisin, the pathogenic gene, is involved in adhesion and transmission between photoreceptors and bipolar cells. Mutations lead to schisis of the macula, associated retinal detachment and vitreous haemorrhages.

Achromatopsia with a prevalence of 1 in 30,000 is a non-progressive complete colour blindness due to loss of cone photoreceptors, presenting with symptoms in early infancy. Patients present with decreased visual acuity absence of colour vision, hemeralopia, nystagmus and photophobia. Mutations in several genes are known to cause the disorder. CNGA3 or CNGB3 related achromatopsia are amenable to gene therapy.

Usher syndrome is a rare genetic disorder caused by mutations in genes involved in the function of the inner ear and retina, presenting with varying combinations of visual loss and sensorineural deafness. The visual loss is due to retinitis pigmentosa with loss of peripheral vision. Usher Type 2 is characterised by moderate to severe hearing loss at birth and later onset of night blindness, retaining central vision into adulthood.

Age-related macular degeneration (ARMD) is a complex retinal degenerative disorder where photoreceptor loss in the macular area results in loss of central vision. It is one of the most common causes of irreversible visual impairment with loss of choroidal endothelial cells, retinal pigment epithelium and photoreceptor cells [7–9]. Both dry and wet forms (exudative) of the disease are under consideration for clinical trials.

Gyrate atrophy of the choroid and retina is characterised by progressive visual loss caused by a defect in ornithine aminotransferase (OAT) leading to the accumulation of ornithine, causing retinal thinning. Patients present with poor night vision leading to visual loss, increasing tunnel vision and atrophic patches of the retina.

34.4 Diagnosis of Inherited Retinal Disease

Clinically IRDs present at different ages. They present with decreased vision, night blindness, or photo-aversion. If the IRD presents in early life and is of a severe nature nystagmus is noted. As treatment hinges on an accurate diagnosis it is important to identify the phenotype correctly. Detailed clinical examinations including family history and pedigrees, associated medical history, serial clinical photography, ocular coherence tomography (OCT) fundus fluorescein angiography, retinal autofluorescence and electrodiagnostics in addition to genotyping is essential.

With the advent of better psychophysical testing, high-resolution coherence tomography and scanning laser ophthalmoscopy a more accurate clinical diagnosis is achieved.

It is important to identify hitherto treatable inherited retinal conditions, i.e., gyrate atrophy using enzyme replacement and diets low in ornithine, Refsum disease, a leukodystrophy with pigmentary retinopathy wherein dietary phytanic acid restriction helps slow this autosomal recessive lipoprotein disorder. Abetalipoproteinemia with pigmentary retinopathy is treated with injections of fat-soluble vitamins.

Due to the heterogeneous nature of IRDs the gene implicated may be the same, however, the phenotypes may be different. Variable penetrance and expressivity in addition to intra-familial phenotypic variability in some disorders, necessitate an accurate genetic diagnosis prior to enrolment in clinical trials.

Molecular genetic diagnosis involves detecting the gene mutation that segregates with the disease in the family. Several DNA microarray chips are available for screening. Both exome and whole genome sequencing are undertaken when no previously known mutation is identified.

34.5 Aims of Gene Therapy

The chief intent in treating IRDs is to restore function or delay deterioration of the disease. The essential aim is to replace the mutated gene with a normal copy [10] or inactivate the gene [11]. With the advent of gene editing it is now possible to introduce the gene, inactivate it or introduce a targeted mutation. Optogenetics creates artificial photoreceptors using gene delivery of light-activated channels or pumps to surviving ganglion cells [12]. Gene replacement therapy has been studied extensively in both animal models and humans. The initial success of gene replacement therapy in knockout mice and dogs led to successful clinical trials in humans with *RPE65* related LCA. Enzyme replacement therapy in gyrate atrophy has been of help in patients.

34.6 Methods

The use of Adeno associated viral vectors in the delivery of gene therapy for eye diseases has revolutionised treatment. This treatment showed improvement in retinal function and visual behaviour in canine models of *RPE65*-related LCA [10]. The retina has been at the forefront of translational gene therapy. The remarkable success of proof of principle, efficacy and safety in clinical trials of *RPE65* related LCA has increased the possibilities of retinal gene therapy in other IRDs.

The eye due to its small size, easy accessibility and some degree of immune privilege has made it possible to study and quantify progress using viral vectors for retinal disease. Adeno-associated Virus (AAV) and lentivirus have been used for retinal gene delivery [13]. AAV vectors are efficient at maintaining sustained transduction of retinal cells. However, they are limited by their small capacity [14]. Lentiviruses have greater capacity when larger genes are used. Viral vectors delivering the target gene is placed in the sub-retinal space using a fine cannula. Injections into the vitreous cavity and the suprachoroidal space have been undertaken [15]. The other eye has often been used as a control in most studies. The safety and efficacy of gene transfer in *RPE65*-related LCA as noted by several investigators in three well-known studies have prompted the further use of these vectors [13, 16, 17]. The CRISPR-Cas system has now overtaken many other methods of DNA targeting *in vivo*. Guide RNA that recognises the target DNA and Cas nucleases that cut the DNA at the precise location are able to offer gene therapy in several *in vivo* studies.

Successful delivery of the *RPE-65* gene using recombinant AAV restored vision in rodents and canines thus paving the way for clinical trials in patients with LCA [10, 18–20].

34.7 Clinical Trials

Clinical studies involve studying the natural history of these rare IRDs and are undertaken in many ophthalmic departments. However, interventional clinical trials are conducted only in a few specific centres for a few specific diseases. Considerable collaborations are in place to enable clinical trials as the number of patients are few and the availability of participant numbers are few too in the early phases of trials. Table 34.1 lists some of the clinical trials for IRDs (https://clinicaltrials.gov/).

Table 34.1 Clinical trials

	IRD	Intervention
1	ESORD	AAV2/2hRPE65
2	Choroideremia	AAV2-REP1
3	X-linked retinitis pigmentosa	AAV8-RPGR
4	*RPE65*-related retinal dystrophy	AAV OPTIRPE65
5	*RPE65*-related LCA	AAV2-Hrpe65v2 Voretigene neparvovec-rzl
6	X-linked retinoschisis	RS1-AAV
7	Achromatopsia	AAV-CNGA3
8	Achromatopsia	AAV CNGB3
9	Gyrate atrophy	Keratinocyte transfer
10	Retinitis pigmentosa	GS030-DP AND medical device: GS030-MD
11	*PDEA*-related RP	PDEA6
12	Neovascular AMD	RX314
13	AMD	AAV2-sFLT01
14	Retinal disease *MERTK* mutations	Raav2-vmd2-hMERTK
15	AMD	Retinostat
16	Stargardt	Lentivirus ABCA4
17	Usher Type1B	Lentivirus MYO7A
18	*RLBP1*-related RP	CPK850
19	*RPGR*-XL RP	AAV8-RPGR
20	*CEP290*-related LCA	EDIT-101 AGN 151587

ABCA adenosine triphosphate binding cassette subfamily A member 4, *AAV* adeno-associated viral vector, *AMD* age-related macular degeneration, *CNGA* cyclic nucleotide-gated channel alpha, *CNGB* cyclic nucleotide-gated channel beta, *ESORD* early onset of severe retinal dystrophy, *MYO* myosin VII A, *MERTK* mer tyrosine kinase, *PDE* phosphodiesterase, *RPE65* retinal pigment epithelium, *REP* Rab escort protein, *RLBP* Retinaldehyde binding protein, *RPGR* retinitis pigmentosa GTPase regulator, *XL* X linked.

34.8 Results

Gene replacement therapy improved visual function in murine and canine models of *RPE65*-related LCA, it also improved electroretinography, pupillometry and flash-evoked cortical potentials in the dark-adapted state. This was sustained for several years [10]. The clinical results using RPE65 gene therapy in adults initially and children later proved the safety and efficacy of this form of therapy [21]. Post-trial objective measures included nystagmus testing, pupillary light reflex assessment and optical coherence tomography (OCT). Subjective measures included standard tests of visual acuity Goldmann visual field testing and mobility assessment in navigating a standardised obstacle course before and after therapy. Improvement in visual acuity mobility visual behaviour and retinal function after treatment were noted [22].

However, the vector carrying the RPE65 gene enabled transfection of the target cells to induce generation of RPE65 protein but visual restoration was not sustained because retinal degeneration continued as part of the disease process. Following injection of the vector into the sub-retinal space no evidence of systemic dissemination of vector sequences or humoural immune response or cell-mediated immune responses to AAV2 capsid or RPE65 protein were noted in the 3-year follow-up study [17, 23]. No serious adverse effects or systemic effects have been reported. Some adverse outcomes that were observed in a few cases included choroidal effusions, retinal detachment, transient ocular hypertony and ocular hypertension-related to the administration of topical steroids.

Following the initial success of *RPE65*-related LCA studies, the FDA approved voretigene neparvovec (Luxturna) for use in patients with *RPE65*-related LCA and more clinical trials are underway.

Long-term post-treatment follow-up in patients and canine models with LCA showed that gene therapy improved vision but photoreceptor degeneration progressed unabated [17]. The early effect of therapy up to 6–12 months sustains visual improvement but over a period of time there was no consistent improvement in acuity or ERG and a decrease in retinal thickness occurred. The lack of long-term effects of gene augmentation suggests a need for further strategies to improve outcomes. More recently gene editing has become an option for patients with the common *CEP290* splice site mutation where an antisense oligonucleotide (ASO treatment) restores pre-mRNA splicing thereby increasing CEP290 protein necessary for efficient ciliary transport in photoreceptors [24]. Gene replacement therapy trials could also be applicable in LCA caused by mutations in *AIPL1 CEP290 GUCY2D, LCA5* and *RPGRIP* [25, 26]. X-linked RP clinical trials using AAV-mediated gene supplementation are underway in several centers and the safety, tolerability and potency of the study are under evaluation [27]. The end point of a 2-year study in patients with choroideremia who received varying doses of AAV2.RP1 vector surgically delivered into the sub-retinal space via an iatrogenic retinal detachment showed improvement by 4.5 chart letters while the untreated eye declined by 1.5 letters (ETDR letters) Retinal thinning and significant retinal inflammation at 2 weeks were noted in three patients. Sustained visual improvement was maintained for up to 5 years. No systemic immune response or viral replication was noted. Advancement of very slow degeneration measured over 2 years was detected only in the peripheral retina [28, 29]. Several models of achromatopsia have been treated using AAV vectors. In canine models, with *Cngb3* mutations, the vector was introduced by transvitreal sub-retinal injection and improved photopic and functional vision. Clinical trials using Ciliary NeuroTrophic Factor (CNTF) delivered by an encapsulated cell-based device showed no evidence of improved cone function and further decline in rod function was noted [30, 31].

In patients with X-Linked retinoschisis who received gene therapy with the normal gene delivered by AAV vectors, via intravitreal injections, safety of administration, a degree of transient uveitis and no remarkable sustained level of vision were detected [32]. In patients with MERTK-related RP, AAV-mediated gene therapy was deemed safe and a few participants in the trial benefitted as they showed a transient increase in visual acuity [33].

In patients with Stargardt disease, the lentivirus containing a normal copy of the gene was introduced via sub-retinal injections to study efficacy and safety. In an effort to address the accumulation of toxic bisretinoids and lipofuscin in the retina and retinal pigment epithelium, C5 complement inhibitors to reduce inflammation have been tried [34]. Stem cell transplantation and pharmacotherapy with visual cell modulators and complement inhibitors are under evaluation.

Using the human transgene driven by cone-specific promotor fragments packaged in an AAV capsid delivered sub-retinally post vitrectomy and in addition to intraocular implants that released CNTF, it has been possible to further potentiate rescue of photoreceptors in animal models [35].

In vivo experiments using CRISPR/Cas9 technology have yielded some success. However, the need to obviate off-target effects and sustain higher therapeutic ranges still need to be addressed before this technology is more useful in IRD [36].

34.9 Other Therapeutic Approaches

These include pharmacotherapy, cell transplantation, retinal prosthesis and combinations of gene and other therapies to maximise the benefit of treatment.

CNTF sequestered in semipermeable capsules and implanted in the vitreous cavity have maintained cone survival. Combined with gene therapy a delay in retinal degeneration has been noted [37]. Inhibition of specific biochemical and cellular pathways are under evaluation. Targeting the cyclic Guanosine Monophosphate (cGMP) pathway in photoreceptor signal transduction in an attempt to preserve photoreceptors is under evaluation [38]. Oral treatment with QLT, a stable synthetic compound, converted in the body to 9-cis retinal, binds with opsin to form isorhodopsin and activates the phototransduction cascade on exposure to light in *RPE65* and *LRAT*-related LCA, improving visual function [39].

Stem cell transplantation provides mutation independent regenerative therapy. Transplantation of cells serves to replace damaged cells, provide trophic factors to prevent further cell loss and results in a potential route for photoreceptor cell renewal. In using Human embryonic cell-derived stem cells for the treatment of macular degeneration, possible cellular engraftment with sustained improvement in visual acuity was noted [40]. Using patient-specific somatic cells and reprogramming them into pluripotent stem cells to restore functional retinal pigment epithelium and photoreceptors, ameliorates immunologic adverse events, noted with the use of allogenic transplants [41]. When induced pluripotent stem cells (iPSC) cells have been paired with gene editing it is possible to create immunologically matched and genetically corrected cells to replace degenerated tissue, obviating the need for systemic immunosuppression [41].

Restoration of ciliogenesis in *CEP290*-related LCA using *CEP290* gene transfer in cells provides another avenue for gene- and cell-based therapies [42].

The use of visual prosthesis whereby electrical stimulation bypasses damaged nerve endings has been used in the treatment of IRD [43]. This option for treatment in patients with IRDs is not genotype dependent. The plasticity of the visual cortex as evidenced by positron emission tomography in patients with severe visual loss makes it possible to continue this avenue of treatment [44]. Using intact inner retina to transmit impulses to the visual cortex has been possible with retinal prosthesis. Both the crude appreciation of light and the ability to detect motion has been observed in these patients with retinitis pigmentosa [45]. The Argus system works by direct stimulation of the inner retina via epiretinal electrodes. Visual information is gathered by a video camera mounted on external glasses and converted to pixelated images by an external processor. These images are transmitted to the microarray electrode placed surgically in the retina which in turn transmits to the occipital cortex [46, 47]. It has been noted that although the vision obtained following this implantation is not easily quantifiable in terms of improved visual acuity or increased fields it has made the performance of real-world functional vision better [48].

34.10 Conclusions

The past few decades have seen a great surge in gene identification, a greater understanding of biochemical and cellular pathways and the need for better treatment options for patients with heritable retinal disease. Due to the rapid advances in molecular genetics, gene therapy too is keeping close pace with increasing trials in IRD. With the proven safety and efficacy of gene therapy in several clinical trials, more trials are in several phases in different centers. Promising results of gene replacement in *RPE-65* related LCA, choroideremia and retinoschisis, with some restoration of visual function has made it possible to continue with more clinical trials in Stargardt disease, Usher Type 2A, XLRP, achromatopsia, AMD and retinitis pigmentosa. Combining gene, pharmaco and cell therapy are being explored. The greater co-operation of industry with academic units and regulatory bodies has accelerated better treatment options. The active participation of patient and support groups, have furthered greater involvement in clinical trials and advancing research.

Acknowledgement The author would like to thank Debora Marletta of the Institute of Ophthalmology Library University College London, for helping with the bibliography and Suzanne Yzer MD, Rottterdam Eye Hospital, Rotterdam, The Netherlands for the fundus photographs.

Compliance with ethical requirements: No conflict of interest. No procedures were undertaken by the author, neither any animal nor any interventional human studies.

References

1. Retnet. https://sph.uth.edu/retnet/.
2. Wong TY, Zheng Y, Jonas JB, Flaxman SR, Keeffe J, Leasher J, Naidoo K, Pesudovs K, Price H, White RA, Resnikoff S, Taylor HR, Bourne RR. Vision loss expert group of the global burden of disease study. Prevalence and causes of vision loss in East Asia: 1990–2010. Br J Ophthalmol. 2014;98(5):599–604.
3. Berger W, Kloeckener-Gruissem B, Neidhardt J. The molecular basis of human retinal and vitreoretinal diseases. Prog Retin Eye Res. 2010;29(5):335–75.
4. Hartong DT, Berson EL, Dryja TP. Retinitis pigmentosa. Lancet. 2006;368(9549):1795–80.
5. Bunker CH, Berson EL, Bromley WC, Hayes RP, Roderick TH. Prevalence of retinitis pigmentosa in Maine. Am J Ophthalmol. 1984;97(3):357–65.
6. Jolly JK, Xue K, Edwards TL, Groppe M, MacLaren RE. Characterizing the natural history of visual function in choroideremia using microperimetry and multimodal retinal imaging. Invest Ophthalmol Vis Sci. 2017;58(12):5575–58.
7. Songstad AE, Wiley LA, Duong K, Kaalberg E, Flamme-Wiese MJ, Cranston CM, Riker MJ, Levasseur D, Stone EM, Mullins RF, Tucker BA. Generating iPSC-derived choroidal endothelial cells to study age-related macular degeneration. Invest Ophthalmol Vis Sci. 2015;56(13):8258–67.
8. Songstad AE, Worthington KS, Chirco KR, Giacalone JC, Whitmore SS, Anfinson KR, Ochoa D, Cranston CM, Riker MJ, Neiman M, Stone EM, Mullins RF, Tucker BA. Connective tissue growth factor promotes efficient generation of human induced pluripotent stem cell-derived choroidal endothelium. Stem Cells Transl Med. 2017;6(6):1533–154.
9. Chirco KR, Sohn EH, Stone EM, Tucker BA, Mullins RF. Structural and molecular changes in the aging choroid: implications for age-related macular degeneration. Eye (Lond). 2017;31(1):10–25.
10. Acland GM, Aguirre GD, Ray J, Zhang Q, Aleman TS, Cideciyan AV, Pearce-Kelling SE, Anand V, Zeng Y, Maguire AM, Jacobson SG, Hauswirth WW, Bennett J. Gene therapy restores vision in a canine model of childhood blindness. Nat Genet. 2001;28(1):92–5.
11. Farrar GJ, Millington-Ward S, Chadderton N, Humphries P, Kenna PF. Gene-based therapies for dominantly inherited retinopathies. Gene Ther. 2012;19(2):137–44.
12. Duebel J, Marazova K, Sahel JA. Optogenetics. Curr Opin Ophthalmol. 2015 May;26(3):226–32.
13. Maguire AM, Simonelli F, Pierce EA, Pugh EN Jr, Mingozzi F, Bennicelli J, Banfi S, Marshall KA, Testa F, Surace EM, Rossi S, Lyubarsky A, Arruda VR, Konkle B, Stone E, Sun J, Jacobs J, Dell'Osso L, Hertle R, Ma JX, Redmond TM, Zhu X, Hauck B, Zelenaia O, Shindler KS, Maguire MG, Wright JF, Volpe NJ, McDonnell JW, Auricchio A, High KA, Bennett J. Safety and efficacy of gene transfer for Leber's congenital amaurosis. N Engl J Med. 2008;358(21):2240–8.
14. Dong JY, Fan PD, Frizzell RA. Quantitative analysis of the packaging capacity of recombinant adeno-associated virus. Hum Gene Ther. 1996;7(17):2101–12.
15. Peden MC, Min J, Meyers C, Lukowski Z, Li Q, Boye SL, Levine M, Hauswirth WW, Ratnakaram R, Dawson W, Smith WC, Sherwood MB. Ab-externo

AAV-mediated gene delivery to the suprachoroidal space using a 250 micron flexible microcatheter. PLoS One. 2011;6(2):e17140.
16. Bainbridge JW, Smith AJ, Barker SS, Robbie S, Henderson R, Balaggan K, Viswanathan A, Holder GE, Stockman A, Tyler N, Petersen-Jones S, Bhattacharya SS, Thrasher AJ, Fitzke FW, Carter BJ, Rubin GS, Moore AT, Ali RR. Effect of gene therapy on visual function in Leber's congenital amaurosis. N Engl J Med. 2008;358(21):2231–9.
17. Cideciyan AV, Jacobson SG, Beltran WA, Sumaroka A, Swider M, Iwabe S, Roman AJ, Olivares MB, Schwartz SB, Komáromy AM, Hauswirth WW, Aguirre GD. Human retinal gene therapy for Leber congenital amaurosis shows advancing retinal degeneration despite enduring visual improvement. Proc Natl Acad Sci USA. 2013;110(6):E517–2.
18. Dejneka NS, Surace EM, Aleman TS, Cideciyan AV, Lyubarsky A, Savchenko A, Redmond TM, Tang W, Wei Z, Rex TS, Glover E, Maguire AM, Pugh EN Jr, Jacobson SG, Bennett J. In utero gene therapy rescues vision in a murine model of congenital blindness. Mol Ther. 2004;9(2):182–8.
19. Narfström K, Bragadóttir R, Redmond TM, Rakoczy PE, van Veen T, Bruun A. Functional and structural evaluation after AAV.RPE65 gene transfer in the canine model of Leber's congenital amaurosis. Adv Exp Med Biol. 2003a;533:423–30a.
20. Narfström K, Katz ML, Bragadottir R, Seeliger M, Boulanger A, Redmond TM, Caro L, Lai CM, Rakoczy PE. Functional and structural recovery of the retina after gene therapy in the RPE65 null mutation dog. Invest Ophthalmol Vis Sci. 2003b;44(4):1663–72.
21. Jacobson SG, Cideciyan AV, Ratnakaram R, Heon E, Schwartz SB, Roman AJ, Peden MC, Aleman TS, Boye SL, Sumaroka A, Conlon TJ, Calcedo R, Pang JJ, Erger KE, Olivares MB, Mullins CL, Swider M, Kaushal S, Feuer WJ, Iannaccone A, Fishman GA, Stone EM, Byrne BJ, Hauswirth WW. Gene therapy for Leber congenital amaurosis caused by RPE65 mutations: safety and efficacy in 15 children and adults followed up to 3 years. Arch Ophthalmol. 2012;130(1):9–24.
22. Testa F, Maguire AM, Rossi S, Pierce EA, Melillo P, Marshall K, Banfi S, Surace EM, Sun J, Acerra C, Wright JF, Wellman J, High KA, Auricchio A, Bennett J, Simonelli F. Three-year follow-up after unilateral subretinal delivery of adeno-associated virus in patients with Leber congenital Amaurosis type 2. Ophthalmology. 2013;120(6):1283–91.
23. Jacobson SG, Cideciyan AV, Roman AJ, Sumaroka A, Schwartz SB, Heon E, Hauswirth WW. Improvement and decline in vision with gene therapy in childhood blindness. N Engl J Med. 2015;372(20):1920–6.
24. Collin RW, den Hollander AI, Van der Velde-Visser SD, Bennicelli J, Bennett J, Cremers FP. Antisense oligonucleotide (AON)-based therapy for Leber congenital amaurosis caused by a frequent mutation in CEP290. Mol Ther Nucleic Acids. 2012;1:e14.
25. Pawlyk BS, Bulgakov OV, Liu X, Xu X, Adamian M, Sun X, Khani SC, Berson EL, Sandberg MA, Li T. Replacement gene therapy with a human RPGRIP1 sequence slows photoreceptor degeneration in a murine model of Leber congenital amaurosis. Hum Gene Ther. 2010;21(8):993–1004.
26. Kumaran N, Michaelides M, Smith AJ, Ali RR, Bainbridge JWB. Retinal gene therapy. Br Med Bull. 2018;126(1):13–2.
27. Martinez-Fernandez De La Camara C, Nanda A, Salvetti AP, Fischer MD, MacLaren RE. Gene therapy for the treatment of X-linked retinitis pigmentosa. Expert Opin Orphan Drugs. 2018;6(3):167–77.
28. Dimopoulos IS, Hoang SC, Radziwon A, Binczyk NM, Seabra MC, MacLaren RE, Somani R, Tennant MTS, MacDonald IM. Two-year results after AAV2-mediated gene therapy for choroideremia: the Alberta experience. Am J Ophthalmol. 2018;193:130–42.
29. Xue K, Jolly JK, Barnard AR, Rudenko A, Salvetti AP, Patrício MI, Edwards TL, Groppe M, Orlans HO, Tolmachova T, Black GC, Webster AR, Lotery AJ, Holder GE, Downes SM, Seabra MC, MacLaren RE. Beneficial effects on vision in patients undergoing retinal gene therapy for choroideremia. Nat Med. 2018;24(10):1507–12.
30. Zein WM, Jeffrey BG, Wiley HE, Turriff AE, Tumminia SJ, Tao W, Bush RA, Marangoni D, Wen R, Wei LL, Sieving PA. CNGB3-achromatopsia clinical trial with CNTF: diminished rod pathway responses with no evidence of improvement in cone function. Invest Ophthalmol Vis Sci. 2014;55(10):6301–8.
31. Shaikh RS, Reuter P, Sisk RA, Kausar T, Shahzad M, Maqsood MI, Yousif A, Ali M, Riazuddin S, Wissinger B, Ahmed ZM. Homozygous missense variant in the human CNGA3 channel causes cone-rod dystrophy. Eur J Hum Genet. 2015;23(4):473–80.
32. Cukras C, Wiley HE, Jeffrey BG, Sen HN, Turriff A, Zeng Y, Vijayasarathy C, Marangoni D, Ziccardi L, Kjellstrom S, Park TK, Hiriyanna S, Wright JF, Colosi P, Wu Z, Bush RA, Wei LL, Sieving PA. Retinal AAV8-RS1 gene therapy for X-linked retinoschisis: initial findings from a phase I/IIa trial by intravitreal delivery. Mol Ther. 2018;26(9):2282–94.
33. Ghazi NG, Abboud EB, Nowilaty SR, Alkuraya H, Alhommadi A, Cai H, Hou R, Deng WT, Boye SL, Almaghamsi A, Al Saikhan F, Al-Dhibi H, Birch D, Chung C, Colak D, LaVail MM, Vollrath D, Erger K, Wang W, Conlon T, Zhang K, Hauswirth W, Alkuraya FS. Treatment of retinitis pigmentosa due to MERTK mutations by ocular subretinal injection of adeno-associated virus gene vector: results of a phase I trial. Hum Genet. 2016;135(3):327–43.
34. Hussain RM, Ciulla TA, Berrocal AM, Gregori NZ, Flynn HW Jr, Lam BL. Stargardt macular dystrophy and evolving therapies. Expert Opin Biol Ther. 2018;18(10):1049–59.
35. Hassall MM, Barnard AR, MacLaren RE. Gene therapy for color blindness. Yale J Biol Med. 2017;90(4):543–51.

36. Peddle CF, MacLaren RE. The application of CRISPR/Cas9 for the treatment of retinal diseases. Yale J Biol Med. 2017;90(4):533–41.
37. Cayouette M, Gravel C. Adenovirus-mediated gene transfer of ciliary neurotrophic factor can prevent photoreceptor degeneration in the retinal degeneration (rd) mouse. Hum Gene Ther. 1997;8(4):423–30.
38. Tolone A, Belhadj S, Rentsch A, Schwede F, Paquet-Durand F. The cGMP pathway and inherited photoreceptor degeneration: targets, compounds, and biomarkers. Genes (Basel). 2019;10(6):453.
39. Koenekoop RK, Sui R, Sallum J, van den Born LI, Ajlan R, Khan A, den Hollander AI, Cremers FP, Mendola JD, Bittner AK, Dagnelie G, Schuchard RA, Saperstein DA. Oral 9-cis retinoid for childhood blindness due to Leber congenital amaurosis caused by RPE65 or LRAT mutations: an open-label phase 1b trial. Lancet. 2014;384(9953):1513–2.
40. Schwartz SD, Tan G, Hosseini H, Nagiel A. Subretinal transplantation of embryonic stem cell-derived retinal pigment epithelium for the treatment of macular degeneration: an assessment at 4 years. Invest Ophthalmol Vis Sci. 2016;57(5):ORSFc1–9.
41. Schwartz SD, Tan G, Hosseini H, Nagiel A. Let there be light: gene and cell therapy for blindness. Hum Gene Ther. 2016;27(2):134–47.
42. Burnight ER, Wiley LA, Mullins RF, Stone EM, Tucker BA. Gene therapy using stem cells. Cold Spring Harb Perspect Med. 2014;5(4):017434.
43. Margalit E, Maia M, Weiland JD, Greenberg RJ, Fujii GY, Torres G, Piyathaisere DV, O'Hearn TM, Liu W, Lazzi G, Dagnelie G, Scribner DA, de Juan E Jr, Humayun MS. Retinal prosthesis for the blind. Surv Ophthalmol. 2002;47(4):335–56.
44. Sadato N, Okada T, Kubota K, Yonekura Y. Tactile discrimination activates the visual cortex of the recently blind naive to Braille: a functional magnetic resonance imaging study in humans. Neurosci Lett. 2004;359(1–2):49–52.
45. Weiland JD, Humayun MS. Retinal prosthesis. IEEE Trans Biomed Eng. 2014;61(5):1412–24.
46. Luo YH, da Cruz L. The Argus(®) II retinal prosthesis system. Prog Retin Eye Res. 2016;50:89–107.
47. Luo YH, Fukushige E, Da Cruz L. The potential of the second sight system bionic eye implant for partial sight restoration. Expert Rev Med Devices. 2016;13(7):673–8.
48. Dagnelie G, Christopher P, Arditi A, da Cruz L, Duncan JL, Ho AC, Olmos de Koo LC, Sahel JA, Stanga PE, Thumann G, Wang Y, Arsiero M, Dorn JD, Greenberg RJ. Argus® II study group. Performance of real-world functional vision tasks by blind subjects improves after implantation with the Argus® II retinal prosthesis system. Clin Experiment Ophthalmol. 2017;45(2):152–9.

Retinal Surgical Techniques for Gene Therapy

35

Manickam Nick Muthiah, Sui Chien Wong, Michel Michaelides, and James W. Bainbridge

35.1 Introduction

Recent successes in trials of gene therapy for *RPE65* Leber Congenital Amaurosis (LCA) [1–8] have led to the first United States Food and Drug Administration (FDA) and European Medicines Agency (EMA)-approved gene therapy for inherited eye disease, voretigene neparvovec (Luxturna, Spark Therapeutics, Philadelphia, Pennsylvania), a recombinant adeno-associated virus (rAAV) vector containing the cDNA for *RPE65* [9].

The efficacy of this novel therapy depends on an appropriate surgical technique for administration to the retina. Intravitreal delivery of AAV vectors can result in transduction of ganglion cells but targeting of the outer retina is currently relatively inefficient.

M. N. Muthiah (✉)
Bristol Eye Hospital, Bristol, UK

Moorfields Eye Hospital and UCL Institute of Ophthalmology, London, UK

S. C. Wong
Moorfields Eye Hospital, Great Ormond Street Hospital and Royal Free Hospital, London, UK
e-mail: chien.wong1@nhs.net

M. Michaelides · J. W. Bainbridge
Moorfields Eye Hospital and UCL Institute of Ophthalmology, London, UK
e-mail: michel.michaelides@ucl.ac.uk; j.bainbridge@ucl.ac.uk

A. Jain et al. (eds.), *Cutting-edge Vitreoretinal Surgery*, https://doi.org/10.1007/978-981-33-4168-5_35

Intravitreal (IVT) injection [10] is technically simple to perform but targeting of retinal cells is limited by significant dilution of vector suspension within the vitreous gel, and by the anatomical barriers of the posterior hyaloid and inner limiting membranes. Delivery of AAV vector under the inner limiting membrane (ILM) can enhance targeting of cells in the outer retina, but this does not match the efficiency of subretinal delivery for targeting of photoreceptor and retinal pigment epithelial (RPE) cells [11]. In the non-human primate, IVT injection can result in significant extraocular dissemination of rAAV to the systemic circulation and the lymphatic system [12], which may partly account for the increased frequency of intraocular inflammation associated with IVT compared to subretinal AAV delivery. The recent phase 1/2a clinical trial for X-linked retinoschisis (*RS1* gene) with intravitreal injection of adeno-associated virus (AAV8-*RS1*) (NCT02317887) also resulted in dose-related intraocular inflammation [13]. Another X-linked retinoschisis gene therapy trial (NCT02416622) with IVT delivery was also pro-inflammatory and showed no efficacy [14]. Therefore, the immunogenic response triggered following intravitreal delivery of viral vector could attenuate any potential therapeutic response.

For reliable and efficient targeting of photoreceptors or RPE cells, currently available vectors are delivered subretinally, see Fig. 35.1. Injection into the potential space between photoreceptor

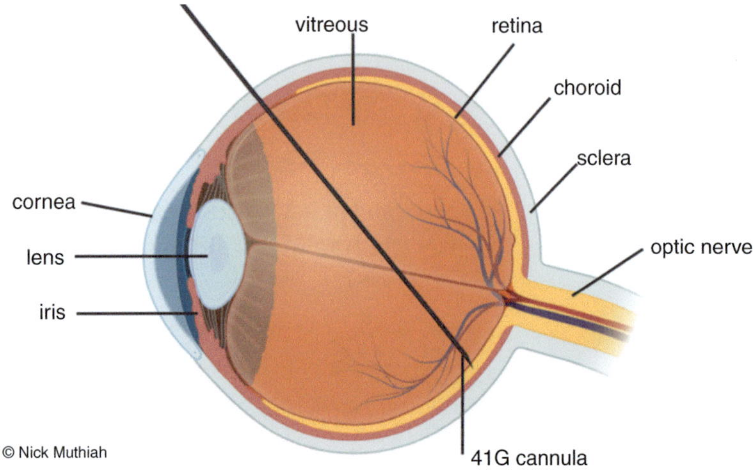

Fig. 35.1 Illustration of 41G cannula advanced into the subretinal space for gene delivery to outer retina

cells and the underlying RPE cells generates a bleb of vector suspension, the limits of which define the extent of the outer retina directly exposed to vector particles. Precision is required to ensure effective administration of vector to the target cells, while minimising harm to the neurosensory retina owing to stretching and protracted separation from the underlying RPE/choroid.

35.2 Imaging

35.2.1 Pre-operative Imaging

Since gene supplementation therapy can benefit only viable target cells these should be identified and mapped appropriately prior to vector administration. The area of viable outer retina can be most readily identified pre-operatively by optical coherence tomography (OCT) and fundus autofluorescence (FAF) imaging. Adaptive optics (AO) imaging can also help assess the extent and location of viable RPE cells, photoreceptor outer segments and inner segments [15–17].

35.2.2 Intra-operative Imaging

Intraoperative optical coherence tomography (*i*OCT) can provide valuable real-time imaging of the retina [18, 19], to confirm accurate localisation of vector delivery and the extent of the vector bleb, see Fig. 35.2. *i*OCT has been employed in locating the site of retinotomy when balanced salt solution and viral vector injections are to be administered through the same site as the site can self-seal or if it remains open at end of procedure, to reduce the risk of macular hole in a thinned retina during subretinal injection, to ensure the posterior hyaloid membrane is fully detached prior to the insertion of subretinal cannula through the inner limiting membrane, to assess reflux post-vector injection and to assess for presence of air bubble subretinally [19–21]. Head-up displays on new microscope platforms enable a surgeon to visualise changes occurring at the level of a retinal lamellae in real time, thereby reducing the risk of tissue trauma and incorrect target location during delivery of vector.

35.2.3 Post-operative Imaging

The outer retina is assessed post-operatively by optical coherence tomography (OCT) and fundus autofluorescence (FAF) imaging to assess for early changes at the outer lamellar layers; anticipated early absorption of subretinal vector and to identify any potential adverse events, i.e. retinal thinning, macular hole, presence of subretinal fluid, localised neurosensory detachments and the state of RPE, i.e. atrophy [6, 22]. AO imaging

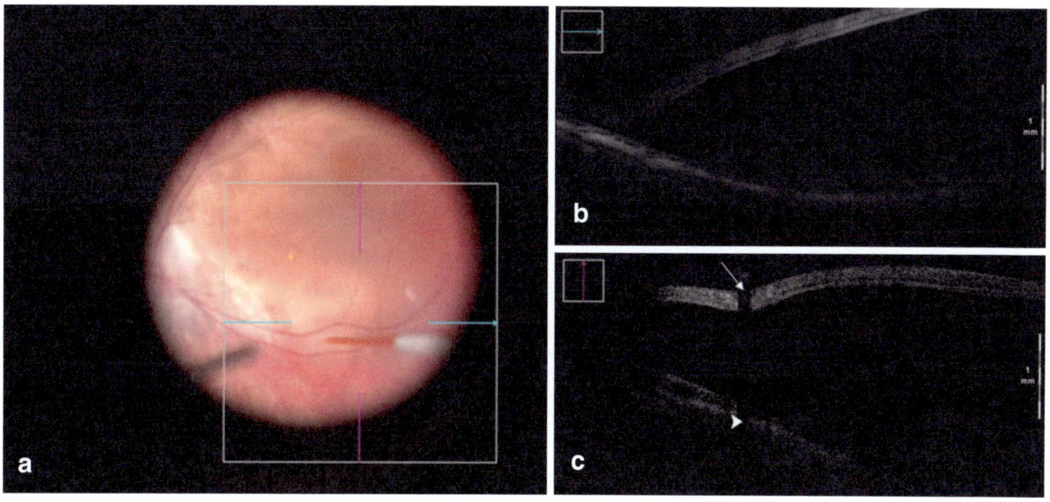

Fig. 35.2 *i*OCT image-guided subretinal delivery. (**a**) Real-time fundus image showing the overlay of OCT scan: vertical (purple) and horizontal (blue) lines where the OCT scan is captured intra-operatively. (**b**) Horizontal OCT scan demonstrating subretinal bleb. (**c**) Vertical OCT scan demonstrating the retinal entry point (arrow—retinotomy) and shadow from 41G subretinal cannula (arrowhead)

system enables post-operative assessment of treatment outcomes, to identify rescue of photoreceptors at an individual cell level [23, 24].

35.3 Anaesthesia

Care should be taken to minimise unplanned movements during vector administration because this presents a risk of harm from stretching of the retinotomy with consequent unintended reflux of vector suspension into the vitreous cavity. General anaesthesia is helpful in controlling for this but periocular (sub-Tenon's or peribulbar) anaesthesia are alternatives for a patient with predictable compliance.

35.4 Subretinal Gene Delivery

The *in vivo* development of vectors for retinal gene therapy has relied mainly on experimental work in mice, using predominantly an *ab externo* (trans-scleral) approach for subretinal injection [25–27]. Preclinical evaluation in larger animals have identified a substantial risk of vector reflux and estimated a 10% risk of harm from iatrogenic retinal perforation [26].

Subretinal injection of vector may be preceded by an injection of a small volume of fluid (balanced salt solution) to establish a small bleb (often referred to as a 'pre-bleb') in the intended tissue plane, into which the vector can subsequently be administered. This technique may reduce the volume of vector introduced unintentionally into the vitreous cavity or deep retinal layers, and preserve vector for administration to the target area [1].

To facilitate generation and propagation of the subretinal bleb, the vitreous cavity infusion pressure can be reduced (e.g. to 10 mmHg). Measures to protect the neurosensory retina against undue stretch include capping the injection pressure (e.g. at 10 PSI) and minimising the height and duration of the bleb formed [28]. One or more retinotomies may be used to administer vector to the target retina—which may also help to reduce excess stretch and/or height of detachment. Fluid–air exchange can be used to extend a bleb across a target area if this is not otherwise achievable by injection of a greater volume of vector suspension.

35.4.1 Surgical Steps for Subretinal Gene Delivery

It is critical that the surgeon follows specific instructions as per gene therapy manufacturer.

The eye is cleaned and draped.

Superotemporal, superonasal and inferonasal conjunctival peritomies are made for trocar insertion. 25G trocars are inserted at a distance from the limbus according to age. Wide-angle viewing system is centred on disc. High-speed cutters are used. Posterior vitreous detachment (PVD) is induced.

AAV vector is thawed and diluted if appropriate in theatre under sterile conditions according to the manufacturer's instructions. The vector for injection (take into consideration the dead space) is drawn into a syringe with subretinal 41G cannula.

Infusion pressure is set at 5 mmHg. Subretinal injection is given via retinotomy site according to the target area (e.g. superotemporal arcade) to create bleb. Injection pressured is controlled using automated fluid injection with foot-pedal control (ideally under *i*OCT guidance). The area and extent of bleb (including involvement of the fovea) can be controlled by the volume injected and subsequent injection of air if appropriate, see Fig. 35.3.

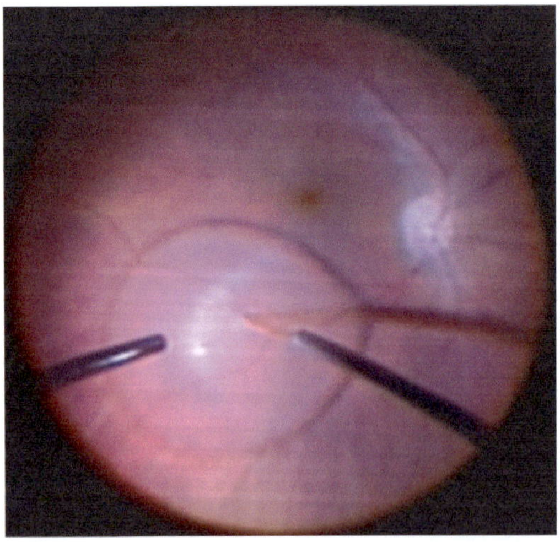

Fig. 35.3 Subretinal bleb following injection with a 41G cannula

Retinal periphery is examined 360° to look for any retinal break. Vitreous cavity fluid is washed out to minimise the persistence of refluxed vector. Scleral ports are closed with 7/0 or 8/0 vicryl followed by conjunctival closure.

35.5 Surgical Complications of Transvitreous Subretinal Surgery

Surgical complications of transvitreous subretinal injection of viral vector include unplanned retinal detachment owing to persistent retinotomies or iatrogenic peripheral retinal breaks. Full-thickness macular hole has been reported, intra-operatively and post-operatively [2, 29]. Thinning of the outer retina has been described [6, 30], but can be minimised with careful attention to surgical technique; as evidenced by data showing stability of foveal thickness in a Phase I/II trial investigating an optimised viral vector for *RPE65*-associated LCA (NCT 02781480) [31]. An uncommon but significant sight-threatening risks with either IVT or subretinal injection is endophthalmitis, with rates of 0.021% to 0.05% in the former [32, 33]. *One* instance of bacterial *Staphylococcus epidermidis* endophthalmitis has been reported following subretinal injection of rAAV vector in another *RPE65* trial [7]. Cataract is a predictable longer-term consequence of vitrectomy surgery [7], and may develop more rapidly in the context of retinal degeneration.

35.6 New Surgical Developments

Alongside the improvements in intra-operative imaging to achieve precision delivery of the AAV vector to the subretinal space, the potential of robotic assistance to improve the surgical precision of vector delivery by mechanically stabilising the introduction and holding position of the subretinal cannula is being evaluated with PRECEYES Surgical System (Preceyes BV, Eindhoven, Netherlands) [34–37].

Various devices and routes of gene delivery to the outer retina have been studied over the years.

Recent developments in microneedles [38, 39], could potentially enable a reliable trans-scleral route for subretinal gene delivery.

Suprachoroidal route of injections of RGX-314 (AAV8 viral vector expressing anti-VEGF Fab) have recently been found to achieve equivalent transgene expression of anti-VEGF Fab in retina and RPE along with similar reduction in VEGF-induced vascular leakage as subretinal injections in animal models [40].

Regenxbio has been running a Phase I/II, dose-escalation study of subretinal RGX-314 to evaluate the safety and tolerability in patients with neovascular age-related macular degeneration (AMD) previously treated with anti-VEGF drugs (NCT03066258), with promising preliminary results [41, 42]. It is currently preparing to start suprachoroidal delivery trials for neovascular AMD and diabetic retinopathy in 2020 [43]. A more posterior delivery of therapeutic agents with greater exposure to retina and RPE was noted in another preclinical study employing this route [44]. In the past, researchers have inserted an iTrack microcatheter (iTrack 400, iScience Interventional Corporation, Menlo Park, CA, USA) into the suprachoroidal space to deliver a combination of triamcinolone and bevacizumab submacularly in a clinical trial of 21 patients with neovascular AMD [45]. In this study, one eye had a transient increase in intraocular pressure at 3 months follow-up and two eyes had progression of nuclear sclerotic cataract, these risks were most likely to be secondary to the triamcinolone rather than the procedure itself. The benefits outweigh the risks with suprachoroidal route in that it is potentially a safer approach not requiring posterior segment (vitrectomy) surgery and the procedure could be delivered in an out-patient setting.

Finally, transchoroidal approach has also been studied in animal models, though the risk of entering the choriocapillaris layer is not without significant risks as firstly it is not under direct visualisation and secondly in this highly vascular bed the risk of inducing an immune response is high [46].

35.7 Future of Gene Therapy

The promise of gene therapy is not just confined to the field of inherited retinal degenerations. It can also be utilised to tackle the increasing socio-economic burden of neovascular AMD and diabetic retinopathy associated with current long-term requirement for regular intravitreal anti-VEGF injections in these patients. The potential increase in gene therapy for these therapeutic areas, new targets along with the need to develop safer viral vector delivery systems to ensure effective expression of the genes necessitates an urgent need to investigate all routes of vector delivery; subretinal, intravitreal and suprachoroidal and develop new devices to ensure success during clinical trials.

Vitreoretinal surgeons delivering these gene therapies can ensure success for individual patients by pre-planning surgery with accurate OCT, FAF and AO retinal image mapping and using intra-operative OCT image guidance for precision delivery of the viral vector.

References

1. Bainbridge JW, Smith AJ, Barker SS, et al. Effect of gene therapy on visual function in Leber's congenital amaurosis. N Engl J Med. 2008;358(21):2231–9.
2. Maguire AM, Simonelli F, Pierce EA, et al. Safety and efficacy of gene transfer for Leber's congenital amaurosis. N Engl J Med. 2008;358(21):2240–8.
3. Maguire AM, High KA, Auricchio A, et al. Age-dependent effects of RPE65 gene therapy for Leber's congenital amaurosis: a phase 1 dose-escalation trial. Lancet. 2009;374(9701):1597–605.
4. Jacobson SG, Cideciyan AV, Ratnakaram R, et al. Gene therapy for leber congenital amaurosis caused by RPE65 mutations: safety and efficacy in 15 children and adults followed up to 3 years. Arch Ophthalmol. 2012;130(1):9–24.
5. Cideciyan AV, Jacobson SG, Beltran WA, et al. Human retinal gene therapy for Leber congenital amaurosis shows advancing retinal degeneration despite enduring visual improvement. Proc Natl Acad Sci USA. 2013;110(6):E517–25.
6. Bainbridge JW, Mehat MS, Sundaram V, et al. Long-term effect of gene therapy on Leber's congenital amaurosis. N Engl J Med. 2015;372(20):1887–97.
7. Bennett J, Wellman J, Marshall KA, et al. Safety and durability of effect of contralateral-eye administration

of AAV2 gene therapy in patients with childhood-onset blindness caused by RPE65 mutations: a follow-on phase 1 trial. Lancet. 2016;388(10045):661–72.
8. Russell S, Bennett J, Wellman JA, et al. Efficacy and safety of voretigene neparvovec (AAV2-hRPE65v2) in patients with RPE65-mediated inherited retinal dystrophy: a randomised, controlled, open-label, phase 3 trial. Lancet. 2017;390(10097):849–60.
9. Food and Drug Administration. FDA approves novel gene therapy to treat patients with a rare form of inherited vision loss. 2017. https://www.fda.gov/NewsEvents/Newsroom/PressAnnouncements/ucm589467.htm. Accessed 31 Dec 2019.
10. Boyd RF, Sledge DG, Boye SL, et al. Photoreceptor-targeted gene delivery using intravitreally administered AAV vectors in dogs. Gene Ther. 2016;23(2):223–30.
11. Boye SE, Alexander JJ, Witherspoon CD, et al. Highly efficient delivery of adeno-associated viral vectors to the primate retina. Hum Gene Ther. 2016;27(8):580–97.
12. Seitz IP, Fischer MD, Michalakis S, Wilhelm B, Kahle N, Zrenner E. rAAV8 biodistribution and shedding after subretinal injection in non-human primates. Invest Ophthalmol Vis Sci. 2016;57:4025.
13. Cukras C, Wiley HE, Jeffrey BG, et al. Retinal AAV8-RS1 gene therapy for X-linked retinoschisis: initial findings from a phase I/IIa trial by Intravitreal delivery. J Am Soc Gene Therapy. 2018;26(9):2282–94.
14. AGTC. AGTC announces topline interim six-month data from phase 1/2 X-linked retinoschisis clinical study; termination of biogen collaboration. 2018. http://ir.agtc.com/node/9661/pdf. Accessed 31 Dec 2019.
15. Sundaram V, Wilde C, Aboshiha J, et al. Retinal structure and function in Achromatopsia: implications for gene therapy. Ophthalmology. 2014;121(1):234–45.
16. Langlo CS, Patterson EJ, Higgins BP, et al. Residual Foveal cone structure in CNGB3-associated Achromatopsia. Invest Ophthalmol Vis Sci. 2016;57(10):3984–95.
17. Patterson EJ, Kalitzeos A, Kasilian M, et al. Residual cone structure in patients with X-linked cone Opsin mutations. Invest Ophthalmol Vis Sci. 2018;59(10):4238–48.
18. Ehlers JP, Dupps WJ, Kaiser PK, et al. The prospective intraoperative and perioperative ophthalmic ImagiNg with optical CoherEncE TomogRaphy (PIONEER) study: 2-year results. Am J Ophthalmol. 2014;158(5):999–1007.
19. Vasconcelos Junior H, Yang P, Pennesi ME, Lujan BJ, Lauer AK. An analysis of intraoperative optical coherence tomography findings in subretinal gene therapy surgery. Invest Ophthalmol Vis Sci. 2019;60(9):6399.
20. Gregori NZ, Lam BL, Davis JL. Intraoperative use of microscope-integrated optical coherence tomography for subretinal gene therapy delivery. Retina. 2019;39:9–12.
21. Xue K, Groppe M, Salvetti AP, MacLaren RE. Technique of retinal gene therapy: delivery of viral vector into the subretinal space. Eye. 2017;31(9):1308–16.
22. Le Meur G, Lebranchu P, Billaud F, et al. Safety and long-term efficacy of AAV4 gene therapy in patients with <em>RPE65</em> Leber congenital Amaurosis. Mol Ther. 2018;26(1):256–68.
23. Talcott KE, Ratnam K, Sundquist SM, et al. Longitudinal study of cone photoreceptors during retinal degeneration and in response to ciliary neurotrophic factor treatment. Invest Ophthalmol Vis Sci. 2011;52(5):2219–26.
24. Muthiah MN, Keane PA, Zhong J, et al. Adaptive optics imaging shows rescue of macula cone photoreceptors. Ophthalmology. 2014;121(1):430–1.
25. Peden MC, Min J, Meyers C, et al. Ab-externo AAV-mediated gene delivery to the suprachoroidal space using a 250 micron flexible microcatheter. PLoS One. 2011;6(2):e17140.
26. Smet MD, de Wyse S, Vezina M, Conston S, Sachs C, Popma SH. Repeated Ab-externo catheterization of the sub-retinal space using a microcatheter for targeted delivery of a cell therapy product in a pig model. Invest Ophthalmol Vis Sci. 2012;53:5844.
27. Fischer MD, Goldmann T, Wallrapp C, et al. Successful subretinal delivery and monitoring of MicroBeads in mice. PLoS One. 2013;8(1):e55173.
28. Fischer MD, Hickey DG, Singh MS, MacLaren RE. Evaluation of an optimized injection system for retinal gene therapy in human patients. Hum Gene Ther Methods. 2016;27(4):150–8.
29. Campochiaro PA, Lauer AK, Sohn EH, et al. Lentiviral vector gene transfer of Endostatin/Angiostatin for macular degeneration (GEM) study. Hum Gene Ther. 2017;28(1):99–111.
30. Jacobson SG, Acland GM, Aguirre GD, et al. Safety of recombinant adeno-associated virus type 2-RPE65 vector delivered by ocular subretinal injection. Mol Ther. 2006;13(6):1074–84.
31. Michaelides M, Kumaran N, Georgiadis T, et al. Results of a phase 1/2 trial of an optimized gene therapy in adults and children with retinal dystrophy associated with bi-allelic variants in RPE65. Paper presented at the Retina Society. 2019. https://www.retinasociety.org/content/documents/retina_society_2019_program_london_v5.pdf. Accessed 19 Apr 2020.
32. Bhavsar AR, Ip MS, Glassman AR. Drcrnet, the SSG. The risk of endophthalmitis following intravitreal triamcinolone injection in the DRCRnet and SCORE clinical trials. Am J Ophthalmol. 2007;144(3):454–6.
33. Dossarps D, Bron AM, Koehrer P, Aho-Glele LS, Creuzot-Garcher C, Net F. Endophthalmitis after Intravitreal injections: incidence, presentation, management, and visual outcome. Am J Ophthalmol. 2015;160(1):17–25.
34. Meenink T, Naus G, de Smet M, Beelen M, Steinbuch M. Robot assistance for micrometer precision in vitreoretinal surgery. Invest Ophthalmol Vis Sci. 2013;54(15):5808.

35. de Smet MD, Meenink TCM, Janssens T, et al. Robotic assisted cannulation of occluded retinal veins. PLoS One. 2016;11(9):–0162037.
36. de Smet MD, Stassen JM, Meenink TCM, et al. Release of experimental retinal vein occlusions by direct intraluminal injection of ocriplasmin. Br J Ophthalmol. 2016;100(12):1742–6.
37. Edwards TL, Xue K, Meenink HCM, et al. First-in-human study of the safety and viability of intraocular robotic surgery. Nature Biomed Eng. 2018;2:649–56.
38. Patel SR, Lin AS, Edelhauser HF, Prausnitz MR. Suprachoroidal drug delivery to the back of the eye using hollow microneedles. Pharm Res. 2011;28(1):166–76.
39. Jiang J, Moore JS, Edelhauser HF, Prausnitz MR. Intrascleral drug delivery to the eye using hollow microneedles. Pharm Res. 2009;26(2):395–403.
40. Ding K, Shen J, Hafiz Z, et al. AAV8-vectored suprachoroidal gene transfer produces widespread ocular transgene expression. J Clin Invest. 2019;129(11):4901–11.
41. AAO. 2019 daily. Gene therapy for wet AMD? 2019. https://www.aao.org/eyenet/academy-live/detail/gene-therapy-wet-amd-3. Accessed 17 Apr 2020.
42. REGENXBIO. REGENXBIO announces additional positive interim phase I/IIa trial update for RGX-134 for the treatment of wet AMD at the American Academy of Ophthalmology 2019 annual meeting. 2019. https://www.prnewswire.com/news-releases/regenxbio-announces-additional-positive-interim-phase-iiia-trial-update-for-rgx-314-for-the-treatment-of-wet-amd-at-the-american-academy-of-ophthalmology-2019-annual-meeting-300937385.htm. Accessed 17 Apr 2020.
43. REGENXBIO. REGENXBIO reports continued progress across programs in year-end 2019 corporate update. 2020. https://www.prnewswire.com/news-releases/regenxbio-reports-continued-progress-across-programs-in-year-end-2019-corporate-update-300983973.html. Accessed 17 Apr 2020.
44. Habot-Wilner Z, Noronha G, Wykoff CC. Suprachoroidally injected pharmacological agents for the treatment of chorio-retinal diseases: a targeted approach. Acta Ophthalmol. 2019;97(5):460–72.
45. Tetz M, Rizzo S, Augustin AJ. Safety of submacular suprachoroidal drug administration via a microcatheter: retrospective analysis of European treatment results. Ophthalmologica. 2012;227(4):183–9.
46. Bennett J, Chung DC, Maguire A. Gene delivery to the retina: from mouse to man. Methods Enzymol. 2012;507:255–74.

Part XI

Miscellaneous

Surgical Management of Retinopathy of Prematurity

36

Komal Agarwal, Sushma Jayanna, and Subhadra Jalali

36.1 Introduction

Retinopathy of prematurity (ROP) is becomming one of the leading causes of blindness in children in our country and in the developing world. Screening of premature neonates as per the National guidelines of various countries, is mandatory to identify on time the vision-threatening ROP. Early stages of ROP can be well managed by laser photocoagulation. Surgical approach becomes a mandate in ROP once tractional retinal detachment sets in.

Surgical management of ROP has been evolving over decades. Once considered as an inoperable disease, tractional retinal detachments in ROP are now well managed due to both better instrumentation and also changing expectations of surgical outcomes. This chapter aims to review goals, techniques, and advancements in the surgical management of ROP.

36.2 Applied Anatomy and Instrumentation [1, 2]

Poorly developed structures and size and shape differences of the infantile eye when compared to adults, needs to be understood to face multiple challenges in infantile eye VR surgeries. Since the pars plana in infants of less than 6 month age is incompletely developed, the usual adult entry site of 4 mm from limbus will damage the retina. An anterior entry, usually 1.0–1.5 mm from limbus is advised (Fig. 36.1). A more anterior entry through iris root or through limbus into anterior chamber is preferred when handling case of Stage 5 retinopathy of prematurity (ROP), where the retinal

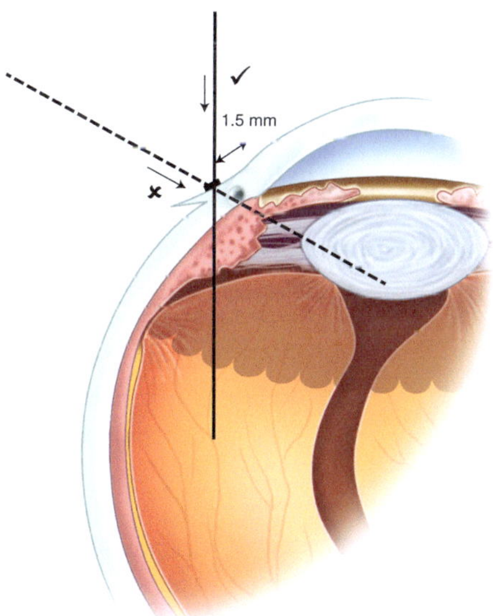

Fig. 36.1 Diagrammatic representation showing the entry site 1.0–1.5 mm from limbus with more vertically oriented ports. Silicone band at the base of the cannula avoids complete penetration of instruments. Angulated usual entry would touch the lens as shown

K. Agarwal · S. Jayanna · S. Jalali (✉)
L V Prasad Eye Institute, Hyderabad, India
e-mail: drkomalagarwal@lvpei.org; drsushma@lvpei.org; subhadra@lvpei.org

A. Jain et al. (eds.), *Cutting-edge Vitreoretinal Surgery*,
https://doi.org/10.1007/978-981-33-4168-5_36

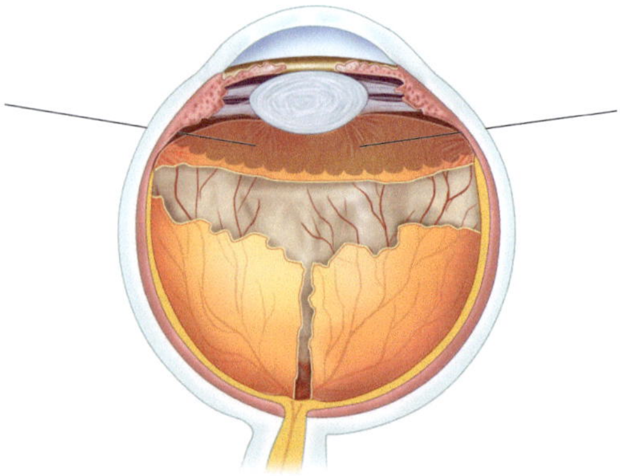

Fig. 36.2 Horizontal entry through iris root into the lens during Stage 5 ROP surgery because retinal folds are present at the usual entry site

folds will be lying much anterior even to the retrolental plane (Fig. 36.2). In some advanced cases, the lens is also displaced anteriorly. Sites of entry: entry at 3'clock and 9'clock hours provide maximum space in these eyes with narrow palpebral fissures; inadvertent damage to long posterior ciliary nerves and vessels does not happen as they enter the globe much posterior to 1.0 mm from limbus. These entry meridians avoid lens and retinal touch with improved access. A more vertical entry is preferred to prevent lens touch, because the lens is quite large in these eyes vis-à-vis the size of the vitreous cavity (Fig. 36.1). Lateral canthotomy may be needed in some eyes.

The Vitreous in neonates and infants is densely adherent to surface of retina, making PVD induction much difficult. Also, it is a relatively immature gel and feels blubbery and very thick while cutting with cutter. Fetal hyaloid vasculature and Tunica vasculosa lentis usually regress from 18 to 35 weeks of gestation respectively. A significant number of ROP eyes with tractional retinal detachment have persistent fetal vasculature stalk which provides a scaffold around which the retinal tissues "curl around." Removal of this stalk is one of the surgical goals in Stages 5 and 4 B, ROP surgeries.

Cornea is much steeper in neonates and smaller in size, with the maximum horizontal diameter of 9–10.5 mm and a vertical diameter of 9.9–10.5 mm. The axial length of neonatal eye ball is approximately 16.5–17.5 mm. Using surgical instruments designed for adult eye in such small eyes is difficult. Small size and more steep base of the viewing lenses or using a BIOM help in better visualization. Similarly, instruments designed for infantile eyes can be used, which would be of smaller length. As an alternative, we use a trimmed silicone band at the base of the trocar to shorten the effective length inside the eye (Fig. 36.1). Neonatal sclera is much pliable and less tensile compared to adults, and hence either one should suture sclerotomy ports or have a different type of entry for sutureless surgeries. Cut through of sclera/cornea with trocar or sutures can occur-tiny bites and delicate handling are needed. Other instruments designed for infantile retinal surgeries include 23 G cannula or scalp vein needle alone serving as infusion tip, infusion spatula, infusion forceps, retractable lighted picks, irrigating, and illuminated pick and wide-angle high-flow light pipe. Advantage of using large gauge instruments include easy removal of stiffer proliferative tissues through large-sized ports, whereas small gauge ports are more safer, which can be freely moved behind the large lens. While doing lens sparing vitrectomy, only a limited area inside the eye can be reached safely (Fig. 36.3).

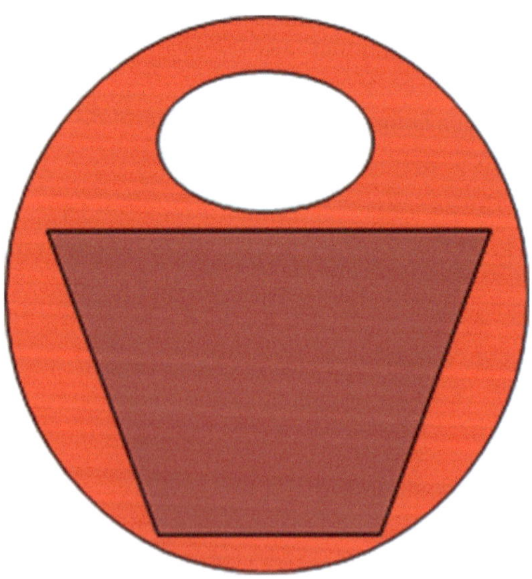

Fig. 36.3 The area inside the eyeball available during safe lens-sparing vitrectomy

36.3 Pathophysiology

Retinal detachments in ROP are mainly due to progressive vitreous traction, which distorts and stretches the infantile elastic retina, causing a tractional retinal detachment (TRD). This traction starts developing at the edge of the vascular and avascular retina/ridge. Glial proliferation occurs at the posterior cortical vitreous and the retinal surface. Inflammatory mediators play a crucial role at this stage leading to vitreous condensation and contraction. Contraction of this causes the ridge and the surrounding retina to tent and lift causing retinal elevation. Retinal tissues are healthy and vascularized behind the ridge and do not have ischemia and hence are very viable. Anterior avascular retina also gets vascularized in many eyes subsequently. Further contraction and elastic nature of the *neonatal* retina, that allows retina to stretch to larger surface area, facilitates anterior placement of these retinal folds till the vitreous cavity is decreased to minimum. Also, proliferation of the persistent fetal vasculature from the disc acts as a scaffold worsening the tractional detachment and causing a funnel centrally. Proliferation along the rudimentary anterior hyaloid along the posterior lens surface forms a retrolental membrane that along with the peripheral ridge causes a circumferential trough. TRDs are progressive in nature in most eyes. Unlike typical PVR, there are no RPE cells and metaplasia seen due to absence of retinal breaks in most of the eyes.

Various vectors are responsible for different configurations seen in tractional detachments of ROP (Fig. 36.4). These are:

1. Ridge to ridge
2. Ridge to lens
3. Ridge to ciliary body
4. Ridge to optic disc or posterior retina
5. Ridge to anterior retina
6. Intrinsic vector forces to the retina worsened by the persistent fetal vasculature stalk

Transection of these vector forces to the extent possible, without creating any retinal tear, is the mainstay to settling these complex retinal detachments.

Besides TRD, there can be other types of coexisting detachments including exudative detachments and very rarely rhegmatogenous detachments that may be seen in acute phase rarely, though mostly they are seen in older years of age.

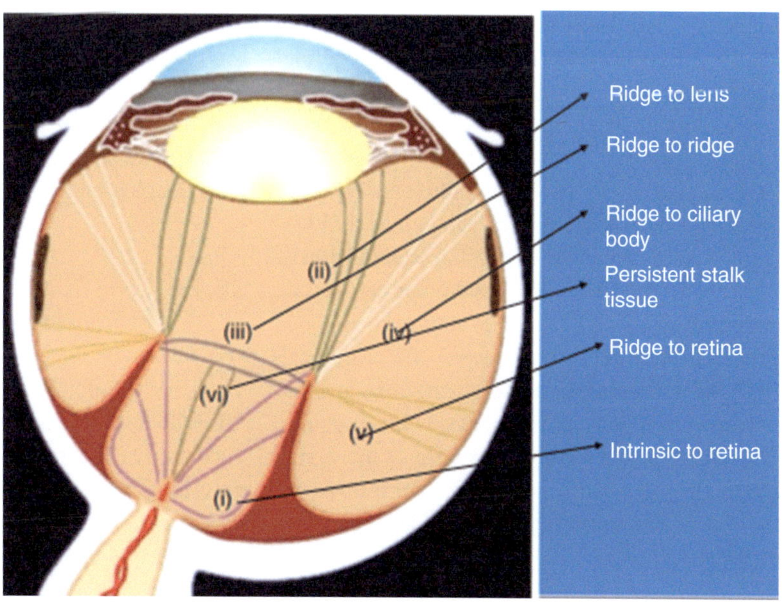

Fig. 36.4 Vector forces causing the tractional retinal detachment, that need removal

36.4 Goals, Indications, Techniques, and Outcomes of Management [3–7]

Indications for vitreoretinal surgical management in ROP are limited and specific. These are:

1. Progressive Stages 4A and 4B ROP tractional retinal detachments
2. Stage 5 ROP
3. Non-resolving vitreous hemorrhage
4. Rhegmatogenous retinal detachments

Goals in the surgical management of ROP are widely different from rhegmatogenous retinal reattachment surgeries in adults. It is critical to remove major points of traction, taking care not to cause any retinal break. Surgery for Stage 4 A aims at complete retinal reattachment with no or minimal macular distortion. Partial retinal reattachment with prevention of further tractional elevation is the goal in surgery for Stage 4B. Complete Retinal reattachment is difficult after surgery for Stage 5 ROP. Only a few surgeons realize that Stage 5 ROP TRD eyes need surgery also early enough because they are also progressive in nature. In such cases, one aims for attachment of posterior pole and as much as peripheral retina as possible, without causing a break. Untreated ROP detachments may progress sooner or later. Eyes with stable cicatricial ROP can be observed if there are no active tractional elements present.

Functional Visual recovery and success deteriorate rapidly with advanced stages of ROP. Stage 4 A ROP has universally good outcomes with most babies achieving 20/50 or better vision. Stage 4 B eyes often attain vision of 20/800 to 20/400 with stable retinal status. Ambulatory vision to some level of form vision is expected after successful surgery for a Stage 5 ROP. Myopic glasses are often needed in most vitrectomized lens sparing eyes while aphakic glasses are needed after successful Stage 5 surgeries. It is therefore very important to counsel the caregivers regarding the expected outcomes of surgery.

36.4.1 Scleral Buckle in Acute ROP Detachments

A 240 band encircling element is useful to reattach few selected eyes of Stage 4 A ROP. The anatomical configurations that are best suited include Stage 4 A and very early Stage 4 B detachments where the traction is peripheral and circumferential without any anterioposterior component. Band is placed at the highest site of retinal elevation, often temporally more posterior to equator, while the nasal side of buckle would then be placed obliquely, more anteriorly than equator to get a good grip on the globe and counter the traction effectively. Anterior chamber paracentesis is usually needed to keep IOP low. Care should be taken while handling the fragile extraocular muscles as they can get detached by any extra forceful maneuver. Either sutures or tunnels can be used to secure the element to the sclera. The elements were earlier removed after a year of age of baby, due to the possibility of intrusion into a growing eye. Re-detachment can occur in some eyes after buckle removal. More recently, the trend is only to divide the belt buckle and not remove. Some patients may not return for band excision and we have experienced no complication from retained bands in a large majority of such eyes. During band excision, the band is seen to be in a more posterior position and often not tightly invaginating into the globe, as if the growing globe has escaped out. Postoperatively after 6–8 h, we prefer to remove the bandage and instill a drop of anti-glaucoma medication to keep IOP low and avoid any chance of retinal artery occlusion.

36.4.2 Lens Sparing Vitrectomy in Stages 4A and 4B

The two techniques available for Stages 4A and 4B ROP are scleral buckling and lens sparing vitrectomy. Due to various tractional vectors as described above, lens sparing vitrectomy is the procedure of choice. However, selected cases having limited peripheral traction without a central fetal vasculature tractional component can be managed well with an encircling buckle element. Rhegmatogenous detachments are always best managed by buckling procedures and sometimes by adult types of vitrectomy procedures.

36.4.2.1 Preoperative Ocular Evaluation

A thorough preoperative evaluation "under General anesthesia" is a necessity before surgery. The extent of the detachment should be thoroughly checked before making the incision. Tractional detachments in ROP are complicated by distorted retina that is pulled forward, sometimes to just behind the lens. This results in narrowing of the space for surgical entry. It is, therefore, important to evaluate such anterior traction and folds by careful indirect Ophthalmoscopy and peripheral scleral depression, and modify the placement of sclerotomy sites in order to avoid iatrogenic retinal breaks. Corneal clarity, lens status, and intraocular pressure should be noted before planning the surgery. Aggressive and active tractional detachments can present with iris neovascularization that might lead to both intraoperative and postoperative complications. This should, hence be evaluated before surgery.

36.4.2.2 Timing of the Surgery

Balancing the time of the surgery is critical to achieving favorable outcomes in ROP. Various authors recommend planning a surgery at around the term date (36–38 weeks). Decreased VEGF levels during this period with reduced vascularity decreases the risk of intraoperative bleeding and postoperative re-proliferation. Risk of general anesthesia due to prematurity, anemia, low birth weight, PDA, and an immature lung function is also decreased at this age.

We, however, believe that a prompt treatment is required to prevent progression of Stage 4A disease to achieve best visual outcomes (Fig. 36.5). A preoperative laser photocoagulation to the avascular retina helps to reduce the

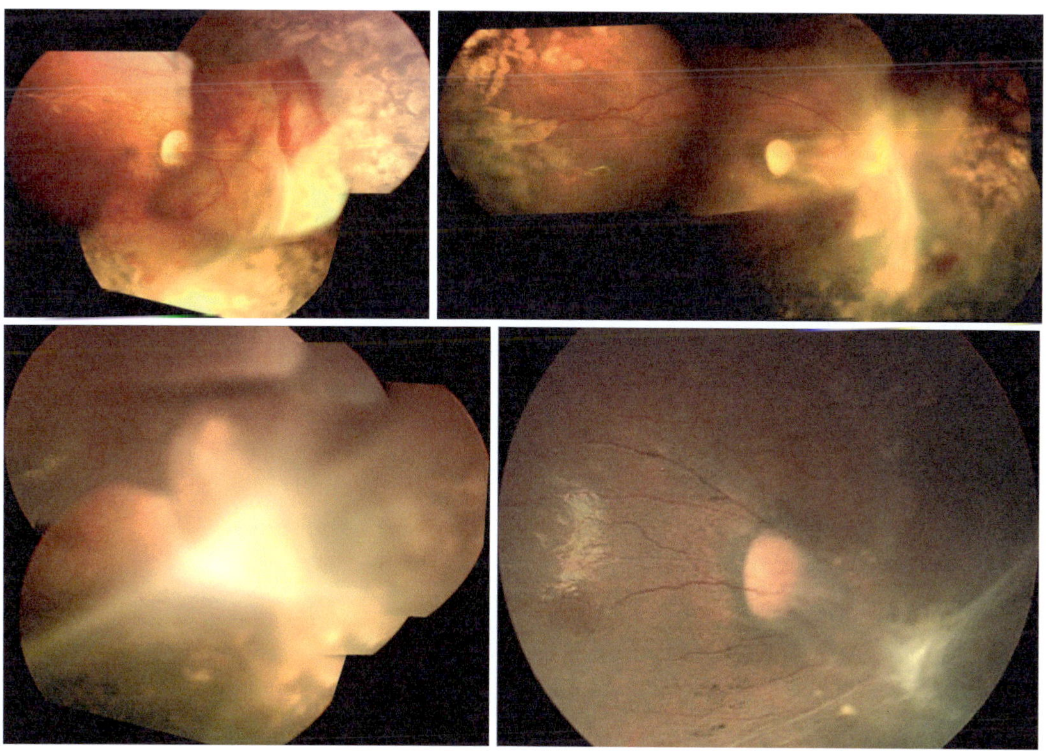

Fig. 36.5 Progressive tractional detachment within 10 days, from nasal side ultimately threatening macular area (first three photos) and result of lens sparing vitrectomy (bottom right). On hind sight, surgery at onset of the nasal side tractional RD (upper left) would have been better

plus and the vascularity of the membranes. It also decreases the risk of intraoperative breaks. The use of anti-VEGF agents to reduce vascularity in Stage 4 is controversial as it may lead to "crunch" phenomena and progression to a combined detachment. However, in selected cases after the fitness for anesthesia is obtained, anti-VEGF injection can be given a day prior to surgery in cases with severe vascular conditions.

36.4.2.3 Steps

Trese described lens sparing 2-port vitrectomy for Stage 4 ROP in 1992. He used a dual endoilluminator-infusion system with a vitrectomy cutter, hence eliminating the need for a third sclerotomy. This decreased the chances of iatrogenic lens touch, but was limited due to difficult maneuvering during pre-equatorial dissection.

With the advent of small gauge systems, a sutureless three-port vitrectomy is the standard of care. Both 23 or 25G systems can be used. Following steps should be performed while managing a Stage 4 ROP:

1. Sclerotomy sites should be decided after a thorough preoperative evaluation of the fundus under anesthesia. The circumferential and the anteroposterior extent of the detachment and the anterior vitreous space should be taken into consideration before deciding sclerotomy sites.
2. Sclerotomies are made 1.0 mm behind the limbus through the pars plicata. Pars plana region is avoided, as it is underdeveloped in preterm infants. The direction of the entry should be parallel to the visual axis, i.e., perpendicular to the scleral surface in order to avoid lens touch (Fig. 36.1). The common entry sites are 3 and 9 0 clock positions for the active hands and inferotemporal for the infusion. As the conjunctiva is adherent so close to the limbus, conjunctival mobilization is from posterior to anterior while entering the eye. That is, the 1.0-mm of bulbar conjunctiva is pulled onto the cornea anterior to the limbus during entry and while closure of sutureless sclerotomy, this is reposited back posteriorly.
3. Initial core vitrectomy is done always starting from the disc or posterior pole as much as possible. This gives a good safety against touching the relatively large-sized lens that can happen if we start anteriorly. Careful vitrectomy is then done to transect all the vector forces causing the detachment. Retinal breaks should be carefully avoided by avoiding "vitreous pulling" or high suction to create PVD. Viewing systems include non-contact and contact wide-field systems, based on surgeons' preference. Small gauge pediatric surgical sets are also now available. We use some sort of bolster of a silicone band on the outside of the cannula to make its intraocular part shorter by a mm or so and hence avoid lens and peripheral retinal touch (Fig. 36.1).
4. Posterior vitreous detachment (PVD), is extremely difficult but not impossible, in infants due to tightly adherent posterior cortical vitreous. An active attempt for PVD can be avoided in most surgeries for ROP. Triamcinolone to visualize vitreous or assist in PVD is used by some. We found that in most cases the vitreous is yellow-tinged and blubbery due to inflammatory and hematological components and is hence easy to visualize even without any adjuncts.
5. Partial or complete fluid air exchange is done after vitrectomy. Suturing is not required in 25G and 23G ports. 20G ports can be sutured with 8-0 or 10-0 absorbable vicryl.
6. Subconjunctival dexamethasone is an option as vitreous studies show significant inflammatory mediators.
7. Stage 4 B ROP detachments can have a lens sparing surgery as above after altering port entry sites, mostly to nasal side. Some eyes with more advanced TRD are approached with lens removal surgery similar to Stage 5 ROP eyes.
8. While closing the eyelids, after putting the mandatory Betadine eye drops, in sutureless surgery be careful not to "press" underlying eyeball that can happen because the overlying lids are very thin. Hold the lid margins alone and close gently with a tight bandage. This prevents hypotony at end of surgery.

36.4.3 Lensectomy-Vitrectomy for Stages 4B and 5 ROP

The goal of the surgery in Stage 5 is to achieve as much retinal reattachment as possible without creating a retinal break. Residual tractional retinal detachment folds are expected post surgery. To minimize the chances of retinal break, an anterior approach is preferred by most surgeons, hence mandating the removal of the lens.

36.4.3.1 Preoperative Ocular Evaluation (Figs. 36.6, 36.7, 36.8, 36.9, and 36.10)

Stage 5 ROP is characterized by total tractional retinal detachment. This can be of the following configurations:

1. Open funnel: Both anterior and posterior parts of retinal folds can be visualized.
2. Narrow anterior funnel: Minimal part of anterior funnel is open making visibility of posterior tissues difficult. Posteriorly open is seen on USG or intraoperative.
3. Narrow posterior funnel: Anterior part of funnel is open and retina is visible.
4. Closed funnel: No retinal tissue is visible.

Determining the configuration helps in planning as well as prognosticating the surgery. Open funnel detachments have much better outcomes than closed funnel detachments. A preoperative ultrasonography and good indirect

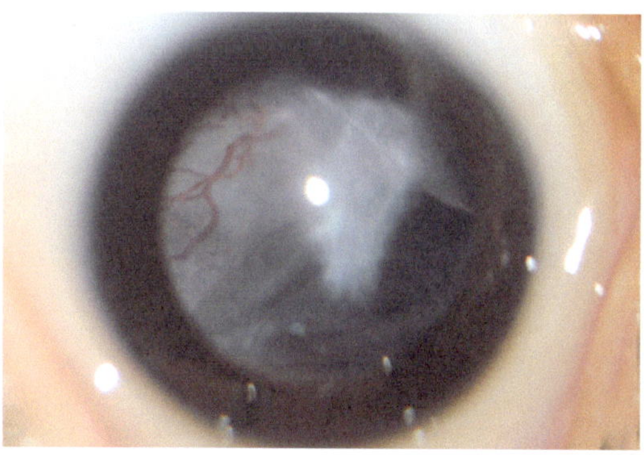

Fig. 36.6 Anteriorly and posteriorly open funnel TRD where retinal tissue is seen only partly involving the retrolental pupil area

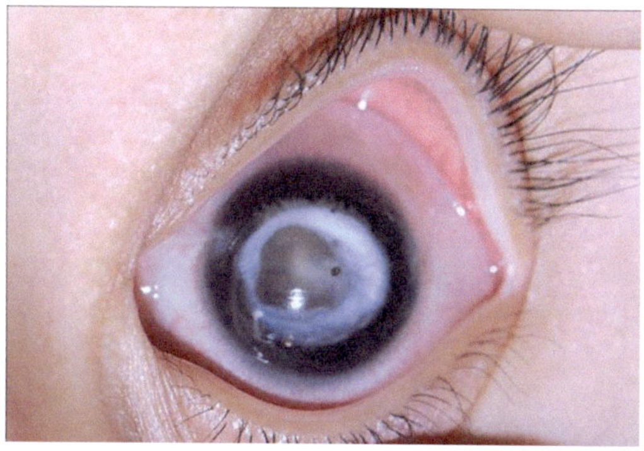

Fig. 36.7 Same eye as in Fig. 36.6, 6 months after surgery showing retinal reattachment centrally. Functional vision of this baby is seen in Fig. 36.16

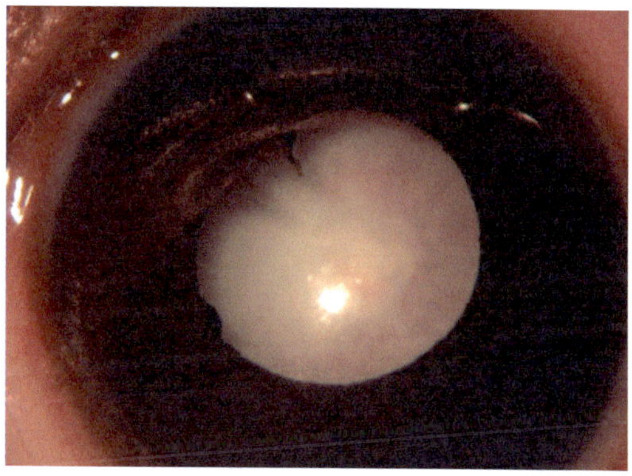

Fig. 36.8 Anteriorly open funnel of retinal vessels with posterior closure (central dense white gliotic tissue) seen under the microscope

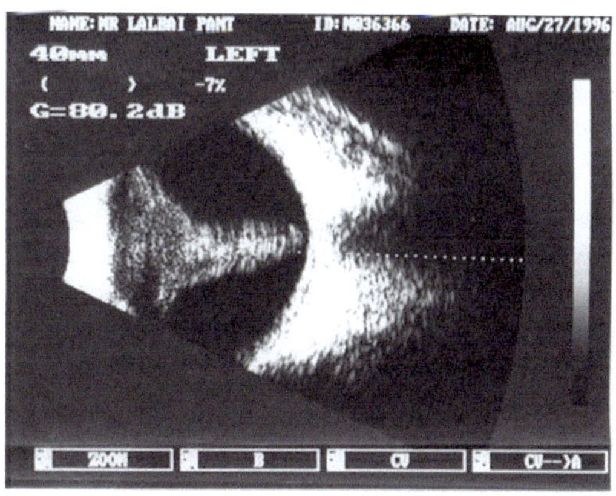

Fig. 36.9 Ultrasound of the same eye as in Fig. 36.8 showing open funnel anteriorly and relatively narrow funnel posteriorly

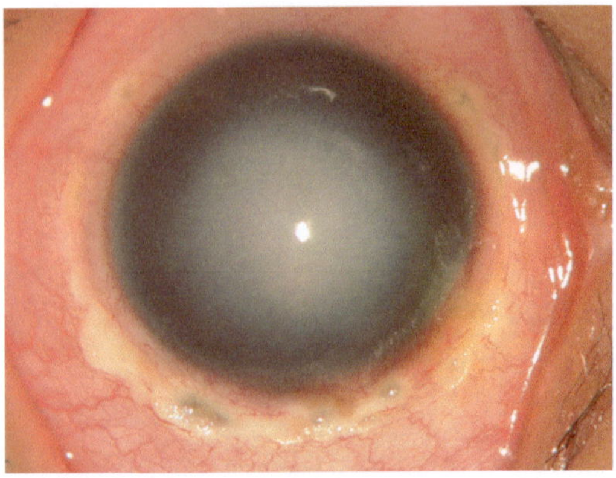

Fig. 36.10 Untreated Stage 5 eyes have progression of pathology and develop corneal scarring from lens-corneal touch (resembles and can be mistaken for Peters' anomaly), often causing secondary glaucoma. Scars of TSCPC (Transconjunctival cyclophotocoagulation) are seen

Ophthalmoscopy is necessary to determine the same. Subretinal hyper-reflective echoes due to lipids or blood suggest chronic detachment and are a poor prognostic indicator. Intraocular pressure measurement must be done for hypotony or glaucoma.

Corneal haze due to increased intraocular pressure, or lens–corneal touch in late Stage 5 disease pose surgical difficulty intraoperatively. These surgeries can be planned as staged procedures—first removing the lens corneal touch with lensectomy and later after cornea clears, in 4–6 weeks, vitrectomy and peeling of membranes for retinal reattachment. Iris neovascularization and/or presence of dilated and tortuous retinal vessels behind the retrolental membrane need to be addressed before surgery, often by anti-VEGF injection.

In advanced cases of corneal scarring, including secondary to hydrops from constant eye poking, an open sky vitrectomy combined with penetrating keratoplasty provide some ambulatory vision in few cases (Figs. 36.11, 36.12, 36.13, 36.14, and 36.15).

36.4.3.2 Timing of the Surgery

Unlike Stage 4 ROP, surgery of Stage 5 requires extensive dissection of preretinal membranes. This requires minimal vascular proliferation in order to minimize intraoperative bleed and facilitate dissection. Presence of iris neovascu-

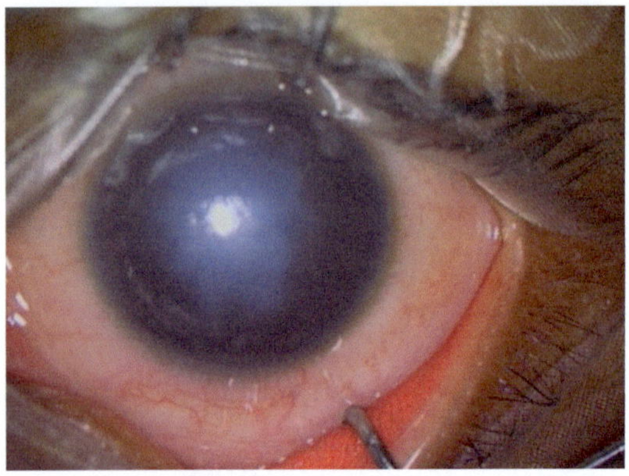

Fig. 36.11 At presentation, ROP Stage 5 with corneal opacity, corneolenticular touch, and flat AC

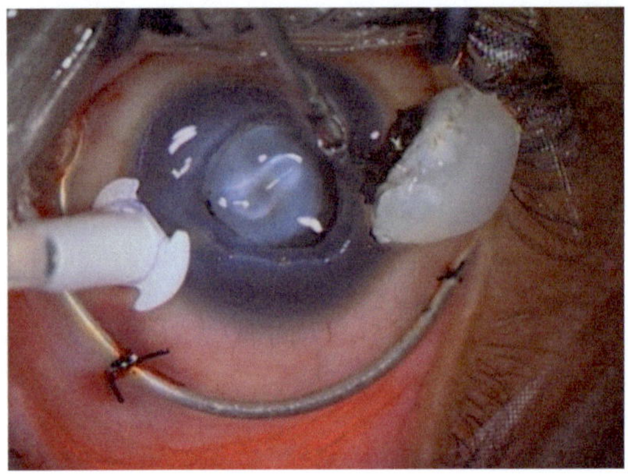

Fig. 36.12 After trephining corneal button, removal of dense cataract and part of adherent iris, retrolenticular fibroplasia is visible as a white membrane, which is stuck to retina behind (not visible at this stage). Note Felingra ring and 20 Gauge sutured cannula

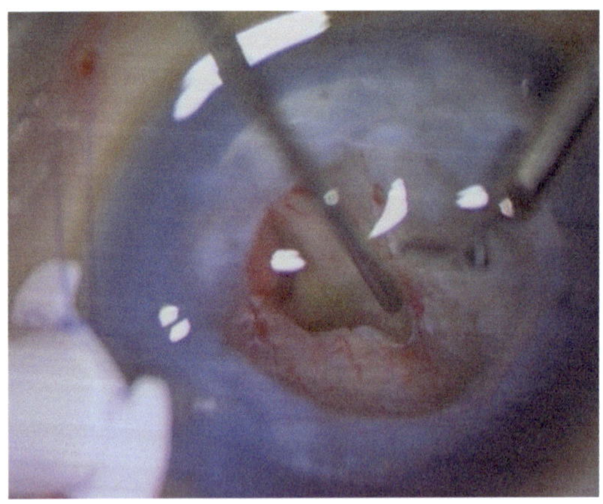

Fig. 36.13 Open sky vitrectomy using coverslip, viscoelastic, and modern, Treses' irrigating spatula (instrument to the right)—yellow area visible is the macula

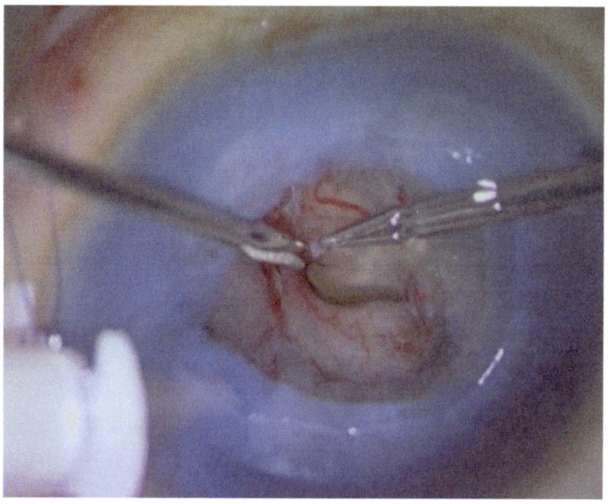

Fig. 36.14 Reaching up to the "stalk" on the disc that is "cut" to open the retina "funnel"—nearly bloodless surgery!

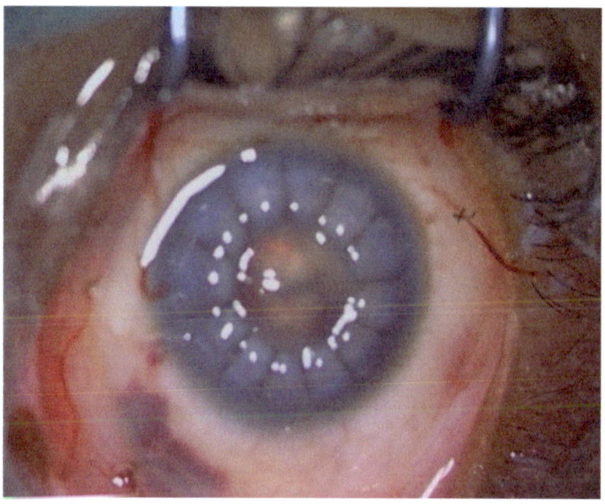

Fig. 36.15 Eye appearance at end of surgery. The opened retinal funnel is seen through a clear well centered corneal graft

larization or plus disease should be carefully evaluated for. Some groups prefer intracameral anti-VEGF injection to reduce vascularity before surgery instead of observation for few weeks.

36.4.3.3 Steps

Anterior approach is preferred for Stage 5 ROP in view of severe distortion and pulling of the retina anteriorly. Multiple approaches have been tried in order to facilitate membrane dissection including open sky vitrectomy, 2 port vitrectomy or a 3 port vitrectomy with similar outcomes. Choice of the procedure depends on surgeon's preference and anatomical situation.

1. Limbal approach is preferred for instrument introduction. Some surgeons prefer making Sclerotomies 0.5 mm behind the limbus after limited conjunctival peritomy. Unlike in lens sparing vitrectomy, entry is horizontal and aimed into the lens substance, since retinal tissues are present just behind the lens (Fig. 36.2).
2. Insufficient pupillary dilatation can be handled by iris hooks (preferred) or sphincterotomy or iris removal.
3. Endocapsular lensectomy can be performed followed by cutting the anterior lens capsule. The posterior capsule should be peeled next using an end gripping forceps. Firm grasping of capsule involving one-third of it from equator to posterior pole helps in removing it at once. Residual capsule if left behind can cause retinal and iridial adhesion leading to failed opening of retinal funnel in Stage 5 ROP surgery. Removal of posterior capsule is also necessary to prevent preretinal proliferation over the ciliary body that eventually can cause intractable hypotony.
4. The central/retrolental membrane is then opened in the area of least retinal apposition in a cruciate manner. It can be done using trocars or 23G needles (for example, needle of scalp vein sets bent appropriately in the middle). Each flap is then extended by dissection using spatula/scissors/forceps till the periphery taking care of the areas of retinal apposition and preventing retinal breaks. This is best done using a bimanual technique under direct visualization of the microscope.
5. Multiple sheets of preretinal membranes are expected to be tightly adherent to the retinal surface throwing it into troughs and folds. Sometimes it might be difficult to separately identify the underlying retinal surface under microscope illumination. Endoilluminator directed to corneal surface or into anterior vitreous cavity, can be used during such times.
6. Preretinal membranes are peeled and removed using bimanual dissection in layers. Opening of the funnel is the desirable end-point. These

should also be freed from ciliary attachment in the periphery. Special care should be taken to avoid retinal breaks. Bleeders can be touched gently with intraocular diathermy without retinal injury.

7. Viscoelastic like healon or methylcellulose can be injected in the funnel to open it further. This aids dissection and helps in removal of posterior membranes and persistent fetal vasculature remnants.
8. These eyes do not need intraocular gas or silicone oil or laser retinopexy as there is no PVR and no retinal break. Air tamponade is sufficient and rarely viscoelastic is left behind as a temporary tamponade.
9. Partial or complete fluid–air exchange is done. Sclerotomy sites are preferably sutured with 8-0 or 10-0 vicryl.

36.5 Complications

1. *Iatrogenic retinal break*: The retinal reattachment rate declines significantly in presence of a retinal break in both Stage 4 and Stage 5 ROP. In the inadvertent event of a break, oil or gas tamponade after removing all traction around the break and laser around the break can be tried. These steps are successful when break was in an area devoid of vitreous and not in the retinal fold.
2. *Intraoperative and postoperative bleeding:* Unlasered peripheral avascular retina or perfused fibrovascular proliferation increase the chance of intra- or postoperative bleeding and also postoperative NVI and NVG. The bleeds usually resolve over 1–2 weeks. Non-removing postoperative bleed increases the risk of PVR and re-detachment and may need vitreous lavage or rarely also responds to anti-VEGF injection. Intraoperative and preoperative laser to all avascular retina is mandatory.
3. *Hypotony:* Immediate postoperative hypotony can happen because of leaking sclerotomy ports. Due to low scleral rigidity in neonates, suturing of any leaking scleral/limbal ports is preferred. Late postoperative hypotony can be caused due to re-proliferation over ciliary body or rhegmatogenous detachment. This can cause phthisis.
4. Cataract: Development of cataract is not uncommon. This can be seen mostly due to intraoperative lens touch and manifests between a week or a month or so after vitrectomy surgery. Rarely this is seen as a feathering of posterior lens substance if there is intraocular air that is in contact with the lens because postop prone position was not maintained. Rarely it is due to a developmental cataract or post silicone oil cataract that manifests delayed postoperatively. Intraoperative lens touch is detected during surgery in retroillumination as a small or large dimple in the red reflex from fundus. Small opacities can be managed by mydriatics; more opaque lenses need surgery.
5. *Glaucoma:* Postoperative glaucoma is common and increases with increase in stage of ROP. Development of peripheral anterior synechiae, distortion of anterior segment anatomy, preexisting closed angles, preexisting primary congenital glaucoma, steroid responsiveness, intraocular inflammation, and rarely pupillary block can cause glaucoma in these infants. It can be controlled by adding antiglaucoma medications. Rarely surgical interventions like peripheral iridectomy, filtering, or valve surgery are required.
6. *Endophthalmitis:* It is a known complication of any intraocular surgery. Postoperative wound leak and hypotony besides undetected Nasolacrimal duct obstruction with lacrimal sac infections can predispose to infection. Reports of endophthalmitis after ROP surgery are fortunately extremely rare.

36.6 Advances

1. *Abinterno Incisions:* In this technique, after making the sclerotomy, a microvitreoretinal blade is used. It is inserted carefully posterior

to the lens and anterior to the retinal folds. The blade is then gently rotated using sclerotomy as the pivot till the clock hours possible. This helps to transect the tractional vectors extending anteriorly to the ciliary body. Relieving this traction helps the retina to fall behind and provides adequate space for further dissection. Sweeping of the blade across the equator of the lens should be avoided to avoid lens touch. This is especially useful in some of the early Stagev4 A and 4 B TRD.

2. *Plasmin assisted vitrectomy:* Ocriplasmin and human-derived plasmin enzyme have been used to induce posterior vitreous detachment during vitrectomy for various surgeries. Since there is a strong attachment of posterior hyaloid to the retina in neonates, PVD induction is best avoided using traditional techniques. Incomplete regression of primary hyaloid, atrophic and thin retina, and poor development of angle structures and pars plana make this further difficult. Although the data of plasmin-assisted vitrectomy in ROP is retrospective and limited, it opens new avenues for further improvisation in vitrectomy techniques.
3. Endoscopic ROP surgery: More recent attempts are being made to use endoscope guided ROP surgery.

36.7 Late-Onset Rhegmatogenous Retinal Detachments

These occur due to either Myopia-related retinal pathologies or due to vitreoretinal traction abnormalities. Both are more likely to happen in eyes that did not receive early and good therapy at the appropriate stage of ROP when best outcomes are achieved (high-risk prethreshold ROP and early stages of APROP). Both spontaneously regressed Threshold ROP and advanced postop cases are more at risk for late-onset retinal detachments. Scleral buckling is a preferred technique. Rarely, Vitrectomy techniques, as in adults are used with three important caveats: (1) Select entry site after careful peripheral retinal examination; (2) Avoid large retinectomy and be gentle in vitreous removal—partial vitreous removal may have to be accepted in some areas if they are not adjacent to a break. (3) Use air/gas/oil infusion very gently at low pressure as breaks can appear with forceful entry.

36.8 Postoperative Care

Surgery is only the first step to achieve visual goals in these babies. Eye drops are prescribed for 4–6 weeks and include mydriatics like homatropine and topical steroids. Antiglaucoma eye drops include latanoprost, Dorzolamide, or Brinzolamide. Timolol or Brimonidine like drops are avoided due to systemic toxicity. Postoperative positioning is important. Babies are kept prone for 3–5 days and then in propped up position. Arm restraints are better than eye shields and parents are encouraged to provide toys and vision stimulating colorful surroundings to tackle amblyopia. This also provides early intervention stimulation for eye and brain coordination promoting motor and cognitive development. One week postoperative, babies are referred to Vision and developmental therapists. Aphakic glasses (from +16.00 to +20.00D sphere or so) are started and these are refined in 4–6 months as the retina settles and media clarity allows proper refraction in aphakic eyes. Usually, they require +24.00 D sphere or more. Contact lenses can be used. Phakic eyes are refracted at 4 weeks and every 4 monthly thereafter. They develop progressive Myopia of significant magnitude very quickly after vitrectomy, but usually stabilizes by 3–4 years of age. Unilateral operated cases also need patching therapy for amblyopia and anisometropia (much shorter duration daily sessions in these tiny babies that are at higher risk for developing reverse amblyopia in the good eye). Close working with a pediatric-oriented Ophthalmologist can help guide glass prescriptions, refractions, and proper amblyopia management besides any Squint that develops in some patients. Typical postop prescription:

- Prone for 2–5 days, and then propped up.
- Tobramycin e/d 3 t/d.
- Betamethasone or Fluorometholone or Loteprednol e/d 3–4 t/d and tapered weekly. Stronger steroids like Prednisolone if lens was removed.
- Homide e/d 3 t/d (1 week in lens sparing eyes and 4–8 weeks in lens removed eyes.
- Drozolamide e/d 2/d (all lensectomy cases) till IOP can be recorded.
- No eye patch after 12 h.
- Arm restraints explained.
- Visual stimulation exercises/aphakic glasses from day 7 postop.
- Avoid eye rubbing/poking behavior.

Successful surgical care in ROP, especially in acute ROP where each day of delay counts and baby is fragile, is a team effort. The Team leader is the Ophthalmic surgeon who brings everyone together to the center of the most important person in the team, that is, the premature baby. Each member of this team needs motivation, compassion, energy, and high skills besides high-quality equipment and infrastructure to deliver the best in this critical situation. Team includes retinal Surgeon (Team Leader), assistant surgeon—fellow doctors—trainees, surgical counselor, parents and extended family, neonatal anesthesiologist, neonatologist, trained neonatal nurses, trained surgical nursing staff and anesthesia technicians, low vision and rehabilitation specialists, pediatric-oriented Optometrists and Ophthalmologists, Opticals that cater to small babies, and dedicated Eye Health care managers. Bilateral simultaneous surgery for ROP are routinely done in many centers including ours and are an acceptable risk when weighed against the possible poor surgical and anesthesia outcome of sequential surgery especially in progressive Stage 4 A active phase disease [8]. To build this team takes some time but once everyone is together, wonderful results are obtained (Fig. 36.16).

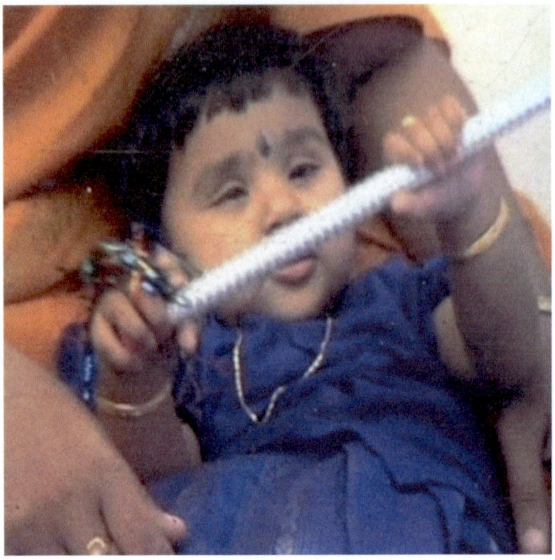

Fig. 36.16 Baby trying to look and fixate at the nearby object 6 months after Stage 5 ROP surgery in Fig. 36.7 (with permission of parents)

References

1. Hartnett ME, editor. Pediatric retina. Berlin: Lippincott Williams & Wilkins; 2005.
2. Gunton KB, Nelson LB, Olitsky SE. Neonatal ophthalmology: ocular development in childhood. In: Harley's pediatric ophthalmology. 4th ed. Philadelphia: Lippincott Williams & Wilkins; 2005. p. 66–52.
3. Trese MT, Droste PJ. Longterm postoperative results of a consecutive series of stage 4 and 5 ROp. Ophthalmology. 1998;105:992–7.
4. Trese MT. Scleral buckle for ROP. Ophthalmology. 1994;101:23–6.
5. Gopal L, Sharma T, et al. Surgery for stage 5 ROP: the learning curve and evolving technique. Ind J Ophthalmol. 2000;48:101–6.
6. Shah PK, Narendran V, et al. Anatomic and visual outcomes of stage 4 and 5 retinopathy of prematurity. Eye. 2009;23:176–80.
7. Hirose T, Katsumi O, Mehta MC, et al. Vision in stage 5 ROP after retinal reattachment by open-sky vitrectomy. Arch Ophthalmol. 1993;111:345–9.
8. Yonekawa Y, et al. Immediate sequential bilateral pediatric vitreoretinal surgery. An international multicentre study. Ophthalmology. 2016;123:1802–8.

37 Management of Posteriorly Dislocated Nucleus and Intraocular Lens

Preetam Samant, Kamal Dedhia, Hasanain Shikari, and Neha Jain

37.1 Introduction

Loss of a part or the whole lens nucleus into the vitreous cavity during cataract surgery is termed nucleus drop. The incidence ranges from 0.3% to 1.1% [1, 2]. If left unmanaged, posteriorly dislocated nucleus can lead to uveitis, cystoid macular edema (CME), elevated intraocular pressure, corneal edema, vitreous hemorrhage, retinal tears, and detachment leading to significant visual loss. Therefore, the nucleus should be removed either at the time of surgery or as a secondary procedure. Other causes of posteriorly dislocated nucleus include trauma and other congenital causes.

Posterior dislocation of the IOL is an uncommon complication of cataract surgery and Nd:YAG posterior capsulotomy, with a frequency of 0.2–1.8% [3]. Although they usually do not cause any significant inflammation, their removal is necessary before implanting a secondary IOL for visual rehabilitation.

37.2 Predisposing Factor

37.2.1 Complication of Intraocular Surgery

The dropped nucleus is a complication that presented due to the advent of modern phacoemulsification cataract surgery (https://crstodayeurope.com/articles/2013-julaug/practical-management-of-a-dropped-nucleus/). Compared to extracapsular cataract extraction or small incision cataract surgery, where the posterior-to-anterior pressure gradient results in forward and outward movement of the cataractous lens, in modern phaco surgery, the sealed surgical wound with fluid administration to maintain the anterior chamber results in an anterior-to-posterior pressure gradient which can push the crystalline lens or nucleus/nuclear fragment downward in case of zonular or capsular bag compromise (https://crstodayeurope.com/articles/2013-julaug/practical-management-of-a-dropped-nucleus/).

Sculpting during phacoemulsification is one of the leading causes of stress on the capsule and zonules [4]. Improper settings or mode during phacoemulsification can cause the lens nucleus to shift and rock within the bag potentially

Electronic Supplementary Material The online version of this chapter (https://doi.org/10.1007/978-981-33-4168-5_37) contains supplementary material, which is available to authorized users.

P. Samant (✉) · K. Dedhia
The Eye Associates, Mumbai, India

H. Shikari
Arete Clinic, Mumbai, India

N. Jain
Dr. Agarwal Eye Hospital, Hyderabad, India

A. Jain et al. (eds.), *Cutting-edge Vitreoretinal Surgery*,
https://doi.org/10.1007/978-981-33-4168-5_37

resulting in compromised capsular integrity. Insufficient phaco power and or excessive movement of the phaco-tip during emulsification of the nucleus can cause capsular compression distally while stretching of the zonules underlying the phaco tip proximally. Slow pulsing power or high vacuum during sculpting can result in nucleus jumping toward the phaco tip causing capsular compression proximally and zonular stretching distally.

Preoperative risk factors include one or a combination of small pupil size, deep set eyes, corneal scarring or compromise, pseudoexfoliation of lens capsule with zonular weakness, posterior polar cataracts, traumatic cataract, hard nucleus, mature or hypermature cataract, vitrectomized eyes or in eyes post multiple intravitreal injections of anti-VEGF.

Intraoperative risk factors that result in posterior capsular rupture (PCR) and dropped nucleus include visible tears in posterior capsule arising due to small capsulorrhexis with anterior capsular block during hydrodissection, radial extension of capsulorrhexis, equatorial or posterior rupture of capsule by phacoemulsification handpiece tip or sharp instrument, and rarely following zonular dialysis larger than 3 clock hours and intraoperative floppy iris syndrome.

Cadaveric studies have demonstrated the role of vitreous in the downward movement of the nucleus or nuclear fragment. Older patients with syneretic vitreous are at a greater risk for nucleus drop compared to patients with undisturbed vitreous that can support the nucleus in case of capsular compromise or PCR preventing the downward passage of nucleus/fragment [4]. Additionally, high vacuum settings that result in high aspiration flow rates and post-occlusion surge can disturb the vitreous supporting the nucleus by drawing it toward the phaco tip resulting in nucleus drop [4]. The turbulence created by phacoemulsification also contributes to vitreous instability and loss of support [4].

The intraocular lens malposition can range from simple decentration (not requiring any further intervention), to complete luxation into the posterior segment (Fig. 37.1). Early dislocation may occur intraoperatively or within 3 months of surgery. It is usually a result of PCR or zonular dialysis with inadequate fixation within the capsular bag or in sulcus or instability of the IOL–bag complex (Fig. 37.2).

Nd:YAG capsulotomy may result in posterior dislocation of the IOL into the vitreous. In the

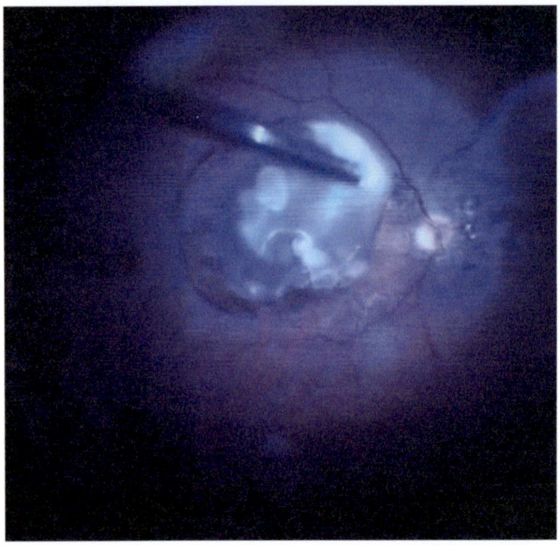

Fig. 37.1 Intraoperative image showing nucleus drop during a cataract surgery with a cutter being used to remove the vitreous

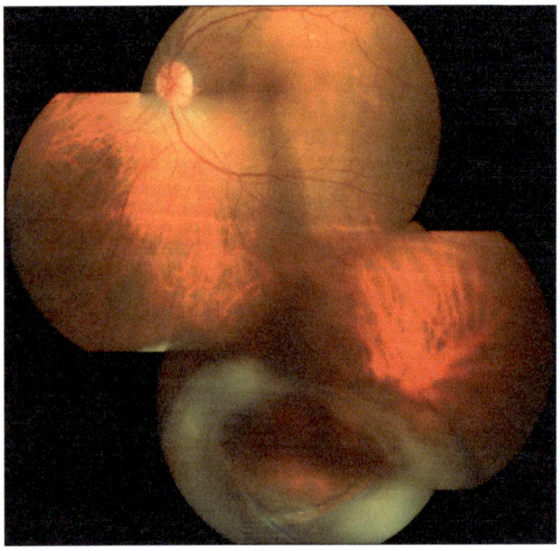

Fig. 37.2 Montage fundus image of the left eye showing posteriorly dislocated IOL with the capsular bag lying inferiorly

author's experience, this is more common with large posterior capsular openings, early capsulotomy postoperatively, and in cases of plate-haptic IOLs.

Late dislocation of IOL occurs more than 3 months after cataract extraction and is a result of zonular compromise since the IOL is implanted within the capsular bag. Risk factors include, but are not limited to pseudoexfoliation syndrome, trauma, and prior vitreous surgery [5]. Trauma can also result in zonular dehiscence with dislocation of IOL–bag complex either anteriorly or posteriorly into the vitreous substance. Axial myopia is also associated with IOL dislocation mainly since it predisposes to zonular weakness; also, since this population is predisposed to retinal detachment, vitreous surgery may further cause weakening of the zonular–capsular bag complex [5].

37.2.2 Traumatic Dislocation

Dislocation or subluxation of the crystalline lens occurs commonly post ocular trauma. Traumatic dislocation commonly occurs dues to direct blunt injury to the globe by a cricket or tennis ball as well as blunt trauma to the head or orbit [6]. If trauma is minor then other underlying predisposing conditions such as Marfan's syndrome should be suspected [7]. Ocular trauma may be associated with other injuries such as retinal detachment, intraocular foreign body, sclerocorneal laceration, etc. and hence may make management difficult.

37.2.3 Congenital Factors

Marfan's syndrome is the most common cause of inherited ectopia lentis, with lenticular dislocation being the most frequent ocular manifestation observed in approximately 75% of patients with Marfan's (usually bilateral and most often in the superotemporal direction) [8, 9]. Homocystinuria is the second most common cause of inherited ectopia lentis; lens dislocation presenting in 90% of patients, bilateral and inferior or nasal dislocation in 60% cases, Weil–Marchesani syndrome, Ehlers–Danlos syndrome, hyperlysinemia, and sulfite oxidase deficiency are other congenital etiologies associated with ectopia lentis [10].

37.3 Evaluation of Patients

Patients with dropped nucleus or IOL will provide a history of cataract surgery and may be referred by an anterior segment surgeon or general ophthalmologist.

External ocular examination should be performed with refraction if required to assess refractive error and keratometry to assess corneal astigmatism. Slit-lamp examination is performed to evaluate the position of crystalline lens/IOL, identify phacodonesis or presence of intact anterior capsulorrhexis margin, iris anatomy, and pupil size and integrity (to facilitate secondary IOL implantation). Intraocular pressure should be measured to rule out secondary glaucoma. A subsequent dilated retinal examination should be performed to look for complications arising out of trauma, nucleus drop, and vitreous traction.

A patient with ectopia lentis may present with complaints of painful red eye (secondary to trauma), diminished vision for distance (secondary to astigmatism or myopia), or monocular diplopia. A detailed history is warranted to rule out trauma and/or systemic disease associations.

Imaging studies are not usually warranted. However, in cases with significant trauma with hyphema/vitreous hemorrhage or corneal compromise secondary to previous cataract surgery, a B-scan ultrasonography may be performed to assess for the posterior segment integrity and presence or absence of retinal detachment. Anterior segment OCT and UBM imaging may be performed to assess zonular integrity and image angle structures. An A-scan biometry should be performed to determine the axial length and power of IOL that needs to be implanted.

37.4 Management

It is important to note that the underlying principle of complication management in any surgical setting must be to reduce the risk of further complications. Although the nucleus may sit on the vitreous, it may not be safe to deal with it in that position, as surgical maneuvers disrupt the vitreous or cause retinal traction, increasing the risk of retinal complications. Lens nucleus is usually less tolerated than lens epinucleus, which in turn is less tolerated than lens cortex (lens fragments smaller than 2 mm may resolve on their own, and one can consider medical management with topical corticosteroids and glaucoma treatment as needed for these pieces).

37.4.1 Anterior Segment Management at the Time of Cataract Surgery

In view of PC Tear, reassess the situation, move the nuclear fragments to a safe position and then remove the second instrument. An ophthalmic viscosurgical device (OVD), preferably dispersive, can then be injected in the anterior chamber. OVD tamponades the vitreous, supports the nucleus, allowing the phaco needle to be withdrawn without letting the vitreous surge forward toward the wound. Surgeon can perform bimanual vitrectomy through two paracenteses with a low bottle height and high cut-rate, triamcinolone acetonide can be used for visualization. This allows further surgical maneuvers to be performed in a vitreous-free environment, reducing or eliminating vitreous traction. It is usually a good idea to debulk the anterior vitreous from behind the posterior capsule to discourage the vitreous from prolapsing forward during further maneuvers. Teixeira et al. [11] examined the effects of vitrectomy on retinal traction through a pars plana approach in vitro and found that traction is directly related to the vacuum and inversely related to the cut-rate and distance from the retina; these principles can be applied to anterior vitrectomy. The settings should therefore be low vacuum (100–150 mmHg) and the highest cut-rate possible.

37.4.2 The Optimal Timing of Vitrectomy

The optimal timing of vitrectomy has been a matter of debate and also varies from case to case. To avoid progressive lens-induced inflammation, the best time for vitrectomy is at the same sitting as the cataract surgery [12]. This may not be possible due to the unavailability of a vitreoretinal surgeon. A delay in vitrectomy of more than 3 weeks could cause an increased incidence of chronic glaucoma [13]. Another study failed to demonstrate a statistical difference between the time of surgery and the final visual outcome or incidence of glaucoma [14]. A delay may be necessary to reduce corneal edema and intraocular inflammation prior to undertaking secondary surgery. In cases in which retained lens material is abutting the cornea, IOP is uncontrolled with medical management, or if early retinal detachment is noted on clinical examination or ultrasonography, the surgeon may not have the luxury of waiting to pursue a PPV.

37.4.3 Evaluation by Vitreoretina Surgeon

Initial evaluation should focus on signs of intraocular inflammation, infection, and increased IOP and they should be managed appropriately. Cornea may be edematous due to inflammation or raised IOP. In such cases, it may be preferable to treat the patient with topical steroids and IOP lowering agents before the second procedure.

37.4.4 Surgical Procedure

37.4.4.1 Securing Anterior Chamber

The anterior chamber should be secured. The wound should be checked and sutured if required to prevent opening up during vitrectomy. Anterior chamber should be cleared of any vitreous or cortical matter, if present, by passing the cutter through the posterior capsule (old wounds should not be used to pass the cutter). Preservation of as much of the anterior and posterior capsule as possible should be done for secondary IOL implantation. Assessment of the nuclear status, amount, and type of retained lens material should then be done.

37.4.4.2 Pars Plana Vitrectomy

The underlying principle of PPV for displaced nuclear fragments is to perform a complete vitrectomy, including removal of vitreous base as far as possible, employing a standard three-port pars plana approach with a conventional 20-gauge system or a smaller-gauge sutureless system (23 or 25 or 27 gauge).

Pars plana vitrectomy for retained lens material begins with a thorough anterior (if needed for visualization) and posterior core vitrectomy to release any vitreous adhesions around the lens and retinal surface. Preservative-free triamcinolone can be utilized to facilitate visualization and complete removal of vitreous strands. Posterior vitreous detachment should be induced if not already present to reduce the risk of postoperative retinal tears, although occasionally a large complete crystalline lens atop the posterior hyaloid may make induction technically more difficult. A very adherent hyaloid may be managed with a bimanual technique. A 25- or 29-gauge chandelier can be introduced separately. A 29-gauge chandelier provides adequate illumination and does not leak when removed. The wound frequently requires suturing after the removal of a 25-gauge chandelier. A pick can then be used in conjunction with the soft tip to detach the hyaloid. Another option when a 20-gauge sclerotomy is needed for the fragmatome is to use a 20-gauge lighted pick with the 23-gauge soft tip. The retinal surgeon should avoid the temptation to pursue lens material with aspiration before complete removal of the core vitreous, as the vitreous may become incarcerated and induce retinal breaks. Peripheral vitrectomy around the ports should be performed.

37.4.4.3 Removal of the Lens Fragment

Once vitrectomy is over, attention is directed on the removal of the lens material. Depending upon the nuclear fragment, whether it is soft or hard, either vitreous cutter or fragmatome can be used. Vitrectomy probe can be used for the efficient removal of smaller nuclear, epinuclear, and cortical pieces. In cases with larger nuclear fragments, more efficient removal can be undertaken, utilizing either a 19-gauge fragmatome or a phacoemulsification probe.

Occasionally, very dense nuclear fragments may be removed using manual extraction. Once a fragment is brought into the mid-vitreous using suction, the tip of the fragmatome is embedded into the fragment by giving a short burst of ultrasound energy. The fragment is then transferred to the anterior chamber and removed by enlarging the corneal incision or creating a scleral tunnel [15].

The surgeon may choose to employ a 20-, 23-, 25-, or 27-gauge system for PPV, bearing in mind that smaller-gauge cutters are more likely to encounter difficulty in the removal of larger lens nuclear fragments without the assistance of a fragmatome or phacoemulsification probe.

One of the most important steps of the procedure is a 360° exam with scleral depression to remove any residual lens material and check for peripheral breaks. One must carefully remove almost every small piece in the vitreous base area. If they are not removed, these pieces can lead to residual persistent chronic inflammation with cystoid macular edema (CME). Breaks should be treated carefully with three contiguous rows of endolaser photocoagulation. A retinal detachment related to breaks may prevent good laser uptake, and fluid–air exchange may be required with complete flattening of the retina for good laser treatment. Careful shaving of the vitreous base is required if any break related retinal detachment is seen, and the patient may require intraocular gas.

37.4.4.4 Fragmatome

A fragmatome, which is similar to a phaco probe without an infusion sleeve, cannot cut vitreous. So, a complete vitrectomy must be performed prior to introducing the fragmatome into the eye. This can be aided by triamcinolone staining, particularly if visibility is limited. Either of the superior ports can be removed, or a separate, fourth sclerotomy can be created for fragmatome.

A local conjunctival peritomy is created, wet-field cautery can be applied as needed for scleral hemostasis, and a 20-gauge micro incisional vitreoretinal blade is utilized to create a 19-gauge sclerotomy.

Once again, it is critical to ensure that the area chosen for the creation of this sclerotomy is cleaned of vitreous gel prior to this step to avoid vitreous dragging and potential retinal breaks.

Also, because there is no counter-resistance by the capsular bag, it is essential to use a pulse or micropulse setting on the fragmatome as the nucleus has a tendency to shoot away from fragmatome tip when using continuous mode. The power of the fragmatome should be set to low, perhaps 20% of normal. If the fragmatome needle drills into the nucleus, the surgeon can use the endoilluminator to push off the nucleus—or use it bimanually to crush the nucleus into the port or chop it in a cartwheel fashion. When the nucleus has been engaged by aspiration only, it should be lifted away from the retina in the mid vitreous cavity. Once safely away from the retina, ultrasound energy should be delivered on maximum to commence phaco fragmentation. Also, whether utilizing the phacoemulsification probe or the fragmatome, the surgeon must remember that the bore of the ultrasound instrument is larger than the infusion line, especially when employing a small-gauge vitrectomy platform. This difference in size can result in the aspiration "outrunning" the infusion line when the tip of the phacoemulsification instrument is not engaged with lens material and collapse of the vitreous cavity and potential iatrogenic trauma.

37.4.4.5 Perfluorocarbon Liquid

When the lens fragment is located near the macula, perfluorocarbon liquid (PFCL) may be used to float the lens away from the retina to protect the macula from the vitrector or fragmatome manipulation of the fragment [16–18]. Prior to closure, it is important to remove all PFCL to prevent ocular toxicity. The majority of displaced nucleus fragments can be dealt with safely in the posterior segment, with the PFCL acting only as a cushion to the macula while nuclear fragments are addressed with the fragmatome. If PFCL is not used, and manipulation must occur at the posterior pole, the surgeon should rotate the globe such that macular contact during phacoemulsification is minimal [19]. The PFCL is not an absolute necessity for retrieval of retained lens fragments but is well suited to cases with co-existing retinal breaks and detachments.

37.4.4.6 Small-Gauge Instrumentation

Although the conventional 20-gauge system can be used for lens fragment removal, many surgeons have been moving toward smaller-gauge instrumentation to reduce operative and healing times, postoperative discomfort, and refractive changes. The 23G cutter can be used to remove smaller fragments at a relatively low cut rate and higher vacuum settings. However, it may not be useful in removing larger pieces or hard nuclear fragments [20]. As no 23-gauge phacofragmatome is currently available for use, the 23-gauge sclerotomy port can be enlarged to accommodate a 20-gauge phacofragmatome avoiding the need for an additional incision during the procedure. However, the use of the larger-gauge phacofragmatome with smaller-gauge vitrectomy systems can create infusion/outflow mismatch leading to hypotony and more vitreous traction if care is not taken to raise infusion pressures to match egress. There are 20/25-gauge and 20/23-gauge adaptors available that can be inserted into a 20-gauge wound after the nucleus or IOFB removal so that the rest of the procedure could continue using small-gauge dynamics.

37.4.5 Difficult Situations

37.4.5.1 Concurrent Retinal Detachment and Dropped Nucleus

Mobile retina can cause problems while trying to perform fragmatome extraction of the nucleus. In this case, PFCL needs to be inserted to stabilize the retina. The perfluorocarbon liquid bubble displaces the subretinal fluid through the retinal breaks reattaching the retina and, at the same time, serves as a cushion between the nucleus and the retina. IOL should be inserted prior to air exchange (with posterior segment filled with heavy liquid) using OVD in the anterior chamber. OVD should be removed before performing air exchange as it is difficult to do this after air has been inserted. In the case of complicated RD silicone oil /heavy liquid exchange can be done.

In the case of unstable IOL in presence of intraocular gas, it is better to have IOL sandwiched by gas, that is gas in the anterior and posterior segment. The presence of gas solely in the posterior segment can push the lens forward causing optic capture. If there is no capsular support for the IOL, one can plan an anterior chamber IOL iris claw lens or scleral fixated IOL; either in the same sitting or as a second procedure at a later date. When performed in the same sitting, the presence of gas can lead to the possibility of dislocation, corneal touch, and displacement from the visual axis.

37.4.5.2 Dropped Nucleus Associated with Choroidal Hemorrhage

After removing the nucleus, the eye should be filled with silicone oil. Secondary IOL should be planned at a later date after the choroidals resolve and silicone oil has been removed

37.4.5.3 Management of Traumatic Dislocated Lens

Corneal scarring or sutures may impair visualization. Combination surgery with an anterior-segment surgeon with placement of a temporary keratoprosthesis may be required. Endoscopic-assisted vitrectomy, if available, may be beneficial for repair of pediatric traumatic retinal detachment with media opacity or exploration in the case of suspected intraocular foreign body.

37.4.6 Removal of Dropped IOL

Complete vitrectomy is performed with clearing of vitreous around the IOL. Levitation of the IOL into the anterior chamber can be performed using end-gripping intraocular vitrectomy forceps. Chandelier illumination can be used to facilitate bimanual surgery.

Flexible IOLs can be cut with an IOL cutter in the anterior chamber under dispersive viscoelastic cover and removed via a corneal or sclerocorneal incision. Care must be taken to avoid trauma to the cornea, iris, and angles.

Rigid IOLs are usually removed through a larger scleral tunnel or sclerocorneal incision.

Perfluorocarbon liquids are very useful if a retinal detachment is also present. It serves as a cushion between IOL and retina, thus protecting the retina from potential damage from IOL impact during surgical manipulation. If a silicone plate lens is dislocated, special care with the use of perfluorocarbon liquids is necessary. It has been reported that these lenses often "skate or glide" on the bubble across the retina. In addition, perfluorocarbon liquids make the grasping of the IOL somewhat more difficult by making the IOL more slippery. If the retina is not detached, the use of perfluorocarbon liquids probably is not necessary

37.5 Outcome

Eyes with dropped nucleus or dropped IOL recover good visual acuity post vitrectomy and secondary IOL implantation. However, in cases complicated with retinal detachment or corneal decompensation, visual rehabilitation may be delayed or compromised. Other possible complications adversely affecting final visual acuity may be the presence of choroidals or cystoid macular edema (which may present as a delayed complication). Scott et al. [21] demonstrated that patients with dropped nucleus operated early with pars plana vitrectomy showed better visual recovery than in those with delayed salvage and vitrectomy. The postoperative risk of uveitis, rise in IOP, and retinal detachment were also significantly reduced in patients who underwent early vitrectomy post cataract surgery [22].

37.6 Conclusion

With modern surgical advancements, the increased risk of a dropped nucleus or IOL is counteracted by a comparable improvement in our ability to perform pars plana vitrectomy. This coupled with the use of various supportive mechanisms such as perfluorocarbon liquids, gas, and oil as well as better visualization techniques with non-contact biomicroscopy and prosthetic corneas has allowed better visual recovery even in complicated cases. Appropriately timed placement of secondary intraocular lens by iris fixation, scleral suturing, or haptic externalization and glue fixation has also dramatically improved visual outcomes while preserving corneal endothelial integrity.

References

1. Leaming DV. Practice and preferences of ASCRS members – 2003 survey. J Cataract Refract Surg. 2004;3:892–900.
2. Pande M, Dabbs TR. Incidence of lens matter dislocation during phacoemulsification. J Cataract Refract Surg. 1996;22:737–42.
3. Gross JG, Kokame GT, Weinberg DV. In-the-bag intraocular lens dislocation. Am J Ophthalmol. 2004;137(4):630–5.
4. Osher RH, Yu BC, Koch DD. Posterior polar cataracts. A predisposition to intraoperative posterior capsular rupture. J Cataract Refract Surg. 1990;16:157–62.
5. Shingleton BJ, Yang Y, O'Donoghue MW. Management and outcomes of intraocular lens dislocation in patients with pseudoexfoliation. J Cataract Refract Surg. 2013;39(7):984–93.
6. Harley RD, Nelson LB, Olitsky SE. Harley's pediatric ophthalmology. Philadelphia: Lippincott Williams & Wilkins; 2005. p. 225.
7. Jarrett WH. Dislocation of the lens. A study of 166 hospitalized cases. Arch Ophthalmol. 1967;78(3):289–96.
8. Wakita M, et al. Statistical analysis of Marfan's syndrome. Nippon GankaGakkaiZasshi. 1989;93(6):682–90.
9. Maumenee IH. The eye in the Marfan syndrome. Trans Am Ophthalmol Soc. 1981;79:684.
10. Marin S. Inherited eye diseases: diagnosis and clinical management. New York: MP Dekker; 1991. p. 131–2.
11. Teixeira A, Chong LP, Matsuoka N, et al. Vitreoretinal traction created by conventional cutters during vitrectomy. Ophthalmology. 2010;117(7):1387–92.
12. Smiddy WE, Flynn HW Jr. Management of retained lens nuclear fragments and dislocated posterior chamber intraocular lenses after cataract surgery. Semin Ophthalmol. 1993;8:96–103.
13. Emery JM, McIntyre DJ. Extracapsular cataract surgery. St. Louis: CV Mosby; 1983. p. 340–58.
14. Gilliland GD, Hutton WL, Fuller DG. Retained intravitreal lens fragments after cataract surgery. Ophthalmology. 1992;9:1263–7.
15. Agarwal A. Management of phaco complications: newer techniques. Philadelphia: JP Medical Ltd; 2014.
16. Wallace RT, McNamara JA, Brown G, Benson W, Belmont J, Goldberg R, et al. The use of perfluorophenanthrene in the removal of intravitreal lens fragments. Am J Ophthalmol. 1993;116:196–200.
17. Rowson NJ, Bacon AS, Rosen PH. Perflourocarbon heavy liquids in the management of posterior dislocation of the lens nucleus during phacoemulsification. BrJ Ophthalmol. 1992;76:169–70.
18. Movshovich A, Berrocal M, Chang S. The protective properties of liquid perflourocarbons in phacofragmentation of dislocated lenses. Retina. 1994;14:457–62.
19. Villegas VM, Gold AS, Wildner A, Ehlies F, Murray TG. Retinal management of dropped lens as a complication of phacoemulsification. Retin Physician. 2014;11(3):44–7.
20. Koh KM, Kim HS, Cho HJ, et al. Surgical outcomes of 23-gauge vitrectomy for the management of lens fragments dropped into the vitreous cavity during cataract surgery. Saudi J Ophthalmol. 2014;28:253–6.
21. Scott IU, et al. Clinical features and outcomes of pars plana vitrectomy in patients with retained lens fragments. Ophthalmology. 2003;110:1567–72.
22. Salehi A, et al. Visual outcome of early and late pars plana vitrectomy in patients with dropped nucleus during phacoemulsification. J Res Med Sci. 2011;16:1422–9.

Management of Suprachoroidal Hemorrhage

38

Ehab El Rayes and Mahmoud Leila

38.1 Introduction

Since the first description of choroidal hemorrhage developing during cataract surgery in the late eighteenth century, suprachoroidal hemorrhage (SCH) continues to retain the notoriety of being the most fearsome complication in ophthalmic surgery. It is a complication that combines insidious onset, often explosive course, difficult management, and morbid visual outcome [1, 2]. Accordingly, the cornerstone of managing SCH constitutes an in-depth understanding of the pathophysiology of SCH and of the risk factors leading to its occurrence, preoperative identification of patients at high-risk and adequate knowledge, and skill acquisition of the various techniques used in managing such complication.

Electronic Supplementary Material The online version of this chapter (https://doi.org/10.1007/978-981-33-4168-5_38) contains supplementary material, which is available to authorized users.

E. El Rayes (✉) · M. Leila
Retina Department, Research Institute of Ophthalmology, Giza, Egypt

A. Jain et al. (eds.), *Cutting-edge Vitreoretinal Surgery*,
https://doi.org/10.1007/978-981-33-4168-5_38

38.2 Anatomic Background

Normally, the suprachoroidal space is a potential space containing approximately 10 μl of fluid that functions as a gliding platform for the choroid to move smoothly against the inner sclera during accommodation. The movement of the choroid over the sclera is checked by the scleral spur anteriorly, the optic nerve head posteriorly, and the perforating vessels and nerves traversing the sclera into and outside the eye. The choroid is also tethered to the sclera at the ampullae of the vortex veins. The thin film of fluid normally present in the suprachoroidal space is derived from the aqueous of the anterior chamber that enters the suprachoroidal space through a siphon-effect produced by the tone of the ciliary muscles and later on exits the suprachoroidal space through the uveoscleral outflow. Normally, the rate of fluid outflow exceeds that of fluid inflow; hence, the choroid and sclera remain in close apposition. The tangential sheets of collagen fibrils that anchor the outer surface of the choroid and ciliary body to the underlying sclera during accommodation can withstand pressure applied by a minimal amount of blood or serous effusion in the suprachoroidal space. However, large shearing force exerted by heavy bleeding or fluid accumulation will stretch these fine fibrils beyond their respective point of maximum stress until they eventually snap giving way to the accumulating blood or fluid [1, 3].

38.3 Pathogenetic Mechanisms of SCH

The pathogenetic cascade of SCH is initiated by hypotony, which will induce the rupture of a short or long posterior ciliary artery (arteries), by either one of two mechanisms or both mechanisms in tandem. Firstly, a severe drop in the intraocular pressure (IOP) will relieve the vascular wall from the outside force preventing its sudden expansion due to the unopposed force of systemic blood pressure leading to the rupture of a weak or necrotic vessel wall. Secondly, in the event of a drop of IOP, the choroidal transmural venous pressure increases, which favors extravasation of fluid from the choroidal veins into the suprachoroidal space. The final chain of the cascade ensues when the movement of albumin from the suprachoroidal space across the sclera is hampered due to extremely low IOP with consequent increase in the oncotic pressure beyond that of the plasma favoring more accumulation of fluid and a vicious circle sets on. Eventually, an excessive amount of fluid will accumulate and lead to the shearing-off of the posterior ciliary vessel(s) as they exit the sclera where they are most vulnerable [1, 3, 4]. Another infrequent mechanism of developing SCH is through obstruction of the venous outflow from the vortex veins, for instance by an overtightened scleral buckle with subsequent severe back pressure inflicted upon the choroidal veins [1, 5].

38.4 Risk Factors of SCH

A variety of ocular and systemic factors can put the patient at high risk of developing SCH. These factors will either produce direct weakening of the vessel wall or will set the stage for the vessel wall to rupture, eventually precipitating SCH particularly if one or more factors co-exist. Long-standing systemic hypertension, arteriosclerosis, vasculitis, and advanced age cause weakening of the vessel wall. High axial myopia is associated with less scleral rigidity, hence less support to the posterior ciliary arteries as they traverse the sclera. High axial hyperopic or nanophthalmic eyes have abnormally increased scleral thickness, which diminishes the uveoscleral outflow of aqueous and the scleral permeability to albumin leading to high albumin concentration in the suprachoroidal space. An aphakic patient would be relatively more susceptible to develop SCH as the absence of the crystalline lens and zonular system would allow more readily separation of the uvea from the sclera in the advent of choroidal effusion, eventually leading to over-stretch and rupture of the posterior ciliary arteries. Certain peri- or intraoperative conditions that are either patient-related or iatrogenic can accentuate the perilous effect of underlying systemic or ocular factors to precipitate SCH. Increased IOP due to excessive volume of retrobulbar anesthesia, uncontrolled glaucoma, or inadequate lid akinesia will increase the odds of rupture posterior ciliary artery upon decompression of the globe during ab-externo incision or sclerotomy creation. Conversely, increased episcleral venous pressure due to coughing, vomiting, Valsalva maneuver, and bucking effect associated with general anesthesia will increase the likelihood of rupture posterior ciliary artery intraoperatively or in the immediate postoperative period. Patients with tachycardia, blood dyscrasias, poor coagulation profile, or those on active anticoagulant therapy are at a special risk of uncontrolled bleeding [1, 6–9].

38.5 Prophylactic Measures in High-Risk Patients

Preoperatively, all patients must receive thorough systemic and ocular evaluation to identify the fore-mentioned risk factors and deploy the respective prophylactic measures. Systemic risk factors as uncontrolled hypertension, poor glycemic control, coagulation disorders, and tachycardia require liaison with the internist, cardiologist, and anesthesiologist for adequate control of these conditions prior to surgery and for discontinuation of anticoagulants before surgical intervention in order to bring down the international normalized ratio (INR) of the patient at the time of surgery to the lower limit of the therapeutic range. The optimal INR value at the time of surgery is 1.1, though surgery could be performed once INR is <2. In cases of high IOP, pressure-lowering agents as intravenous (IV) hyperosmotic agents as mannitol or systemic carbonic anhydrase inhibitors should be administered. Local anesthesia combined with sedating agents is generally preferable to general anesthesia whenever feasible. At the conclusion of surgery, all incisions must be closed watertight to avoid postoperative hypotony and inflammation [1, 6, 10, 11].

38.6 Incidence and Clinical Presentation of SCH

SCH is usually associated with ophthalmic surgery, either intraoperatively or during the postoperative period. SCH has been reported in association with glaucoma filtration surgery and aqueous drainage devices (0.7%), penetrating keratoplasty (PKP); (0.3%), cataract surgery (0.2–0.06%), and vitreoretinal surgery (0.17–1.9%). Less commonly, SCH develops secondary to blunt or penetrating trauma or even spontaneously.

38.6.1 Acute SCH

Intraoperative SCH is characterized by a more dramatic presentation compared to delayed postoperative SCH. Typically, procedures with large wound dimensions as in conventional extracapsular cataract extraction (ECCE), or PKP especially in the advent of protracted surgical time, are associated with severe prolonged hypotony. This would lead to the rapid progression of SCH that could be massive enough to cause the apposition of the retinal surfaces and even extrusion of the entire intraocular contents through the open wound. The classic clinical scenario in intraoperative SCH starts with suddenly increased IOP, iris prolapse with increasing dimming of the red reflex, development of a progressive black mound behind the pupillary plane, followed by vitreous loss and eventually extrusion of the intraocular contents. The briskly timing of these events and eventual prolapse of intraocular tissue through the wound account for the term *expulsive* SCH. Advances in surgical techniques and instrumentation in surgical ophthalmology especially in the field of cataract surgery with the introduction of phacoemulsification technology have greatly diminished the incidence of SCH and the extent of SCH. Acute SCH during vitreoretinal surgery is usually not related to hypotony, as the latter does not usually occur especially with modern small-gauge vitrectomy techniques with valved trocar cannulas due to the closed system platform which provides stable IOP throughout the entire procedure. SCH during vitrectomy is usually caused by inadvertent direct mechanical injury of the choroid by surgical instruments, for instance, while performing fluid–air exchange or during membrane peeling or retinectomy maneuvers. Heavy intensity endolaser especially long-wavelength lasers, excessive cryotherapy, or overtightened scleral buckle could also result in acute SCH [1, 12–17].

38.6.2 Delayed SCH

The incidence of delayed SCH is tenfold greater than that of the acute type. The condition is precipitated by prolonged hypotony with wound leak and inflammation, which are frequently associated with glaucoma filtration surgery, especially when using aqueous drainage devices. The time of presentation is usually 1–4 days after surgery. The patients start experiencing intense ocular pain. Pain is caused by stretching of the long ciliary nerves traversing the suprachoroidal space. Examination will reveal high IOP, and shallow anterior chamber due to blockage of the filtration site either by back pressure of progressive choroidal detachment or due to forward rotation of the iris–lens diaphragm. The red reflex is dull and a black mound is seen behind the pupil. In delayed SCH there is no extrusion of the intraocular contents except if dehiscence of the surgical wound occurred [18, 19].

38.7 Management of SCH

38.7.1 Immediate Intraoperative Measures in Acute SCH

The key management of acute SCH is combating hypotony by immediate restoration of the IOP to tamponade bleeding from the posterior ciliary arteries and breaking down the vicious circle that perpetuates progression to expulsive SCH. In the setting of a large incision dimension, rapid suturing of the wound is needed. Release of eye speculum is advised to avoid exerting pressure on the wall of the globe. Once all prolapsed tissue is repositioned and the wound is secured, reformation of the anterior chamber by air or saline is done. The anesthesiologist could administer sedating agents and systemic hypotensive agents to lower the systolic blood pressure. IV mannitol helps reducing the intraocular volume. Performing drainage sclerotomies should be reserved as a last resort, and exclusively performed in cases the prolapsed tissue through the wound could not be repositioned due to extremely high-back pressure and despite deploying the above-mentioned measures. Drainage sclerotomy would increase the risk of retinal or uveal tissue incarceration due to high IOP. Moreover, sclerotomies could induce more hypotony, hence stimulating re-bleeding. Finally, attempting drainage sclerotomy might be an unwarranted risk as bleeding from the posterior ciliary artery is known to undergo rapid clotting [1, 20, 21].

38.7.2 Drainage of SCH

38.7.2.1 Indications

Drainage of SCH might not be necessary, especially in sectorial SCH away from the posterior pole. In these cases, cycloplegia and analgesics are useful to control the pain. Topical steroids are usually sufficient to control the inflammation [1]. Drainage is indicated in the presence of massive SCH causing apposition of the inner retinal surfaces; the so-called kissing choroidals, hemorrhage involving the macular area, the presence of retinal detachment, vitreous hemorrhage, very high IOP not responsive to medical therapy, flat anterior chamber with corneo-lenticular touch or intractable pain.

38.7.2.2 Timing

If a second surgery to drain the SCH is indicated, we should wait for 10–14 days, which is the time required for the blood clot to undergo liquefaction for easy extrusion through the sclerotomy and minimal manipulation of the suprachoroidal space to express the clotted blood. During that period, the evolution of SCH should be closely monitored by biomicroscopic examination and by ultrasound (Figs. 38.1 and 38.2). In the case of massive SCH, ultrasound during the following few days will show the characteristic features of

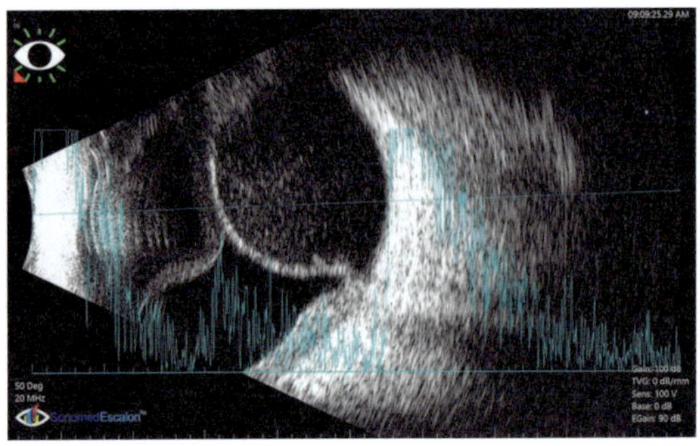

Fig. 38.1 Combined A- and B-scan ultrasonography of hemorrhagic choroidal detachment. B-scan revealed markedly elevated dome-shaped appearance with fine amorphous echoes in the suprachoroidal space "moderate hemorrhage." A-scan revealed a 100% high double spike (retina and choroid)

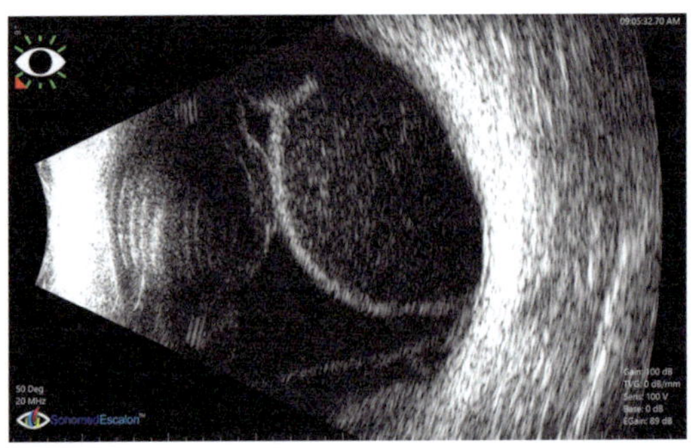

Fig. 38.2 B-scan of the same patient revealed subretinal hemorrhage in the peripapillary area with a retinal detachment extending peripherally in the lower quadrant with mild subretinal hemorrhage

bullous choroidal detachments in close apposition in the posterior chamber (kissing choroidals) with dense SCH. The choroidal detachments yield a characteristic highly reflective double-peak spike followed by a trail of lower internal reflectivity spikes originating from the blood clot. As the blood clot undergoes liquefaction, the height of the choroidal bullae recedes and the suprachoroidal space shows fine dispersed dot opacities with minimal reflectivity originating from liquefied blood. Ultrasound will help the selection of the best quadrant(s) to perform sclerotomy guided by the height of the choroidal detachment. Whenever ultrasonography reveals retinal detachment or involvement of the macular area with hemorrhage, the surgeon should consider earlier intervention for optimum visual outcome [22–25].

38.7.2.3 Surgical Technique

At the start of surgery, the surgeon should close any identifiable wound leaks. Subsequently, an anterior chamber (AC) maintainer or 25-gauge infusion cannula is placed in the anterior chamber. The IOP is set at 30 mmHg. Limited peritomy and bridling of the recti muscles are performed in the quadrant(s) chosen for sclerotomy guided by preoperative ultrasound. A radial sclerotomy 2–3 mm long is performed at 6–8 mm posterior to the limbus parallel to the rectus muscle and extending posteriorly from the equator but anterior to the vortex veins. Initially, the blood is drained only partially to avoid excessive hypotony. Supplemental digital content 1 demonstrates the surgical technique for drainage of SCH. Afterward, PPV is performed, sometimes along with injection of perfluorocarbon liquid which helps in displacing the suprachoroidal blood away from the posterior pole and through the open sclerotomy. The extruded blood is typically dark in color and mixed with small pieces of the clot. At the conclusion of surgery, the retina is evaluated. Gas or silicone oil tamponade is required in cases of retinal detachment or retinal breaks [25, 26]. Some authors advocate the injection of tissue plasminogen activator into the suprachoroidal space to help dissolving the clot [26–29]. It is worthy of note that residual SCH might cause tamponade under-fill weeks after surgery when SCH is completely absorbed [30]. Another technique consists of inserting a 20/25 gauge trocar cannula system into the suprachoroidal space through a beveled incision at 7 mm posterior to the limbus in 1 or 2 quadrants according to the maximum height of choroidal detachment. The trocar cannula system is inserted almost parallel to the sclera to avoid damage to the retina or the uveal tissue. After drainage, the cannula is removed and the conjunctiva over the incision site is cauterized. PPV is performed only in cases of concomitant vitreous hemorrhage, retinal incarceration, or retinal detachment. This technique is especially useful in cases of scarred conjunctiva or scleral thinning [31]. Rossi et al. [30] proposed the insertion of non-valved trocar cannulas at 3.5 mm from the limbus into the suprachoroidal space. Once the infusion line connected to the AC maintainer cannula was opened, the suprachoroidal blood would start egressing through the cannulas, with progressive recession of the choroidal detachment. That was followed by a 23-gauge core vitrectomy using limbal access for the cutter and light probe. Often, that procedure was sufficient for almost complete drainage of SCH. Once the egress of blood stopped from the cannulas, the cannulas were checked through the pupil to ensure vitreous access, and the light probe and cutter were inserted through the pars plana, while maintaining the AC infusion line to drain any additional choroidal blood through the third cannula. Obviously, Rossi's technique could only be performed in aphakic or pseudophakic patients.

38.8 Prognosis

Factors heralding poor visual outcome after an episode of SCH include retinal detachment, breakthrough of suprachoroidal blood into the subretinal space or the vitreous, and incarceration of retinal or uveal tissue. In absence of these events, the patient can achieve favorable visual outcomes [1, 7–12].

38.9 Conclusion

SCH remains a serious complication in ophthalmic surgery, even though technological advances in surgical techniques and machinery have reduced its occurrence. Due to the frequent morbid visual outcome of SCH, identification of patients at high risk of developing SCH, and deploying the necessary prophylactic measures, both pre- and intraoperatively is of the essence. Surgical intervention to drain SCH can achieve good results if properly executed and appropriate timing for surgical intervention and surgical technique were selected.

References

1. Chu TG, Green RL. Suprachoroidal hemorrhage. Surv Ophthalmol. 1999;43(6):471–86.
2. Payne JW, Kameen AJ, Jensen AD, Christy NE. Expulsive hemorrhage: its incidence in cataract surgery and a report of four bilateral cases. Trans Am Ophthalmol Soc. 1985;83:181–204.
3. Brubaker RF, Pederson JE. Ciliochoroidal detachment. Surv Ophthalmol. 1983;27(5):281–9.
4. Jackson TL, Hussain A, Salisbury J, Sherwood R, Sullivan PM, Marshall J. Transscleral albumin diffusion and suprachoroidal albumin concentration in uveal effusion syndrome. Retina. 2012;32(1):177–82.
5. Zauberman H. Expulsive choroidal hemorrhage: an experimental study. Br J Ophthalmol. 1982;66:43–5.
6. Speaker MG, Guerriero PN, Met JA, Coad CT, Berger A, Marmor M. A case-control study of risk factors for intraoperative suprachoroidal expulsive hemorrhage. Ophthalmology. 1991;98:202–10.
7. Yang SS, Fu AD, McDonald HR, Johnson RN, Ai E, Jumper JM. Massive spontaneous choroidal hemorrhage. Retina. 2003;23:139–44.
8. Nguyen HN, Nork TM. Massive spontaneous suprachoroidal hemorrhage in a young woman with cystic fibrosis and diabetes mellitus on anticoagulants. Retin Cases Brief Rep. 2012;6:216–8.
9. Elagouz M, Stanescu-Segall D, Jackson TL. Uveal effusion syndrome. Surv Ophthalmol. 2010;55(2):134–45.
10. Lip GYH, Durrani OM, Roldan V, Lip PL, Marin F, Reuser TQ. Peri-operative management of ophthalmic patients taking antithrombotic therapy. Int J Clin Pract. 2011;65(3):361–71.
11. Hamilton RC, Loken RG. Anesthesia for cataract surgery. In: Steinert RF, editor. Cataract surgery: techniques, complications, & management. 1st ed. Philadelphia: Saunders; 1995. p. 68–103.
12. Ling R, Cole M, James C, Kamalarajah S, Foot B, Shaw S. Suprachoroidal haemorrhage complicating cataract surgery in the UK: epidemiology, clinical features, management, and outcomes. Br J Ophthalmol. 2004;88(4):478–80.
13. Ingraham HJ, Donnenfeld ED, Perry HD. Massive suprachoroidal hemorrhage in penetrating keratoplasty. Am J Ophthalmol. 1989;108(6):670–5.
14. Price FW Jr, Whitson WE, Ahad KA, Tavakkoli H. Suprachoroidal hemorrhage in penetrating keratoplasty. Ophthalmic Surg. 1994;25(8):521–5.
15. Chandra A, Xing W, Kadhim MR, Williamson TH. Suprachoroidal hemorrhage in pars plana vitrectomy. Risk factors and outcomes over 10 years. Ophthalmology. 2014;121:311–7.
16. Tabandeh H, Flynn HW Jr. Suprachoroidal hemorrhage during pars plana vitrectomy. Curr Opin Ophthalmol. 2001;12(3):179–85.
17. Reibaldi M, Longo A, Romano MR, Cennamo G, Mariotti C, Boscia F, Bonfiglio V, Avitabile T. Delayed suprachoroidal hemorrhage after pars plana vitrectomy: five-years results of a retrospective multicenter cohort study. Am J Ophthalmol. 2015;160(6):1235–42.
18. Tuli SS, WuDunn D, Ciulla TA, Cantor LB. Delayed suprachoroidal hemorrhage after glaucoma filtration procedures. Ophthalmology. 2001;108:1808–11.
19. Jeganathan VSE, Ghosh S, Ruddle JB, Gupta V, Coote MA, Crowston JG. Risk factors for delayed suprachoroidal hemorrhage following glaucoma surgery. Br J Ophthalmol. 2008;92(10):1393–6.
20. Ruderman MJ, Rosenberg LF, Krupin T. Anterior segment surgery. In: Krupin T, Kolker AE, Rosenberg LF, editors. Complications in ophthalmic surgery. 2nd ed. St. Louis: Mosby; 2000. p. 37–55.
21. Sukpen I, Stewart JM. Acute intraoperative suprachoroidal hemorrhage during small-gauge pars plana vitrectomy. Retin Cases Brief Rep. 2018;12:S9–S11.
22. Lakhanpal V. Experimental and clinical observations on massive suprachoroidal hemorrhage. Trans Am Ophthalmol Soc. 1993;91:545–62.
23. Dibernardo C, Schachat A, Fekrat S. Choroid. In: Ophthalmic ultrasound. A diagnostic atlas. 1st ed. New York: Thieme; 1998. p. 67–76.
24. Learned D, Eliott D. Management of delayed suprachoroidal hemorrhage after glaucoma surgery. Semin Ophthalmol. 2018;33(1):59–63.
25. Garcia-Arumi J. Massive suprachoroidal hemorrhage. In: Ryan SJ, editor. Retina. 6th ed. Philadelphia: Saunders; 2018. p. 2371.
26. Kadonosono K. Suprachoroidal hemorrhage during cataract surgery. In: Ryan SJ, editor. Retina. 6th ed. Philadelphia: Saunders; 2018. p. 2371.
27. Fei P, Jin HY, Zhang Q, Li X, Zhao PQ. Tissue plasminogen activator-assisted vitrectomy in the early treatment of acute massive suprachoroidal hemorrhage complicating cataract surgery. Int J Ophthalmol. 2018;11(1):170–1.

28. Matsumoto K, Matsumoto CS, Shinoda K, Watanabe E, Mizota A. Tissue plasminogen activator-assisted vitrectomy for ruptured eye with suprachoroidal hemorrhage. Case Rep Ophthalmol. 2012;3(2):258–61.
29. Kunjukunju N, Gonzales CR, Rodden WS. Recombinant tissue plasminogen activator in the treatment of suprachoroidal hemorrhage. Clin Ophthalmol. 2011;5:155–7.
30. Rossi T, Boccassini B, Iossa M, Lesnoni G, Tamburrelli C. Choroidal hemorrhage drainage through 23-gauge vitrectomy cannulas. Retina. 2010;30:174–6.
31. Rezende FA, Kickinger MC, Li G, Prado RF, Regis LGT. Transconjunctival drainage of serous and hemorrhagic choroidal detachment. Retina. 2012;32:242–9.

Keratoprosthesis in Vitreoretinal Surgery

39

Nikoloz Labauri, Tekla Mamageishvili, and Ana Vachiberidze

39.1 Introduction

Corneal transplantation is the *most common* type of allogeneic transplantation counting approximately 100,000 procedures every year [1] done worldwide with a success rate of 80% graft survival within 5 years. However, there are many different clinical entities where corneal allografts are commonly rejected. In limbal stem cell failure, after chemical or thermal burns, in autoimmune diseases such as Steven–Johnson syndrome and cicatricial pemphigoid corneal transplantation success rate is less than 25% and correspondingly visual prognosis is very poor [2]. In such severe diseases, an alternative to corneal allografts should be considered such as artificial cornea referred to as Keratoprosthesis (Kpro). Nowadays, the best candidates for Kpro are those patients who are having autoimmune-related corneal opacity, chemical injury, or corneal allograft failure. In 1789, Pellier de Quengsy was the first who suggested a keratoprosthesis to replace an opaque natural corneal tissue [3].

39.1.1 Types of Keratoprosthesis

There are two main types of Kpro: (1) Permanent keratoprosthesis which is used to exchange biological tissue with an artificial tissue for life long, such as osteo-odonto-keratoprosthesis [4] (OOKP), the AlphaCor™ artificial cornea [5], and the Boston keratoprosthesis (KPro™) [6] and (2) Temporary keratoprosthesis (TKP), is used for temporary purposes *either* to replace the opaque cornea to better visualize the retina during vitrectomy and at the end replace it with a regular corneal allograft *or* TPK application in a procedure called "Bilateral Corneal Autotransplantation," where corneal tissue is to be exchanged between both eyes of the patient in the same time and once the graft is taken from donor eye it is closed by temporary Kpro until surgery is undergoing on the fellow eye. At the end, temporary keratoprosthesis is removed and opaque cornea taken from the fellow eye is transplanted (Fig. 39.1).

The first use of TKP during Pars plana vitrectomy (PPV) was described by Landers et al. in 1981 [7]. Landers TKP was made by PMMA and had a 5-mm length. Another invention was done by Eckardt [8] in 1987, who proposed a 7 mm disposable TPK made by silicone material. However, Eckardt's device has become cloudy during fluid–air exchange and silicone was irresistible for multiple suture trucks [9]. Nowadays we commonly use Landers PMMA TPKs with two main modifications. One is truncated with a 1-mm cylinder protruding to the anterior chamber with a mushroom-shaped corneal surface of a diameter 15.5 mm and 6 suture holes in the

N. Labauri (✉) · T. Mamageishvili · A. Vachiberidze
Davinci Eye Hospital, Tbilisi, Georgia

A. Jain et al. (eds.), *Cutting-edge Vitreoretinal Surgery*,
https://doi.org/10.1007/978-981-33-4168-5_39

periphery and another is the latest modification so-called trunkless TKP [10] (Fig. 39.2). This latest has an advantage in the sizing of corneal recipient graft. When TPK with trunk is used, the recipient has to be trephined not less than 8.0 mm in diameter to allow fitting of the trunk through the corneal opening, compare to trunkless TKP, which does not have this limitation and can be used at any recipient corneal size. Besides, the trunkless TPK is much easier to suture and it maintains a water seal condition as perfectly as it does the TPK with a trunk. Landers device is reusable, durable, and has anterior convexity to better visualize posterior pole as well as retinal periphery during vitrectomy procedure. In addition, there are some models which have in-built metallic infusion lines to further facilitate vitrectomy procedure and make sure that iatrogenic choroidal detachment will not happen in case of inadvertent suprachoroidal trocar placement.

39.2 Surgical Steps

When TKP is planned in combination with posterior pole surgery, some consecutive steps have to be followed by the operating surgeon. At the beginning infusion trocar placement is to

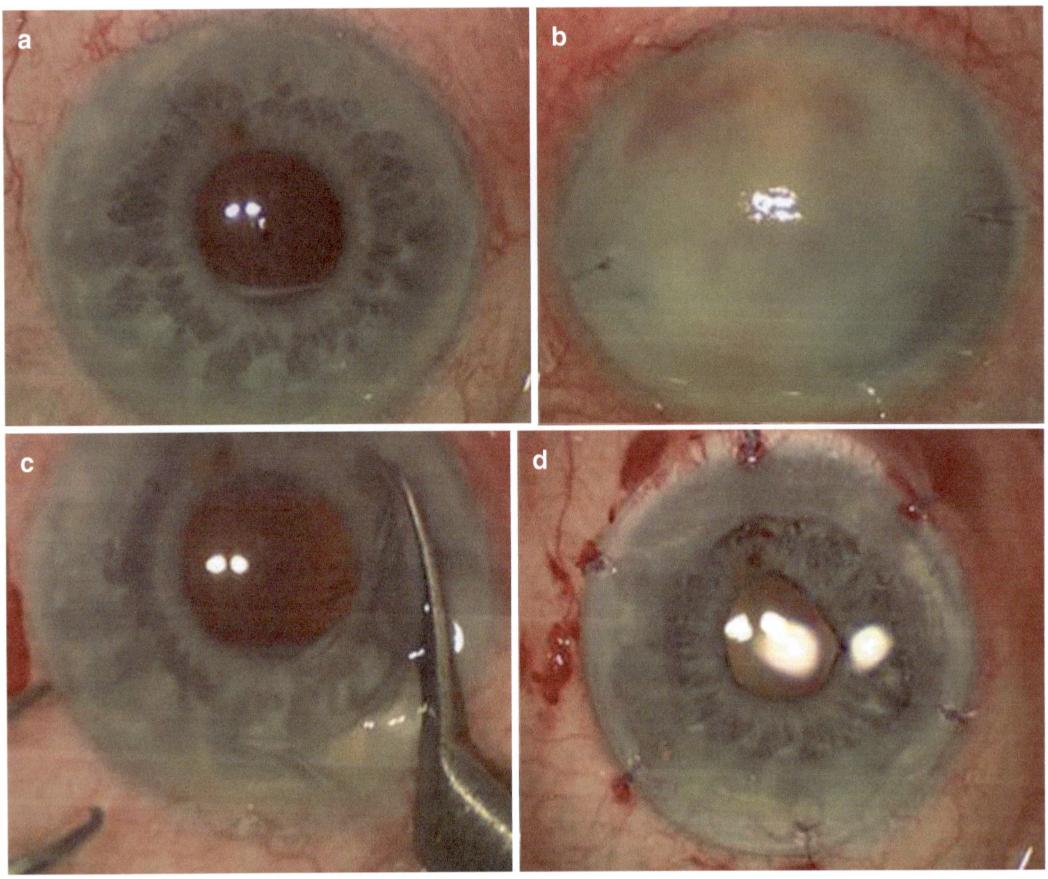

Fig. 39.1 Demonstrates the use of TPK in bilateral autokeratotransplantation where donor is the Left eye (**a**) having absolute glaucoma but optically clear cornea and recipient is the Right eye (**b**) where the cornea is hazy due to complicated cataract surgery. Donor cornea is harvested from the left eye first (**c**) and TPK is used (**d**) to restore the integrity of the globe until it receives a hazy corneal transplant from the right eye at the very end of the procedure. After donor cornea is stored and prepared for transplantation, hazy cornea is trephined in the right eye (**e**) followed by autotransplantation of optically clear cornea (**f**). As a last step, we are back to the left eye, where TPK is removed (**g**) and hazy cornea harvested from the right eye is transplanted (**h**) (Courtesy of Nikoloz Labauri, MD)

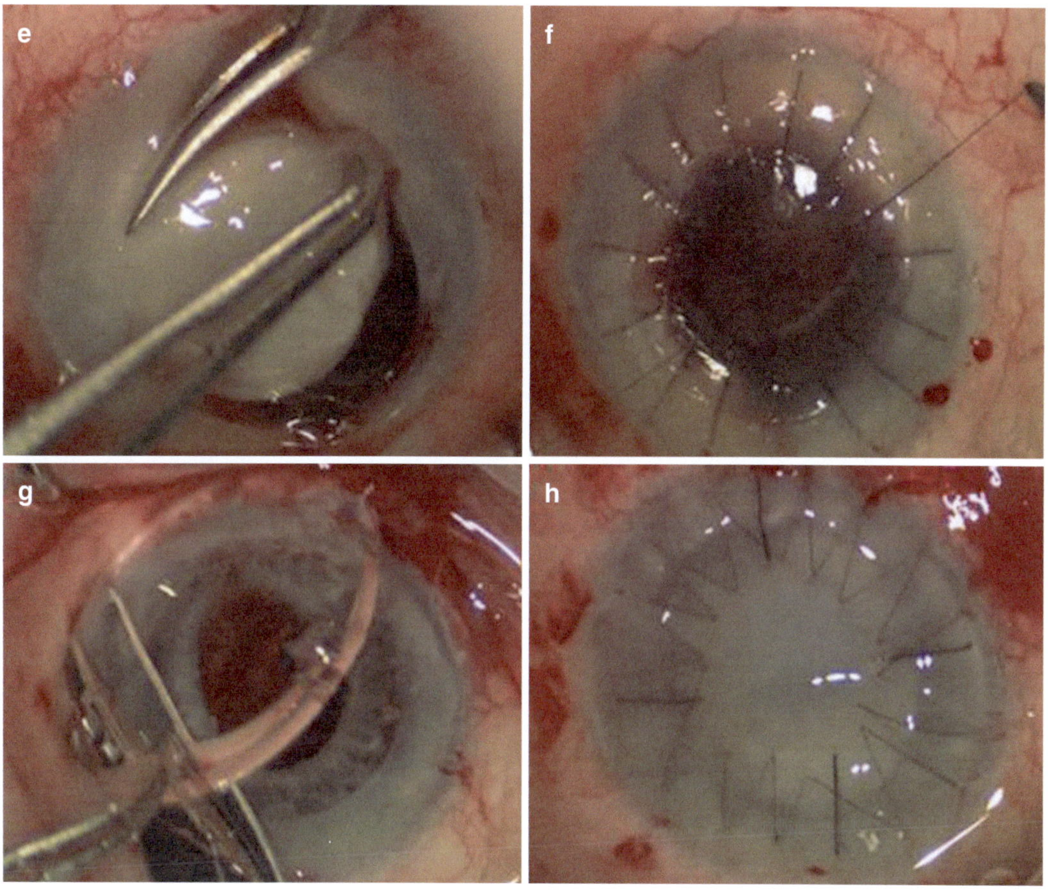

Fig. 39.1 (continued)

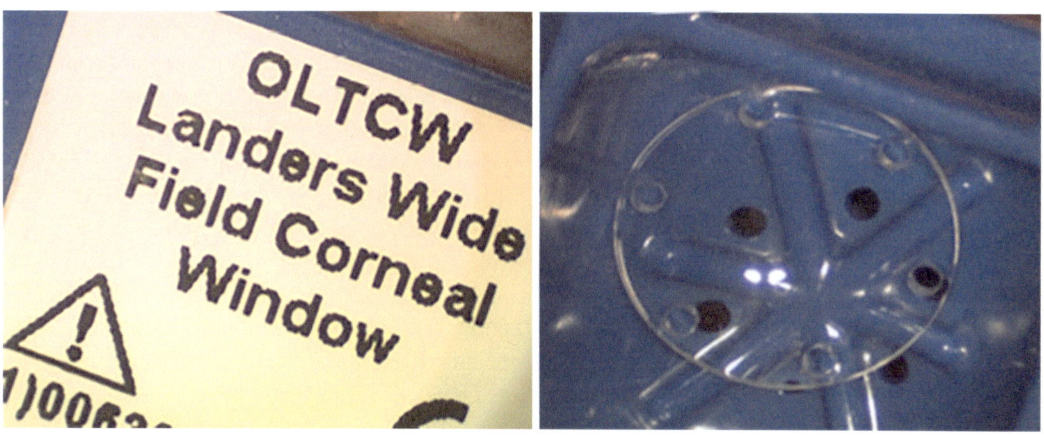

Fig. 39.2 Shows trunkless Landers temporary keratoprosthesis (TPK) model—OLTCW

be performed followed by corneal trephination and TKP suturing. The infusion line is turned on after the operating surgeon makes sure that the infusion cannula is properly positioned into the vitreous cavity. Once the infusion is turned on and the globe is reformed other trocars should be placed into the appropriate quadrants. For the TKP fixation, we use 7-0 Vycril absorbable sutures to fixate it onto the sclera, and sutures are passed across the intact conjunctiva. Care should be taken to not to insert trocars far posterior from the limbus to avoid iatrogenic retinal damage. Before we start vitrectomy the lens status should be carefully evaluated. If the eye is phakic we need to proceed with open sky extracapsular lens extraction trying not to damage the posterior capsule since this latest is necessary to prevent silicone oil or gas migration into the anterior chamber. If the eye is pseudophakic or aphakic we need to proceed directly with routine vitrectomy surgery. We usually advocate not to implant an IOL during the first procedure and to plan a secondary IOL implantation after silicone oil and corneal sutures are removed to better calculate the appropriate IOL power. Anterior chamber IOLs we usually remove before proceeding with vitrectomy and if the eye is aphakic inferior peripheral iridectomy (PI) is to be performed at the initial stage. After the vitrectomy is completed and the retina is attached, the surgeon should focus on the tamponading agent and select a proper step when he or she should perform corneal allotransplantation. Usually, we advocate to remove the TKP and suture the donor cornea on air-filled eye. Sometimes if silicone tamponade is planned oil can be injected to fill at least half of the vitreous cavity. This may help a bit to maintain the shape of the globe and at the end after the corneal transplantation is finished silicone oil fill is accomplished. It should be noted that after TKP is removed, corneal transplantation will be performed in extremely hypotonic conditions and will cause some trouble while suturing a graft to the host tissue. This step needs to be done as quickly as possible or at least four cardinal sutures in each quadrant to allow incoming air to restore intraocular pressure and avoid a complication such as suprachoroidal hemorrhage. Double Flieringa ring may help in these situations, which also has to be sutured at the very beginning of the procedure. For suturing the graft we use 10-0 Nylon suture with 16 interrupted suture bites. Once corneal transplantation is completed and air is maintaining eye pressure, we accomplish silicone oil fill, or in case of gas tamponade, first remove trocar cannulas and end up with air–gas exchange. Care should be taken to avoid silicone oil bubble migration into the anterior chamber at the final stage and we recommend to use the biplanar closure technique to seal the sclerotomy wounds in case of leakage [11].

Postoperative care has to be started right after the surgery with intravenous prednisolone (500–800 mg) transfusion to better control the postoperative inflammation. Eye drops such as antibiotics, steroids, lubricants, cycloplegics and if needed pressure lowering medications should be started within less than 24 h after surgery.

39.3 Viewing System

Another scenario is what wide-angle viewing system is the best to use with TKP to better visualize the retina. In fact, both contact and noncontact systems are successfully used with TPK. The same is true with permanent keratoprostheses. Sometimes when contact systems are used a large-size contact lens can be applied to the surface of TKP to make its surface more regular and facilitate the lens holding by a surgical assistant. We use Volk wide-angle indirect contact lenses for peripheral as well as for macular work. Among permanent keratoprosthesis, there are some types through which visualization of peripheral retina is extremely limited, because of the architecture of the prosthesis itself, such as OOKP, Pintucci Krpos, etc. These devices are having smaller window diameter as well as the long optical body which significantly alters the surgeon's view (Fig. 39.3).

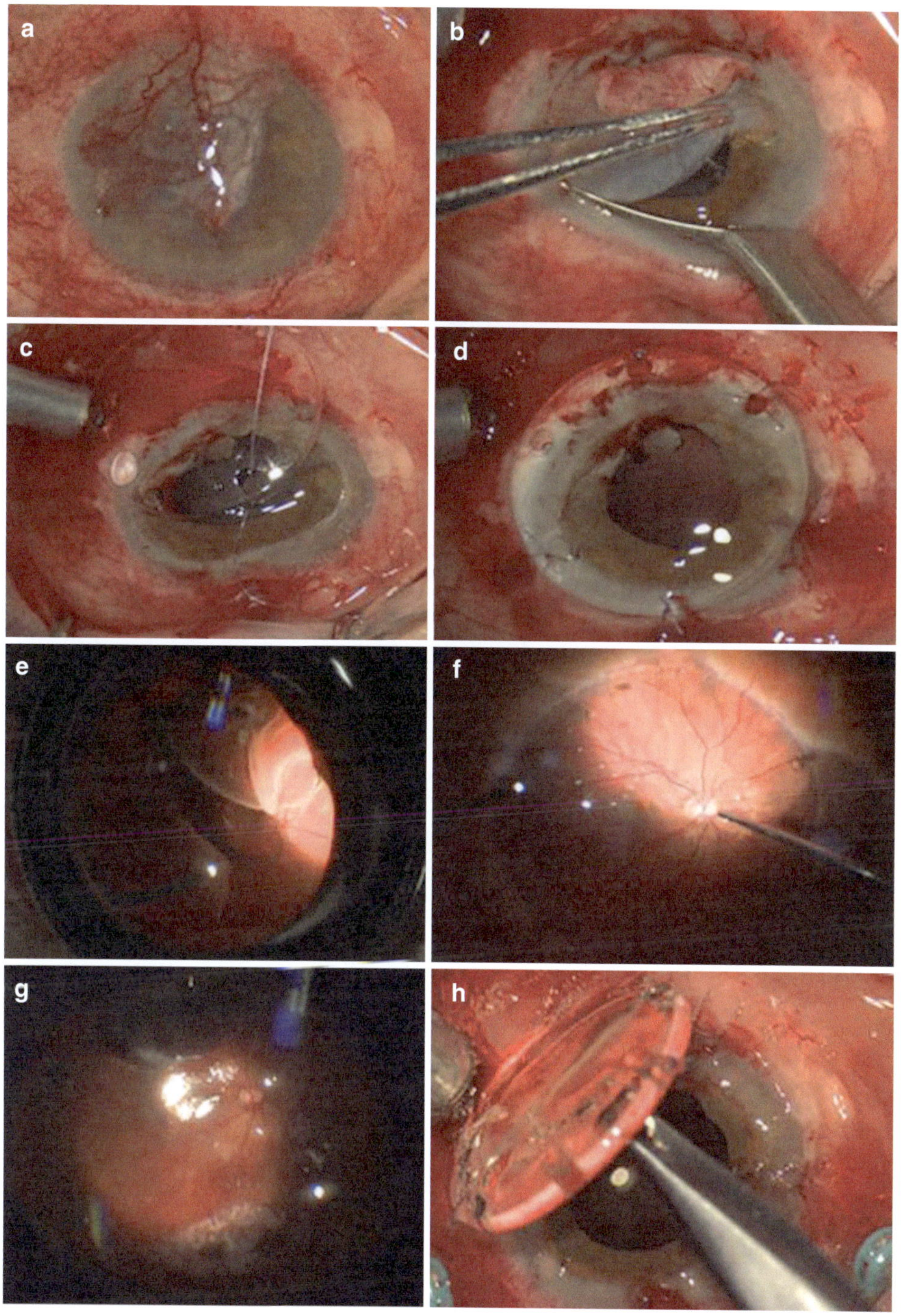

Fig. 39.3 Demonstrates the stepwise approach of combined TPK and PPV for the patient having perforating corneal trauma (corneal wound was closed using multiple sutures and conjunctival autograft (**a**) to achieve water seal condition) and coexisting retinal detachment with multiple breaks. Damaged cornea was trephined in 8.0 mm and cut using corneal scissors (**b**) followed by Landers TPK suturing using 7-0 vycril suture (**c**) with fixation in 5 points (**d**). Posterior pole view during 25G PPV for detached retina using a wide-angle contact lens held onto the surface of TPK (**e**). Perfluorocarbon liquid is used to stabilize the posterior retina (**f**). Laser retinopexy is applied after the fluid–air exchange (**g**). TPK is removed (**h**) and corneal allotransplantation is accomplished under air (**i**) followed by pupilloplasty and air–silicone oil exchange (**j**) (courtesy of Nikoloz Labauri MD)

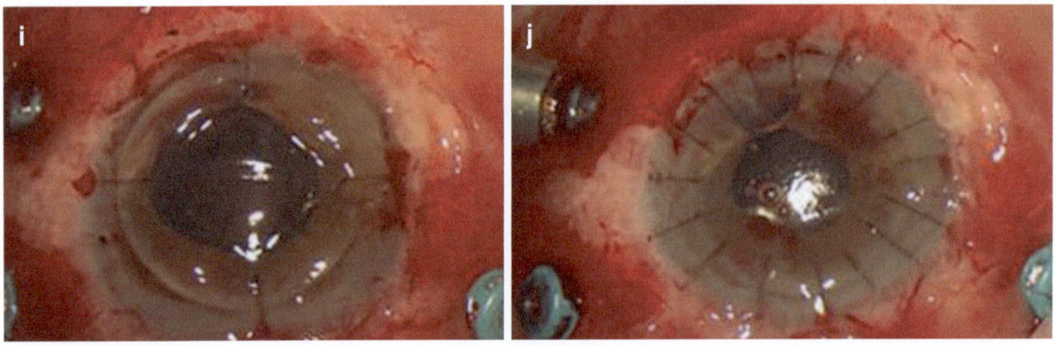

Fig. 39.3 (continued)

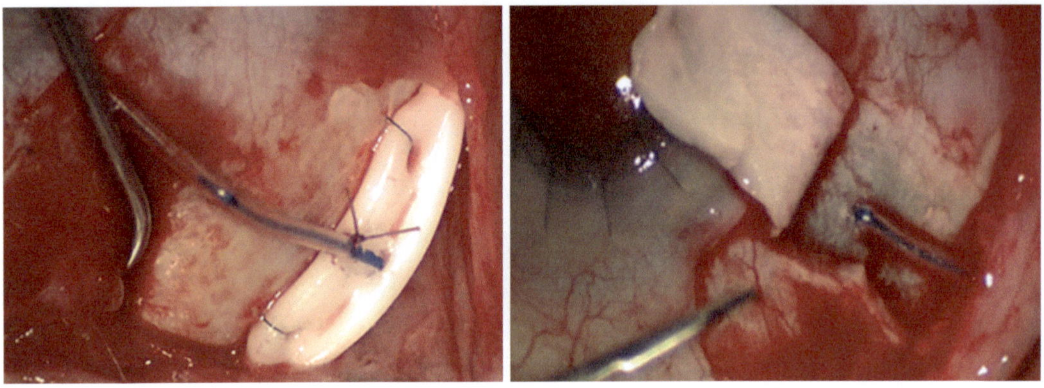

Fig. 39.4 Demonstrates glaucoma tube shunt (Baerveldt BG-101-350) placement through the pars plana to control refractory glaucoma 2 months after the combined TPK-PPV-PKP procedure (Courtesy of Nikoloz Labauri, MD)

39.4 Complications

Complications related to TPK are not many, but if happens sometimes those could have devastating results. As already mentioned, intraoperative complications such as suprachoroidal hemorrhage may happen while suturing the corneal graft under hypotonic conditions. Therefore, keeping low blood pressure during the surgery is recommended and those procedures are preferably done under general anesthesia. Other systemic factors, which may lead to suprachoroidal hemorrhage should be foreseen and addressed appropriately. During the postoperative period, the most common complication is elevated intraocular pressure, which is caused either by anterior angle pathology or high-dose steroid use to avoid graft immune rejection. If anti-glaucoma medications are not sufficient to keep the eye pressure within normal limits, glaucoma surgery using valved or nonvalved tube shunts is advocated (Fig. 39.4). In our clinical series of 22 eyes, we used tube shunts in 16 (72%) cases with a preference of Baerveldt shunt versus Ahmed valve. If silicone oil is removed or gas was used initially we prefer a pars plana placement of the tube instead of into the anterior chamber. Our clinical observation showed that pars plana implants last longer and regulate intraocular pressure much effectively to the tube placed in the anterior chamber. Tube placement into the anterior chamber should be considered when the vitreous cavity is filled with silicone oil.

39.5 Outcome

Anatomical and visual prognosis are strongly dependent on the severity of the disease. Some studies have shown a graft survival rate of 49% and retinal attachment in 90% and 78% of patients in the non-trauma and ocular trauma groups, respectively [12]. Another study by another group has shown visual acuity improvement in some patients as well as corneal survival rate in 30% of cases [13]. Our clinical observation revealed graft survival in 65% (15 out of 22) and visual improvement in 55% (12 out of 22) of cases (unpublished data).

39.6 Conclusion

The development of TKP has provided a new opportunity to salvage the vision of those eyes which require penetrating keratoplasty as well as pars plana vitrectomy for posterior pole pathology at the same time.

References

1. Eye Banking Statistical Report 2007. Eye Bank Association of America.
2. Tugal-Tutkun I, Akova YA, Foster CS. Penetrating keratoplasty in cicatrizing conjunctival diseases. Ophthalmology. 1995;102:576–85. https://doi.org/10.1016/S0161-6420(95)30980-3.
3. Pellier de Quengsy G. Précis ou cours d'operations sur la chirurgie des yeux. Montpellier: Rigaut, Roullet. Paris, Didot, Mequignon; 1789. p. 94.
4. Strampelli B. Osteo-odontokeratoprosthesis. Ann Ottalmol Clin Ocul. 1963;89:1039–44.
5. Chirila TV, Vijayasekaran S, Horne R, et al. Interpenetrating polymer network (IPN) as a permanent joint between the elements of a new type of artificial cornea. J Biomed Mater Res. 1994;28:745–53. https://doi.org/10.1002/jbm.820280612.
6. Dohlman CH, Schneider H, Doane MG. Prosthokeratoplasty. Am J Ophthalmol. 1974;77:694–700. https://doi.org/10.1016/0002-9394(74)90534-0.
7. Landers MB, Foulks GN, Landers DM, et al. Temporary keratoprosthesis for use during pars plana vitrectomy. Am J Ophthalmol. 1981;91(5):615–9. https://doi.org/10.1016/0002-9394(81)90061-1.
8. Eckardt C. A new temporary keratoprosthesis for pars plana vitrectomy. Retina. 1987;1:34–7. https://doi.org/10.1097/00006982-198700710-0008.
9. Narendram V, Kothari AR, Charles S, Saravanan VR, Kreissing I. Principles and practice of vitreo-retinal surgery. New Delhi: Jaypee Brothers Medical Publishers; 2014.
10. Toth CA, Landers MB. A new wide-field temporary keratoprosthesis. Retina. 1993;4:353–5. https://doi.org/10.1097/00006982-199313040-00014.
11. Labauri N, Mamageishvili T, Tsomaia K, Omiadze M. Sutureless biplanar closure of leaking wounds in micro-incision vitreous surgery: A novel technique. Eur J Ophthalmol. 2019;29(1):110–2. https://doi.org/10.1177/1120672118767555.
12. Nowomiejska K, Haszcz D, Forlini C, Forlini M, Moneta-Wielgos J, Maciejewski R, et al. Wide-field landers temporary keratoprosthesis in severe ocular trauma: functional and anatomical results after one year. J Ophthalmol. 2015;2015:1–6. https://doi.org/10.1155/2015/163675.
13. Bové Álvarez M, Arumí CG, Distéfano L, Güell JL, Gris Ó, Mateo C, et al. Comparative study of penetrating keratoplasty and vitreoretinal surgery with Eckardt temporary keratoprosthesis in ocular trauma versus non-trauma patients. Graefes Arch Clin Exp Ophthalmol. 2019;11:2547–58. https://doi.org/10.1007/s00417-019-04420-0.

40 Phaco-vitrectomy

Timothy G. Murray and Victor M. Villegas

40.1 Introduction

Recent advances in microincisional vitrectomy surgery (MIVS) combined with advances in small-incision cataract surgery have enabled the ophthalmic surgeon to provide combined management of cataract and retinal pathology. Progressive understanding of the certainty of cataract progression after pars plana vitrectomy along with the negative impact of early cataract progression on visual acuity outcomes have defined the importance of combined cataract surgery and pars plana vitrectomy in improving surgical outcomes. Multiple authors have described the therapeutic benefits of combined phaco-vitrectomy including decreased incidence of macular edema, decreased postsurgical vitreous traction, optimized visualization of the posterior segment, and decreased the total surgical procedures required for the individual patient [1–3]. Phacoemulsification following vitrectomy carries increased risks of posterior capsular tears, zonular dialysis, and loss of lens particles posteriorly [4]. Combining phacoemulsification with vitrectomy decreases rehabilitation time, risks, and costs associated to a second surgery [5–8]. This chapter will describe the preferred surgical techniques used by the authors during microincisional phaco-vitrectomy.

Electronic Supplementary Material The online version of this chapter (https://doi.org/10.1007/978-981-33-4168-5_40) contains supplementary material, which is available to authorized users.

T. G. Murray
Murray Ocular Oncology and Retina (MOOR), Miami, FL, USA
e-mail: tmurray@murraymd.com

V. M. Villegas (✉)
Department of Ophthalmology, University of Puerto Rico, San Juan, PR, USA

Bascom Palmer Eye Institute, University of Miami Miller School of Medicine, Miami, FL, USA

Department of Surgery, Ponce Health Sciences University, Ponce, PR, USA

40.2 Indications

The most common indication for phaco-vitrectomy in patients with a dense cataract is optimization of visualization during vitrectomy [9]. Avoiding phacoemulsification if a dense cataract is present may hinder optimal surgical outcomes, especially if epiretinal or internal limiting membrane peeling is necessary during MIVS [10]. Patients with preexisting, but early, lenticular changes who are certain to have visual loss due to cataract progression postoperatively are also excellent candidates.

Pediatric patients less than 2 years of age with a clear crystalline lens may benefit from vitrectomy to preserve accommodation during the amblyopic age range. This facilitates amblyopia

A. Jain et al. (eds.), *Cutting-edge Vitreoretinal Surgery*,
https://doi.org/10.1007/978-981-33-4168-5_40

therapy as compared to aphakic correction. Intraocular lens implantation should be avoided if the corneal diameter is less than 9 mm or if active uveitis is present. Family members need to be aware that a second surgery will be warranted in the near future. Older children may benefit from phaco-vitrectomy, especially at the time of silicone oil extraction or if complex pathology is present at the time of primary surgery (e.g., giant retinal tear).

40.3 Dilation and Visualization

Preoperative dilation with both a cycloplegic and sympathomimetic agent is routinely performed. We use 10% phenylephrine in patients without contraindications to achieve optimal mydriasis and visualization of the posterior pole during vitrectomy. Avoidance of long-acting cycloplegic drops may decrease the incidence of posterior synechiae and may also minimize having silicone oil in the anterior segment during the first postoperative week.

The most important part of any surgery is visualization. Without an outstanding view, the simplest parts of the surgery can become extremely challenging. We routinely use noncontact visualization systems such as the Resight 700 (Carl Zeiss Meditec) or the BIOM (Oculus Surgical) for widefield viewing. The biggest advantage of using noncontact systems is the ability to operate without an assistant. They also allow excellent theoretical 130° of visualization and the capability to work in the far retinal periphery without prisms. Furthermore, this technology allows quick exchange from anterior segment surgery to posterior segment visualization.

40.4 Trochars

Transconjunctival, sutureless, trochar vitrectomy systems (23/25/27/29G) have evolved significantly during the last years. Advantages of the 23/25/27/29G systems include improved safety of fewer iatrogenic breaks, reduced operating times, less patient discomfort, less astigmatism, and enhanced visual rehabilitation.

The advent of valved trochars has improved the fluidics of combined phaco-vitrectomy by preventing aqueous reflux through an open cannula [11]. Difficulty introducing instruments such as the soft-tipped extrusion cannula through the valved cannula may be experienced. However, this may be managed by the use of the push–pull technique or displacement of the valved leaflets. The stabilization of the fluid dynamics during surgery outweighs any difficulties especially in complex previously vitrectomized eyes.

Valved systems also help to stabilize IOP during surgery, minimizing the risks of intraoperative and postoperative maculopathy, choroidal detachment, and choroidal hemorrhage. Patients who have undergone refractive cataract surgery with loss of lenticular material may benefit from the minimal refractive changes and enhanced visual rehabilitation following surgery with small-gauge trocar systems.

We typically place the trochars at the beginning of surgery prior to the phacoemulsification due to better globe stability (Fig. 40.1). Alternatively, in Europe, patients undergo complete phacoemulsification with intraocular lens placement prior to placement of the trochars. The infusion cannula is connected but kept off until the phacoemulsification portion of the procedure is completed to decrease posterior pressure during phacoemulsification. Early trochar placement also permits the surgeon to perform a core

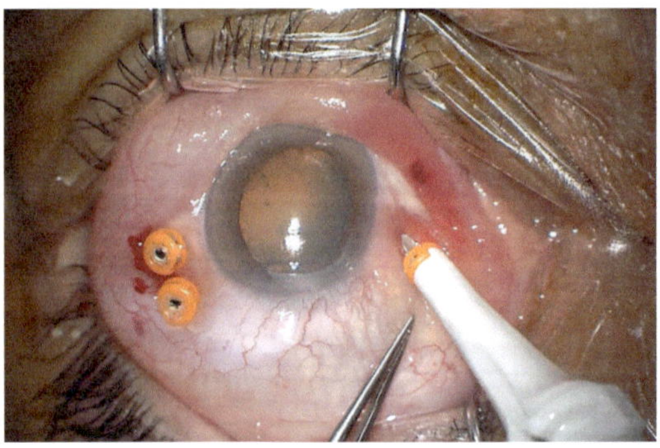

Fig. 40.1 Sclerotomies are made at the beginning of surgery prior to the phacoemulsification due to better globe stability

vitrectomy in cases in which posterior pressure makes the anterior chamber uncomfortably shallow for safe lens manipulation such as in nanophthalmic eyes. In cases of posterior capsular tear, prior placement of the trochars allows quick access to the posterior segment.

40.5 Sclerotomies

Transconjunctival sutureless sclerotomies can be performed routinely during MIVS [11]. This technique decreases operative time, postoperative inflammation, and astigmatism. Conjunctival displacement at the initial incision maximizes that the conjunctiva and scleral wound do not overly. The displacement of the conjunctiva is important for the transconjunctival sutureless technique in order to decrease the possibility of having a vitreous wick in the incision site as well as to prevent access of the tear film into the sclerotomy. In addition, using an oblique trochar wound incision provides added incision stability and reduces postoperative hypotony.

Sclerotomies should avoid conjunctival scars, filtering blebs, tumors, choroidal detachments, bullous retinal detachments, and regions of abnormal pars plana. The placement should maximize the angle for intraocular access and comfort. The inferotemporal trochar should be placed just below the horizontal meridian to reduce the risk of touching the inferior eyelid when manipulating the globe to visualize the inferior retina.

40.6 Corneal Incisions

Corneal incisions should be placed to maximize the surgical approach to the lens while taking into account existing trochar placement and ocular pathology (Fig. 40.2). Choosing the location of the corneal incisions at the steep axis of corneal astigmatism improves astigmatic postoperative correction. Most older adults have against-the-rule astigmatism and benefit from the placement of incisions in the horizontal meridian. A biplanar clear corneal phaco incision with a medium tunnel that starts at the limbus is preferred due to better fluidics, less astigmatism, and increased corneal wound stability. Closure of the phaco wound with 10-0 Nylon prior to the pars plana vitrectomy minimizes the possibility of iris prolapse and anterior segment instability. Stabilization of the anterior segment with viscoelastic prior to the start of vitrectomy minimizes having iris prolapse, lens displacement, and implanted air/gas/silicone oil migration into the anterior chamber during and immediately following surgery.

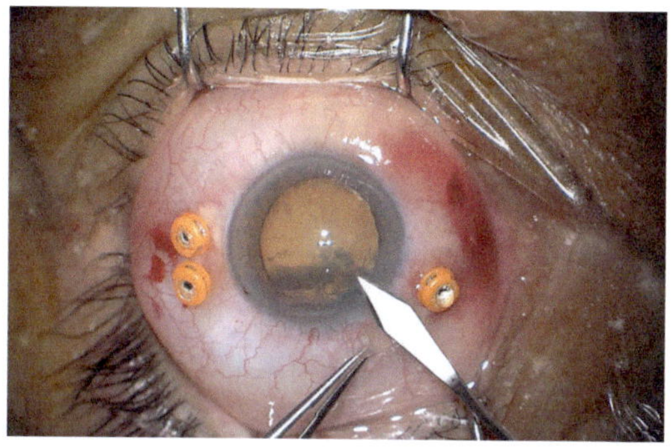

Fig. 40.2 Biplanar corneal incision should be placed to maximize the surgical approach to the lens while taking into account existing trochar placement and ocular pathology

40.7 Capsulorrhexis

The success of phaco vitrectomy is largely dependent on the continuous curvilinear capsulorrhexis. If the red reflex is limited due to vitreous opacity or hemorrhage retroillumination with the endoilluminator inserted through the pars plana cannula can help improve contrast of the anterior capsule. Alternatively, trypan blue may be used to stain the anterior capsule after air infusion into the anterior segment. We prefer a large capsulorrhexis of approximately 6.5 mm to maximize the peripheral view during and after surgery in patients at risk to develop significant posterior capsule opacification (Fig. 40.3). However, a smaller capsulorrhexis may be preferred, especially in cases of toric IOLs, if the posterior capsule is compromised, or a sulcus lens is planned.

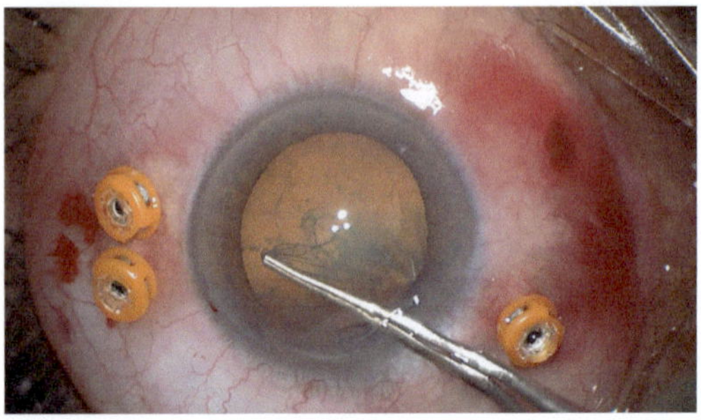

Fig. 40.3 A large capsulorrhexis of approximately 6.5 mm is preferred to maximize the peripheral view during and after surgery in patients at risk to develop significant posterior capsule opacification

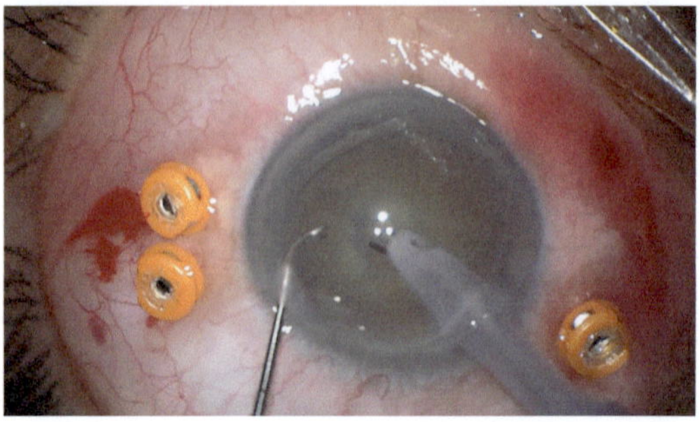

Fig. 40.4 Phacoemulsification with chop technique is preferred in order to minimize ultrasonic energy

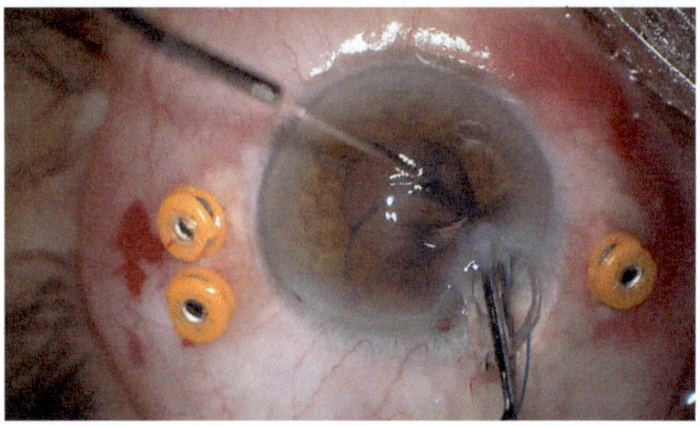

Fig. 40.5 Intraocular lens implantation can be done prior to or after vitrectomy

40.8 Phacoemulsification

Phacoemulsification may be performed before vitrectomy in order to optimize the view of the posterior pole during subsequent vitrectomy. However, in cases where an adequate view is present, cataract extraction may be performed following the vitrectomy. In cases of vitreous hemorrhage, clearing the hemorrhage from the posterior segment in order to elicit an optimal red reflex may also be beneficial. However, phacoemulsification prior to vitrectomy may allow a more peripheral approach, especially in cases such as giant retinal tears, peripheral tumors, or if endocyclophotocoagulation needs to be performed.

Phacoemulsification should be performed at the iris plane when possible to minimize both corneal edema and posterior capsule breaks. We prefer to use a chop technique in order to minimize ultrasonic energy (Fig. 40.4). However, phacoemulsification techniques vary widely and a surgeon's choice of technique may vary depending on the individual clinical presentation. Posterior capsule integrity after nucleus and cortex extraction is critical to maximize the refractive outcomes.

40.9 Intraocular Lens

The intraocular lens can be implanted prior to or after vitrectomy (Fig. 40.5). The intraocular lens should be placed in the capsular bag unless there is any concern about an intact posterior capsule. A three-piece sulcus intraocular lens should be placed if a posterior capsule break is suspected or present.

Silicone intraocular lenses should be avoided. Silicone oil beads and condenses on the surface of the lens when intraocular silicone oil is present [12]. Additionally, during fluid–air exchange, tiny droplets of fluid coat the exposed posterior surface of the silicone intraocular lens and impair the surgeon's view. Because of their physical properties, acrylic intraocular lenses are the preferred choice for most vitreoretinal surgeons.

In some cases of Stage C or above proliferative vitreoretinopathy, uveitis, endophthalmitis, intraocular tumors, and trauma, it may be beneficial to perform a lensectomy with capsulectomy to accomplish decompartmentalization of the eye.

40.10 Small Pupil Management

Incomplete mydriasis may be encountered during surgery due to a wide variety of conditions including neurologic disease, posterior synechia, iris tumors, pseudoexfoliation syndrome, intraocular inflammation, and medication use. Performing combined phaco-vitrectomy with a small pupil can be extremely challenging. Therefore, preoperative diagnosis is important to avoid intraoperative adverse events.

Pharmacological management is an effective way to enhance pupil dilation and stabilization during intraocular surgery, especially in the absence of posterior synechia. Epinephrine (0.3–0.5 ml of 1:1000) may be added to the irrigation or infusion bottle. Similarly, a mixture of phenylephrine 1.5% and xylocaine 1% may be injected into the anterior chamber before adding a viscoelastic agent.

Posterior synechia may be released at the beginning of surgery using an iris spatula or with a cannula while performing viscodissection. In some cases, viscomydriasis may allow enough dilation to proceed with the case after the successful release of posterior synechia.

A surgical approach may be indicated if pharmacologic strategies have failed. Relaxing microsphincterotomies may be performed to enhance dilation intraoperative and postoperatively. Multiple pupil dilators or rings are also commercially available by various manufacturers and may aid mydriasis intraoperatively. Pupil dilators or rings have the benefit that they do not move the iris plane anteriorly and allow easier access to the nucleus and capsular bag. Iris retractors can also be used and allow the largest theoretical pupil diameter while displacing the iris plane anteriorly.

Patients that undergo phaco-vitrectomy with small pupils are at higher risk for delayed healing, corneal edema, intraocular inflammation, and high intraocular pressure. This may be due to various mechanisms including extended surgical time and/or iritis following surgical manipulation of the pupil. Individualized preoperative discussion in small pupil cases may allow improved patient perception of postoperative outcomes. These patients may benefit from extended postoperative use of anti-inflammatory topical medications or intraocular/periocular corticosteroids at the time of surgery.

40.11 Special Considerations

It is important to individualize the surgical approach depending on the pathology encountered. We typically avoid phaco-vitrectomy at the time of rhegmatogenous retinal detachment repair in order to minimize the possibility of the tamponade shifting into the anterior chamber. In cases of macula off rhegmatogenous retinal detachment with dense cataracts, we avoid intraocular lens implantation at the time of primary phaco-vitrectomy for retinal detachment repair because of limited refractive outcomes.

Avoiding intraocular lens implantation becomes particularly important if an encircling scleral buckle is going to be performed due to the variable myopic shift [12]. We routinely perform biometry after rhegmatogenous retinal detachment repair in order to achieve the best possible refractive outcomes. Secondary intraocular lens implantation is performed on a secondary surgery. If silicone oil is present in the posterior segment, we routinely perform phaco-vitrectomy after extraction of the silicone oil in order to avoid unnecessary posterior capsule pressure.

Phakic patients without significant lens opacity who undergo silicone oil tamponade at the time of primary surgery may benefit from vitrectomy only since the crystalline lens helps minimize silicone oil migration into the anterior segment. Phaco-vitrectomy can be delayed until silicone oil removal is performed. Patients with traumatic cataracts in which there is a special concern for zonular dialysis may also benefit from a phaco-vitrectomy approach.

Patients with visually significant cataracts who will undergo macular surgery may benefit the most from phaco-vitrectomy in order to optimize visualization prior to epiretinal membrane peeling, macular endolaser, macular hole repair (Fig. 40.6).

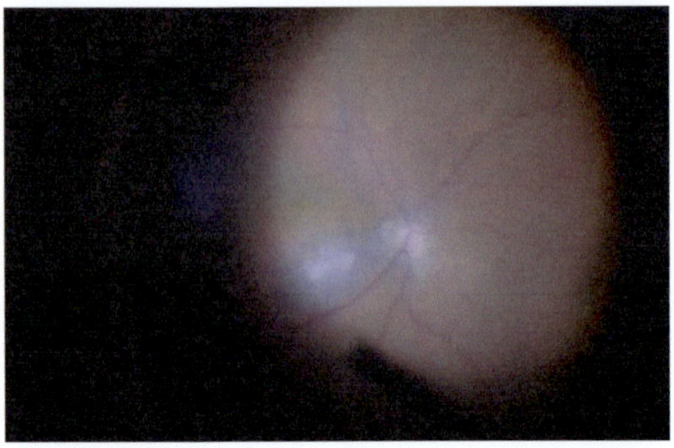

Fig. 40.6 Circumscribed choroidal hemangioma undergoing endolaser photocoagulation

40.12 Safety and Efficacy

A study that evaluated 1052 subjects that underwent combined phaco-vitrectomy for epiretinal membranes or full-thickness macular holes between 1998 and 2017 found the rate of posterior capsule rupture was 2.2% [13]. The most common adverse events were: posterior capsular opacification 10.6%, posterior synechiae 4.2%, uveitis 2.1%, angle-closure glaucoma 1.6%, and rhegmatogenous retinal detachment 1.1%. The study concluded that phaco-vitrectomy was safe in phakic patients with ERM or MH, performed either by training surgeons or faculty. Phaco-vitrectomy avoided the requirement for repeat surgery and was cost-efficient.

Refractive outcomes of phaco-vitrectomy have also recently been investigated [14]. A study that evaluated 50 eyes that underwent combined phaco-vitrectomy and a control group of 50 eyes that underwent cataract surgery alone over a 3-year period was undertaken. The differences in predicted and final refractive errors were not statistically significant between groups. There was no difference in postsurgical astigmatism between groups. No foveal differences were detected in optical coherence tomography.

Phaco-vitrectomy at the time of rhegmatogenous retinal detachment repair has also been investigated [15]. A retrospective study between 2008 and 2014 that evaluated 1690 consecutive cases that were managed with phaco-vitrectomy or vitrectomy alone found the risk for reoperation was 2.67 times higher in the phaco-vitrectomy group compared to the vitrectomy alone group. This may be related to the complexity of pathology in cases that underwent phaco-vitrectomy.

40.13 Complications

The most common complication following phaco-vitrectomy is posterior capsule opacity formation following surgery. YAG laser can be performed 3 months after surgery with a possibly decreased risk of retinal detachment as compared to a non-vitrectomized eye. The risk of retinal detachment is similar to vitrectomy alone. We have not encountered endophthalmitis and hypotony following phaco-vitrectomy. Overall, the risks of surgery are similar to the individual risks of cataract and MIVS surgery.

40.14 Conclusion

Recent improvements in MIVS and small incision cataract surgery have allowed improved outcomes in combined phaco-vitrectomy during the last decade. The ability to perform small incisions in both the anterior and posterior segment has allowed for better fluidic and intraocular pressure control. This technique decreases the need for a second surgery and decreases the total time spent during visual recovery. Utilizing combined phaco-vitrectomy within our institution allows an outstanding success rate with over 95% of our patients having 2-line improvement at 6 weeks post surgery. We have had no cases of hypotony or endophthalmitis. Retinal detachment rates less than 5% in patients with high-risk characteristics for retinal detachment. Phaco-vitrectomy minimizes both the time and expense of visual recovery and the need for additional surgery. We expect this technique to continue to expand due to continual technological improvements that may improve safety and efficacy while ultimately improving anatomic and visual outcomes for these complex patients.

References

1. Parke DW, Sisk RA, Murray TG. Intraoperative intravitreal triamcinolone decreases macular edema after vitrectomy with phacoemulsification. Clin Ophthalmol. 2012;6:1347–53.
2. Sisk RA, Murray TG. Combined phacoemulsification and sutureless 23-gauge pars plana vitrectomy for complex vitreoretinal diseases. Br J Ophthalmol. 2010;94(8):1028–32.
3. Jun Z, Pavlovic S, Jacobi KW. Results of combined vitreoretinal surgery and phacoemulsification with intraocular lens implantation. Clin Exp Ophthalmol. 2001;29:307–11.
4. McDermott ML, Puklin JE, Abrams GW. Phacoemulsification for cataract following pars plana vitrectomy. Ophthalmic Surg Lasers. 1997;28:558–69.
5. Lahey JM, Francis RR, Kearney JJ, et al. Combining phacoemulsification and vitrectomy in patients with proliferative diabetic retinopathy. Curr Opin Ophthalmol. 2004;15:192–6.
6. Androudi S, Ahmed M, Fiore T, et al. Combined pars plana vitrectomy and phacoemulsification to restore visual acuity in patients with chronic uveitis. J Cataract Refract Surg. 2005;31:472–8.
7. Soheilian M, Mirdehqhan SA, Peyman GA. Sutureless combined 25-gauge vitrectomy, phacoemulsification, and posterior chamber intraocular lens implantation for management of uveitic cataract associated with posterior segment disease. Retina. 2008;28: 941–6.
8. Lott MN, Manning MH, Singh J, et al. 23-gauge vitrectomy in 100 eyes: short-term visual outcomes and complications. Retina. 2008;28:1193–200.
9. Demetriades AM, Gottsch JD, Thomsen R, et al. Combined phacoemulsification, intraocular lens implantation, and vitrectomy for eyes with coexisting cataract and vitreoretinal pathology. Am J Ophthalmol. 2003;135:291–6.
10. Lahey JM, Francis RR, Fong DS, et al. Combining phacoemulsification with vitrectomy for treatment of macular holes. Br J Ophthalmol. 2002;86:876–8.
11. Fine HF, Iranmanesh R, Iturralde D, et al. Outcomes of 77 consecutive cases of 23-gauge transconjunctival vitrectomy surgery for posterior segment disease. Ophthalmology. 2007;114:1197–200.
12. Villegas VM, Gold AS, Latiff A, Wildner AC, Ehlies FJ, Murray TG. Phacovitrectomy. Dev Ophthalmol. 2014;54:102–7.
13. Fajgenbaum MAP, Neffendorf JE, Wong RS, Laidlaw DAH, Williamson TH. Intraoperative and postoperative complications in phacovitrectomy for epiretinal membrane and macular hole: a clinical audit of 1,000 consecutive eyes. Retina. 2018;38(9):1865–72.
14. Shi L, Chang JS, Suh LH, Chang S. Differences in refractive outcomes between phacoemulsification for cataract alone and combined phacoemulsification and vitrectomy for epiretinal membrane. Retina. 2018;39(7):1410–5.
15. Loukovaara S, Haukka J. Repair of primary RRD - comparing pars plana vitrectomy procedure with combined phacovitrectomy with standard foldable intraocular lens implantation. Clin Ophthalmol. 2018;12:1449–57.

Artificial Vision and Retinal Prosthesis

41

Marco Mura and Patrik Schatz

41.1 History

Artificial vision tries to recreate a useful form of vision experience bypassing diseased retinal tissue. Inherited retinal diseases such as retinitis pigmentosa are characterized by loss of retinal pigment epithelium and photoreceptors and eventually blindness at young working age creating a big social impact in the life of these patients. For a very long time, different types of treatments have been tried, among them electrical stimulation.

The possibility to cure eye disease with the use of electrical stimulation is quite old. In 1755 for the first time, C. Le Roy described the treatment of blindness using electricity. He used an iron or brass wire tied around the head like a rim of a hat and another to the leg to create a closed circuit. The wires were then connected to an array of Leiden jars. Twelve shocks waves per session were administered. Along with the pain of the stimulation, the patient perceived vivid phosphenes during the treatments performed in several sessions. Unfortunately the patient remained blind.

The first attempts to partially restore vision in blinded eyes by means of a prosthesis connected to the visual pathway date as far back as the second half of the twentieth century.

In 1956, Tassicker invented and implanted the first retina stimulator to be implanted in the subretinal space. The device, which was ultimately implanted between the choroid and sclera of a patient affected by retinitis pigmentosa due to the inability to separate the retina from the retinal pigment epithelium, led to improved confidence in the motility of the patient [1].

A better understanding of the mechanisms responsible for the functioning of the electrical stimulation came from postmortem anatomic studies of patients with retinitis pigmentosa (RP) and age-related macular degeneration. Those studies have demonstrated that both inner retinal cells and ganglion cells may be relatively preserved in these ocular conditions, even though there is considerable photoreceptor cell death [2–6].

Electronic Supplementary Material The online version of this chapter (https://doi.org/10.1007/978-981-33-4168-5_41) contains supplementary material, which is available to authorized users.

M. Mura (✉)
Retina Department, King Khaled Eye Specialist Hospital, Riyadh, Saudi Arabia

Department of Translational Medicine, University of Ferrara, Ferrara, Italy

P. Schatz
Retina Department, King Khaled Eye Specialist Hospital, Riyadh, Saudi Arabia

Department of Ophthalmology, Clinical Sciences, Skane County University Hospital, University of Lund, Lund, Sweden
e-mail: pschatz@kkesh.med.sa

A. Jain et al. (eds.), *Cutting-edge Vitreoretinal Surgery*,
https://doi.org/10.1007/978-981-33-4168-5_41

Stimulation of viable ganglion cells and cells that feed into the ganglion cell layer, therefore, could be used to elicit some form of artificial vision. Determining which neurons in the retina were being activated became the next challenge.

The use of a rat model that experiences early onset photoreceptor degeneration demonstrated that the electrically evoked potentials in the retina were persistent even in the absence of photoreceptors [7]. The extraocular stimulation method also demonstrated the ability to evoke percepts in individuals blinded by RP [8].

Morphometric studies of human retinal degenerations revealed that despite widespread photoreceptor degeneration, a significant portion of the inner retina survived [4, 5]. It was later demonstrated that electrodes placed on the retinal surface could evoke percepts via electrical stimulation in patients suffering from photoreceptor degeneration [9].

41.2 Pathophysiology

Cellular electrical excitability in the retina and visual pathway is an intrinsic property of nervous tissue. Impulses are constantly exchanged between the retina and the visual cortex, even during darkness. When light excites the retina, a series of rapid and well defined electrical responses are evoked from each layer of retina. Visual transduction is the process by which light absorbed by the outer segment of the photoreceptor layer of the retina is converted into electrical energy.

Perceptions of the world are created by the brain from Action Potentials (AP) sent from sensory receptors. Sensory receptors respond to a particular modality of environmental stimuli. Receptors transduce different forms of sensation to nerve impulses that are conducted to the central nervous system (CNS).

In response to stimulus, sensory nerve endings produce a local graded change in membrane potential. If the temporal and spatial summation of all these graded signals is above a certain threshold of excitability the neurons generate an Action Potential (AP).

Because the photoreceptors are convergently interconnected with the downstream convergent bipolar and ganglion cells, the easiest way would be to place a prosthesis subretinally, from the point of physiological signal processing.

From a surgical perspective, it is challenging to place an implant in a subretinal position (complex accessibility of the subretinal space, energy source, etc…).

It is doubtful whether, after replacement of photoreceptors with a subretinal implant, the signals will reach the ganglion cells following the normal pathway, since a photoreceptor degeneration also causes a degeneration of the inner retinal layers. Because of degenerations within the inner plexiform layer, the signal reaching the ganglion cells could be nonspecific.

Therefore some research groups prefer a direct stimulation of ganglion cells by epiretinally localized stimulator electrodes.

From a surgical point of view, standard methods of vitreoretinal surgery can be utilized to a certain extent, and, compared to subretinal implantation, no retinal detachment has to be performed.

41.3 Types of Retinal Prosthesis

Several types of retinal prostheses have been developed or are currently under development (Fig. 41.1). They vary in user interface, light-detection method, signal processing, and microelectrode array placement within the retina. The three main locations for microelectrode array placement are the epiretinal, subretinal, and supra-choroidal space. Epiretinal prosthesis arrays are placed on the ganglion cell surface within the vitreous space. Subretinal prosthesis arrays are placed between bipolar cells and the retinal pigmented epithelium. Supra-choroidal prosthesis arrays are either placed between the choroid and sclera or contained within the sclera. Each of the approaches is similar in that light from the visual scene is captured and transformed into electrical pulses delivered through electrodes to stimulate any remaining viable retinal cells.

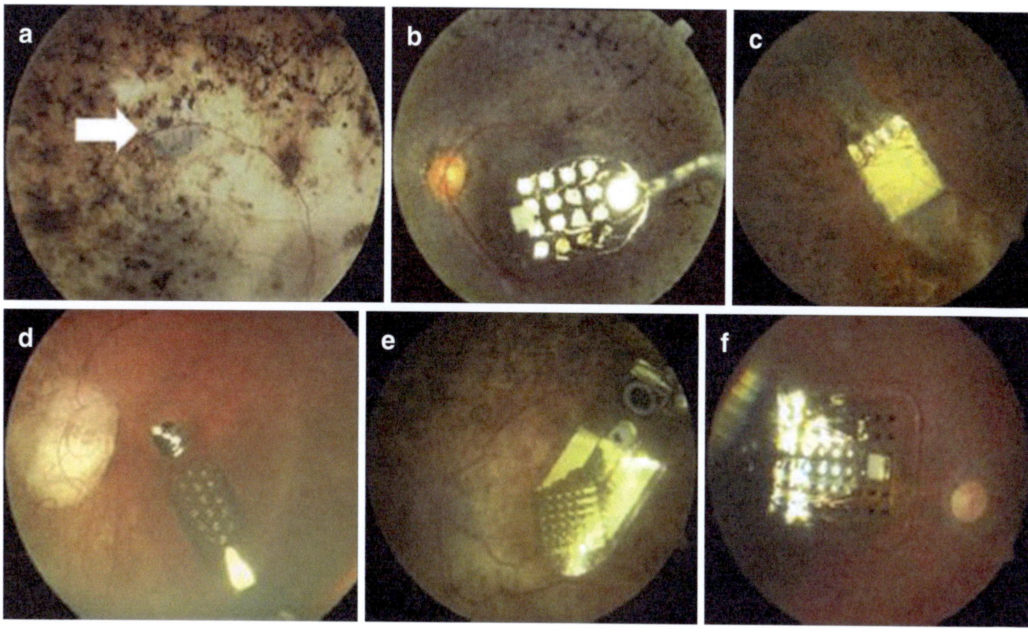

Fig. 41.1 Fundus photographs of all six chronic implants. (**a**) White arrow showing artificial silicon retina (optobionics). (**b**) Argus 1 (Second Sight Medical Products, Inc.). (**c**) Alpha IMS subretinal device (Retinal Implant, GmbH). (**d**) Epi-Ret 25 electrode device. (**e**) Forty-nine electrode epiretinal device (Intelligent Medical Implants). (**f**) Argus 2 (Second Sight Medical Products, Inc.). From Weiland JD et al. Ophthalmology 2011

Table 41.1 provides an overview of the implanted devices mostly in patients with Retinitis pigmentosa. The majority of patients gained more confidence during ambulation and some had better results in terms of improved VA and Visual field. Among them, Argus 2 (second sight) is the only prosthesis FDA and CE approved. Alpha IMS (Retina Implant AG) and Iris 2 (Pixium vision) have both CE mark. Alpha IMS production has been discontinued as per March 2019.

A number of epiretinal and subretinal implants have been developed. Among these, the Argus II Retinal Prosthesis System (Second Sight Medical Products), originally developed by Mark Humayun, MD, Ph.D., and colleagues at the Doheny Eye Center at the University of Southern California, has shown to be able to provide partial restoration of vision to patients blinded from outer retinal degenerative disease in the biggest number of patients worldwide or a detailed description of outcomes from the Argus II Retinal Stimulation System feasibility study, we refer readers to other articles in the literature [10–13].

In brief, most patients implanted with the device showed an improvement in tasks assessing orientation and mobility, spatial-motor localization, and the ability to discern the direction of motion of moving stimuli. Roughly half of the patients did better with the implant on versus off, with an estimated visual field of 20° and one-third of the patients experienced a measurable improvement in visual acuity with the implant. The highest achieved visual acuity ranged from 1.6 logMAR to 2.9 logMAR, with letter reading measured at Snellen 20/1262. Some patients were capable of identifying words with high accuracy.

This chapter outlines our pearls for surgical implantation of the Argus II Retinal Prosthesis System.

Table 41.1 Prosthesis and best functional results

Prosthesis	Patients	Diagnosis	Best result
Argus 2	274	RP, CHM	VF improvements, letter reading, VA 1.8 LogMAR
Alpha IMS	40	RP	Letter reading, VA 1.74 LogMAR
IRIS 2	12	RP	Trials ongoing
Optobionics	30	RP	Visual field and ETDRS improvement
IMI	6	RP	Point discrimination
Epi-Ret	6	RP	–

41.4 The Argus 2 Retinal Prosthesis System

The Argus II epiretinal prosthesis consists of two parts: a device that is surgically implanted on in the eye and an external unit that is worn by the patient. The implanted portion (Fig. 41.2b) consists of a multielectrode array (60 electrodes; 200-μm diameter each) that is secured to the intraocular vitreoretinal surface with a retinal tack (Fig. 41.2a) and a receiving and transmitting coil, a case housing electronics needed for stimulation that is fixed to the scleral surface Fig. 41.2b). The external unit consists of a small camera (510 × 492 pixels resolution; NTSC output), a transmitter mounted on glasses, and a video processor and battery worn on a belt (Fig. 41.3).

The multielectrode array is connected to the case by a metalized polymer cable that penetrates the sclera in the location of the pars plana incision made during implantation. The camera captures video and sends the information to the video processing unit, which converts the image to electronic signals that are then sent to the transmitter on the glasses. The implanted receiver receives these data wirelessly and sends electrical stimulus pulses to the multielectrode array via the polymerized cable. Controlled electrical stimulation depolarizes the remaining retinal neurons. The action potentials travel through the optic nerve and up to higher visual centers, such as the lateral geniculate nucleus, resulting in phosphenes by exciting areas in the visual cortex.

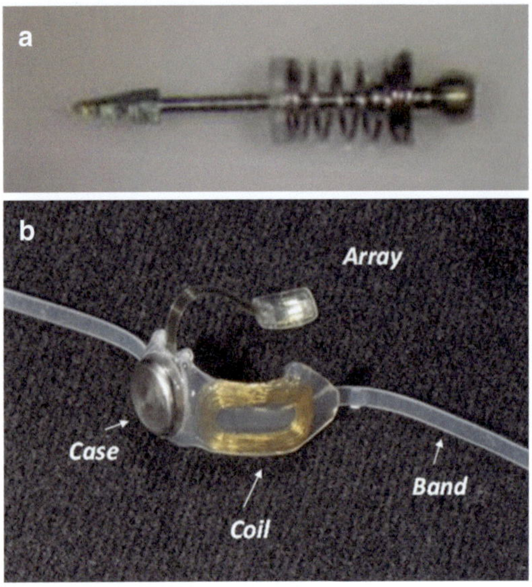

Fig. 41.2 (**a**) Retina Tack. (**b**) Argus 2 implantable portion. Electronic case, transmitting coil, electrodes array, and silicone band are highlighted in the picture

41.5 Surgical Implantation Process

41.5.1 Patient Preparation

Specific surgical and medical handling need to be followed before and during surgical implantation of Argus II retinal prosthesis, in particular:

- Two weeks prior implantation the crystalline lens needs to be removed. The patient is left

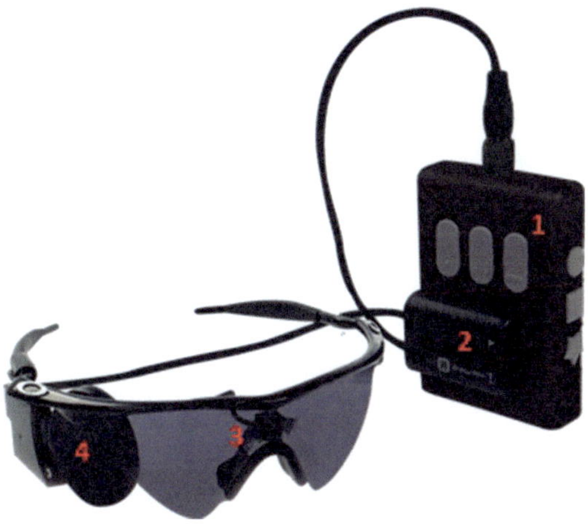

Fig. 41.3 (1) Video processing unit (VPU); (2) battery; (3) glasses with the central camera; (4) receiving coil

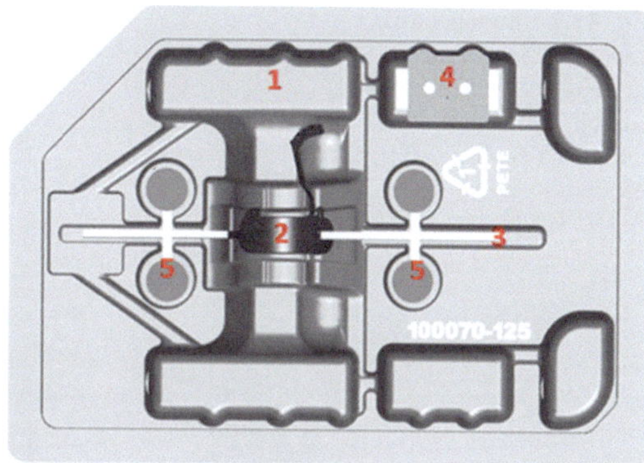

Fig. 41.4 Argus II retinal prosthesis inside holding tray; (1) well, (2) coil and electronic case, (3) silicone band, (4) tack holder, (5) cross bands

aphakic or pseudophakic. In case it is chosen to implant an IOL, posterior capsulotomy is performed.

- Forty-eight hour before surgery the patient is started on oral Fluoroquinolone antibiotics.
- Intraoperatively the following drugs are administered: 8 mg of intravenous dexamethasone (or equivalent), 1 g of Cephazolin (or equivalent first-generation Cephalosporine).
- At the end of the surgical procedure intravitreal Vancomycin 1 mg/0.1 ml and Ceftazidime 2.25 mg/0.1 ml (or equivalents) are injected intravitreally.
- Subconjunctival Cefazolin 100 mg, Dexamethasone 2 mg, Lidocaine 4% 2 ml are injected away from the wound and the device.

41.5.2 Prosthesis Preparation

Using sterile technique the scrubbed nurse opens the implant inner tray by carefully peeling the Tyvek lid off the tray. Carefully remove the plastic cover from the inner tray by pulling the cover straight up and not to the side. The cover has cut-out handles on the side to help with its removal.

Fifty milliliters of sterile saline solution is added to the well of the tray (Fig. 41.4) where the implant is located. The entire implant device, including the electrode array, should be covered with saline. Antibiotics 1 ml of vancomycin (1 mg/0.1 ml) and 1 ml of ceftazidime injection (2.25 mg/0.1 ml) can be added to the saline solution. In this case, the device should soak in it for at least 3–5 min. With the implant under saline, the first impedance measurement needs to be performed to ensure the correct functioning of the prosthesis before implantation. A specific operation room coil (OR Coil) placed in sterile sleeve connected to the video processing unit (VPU) and clinician fitting system (CFS) laptop should be used for this essential step of the surgery (Fig. 41.5). The Argus 2 retinal prosthesis is now ready for eye implantation.

41.5.3 Surgical Technique

Hereunder we describe the implantation technique of Argus II in a right eye.

A 360° conjunctival peritomy is performed in a standard fashion. To avoid dehiscence of the conjunctival wound in the proximity of the implant case, only one radial incision is made, in the inferonasal quadrant. The four recti muscles

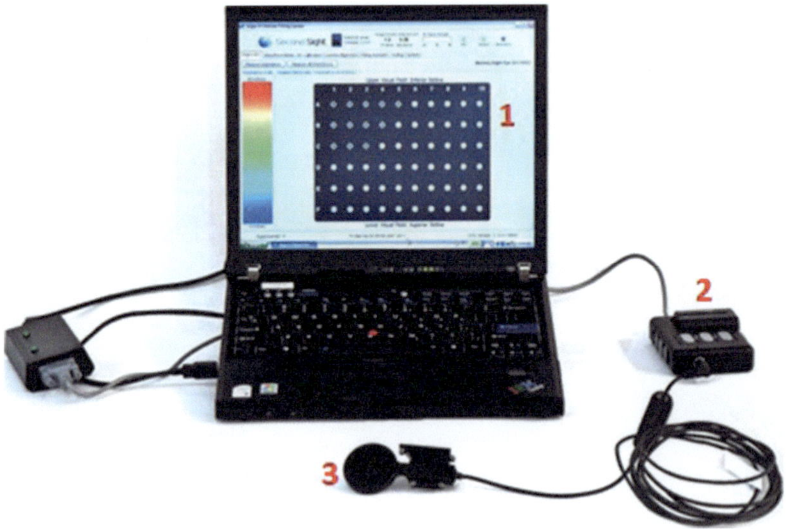

Fig. 41.5 Intraoperative impedance test equipment (1) CFS Laptop with dedicated software; (2) VPU; (3) OR coil

are isolated with 2-0 silk. The episcleral portion of the implant is inserted under the recti muscles and secured onto the sclera with sutures.

First, the receiving coil is inserted under the lateral rectus muscle while the electronic case rests in the supero-temporal quadrant. Then the medial portion of the encircling band is passed under the superior rectus muscle. The lateral portion of the encircling band, connected to the receiving coil, is passed under the inferior and medial recti muscles and secured with a Watzke sleeve to the medial extremity in the supero-nasal quadrant. The correct positioning of the implant and the surgical landmarks are highlighted in Fig. 41.6. Every maneuver must be performed with care not to pinch the silicone shell of the implant or any electronic component, including the multielectrode array, which, at this stage, is hanging outside the eye. To avoid causing damage, the array may be inserted in a small bag created from a cut finger of a surgical glove.

The encirclement band is then sutured with polyester 5-0 suture in all quadrants. The electronic case and the coil are sutured to the sclera with mersilene 6-0, using the special tab holes carved on the silicone shell. The placement of the sutures and, therefore, the positioning of the electronic case on the sclera are performed according to special axial length-related tables, developed to result in correct placement of the multielectrode array on the retinal surface, above the macula (see Table 41.2).

A three-port pars plana vitrectomy is then performed with the aid of a chandelier light. We use the Constellation vitrectomy system (Alcon Inc., Fort Worth, TX), using 25-gage (25+ Series) instruments and valved trocars. The BIOM system (Oculus GmbH, Wezlar, Germany) is used to visualize the retina. After core vitrectomy is performed, triamcinolone acetonide is injected into the vitreous cavity. A posterior vitreous detachment is induced, avoiding excessive traction on the retina. The vitreous cortex is usually very adherent in eyes with RP and normally does not detach further than the midperiphery. If the macular epiretinal membrane is present, it is peeled away from the macula; however, to avoid macular tear, we do not recommend peeling the internal limiting membrane.

Vitreous base shaving is then performed, with particular attention directed to the supero-temporal quadrant. A 5-mm straight sclerotomy in the supero-temporal quadrant is now performed (we use a 15° blade or a 5.1-mm premeasured slit knife). The distance of this sclerotomy from the limbus is calculated according to the axial length-related tables mentioned above. The array is then introduced into the eye by holding it at the level of a special handle located on the distal end of the array and then the electrode cable

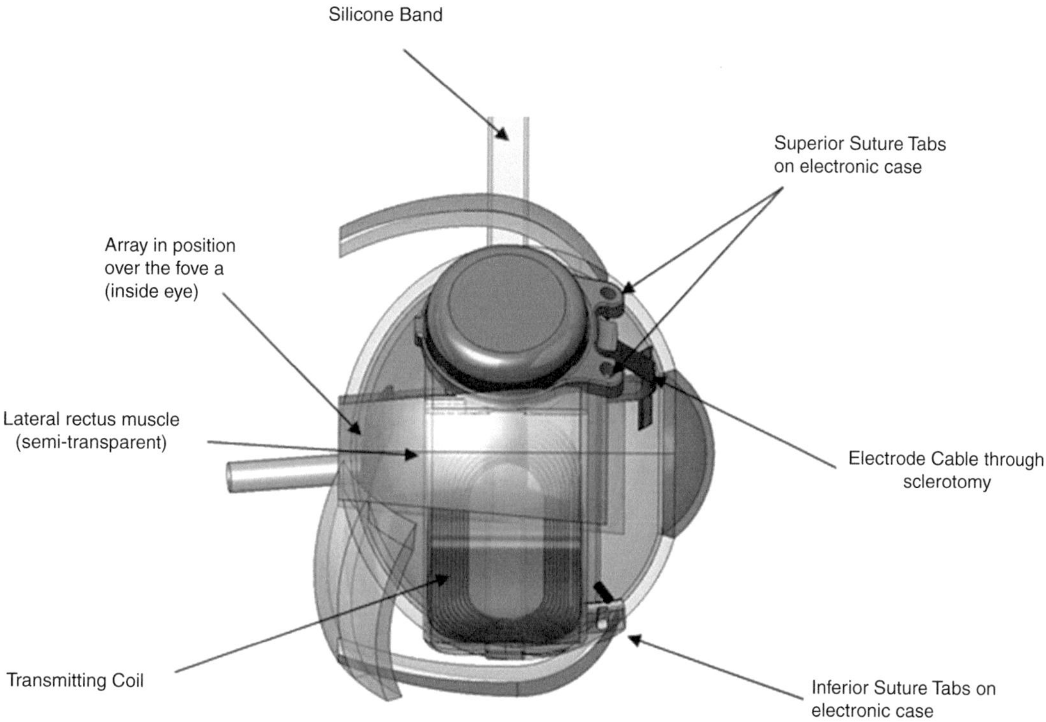

Fig. 41.6 Correct extraocular position of the Argus II retinal prosthesis in right eye implant and surgical landmarks (temporal view)

Table 41.2 Extraocular placement fitting table

Patient axial length range (mm)	Sclerotomy setback (mm)	Superior suture tab(s) hole (mm)	Inferior suture tab hole (mm)
20.5–22.8	3.0	8.0	8.0
22.8–24.2	3.5	7.5	7.5
24.2–25.5	4.0	7.0	7.0
25.5–26.0	4.5[a]	7.0	7.0

[a]Ensure that ora serrata anatomy allows 4.5 mm posterior to limbus sclerotomy

is pushed inside the eye using silicone-tipped forceps (toothed instruments must be avoided). The valved trocars avoid turbulence in the eye and unwanted movements of the array, greatly facilitating this maneuver.

If all previous steps have been performed correctly, the array is now precisely above the macular area and an uniform stimulation of the macular ganglion cells can be elicited. If the array is out of position or twisted, a higher threshold is needed to stimulate the ganglion cells, with consequent potential underperformance of the system.

It is extremely important to know the surgical landmarks on the electrode array to avoid complications (Fig. 41.7). In particular, the surgeon should take extreme care not to touch the array itself. This must be held only on the distal handle for all the surgical manipulations. The retina tack needs to fit precisely in the premade tack hole. Also, particular attention needs to be taken during the suturing of the 5 mm sclerotomy to avoid perforating the silicone electrode cable flanges which are transparent and very poorly visible especially when fluid egresses from the scleral wound.

We then proceed to tack the array to the retina with a bimanual technique. An additional 20-gage sclerotomy is created in the inferotemporal quadrant to introduce the tack tool. The array is held in the desired position (via the distal handle) with an end-gripping forceps while, with the other hand (using special tack forceps via the 20-gage sclerotomy), we proceed to insert the tack in the dedicated hole located at the root of the array. During this maneuver, the intraocular pressure

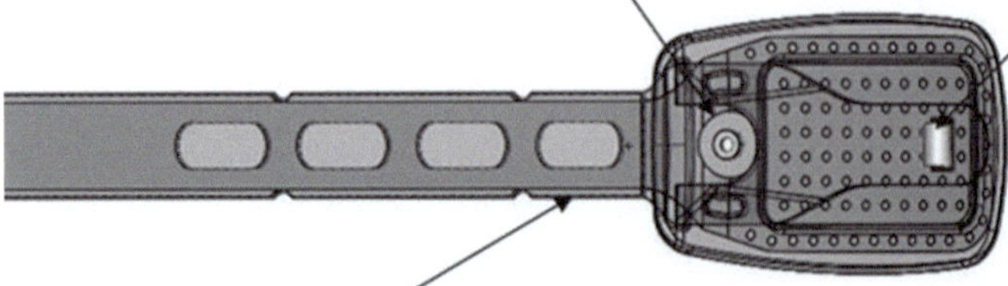

Fig. 41.7 Electrode cable and array surgical landmarks

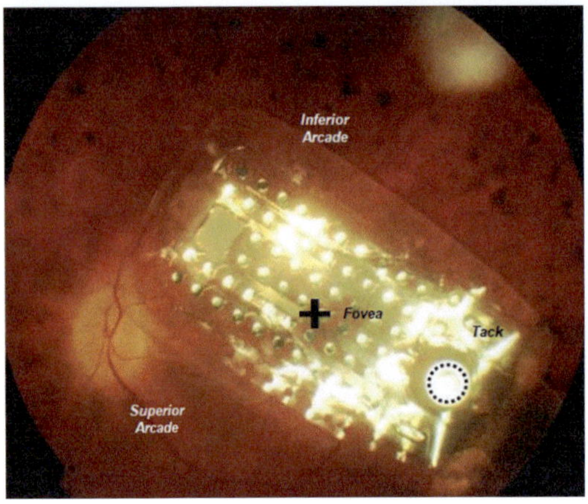

Fig. 41.8 Correct array position and tacking location in the right eye

must be set at 60 mmHg. An indirect sign of a successful tacking is a slight whitening of the retinal surface while pushing on the tack. A new impedance measurement is performed one more time at this stage. Figure 41.8 shows the correct positioning of the array on the retinal surface.

The 20-gage and 5-mm sclerotomies are now carefully sutured with 7-0 vicryl, avoiding damage to the transparent cable connected to the intraocular array. The 25-gage trocars are removed, and the sclerotomies are sutured. The array cable is secured with a mattress suture (passing above it) to avoid movement and extrusion. Processed pericardium is applied on top of the array cable and the anterior edge of the electronic case. The conjunctiva is closed in a standard fashion, and steroids are injected sub-conjuctivally. Last, intravitreal injection of 0.1 mL ceftazidime (2.25 mg/0.1 mL) and vancomycin (1 mg/0.1 mL) is performed (Video demonstration).

41.5.4 Surgical Pearl for Successful Implantation

In conclusion the following pearls will promote success in the challenging case of Argus II retinal prosthesis implantation:

- Perform careful calculation of the distance from the limbus to where the sutures are placed and the 5-mm–long sclerotomy is created.
- Ensure proper instrumentation is used; avoid toothed instruments and use valved trocars.
- Avoid traction on the retina while inducing posterior vitreous detachment.
- Avoid internal limiting membrane peeling.
- Perform careful vitreous removal in the quadrant where the array is to be inserted (supero-temporal).
- Set intraocular pressure to 60 mmHg while inserting the tack.
- Perform careful sclerotomy suturing, avoiding hypotony and endophthalmitis.

41.5.5 Postoperative Follow-Up

Postoperative follow-ups need to be scheduled at day 1, week 1, week 2, week 4, month 3, 6, and 12. Afterward yearly follow-up is recommended.

Postoperative topical antibiotics and steroids are recommended for 4 weeks or until inflammation subsides.

At week 1 the device can be switched on and tested. Intensive rehabilitation and training are mandatory to ensure compliance and usability of the retina prosthesis. Specifically trained and specialized low vision optometrists are pivotal in the post-implantation period.

41.5.6 Complications

The most common complications are reported in Table 41.3 [12–18].

Among them, especially conjunctiva erosion and leakage form the sclerotomy and endophthalmitis are considered serious adverse events and could be minimized with proper surgical handlings.

To minimize conjunctival erosion we perform our conjunctival relaxing incision in the opposite quadrant of the electronic case location and we take particular care in suturing the tenon and conjunctiva separately with vicryl 7-0. Also we cover the exposed parts of the implant (electrode cable and the first third of electronic case) with human processed pericardium which we suture loosely in 4 points with vicryl 7-0. We always suture all sclerotomies ports with vicryl 7-0. The 5 mm sclerotomy we make to introduce the array needs to be closed starting from inside out with two mattress sutures and one single suture (2-2-1 knots) on both sides of the electronic cable, paying extreme care not to punch the silicone flanges of the cable itself as this could result in malfunctioning of the device. Proper closure of the surgical wounds in our opinion is mandatory to avoid leakage and possible endophthalmitis deriving from it.

In the pre- and post-market study a total of three patients required explantation of the device due to technical failure of the prosthesis in two subjects and persistent ocular pain in one subject.

Table 41.3 Device and surgery related serious adverse events in pre- and post-approval studies

Complications	Argus II pre-approval *n* = 30 (%)	Argus II post-approval *n* = 47 (%)
Conjunctival erosion	6.7	9
Endophthalmitis	10	–
Hypotony	10	4
Iatrogenic retinal tears/detachment	10	6[a]
Wound dehiscence	10	–
Dislodged tack	6.7	–
Device explant	3.3	4
Ocular inflammation/episcleritis	4	4

[a]Rhegmatogenous and tractional retinal detachment combined

References

1. Tassicker GE. Preliminary report on a retinal stimulator. Br J Physiol Opt. 1956;13(2):102–5.
2. Weilend JD, Cho AK, Humayun MS. Retinal prostheses: current clinical results and future needs. Ophthalmology. 2011;118(11):2227–37.
3. Weiland JD, Walston ST, Humayun MS. Electrical stimulation of the retina to produce artificial vision. Annu Rev Vis Sci. 2016;2:273–94.
4. Humayun MS, Prince M, de Juan E Jr, Barron Y, Moskowitz M, Klock IB, Milam AH. Morphometric analysis of the extramacular retina from postmortem eyes with retinitis pigmentosa. Invest Ophthalmol Vis Sci. 1999;40(1):143–8.
5. Santos A, Humayun MS, de Juan E Jr, Greenburg RJ, Marsh MJ, Klock IB, Milam AH. Preservation of the inner retina in retinitis pigmentosa. A morphometric analysis. Arch Ophthalmol. 1997;115(4):511–5.
6. Medeiros NE, Curcio CA. Preservation of ganglion cell layer neurons in age-related macular degeneration. Invest Ophthalmol Vis Sci. 2001;42(3):795–803.
7. Potts AM, Inoue J. The electrically evoked response of the visual system (EER). 3. Further contribution to the origin of the EER. Investig Ophthalmol. 1970;9(10):814–9.
8. Potts AM, Inoue J. The electrically evoked response (EER) of the visual system. 2. Effect of adaptation and retinitis pigmentosa. Investig Ophthalmol. 1969;8(6):605–12.
9. Humayun MS, de Juan E, Dagnelie G, Greenberg RJ, Propst RH, Phillips DH. Visual perception elicited by electrical stimulation of the retina in blind humans. Arch Ophthalmol. 1996;114(1):40–6.
10. Finn AP, Grewal DS, Vajzovic L. Argus II retinal prosthesis system: a review of patient selection criteria, surgical considerations, and post-operative outcomes. Clin Ophthalmol. 2018;12:1089–97.

11. Luo YH, da Cruz L. The Argus® II retinal prosthesis system. Prog Retin Eye Res. 2016;50:89–107.
12. da Cruz L, Dorn JD, Humayun MS, Dagnelie G, et al. Five-year safety and performance results from the Argus II retinal prosthesis system clinical trial. Ophthalmology. 2016;123(10):2248–54.
13. Rizzo S, Barale PO, Ayello-Scheer S, Devenyi RG, Delyfer MN, Korobelnik JF, Rachitskaya A, Yuan A, Jayasundera KT, Zacks DN, Handa JT, Montezuma SR, Koozekanani D, Stanga PE, da Cruz L, Walter P, Augustin AJ, Chizzolini M, Olmos de Koo LC, Ho AC, Kirchhof B, Hahn P, Vajzovic L, Iezzi R Jr, Gaucher D, Arevalo JF, Gregori NZ, Grisanti S, Özmert E, Yoon YH, Kokame GT, Lim JI, Szurman P, de Juan E Jr, Rezende FA, Salzmann J, Richard G, Huang SS, Merlini F, Patel U, Cruz C, Greenberg RJ, Justus S, Cinelli L, Humayun MS. Adverse events of the argus II retinal prosthesis: incidence, causes, and best practices for managing and preventing conjunctival erosion. Retina. 2018. https://doi.org/10.1097/IAE.0000000000002394
14. Gedde SJ, Schiffman JC, Feuer WJ, Herndon LW, Brandt JD, Budenz DL. Tube versus trabeculectomy study group. Am J Ophthalmol. 2009;148(5):670–84.
15. Lankaranian D, Reis R, Henderer JD, Choe S, Moster MR. J Glaucoma. 2008;17(1):48–51.
16. Humayun MS, Dorn JD, da Cruz L, Dagnelie G, Sahel JA, Stanga PE, Cidecyan AV, Duncan JL, Eliott D, Filley E, Ho AC, Santos A, Safran AB, Arditi A, del Priore LV, Greenberg RJ, Argus II Study Group. Ophthalmology. 2012;119(4):779–88.
17. Abrams GW, Williams GA, Neuwirth J, Mc Donald HR. Clinical results of titanium retinal tacks with pneumatic insertion. Am J Ophthalmol. 1986;102:13–9.
18. Schaffrath K, Schellhase H, Walter P, Augustin A, Chizzolini M, Kirchhof B, Grisanti S, Weidemann P, Szurman P, Richard G, Greenberg RJ, Dorn JD, Permeggiani F, Rizzo S. One-year safety and performance assessment of the Argus II retinal prosthesis: a post approval study. JAMA Ophthalmol. 2019;137(8):896–902.

Surgical Self-Education 42

S. Natarajan, Lanin Chen, and Astha Jain

The level of education is different in every institution, city, and country. There is a vast range of teaching methods with the advancement in the latest techniques and technology. For example, the camera with a film roll that we used to take photographs has changed and evolved so much over the years. Textbooks were read, saved, and used for generations. We now have a soft copy of textbooks, journals, articles that can be read anywhere, anytime with the use of a smartphone, tablet, laptop, and other devices. It is the era of "digitalization." The Internet has made the world a closer place.

A textbook or an article can only teach one the basics. However, the decision-making or the surgical skill only comes with "self-education." Surgical skills are equally important for a surgeon as medical education and knowledge. The most important task in medical education is to teach problem-oriented thinking and the needed practical ability. Vitreoretinal surgery is complex. The great complexity of vitreoretinal surgery requires an honest assessment of the surgeons' own capabilities. Surgeons doing vitrectomy should have a good stereopsis [1]. It is even important to assess one's temperament. Vitreoretinal surgery requires a calm, rapid, and efficient approach. A surgeon who becomes very tense and inefficient at times of surgical stress cannot do justice to the surgery. Vitreoretinal surgery demands continuous practice and persistence.

Self-education starts from the early days of residency. It is important to have a mentor or many mentors. The physical presence of your mentor is not necessary. With the increasing use of the Internet and social media, it is possible to be updated with your mentor, latest know-how, etc.

Before a beginner operates on a patient, he or she should have practiced multiple number of times on the cadaveric eyes, simulators, other disposables, etc. [2]. Though all institutions may not provide simulators, it is the residents' responsibility to look out for alternatives. The used gloves can be used for practicing various types of sutures. Scleral tunnels can be practiced on tomatoes. A lime can be shaped to simulate an eye and can be used for practicing vitrectomy in the wet lab. Retieye by Aurolab can be used for the practice of laser procedures. Bioniko models are available for ophthalmic stimulator surgeries.

Maintaining preoperative, intraoperative, postoperative notes of patients is important to assess the disease or surgical course. Recording of surgical videos can be a useful learning tool. It is not only important to go through surgical videos by your mentor, senior surgeons, but also

S. Natarajan (✉) · L. Chen
Aditya Jyot Eye Hospital, Mumbai, India

A. Jain
Aditya Jyot Eye Hospital, Mumbai, India

Aditya Jyot Foundation for Twinkling Little Eyes, Mumbai, India

A. Jain et al. (eds.), *Cutting-edge Vitreoretinal Surgery*,
https://doi.org/10.1007/978-981-33-4168-5_42

through recordings of your own surgical videos and of your colleagues. It is more likely that you and your colleague will be having the same difficulty at a particular step than your mentor or senior surgeons. It is of utmost importance to identify your difficulty, discuss it with your colleagues and mentors and to find a better alternative, and practice on the shortcomings.

How does one achieve to become the "best surgeon"? One can only proclaim to be the best surgeon. It is a myth! However, a good surgeon works on the perfection of his or her skills in their daily operating activities.

References

1. Charles S, Calzada J, Wood B. Surgical self-education. In: Vitreous microsurgery. 5th ed. Philadelphia: Wolters Kluwer; 2011. p. 249–51.
2. Eckardt U, Eckardt C. Keratoprosthesis as an aid to learning surgical techniques on cadaver eyes. Ophthal Surg. 1995;26(4):358–9.

Retinal Practice in COVID-19 Era

43

Nibha Mishra and Sandeep Saxena

43.1 Introduction

Coronavirus disease 2019 (COVID-19) is an infectious disease caused by severe acute respiratory syndrome coronavirus 2 (SARS-CoV-2). It was first identified in December 2019 in Wuhan, Hubei, China [1]. The World Health Organization (WHO) declared the COVID-19 outbreak as a pandemic on March 11, 2020. Since then it has infected millions of people around the globe. Fever, cough, fatigue, shortness of breath, and loss of smell and taste are the common symptoms of coronavirus infection [2–4]. While the majority of cases result in mild symptoms, some progress to acute respiratory distress syndrome (ARDS), multi-organ failure, septic shock, and other fatal complications [5, 6]. The time from exposure to onset of symptoms ranges from 2 to 14 days. The standard method of diagnosis is by real-time reverse transcription-polymerase chain reaction (r RT-PCR) from a nasopharyngeal swab [7]. There are no specific antiviral treatments for COVID-19 and the development of a vaccine is still under trial phase. Presently mainstay of management involves the treatment of symptoms, supportive care, isolation, and trial of different antibiotic combinations. Health care workers are the frontline workers in the fight against corona putting them as well as other patients they are treating at risk [8, 9]. As the percentage of SARS-CoV-2-positive cases increases, affected patients or asymptomatic carriers might frequently present to hospitals and clinics. When patients come to an ophthalmologist for ocular examination, they have direct contact with examination equipment. Therefore, strict modifications need to be taken up by ophthalmologists for clinical, diagnostic, and management of eye disorders to decrease the risk of transmission at their level.

43.2 COVID-19 and Ophthalmic Practice—Possible Risks to Patients and Health Care Workers

Coronavirus is mainly transmitted by droplet and aerosol and can remain active on different surfaces for different duration of time [10–13]. In the ophthalmology practice, health care workers may be particularly susceptible to these infections as it requires close contact with the patient. A basic simple slit-lamp examination itself requires close proximity between the patient and ophthalmologist. It has been shown that droplets from a cough or sneeze get propelled for up to 6 m [14], a range that definitely encompasses the

N. Mishra (✉)
Ram Manohar Lohia Institute of Medical Sciences, Lucknow, UP, India

S. Saxena
King George's Medical University, Lucknow, UP, India

A. Jain et al. (eds.), *Cutting-edge Vitreoretinal Surgery*, https://doi.org/10.1007/978-981-33-4168-5_43

distance between the patient and ophthalmologist. Clinical reports have suggested that tears act as a medium of infection. A case series by Loon et al. showed that viral RNA of the SARS-CoV can be detected by reverse-transcription polymerase chain reaction (RT-PCR) from the tears of infected individuals [15], thereby putting ophthalmologists at high risk as the ophthalmologists and instruments used by them come in contact with tears on a daily basis. Thus, it is essential to develop an efficient system of disinfection and personal protective equipment (PPE) protocols for the ophthalmology clinic.

The proximity of patients and doctors during an eye examination, the presence of tears and liquids for anesthesia and dilation, or the potential aerosol or droplets from "air puff" tonometry pose a high risk for transmission [16].

Conjunctivitis has been reported in 0.8–5.2% of COVID-19 patients [4, 17, 18]. Conjunctivitis is a common condition presenting in ophthalmic practice; thus, high vigilance is needed. Direct contact with the ocular surface and mucosal membrane during routine ophthalmic examination may have a risk of infection. Hypercoagulability is a major cause of complications in COVID-19 patients resulting from hyperinflammatory response caused by the SARS-CoV-2 virus [19, 20]. Non-arteritic central retinal artery occlusion has been reported to occur due to the retinal artery being occluded from an atherosclerotic lesion or hypercoagulable state such as with COVID-19 [21].

43.3 General Modifications in the Practice of Ophthalmology: Steps to Decrease the Risk

The Health care system is facing unprecedented times and the only possible way out is reducing the transmission of the coronavirus by flattening the curve of disease transmission [22]. Several modifications have been adopted in the delivery of health care in order to protect the patients visiting hospitals and clinics for treatment. The safety of health care workers is also important for the delivery of uninterrupted services. Several guidelines have been provided and are being modified regularly to develop an efficient low-risk system. Following guidelines are being followed worldwide by ophthalmologists for safe clinical practice.

43.3.1 Triage System

Adopting a triage system of patients is an efficient way of assessing patients needing urgent care. Routine eye care services that can be managed by telemedicine should be discontinued and only emergency eye care services to be provided. Patients coming to an eye clinic are at risk of exposure to COVID-19 infection. Maximum patients attending for eye care belong to the geriatric population suffering from underlying chronic medical conditions such as diabetes and hypertension. Patients with comorbidities are at higher risk of developing complications after acquiring COVID-19 infection. Therefore, it is important to develop an efficient workable system of prioritization of patients needing eye care. Services should continue to be provided to the patients at high risk of visual loss without treatment. Following conditions can be considered as eye emergencies (American Academy of Ophthalmologists (AAO)) [23]:

- Exudative age-related macular degeneration
- Severe diabetic retinopathy
- Acute retinal detachment
- Advanced or rapidly progressive glaucoma
- Severe, active uveitis
- Serious ocular oncology conditions
- Retinopathy of prematurity (screening and treatment)
- Globe rupture or other significant trauma
- Serious ocular infections (microbial keratitis, endophthalmitis)

Triage should be done by trained personnel including an optometrist, ophthalmic technician, or ophthalmologist. Telephonic triaging should be done where possible with respect to the emergency/nonemergency nature of the visit. Preliminary screening can be done regarding possible COVID-19 symptoms or history of contact before giving an appointment. If the condition is considered an emergency, the patient should be given a specific time to report to the clinic/hospital to avoid crowding.

43.3.2 Management of Patients at Eye Care Facility During COVID-19

Several steps need to be taken to provide efficient risk-free services at the level of eye care facility which can be divided into screening, examination, and treatment.

Screening

Every eye care center should set up an entry control and screening facility. Entry of children and the elderly (>65 years) into the hospital should not be encouraged unless they are patients themselves. Proper database should be prepared for all the patients visiting the eye care facility with all demographic details to be taken properly. Every patient should be made to fill a questionnaire prepared for screening everyone presenting at the eye care facility. The questionnaire should include history regarding symptoms that are cold, cough, fever, and respiratory distress, and diarrhea, loss of smell or acute conjunctivitis in patients or attendants or family members. Questions regarding recent travel, occupation, and contact with a COVID-19 patient or a suspected COVID-19 patient and/or their contacts should also be included. Body temperature screening with an infrared noncontact thermometer should be done at the point of entry. The patients and their attendants should wear masks provided and follow proper hand hygiene before entering the examination room with 70% alcohol-based sanitizers. Medical records of all the follow-up patients should be pulled out prior to the patient visit. The waiting area should be kept as empty as possible maintaining the norms of social distancing.

Examination

All possible efforts should be made to minimize patient contact time. Slit-lamp barriers (breath guards or breath shields) made from materials such as acetate sheets, clear plastic, or Perspex should be installed. The patient should also be informed not to speak during the examination and should be encouraged to properly wear the mask as the risk of droplet-based transmission increases during slit-lamp examination. Investigations should be done only if absolutely needed. All aerosol-based procedures including noncontact tonometer (NCT) which has shown to result in micro-aerosol production should be avoided [24, 25]. Use of Tonopen with a disposable tip or Goldmann applanation tonometry (with the cleaning of the applanation cone after every patient) is recommended if IOP measurement is necessary. Refraction can be performed using an autorefractor or a streak retinoscope where mandated. The trial frame and the metal rim of the lenses used should be cleaned with alcohol-based sanitizer after use. Contact lens trial, unless therapeutic, should be avoided. Surfaces and instruments should be cleaned between patients. All instruments and probes used in direct contact with the patient's tear film and ocular surface should be disinfected (using standard protocols) before reuse. For disinfecting 70–75% ethanol or isopropyl alcohol immediately should be used. Instruments having direct contact with the patient's ocular surface such as Goldmann applanation tonometer are disinfected by immersion in either 1:10 diluted bleach solution with sodium hypochlorite or 3% hydrogen peroxide for at least 5 min [26]. Hand hygiene should be performed regularly and after every patient using alcohol-based hand rubs as per the current recommendation by the Centre for Disease Control and Prevention and WHO.

Personal Protective Equipment (PPE) in the form of surgical caps, surgical scrub suits, three-ply surgical masks/N95 masks, and gloves must be provided to the health care workers. The AAO has published a report advising ophthalmologists to wear masks and eye protection when examining patients potentially infected with COVID-19. Few reports have also suggested that when no eye protection was worn, COVID-19 could be transmitted by aerosol contact with conjunctiva [27–29]. Chan et al. recommended the use of PPE for all cases regardless of COVID status, as well as hand hygiene measures and use of gloves, N95 masks, goggles, and gowns.

Treatment
Pharmacy services and optical dispensing should be available maintaining the distancing protocol. All surgeries must be day care unless the medical condition comes under mandatory admission. Defer all procedures and surgeries on a COVID-19 patient until the patient recovers, unless deferral of treatment by 2 weeks has a potential risk for loss of vision, eye, and life. If a procedure or a surgery is mandated, it should be performed in a multispecialty hospital approved for COVID-19 treatment and all the health care workers involved in the procedure/surgery should have full PPE. The role of hydroxyl-chloroquine prophylaxis is debatable but is being given to health care workers attending COVID-19 patients. Local anesthesia should be preferred over general anesthesia for performing surgeries. All universal precautions should be taken with minimum number of staff in the operation theater. Positive ventilation should be avoided in the operation theater during the procedure and for at least 20 min after the patient has left the theater. Protocol-based disinfection of the OT should be done after each surgical procedure (All India Ophthalmological Society—Indian Journal of Ophthalmology Expert Group for COVID-19 Practice Guidelines) [30].

43.4 Modifications in Clinical and Surgical Practices in Retina During COVID Era

43.4.1 Special Challenges Faced

Every specialty in ophthalmology is facing their own challenges during the COVID-19 pandemic. Retinal specialty is also facing unprecedented situations as avoiding close contact with the patient is very difficult during retinal examinations. Most of the retinal disorders are vision-threatening if not treated timely. Also, most of the ophthalmic emergencies fall under this specialty. The retina clinic has a large component of patients who are elderly and with comorbid diseases who are at higher risk of developing severe complications of COVID-19 infection. Thus, retinal specialists have a huge responsibility toward the patients as well as themselves and other health care workers.

43.4.2 Retinal Emergency Care

New measures are being taken in treating retina patients to reduce their exposure to each other and to the medical team. Patients with urgent sight-threatening conditions are being entertained and nonurgent patients are being deferred. Several guidelines are being made by international and national ophthalmic bodies to help retina specialists to provide emergency care by triage of patients. On the basis of the complaint of the patient, we can divide them into urgent, semi-urgent, and nonurgent [31]. Sudden or rapid vision loss, acute onset of flashes, recent onset of metamorphopsia and new cases of ocular tumor, retinopathy of prematurity (ROP), and retinoblastoma are included among urgent and should be promptly treated. Patients with diabetic retinopathy with slow onset of vision loss, exudative age-related macular degeneration, retinal vein occlusion or diabetic macular edema, and recently operated cases can be considered semi-urgent for which appointment can be scheduled. Patients with stable diabetic retinopathy of any stage, stable patients receiving anti-VEGF injections regularly for different indications, and stable post-surgery patients can be deferred.

The American Society of Retina Specialists (ASRS) released guidelines to help retina practices to reduce risk and assure the health and safety of patients during the COVID-19 pandemic. These guidelines were released in March 2020 defining essential visits for patients and categorizing patients into emergent, urgent, and nonurgent, nonelective cases during the pandemic. For emergent surgical indications, the risk of permanent vision loss without early intervention is high whereas for urgent surgical indications, the risk of severe and permanent vision loss without immediate surgery is not as high and treatment can be delayed. Retinal surgeons should monitor urgent indications as they can become emergent, according to the ASRS press release. For nonurgent, nonelective patients, surgery can be delayed without significant risk to further vision. Retinal surgeons should follow nonurgent, nonelective patients, as their condition can worsen and urgency increase [32].

Emergent surgical indications may include:

- Acute retinal detachment—macula attached[1]
- Acute retinal detachment—macula detached in a monocular patient (see Footnote 1)
- Retained lens fragments with elevated intraocular pressure not controlled medically
- Acute endophthalmitis with severe vision loss
- Open globe injury with or without an intraocular foreign body (see Footnote 1)
- Expulsive choroidal hemorrhage (see Footnote 1)
- Dense vitreous hemorrhage in monocular patient
- Exposed/infected scleral buckle or other ocular implants

Urgent surgical indications may include[2]:

- Retinal detachment—macula detached
- Retained lens fragment with medically controlled intraocular pressure
- Vitreous hemorrhage in which a retinal tear or detachment is suspected

Nonurgent, nonelective surgical indications may include[3]:

- Macular hole
- Dislocated intraocular implant lens
- Diabetic vitreous hemorrhage with no macula-threatening retinal detachment
- Retained silicone oil
- Macular epiretinal membrane/vitreomacular traction

43.4.3 Retinal Examination Protocols

The examination and treatment of retinal conditions are done face to face thus involving close contact between the patients and the practitioner. Thus, all the standard protocols mentioned earlier should be followed to minimize the risk of droplet transmission. Patients who are already on follow-ups should be advised home dilation to shorten their visit to the hospital as well as avoiding exposure of health care workers to tears while instilling the drops. Electronic prescriptions can be sent to patients for dilation keeping drug allergies in mind. Dilation of eye in retinal care set-up should be done wearing gloves and a face shield and proper hand hygiene to be followed after every patient. A non-touch technique can be used for putting drops by asking the patient to retract his lid or using disposable cotton-tipped applicator [31].

The use of slit lamp barriers should be done regularly and should be cleaned on regular basis. The retinal examination should be done strictly with an indirect ophthalmoscope and direct ophthalmoscopy and contact lens-based fundus examination should be avoided. Examination should be done using a face shield and protective goggles. The direction of gaze can be instructed by pointing in the direction or gentle tapping to avoid unwanted aerosol generation by talking to the patient. Cotton tipped applicator can be used as a scleral depressor for indentation while examining which should be ideally avoided until needed.

Infants undergoing screening for retinopathy must be placed on a crib with a plastic or polythene sheet covering exposing only the face, with the mother maintaining at least 2 m of distance.

[1]May be urgent depending on location and character.

[2]These indications could be considered emergent if the patient is monocular or extenuating circumstances arise.

[3]These indications could be considered urgent/emergent if the patient is monocular or extenuating circumstances arise.

The examiner screens the baby using indirect ophthalmoscopy or a retinal camera. The barrier sheet used for the crib is replaced or sanitized between successive infants (All India Ophthalmological Society—Indian Journal of Ophthalmology Expert Group for COVID-19 Practice Guidelines) [30].

Mask and PPE etiquette should be followed by all the attending doctors and health care workers. Protections for head, mouth, nose, and eye with a surgical cap, N95 masks, and goggles/face shield should be used by the examiner. Three-ply surgical masks should be worn by patients as well as their attendants. Strict hand hygiene should be followed by the health care workers as well as patients and their attendants using alcohol-based hand rub or by washing with soap and water (minimum 20 s). Clean surfaces and instruments between patients. Masks should be changed every 6 h or immediately when contaminated or wet. The CDC recommended the use of disinfectants specific to COVID-19, including diluted household bleach (five tablespoons of bleach per gallon of water) and alcohol solutions with at least 70% alcohol.

43.4.4 Diagnostic Procedures

Imaging services should be modified shortened imaging protocols in order to provide rapid and minimal contact. Investigations like OCT, OCTA should be ordered on the retina specialist's discretion. OCT should be preferred as they are less time-consuming thus reducing the time of contact. Shared equipment such as the B-scan probes needs strict sterilization protocols as they come in contact with the eye of the patient, should be done when urgent need is there. Fundus Fluorescein Angiography (FFA) and Indocyanine Green Angiography (ICG) should be avoided, unless necessary as they are time taking procedures. All the essential Imaging devices should be placed in different rooms to avoid crowding. Protective shields and regular recommended cleaning of the devices should be done.

43.4.5 Medical Management of Retinal Cases

Several organizations have now produced general guidance for ophthalmologists on managing patients during the pandemic (AAO, ASRS, AIOS). Numerous challenges are being faced by retina specialists both in the field of medical and surgical retina.

43.4.5.1 Retinal Lasers

Retinal lasers to be done for urgent conditions only which includes active proliferative diabetic retinopathy (PDR), ROP, Retinal tears, or breaks (e.g., Horseshoe tears) and laser barrage in macula on RD, subclinical RD, and extrafoveal CNVM. Patients with stable vision and having diabetic macular edema or macular edema due to other causes can be deferred [31, 33–36].

43.4.5.2 Anti-vascular Endothelial Growth Factor (VEGF)

Anti-VEGF therapy is essential for the treatment of certain retinal disorders and has to be administered even monthly in few of them such as macular edema due to diabetic retinopathy, CRVO and exudative age related macular degeneration (AMD). Anti-VEGF therapy should be provided under a modified regimen. Each day different teams of injecting retina specialists and minimum possible paramedical staff should be present, teams scheduled on different days should not meet each other. The Royal College of Ophthalmologists has proposed the following guidelines for administration of anti-VEGF during COVID-19 [37].

Exudative Age-Related Macular Degeneration

For new cases, diagnosis should be confirmed with OCT and OCT-Angiography, if available. Confirmed new wet AMD cases should be treated with a loading phase of three injections of anti-VEGF and then continued on 8 weekly bases with no clinic review. For old cases, 8 weekly anti-VEGF therapy with no clinic review to be followed unless they mention a significant drop in vision at their injection visit. Such patients may need OCT and visual acuity assessments.

Diabetic Macular Oedema

Anti-VEGF injections can be deferred and can be reviewed in the clinic after 4 months. New cases of severe NPDR and active PDR should be treated with anti-VEGF agents and PRP. Virtual review with OCT and wide-field color photography is the preferred option for reviewing patients.

Central Retinal Vein Occlusion (CRVO)

For new patients with macular edema due to CRVO anti-VEGF treatment as per the protocol to be given whereas old patients who had adequately received injections should undergo PRP if needed to reduce the risk of rubeotic glaucoma. Branch retinal vein occlusion is not considered to be sight-threatening, so review can be differed for 4 months.

43.4.6 Indications for Surgery

All elective surgical procedures need to be deferred. Emergency indications have already been discussed for performing retinal surgeries. The American Society of Retinal Surgeons (ASRS) proposed procedures for emergent/urgent conditions enumerated in Table 43.1 [32]

Before operating on any patient they should undergo COVID-19 testing to confirm the status of the patient as per the local regulatory health protocol. All health care workers should follow PPE etiquette and minimal possible staff should be involved in surgical procedures. Donning and doffing areas to be made as per the protocols in the OT premises and proper sequence to be followed for doing the same. It is even advised to perform surgeries with all possible precautions irrespective of COVID-19 status Topical anesthesia and local anesthesia should be preferred where possible. In patient preparation, draping should be done properly to avoid exposure to droplets and aerosols. Five percent povidone-iodine should be instilled in the conjunctival sac 5–10 min as it is virucidal and disinfects the ocular surface and conjunctival cul-de-sac in 15 s. The quickest possible surgical procedure should be performed by an experienced surgeon. Valved cannulas should be used for vitrectomies in order to minimize contact with ocular fluids. Diathermy to be used cautiously as leads to aerosol generation [38]. Vitrectomy should be preferred over scleral buckling. All the instruments, surfaces, and machinery should be properly sterilized following standard protocols. Operation theater should be fumigated regularly. All surgeries must be day care unless the medical conditions strictly mandate admission. If a COVID-19 positive patient is to be operated to salvage vision it should be done in a designated COVID-19 facility. All the health care workers involved in the procedure/surgery should have full PPE and possibly HCQ prophylaxis.

Table 43.1 American Society of Retinal Surgeons (ASRS) proposed emergent/urgent indications and procedures to be performed

Indication	Procedure
Retinal detachment/trauma/intraocular infection/vitreous Hemorrhage/retinal tear/intraocular foreign body	Vitrectomy (MIVS)/scleral buckle
Proliferative diabetic retinopathy/proliferative Vitreoretinopathy/complex preretinal membrane/complex macular pathology or hole	Membrane peeling/ILM peeling
Lens complications acute	Pars plana lensectomy/phacoemulsification
Trauma	Repair open globe
Pediatric/developmentally delayed evaluation (retinoblastoma, trauma, retinal detachment)	Examination under anesthesia (EUA)
Retinal detachment/retinal tear/trauma	Laser indirect retinopexy—complex
Retinal detachment	Pneumatic retinopexy
Trauma/infection/intraocular malignancy	Enucleation
Intraocular malignancy	Ocular brachytherapy

43.4.7 Screening

Early detection and timely treatment are very crucial in both exudative AMD as well as diabetic retinopathy which have been made possible by screening. Regular screening which is the key in both the conditions has become a challenge to retina specialists in the COVID era. Geriatric patients as well as diabetics both are at high risk of developing the COVID infection-related complications.

Age-Related Macular Degeneration Regular appointments of screening should be canceled. Patients should be asked to do home-based monitoring and should be guided to report on a marked drop in vision. Home-based monitoring may include the use of Amsler grid and appointments with specialists using telemedicine. The upcoming home-based remote monitoring on horizon is developing an artificial intelligence-enabled, home-based OCT system for patients with wet AMD [39].

Diabetic Retinopathy The main aim should be reducing the progression and severity of diabetic retinopathy which could be done by controlling the modifiable risk factors like glycemic status and blood pressure. Telemedicine is also an important tool as remote imaging of the fundus can be analyzed by a team of specialists and the course of treatment can be decided upon [40]. Lund et al. recommend that patients who have stable diabetic retinopathy with no urgent or referable indication can have retinal screening at 18–24 months interval during the COVID-19 pandemic [41].

43.4.8 Special Considerations

Intraocular Tumors and Ocular Metastasis As these are vision as well as life-threatening conditions their treatment should continue with all possible precautions. Interdisciplinary cooperation is needed to have all possible investigations and imaging done beforehand and video consultation to be done in order to avoid patients visiting time. Systemic chemotherapy should be continued for intraocular Lymphoma and ocular metastasis. External beam radiation therapy should be preferred. Retinoblastoma treatment for old and new cases should continue as before.

Pediatric Retina Examination of children is a challenge as it is difficult for them to follow precautions like wearing masks and hand hygiene putting both them and health care workers at risk. Special precautions like allowing only a single attendant and distancing protocol should be the mainstay of avoiding infection. For ROP which requires immediate care, the Indian Retinopathy of Prematurity (iROP) Society has formulated guidelines in March 2020 which has been summarized in Table 43.2 [42].

Table 43.2 Suggested ROP follow-up guidelines by the Indian ROP Society during COVID-19 restrictions

Findings	Follow-up and treatment
Immature retina in zone 3 and zone 2 anterior	3–4 weeks or more
ROP in zone 3 and zone 2 anterior	3–4 week
ROP in zone 2 posterior	2 weeks
ROP in zone 1	Urgent/less than a week/treat-laser if disease is amenable. Intravitreal injections can be used but caution to be exercised since follow-up.
Pre-plus	Consider early treatment or early follow-up if the pupil does not dilate well and the media is not clear.
Pre-plus	With good pupillary dilatation and clear media and other low-risk features delay the next screening by an additional 1 week from the current guidelines.
Stage 4A and 4B ROP	Surgery must be performed as soon as the treating ROP specialist feels it is required with adequate precautions taken while providing anesthesia as per prescribed guidelines.
Stage 5 ROP	Surgery is not urgent. Case-to-case based decision must be considered.

43.5 Telemedicine

HK Li first described the use of telemedicine in ophthalmology in 1999 [43]. Telemedicine is defined as the use of information technologies to support health care between participants who are separated from each other. It characterizes a combination of medical expertise and recent technology that delivers medical services over distance. The current new-age technology is well equipped with video-equipped computers, high-resolution cell phone cameras, and fast broadband internet service.

The fight against the COVID 19 virus appears to be a long one and social distancing seems to be the only possible way to flatten the disease curve. Telemedicine can prove to be an apt tool to not only triage the patients needing immediate care but also providing health care inside a safe home environment. Telemedicine provides an opportunity to ophthalmologists in performing their professional responsibilities without being the foci of disease transmission. Telemedicine practice should be widely advertised on social media and other platforms.

43.6 Conclusion

Retina specialists like all other frontline health workers in this COVID era should embrace the present scenario and should move ahead by providing safe and practical eye care services in these unprecedented times. Retinal practice has to follow the new normal. From the above discussion, we can summarize the steps which need to be taken to combat with the easing of the curbs in ever-increasing rate of infection. To begin with, teleconsultation needs to be accepted as the new normal and regular way of reaching out to the patients. As there is a restriction in the number of patients visiting the eye care clinics, we have to increase the working hours so that patients can be provided regular care following all the possible precautions. The cost of PPE and other sanitization measures has to become a part of regular expenditure of hospital establishments. Online training of the residents should also become a part of the new normal.

References

1. Hui DS, I Azhar E, Madani TA, Ntoumi F, Kock R, Dar O, et al. The continuing 2019-nCoV epidemic threat of novel coronaviruses to global health—the latest 2019 novel coronavirus outbreak in Wuhan, China. Int J Infect Dis. 2020;91:264–6.
2. Habibzadeh P, Stoneman EK. The novel coronavirus: a bird's eye view. Int J Occup Environ Med. 2020;11:65–71.
3. Rothe C, Schunk M, Sothmann P, et al. Transmission of 2019-nCoV infection from an asymptomatic contact in Germany. N Engl J Med. 2020;382:970–1.
4. Guan W, Ni ZY, Hu Y, et al. Clinical characteristics of Coronavirus Disease 2019 in China. N Engl J Med. 2020; https://doi.org/10.1056/NEJMoa2002032.
5. Ye Q, Wang B, Mao J. The pathogenesis and treatment of the 'cytokine storm' in COVID-19. J Infect. 2020;80(6):607–13.
6. Murthy S, Gomersall CD, Fowler RA. Care for critically ill patients with COVID-19. JAMA. 2020;323(15):1499.
7. Loeffelholz JM, Tang YW. Laboratory diagnosis of emerging human coronavirus infections - the state of the art. Rev Emerg Microbes Infect. 2020;9(1):747–56.
8. Wang J, Zhou M, Liu F. Reasons for healthcare workers becoming infected with novel coronavirus disease 2019 (COVID-19) in China. J Hosp Infect. 2020;105:100–1.
9. Chang XH, Rebaza A, Sharma L, Dela Cruz CS. Protecting health-care workers from subclinical coronavirus infection. Lancet Respir Med. 2020;8:e13.
10. Li Q, Guan X, Wu P, et al. Early transmission dynamics in Wuhan, China, of novel coronavirus–infected pneumonia. N Engl J Med. 2020;382:1199–207.
11. Kampf G, Todt D, Pfaender S, et al. Persistence of coronaviruses on inanimate surfaces and their inactivation with biocidal agents. J Hosp Infect. 2020;104:246–51.
12. Bourouiba L. Turbulent gas clouds and respiratory pathogen emissions potential implications for reducing transmission of COVID-19. JAMA. 2020. https://doi.org/10.1001/jama.2020.4756.
13. Sahin AR, Erdogan A, Agaoglu PM, et al. 2019 novel Coronavirus (COVID-19) outbreak: a review of the current literature. EJMO. 2020;4:1–7.
14. Xie X, Li Y, Chwang AT, Ho PL, Seto WH. How far droplets can move in indoor environments–revisiting the wells evaporation-falling curve. Indoor Air. 2007;17:211–59.

15. Loon S-C, Teoh SCB, Oon LLE, Se-Thoe S-Y, Ling A-E, Leo Y-S, et al. The severe acute respiratory syndrome coronavirus in tears. Br J Ophthalmol. 2004;88:861–3.
16. Jones RM, Brosseau LM. Aerosol transmission of infectious disease. J Occup Environ Med. 2015;57:501–8.
17. Li X, Wang M, Chen C, et al. Ophthalmologists' strategy for the prevention and control of coronavirus pneumonia with conjunctivitis or with conjunctivitis as the first symptom. Chin J Exp Ophthalmol. 2020;38:276–80.
18. Xia J, Tong J, Liu M, et al. Evaluation of coronavirus in tears and conjunctival secretions of patients with SARS-CoV-2 infection. J Med Virol. 2020;92:589–94.
19. Greven CM, Slusher MM, Weaver RG. Retinal arterial occlusions in young adults. Am J Ophthalmol. 1995;120(6):776–83. https://doi.org/10.1016/s0002-9394(14)72731-x.
20. Panigada M, Bottino N, Tagliabue P. Hypercoagulability of COVID-19 patients in intensive care unit. A report of thromboelastography findings and other parameters of hemostasis. J Thromb Haemost. 2020;18:1738–42. https://doi.org/10.1111/jth.14850.
21. Rotzinger DC, Beigelman-Aubry C, von Garnier C, Qanadli SD. Pulmonary embolism in patients with COVID-19: time to change the paradigm of computed tomography. Thromb Res. 2020;190:58–9. https://doi.org/10.1016/j.thromres.2020.04.011.
22. Anderson RM, Heesterbeek H, Klinkenberg D, Hollingsworth TD. How will country-based mitigation measures influence the course of the COVID-19 epidemic? Lancet. March 2020;395(10228):931–4.
23. American Academy of Ophthalmologists (AAO). List of urgent and emergent ophthalmic procedures. www.aao.org/headline/list-of-urgent-emergent-ophthalmic-procedures.
24. Britt JM, Clifton BC, Barnebey HS, et al. Microaerosol formation in noncontact 'air-puff' tonometry. Arch Ophthalmol. 1991;109:225–8.
25. Li C, Tang Y, Chen Z, et al. Aerosol formation during non-contact "air-puff" tonometry and its significance for prevention of COVID-19. Chin J Exp Ophthalmol. 2020;2020:3.
26. Lam DS, Wong RL, Lai KH, Ko CN, Leung HY, Wing VY, Lau JY, Huang SS. COVID-19: special precautions in ophthalmic practice and FAQs on personal protection and mask selection. Asia Pac J Ophthalmol. 2020;9(2):67–77.
27. American Academy of Ophthalmology. Alert: important coronavirus updates for ophthalmologists. Available: https://www.aao.org/headline/alert-important-coronavirus-context. Accessed 27 Mar 2020.
28. CDC. How coronavirus spreads. https://www.cdc.gov/coronavirus/2019-ncov/prepare/transmission.html. Accessed 27 Mar 2020.
29. Wei LC, Fen LX, Fang JZ. 2019-nCoV transmission through the ocular surface must not be ignored. Lancet. 2020;395:e39.
30. Sengupta S, Honavar SG, Sachdev MS, Sharma N, Kumar A, Ram J, Shetty R, Rao GS, Ramasamy K, Khanna R, Jain E, Bhattacharjee K, Agarwal A, Natarajan S, Lahane TP. Indian J Ophthalmol. 2020;68(5):711–24.
31. Gupta A, Cavallerano J, Sun JK, et al. Evidence for telemedicine for diabetic retinal disease. Semin Ophthalmol. 2017;32:22–8. https://doi.org/10.1080/08820538.2016.1228403.
32. The American Society of Retina Specialists. ASRS releases guidelines to help retina practices navigate COVID-19 pandemic. https://www.asrs.org/clinical/clinical-updates/1962/asrs-releases-guidelines-to-help-retina-practices-navigate-covid-19-pandemic. Accessed March 20, 2020.
33. Chodosh J, Holland GN, Yeh S. Important coronavirus updates for ophthalmologists. https://www.aao.org/headline/alert important coronavirus context. Last accessed on 2020 Apr 04.
34. Romano MR, Montericcio A, Montalbano C, Raimondi R, Allegrini D, Ricciardelli G, et al. Facing COVID 19 in ophthalmology department. Curr Eye Res. 2020;23:1–6.
35. VRSI Webinar on Retina Practice Guidelines in the COVID 19 Era.
36. Eggers M. Infectious disease management and control with povidone iodine. Infect Dis Ther. 2019;8:581.
37. Macular Society. Injection treatment: latest advice from the Royal College of ophthalmologists. https://www.macularsociety.org/injection-treatment-latest-advice-royal-college-ophthalmologists.
38. Coccolini F, Perrone G, Chiarugi M, Di Marzo F, Ansaloni L, Scandroglio I, et al. Surgery in COVID-19 patients: operational directives. World J Emerg Surg. 2020;25:2. https://doi.org/10.1186/s13017-020-00307-2.
39. Loewenstein A. Remote retinal monitoring in the time of COVID-19-decreasing clinic visits keeps patients safer and streamlines care. Retinal Physician. 2020.
40. Kroenke K, Kurt KM. Telemedicine screening for eye disease. JAMA. 2015;313:1666–7. https://doi.org/10.1001/jama.2015.107.
41. Lund SH, Aspelund T, Kirby P, Russell G, Einarsson S, Palsson O, et al. Individualised risk assessment for diabetic retinopathy and optimisation of screening intervals: a scientific approach to reducing healthcare costs. Br J Ophthalmol. 2016;100(5):683–7.
42. Vinekar A, Azad RV, Dogra MR, Jalali S, Bhende P, Narendran V, et al. Retinopathy of prematurity screening and treatment guidelines during the COVID-19 lockdown. 2020. https://sites.google.com/view/irop-society/newsroom?authuser=0. Last accessed on 2020 May 05.
43. Li HK. Telemedicine and ophthalmology. Surv Ophthalmol. 1999;44:61–72.

MIX
Papier aus verantwortungsvollen Quellen
Paper from responsible sources
FSC® C105338

If you have any concerns about our products,
you can contact us on
ProductSafety@springernature.com

In case Publisher is established outside the EU,
the EU authorized representative is:
Springer Nature Customer Service Center GmbH
Europaplatz 3, 69115 Heidelberg, Germany

Printed by Libri Plureos GmbH
in Hamburg, Germany